T0317417

Threats to Homeland Security

Threats to Homeland Security: Reassessing the All-Hazards Perspective

SECOND EDITION

Edited by

Richard J. Kilroy, Jr.

Department of Politics
Coastal Carolina University
Conway, SC, USA

WILEY

Library of Congress Cataloging-in-Publication Data

Names: Kilroy, Richard J., Jr., editor.
Title: Threats to homeland security : reassessing the all hazards perspective / edited by Richard J. Kilroy, Jr., Coastal Carolina University.
Description: Second Edition. | Hoboken, New Jersey : John Wiley & Sons, Inc., [2018] | First Edition: 2008. | Includes index. |
Identifiers: LCCN 2017049073 (print) | LCCN 2017054834 (ebook) | ISBN 9781119251965 (pdf) | ISBN 9781119251989 (epub) | ISBN 9781119251811 (Paper)
Subjects: LCSH: Terrorism–United States–Prevention. | National security–United States. | Civil defense–United States. | Emergency management–United States.
Classification: LCC HV6432 (ebook) | LCC HV6432 .T568 2018 (print) | DDC 363.3250973–dc23
LC record available at https://lccn.loc.gov/2017049073

Cover design by Concept courtesy of Maggy Kilroy, Suss Creative
Cover image: Background: Courtesy of NOAA;
        Chessboard © Rafe Swan/Gettyimages
        (Chess pieces)
        Army man © 4×6/Gettyimages
        Ship, Courtesy of the U.S. Coast Guard
        Terrorists, Iraqi insurgents with guns, 2006 by بدر الإسلام is licensed under CC BY-SA
        Gas mask by Rodrix Paredes is licensed under CC BY
        Red Cross truck, Photo by George Armstrong - Apr 30, 2011 - Location: Birmingham, AL
        Hacker, Anonymous – CeBIT 2016 00 by Frank Schwichtenberg
        FEMA, Photo by Patsy Lynch - Oct 12, 2017 - Location: Orlando, FL
        Missile, Steve Herman / VOA News 26 July, 2013 Pyongyang

Set in 11/13pt Berkeley by SPi Global, Pondicherry, India

10 9 8 7 6 5 4 3 2 1

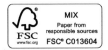

CONTENTS

NOTES ON CONTRIBUTORS

What made this book unique among homeland security texts when it was first published in 2008 was the truly interdisciplinary nature of the work, based on the academic and practical experiences of the authors who contributed chapters. The same holds true in 2018. Each author contributed their own perspectives while at the same time providing continuity of structure and format in order to support the overall goal of providing a reassessment of the "all-hazards" perspective. The authors of the revised text represent diverse academic disciplines in political science, public administration, security studies, engineering, and emergency planning. Some authors also bring practitioner experience in fields related to homeland security, such as emergency management, security management, military and homeland defense planning, intelligence, critical infrastructure protection, and public policy. The end result of the second edition of *Threats to Homeland Security* is a much richer, educational contribution to the broader field of homeland security studies as it currently exists today, as well as how it will likely evolve in the future.

Dr Jonathan M. Acuff is assistant professor of Intelligence and National Security Studies in the Department of Politics at Coastal Carolina University in Conway, SC. His research and teaching interests include security studies, military innovation, strategy, and intelligence analysis. A former Army Reserve Officer, Acuff was a military analyst for the National Bureau of Asian Research in Seattle, Washington, where he worked on funded research projects for the Department of Homeland Security, US Pacific Command, and the Strategic Asia Program. He received his PhD in Political Science from the University of Washington.

Dr Christopher J. Ferrero is assistant professor of Intelligence and National Security Studies in the Department of Politics at Coastal Carolina University. He focuses on the proliferation of weapons of mass destruction (WMD) as well as Middle East politics. Prior to joining Coastal Carolina in 2016, Dr Ferrero held positions at the University of Virginia, Seton Hall University, and Syracuse University. From 2002 to 2006, he served as a WMD analyst for the Departments of State and Defense, primarily on ballistic missile proliferation and missile defense. He has appeared as a source for media outlets including NBC News and the Australian Broadcasting Corporation. He received his PhD in Foreign Affairs from the University of Virginia in 2011.

Dr Joseph Fitsanakis is associate professor of Intelligence and National Security Studies in the Department of Politics at Coastal Carolina University in Conway, SC. Before joining Coastal, he founded the Security and Intelligence Studies program at King University, where he also directed the King Institute for Security and Intelligence Studies. Dr Fitsanakis has written extensively on subjects such as international espionage, intelligence tradecraft, counterintelligence, wiretapping, cyber espionage, transnational crime, and intelligence reform. He is a frequent contributor to international news media and senior editor at intelNews.org, an ACI-indexed scholarly blog that is cataloged through the US Library of Congress. He received his PhD from the Department of Politics and International Relations at the University of Edinburgh in the United Kingdom.

Dr Chad S. Foster is assistant professor in the Homeland Security Program at Eastern Kentucky University in Richmond, KY. He instructs and oversees courses that support the disaster management concentration in the program. He earned a Bachelor of Science degree from the US Military Academy and graduate-level degrees in public administration and urban and public affairs from the University of Louisville.

Dr Richard J. Kilroy Jr. is assistant professor of Intelligence and National Security Studies in the Department of Politics at Coastal Carolina University in Conway, SC. He teaches courses related to intelligence analysis, intelligence operations, homeland security, and Latin American security issues. He is also a retired Army Intelligence and Foreign Area Officer who has served in various positions planning and implementing national and homeland security policy, to include standing up the Department of Defense's new US Northern Command after 9/11. His PhD is in foreign affairs from the University of Virginia.

Mr Steven Kuhr is head of Emergency Management and Continuity at Colorado Springs Utilities, which is among of the nation's largest utility public enterprises. Colorado Springs Utilities operates critical infrastructure across 11 Colorado counties. In this capacity Steven leads a team responsible for a comprehensive crisis management program by integrating the practices and principles of the emergency management, homeland security, and enterprise continuity domains for four utility sectors—electricity, natural gas, water, and wastewater services—for the City of Colorado Springs and a number of communities across the Pikes Peak Region. He is also an adjunct professor for the College of Security Studies at Colorado Technical University and a member of the Board of Directors of the InfraGard Denver Members Alliance. He has an extensive portfolio of emergency management and homeland security experience at the local, state, and private sector levels that spans three decades. He holds a Bachelor of Science in Emergency Management Administration from the State University of New York and a Master of Science in Homeland Security Management from the Homeland Security Management Institute at Long Island University.

Dr Daniel Masters is associate professor of international studies at the University of North Carolina at Wilmington. His area of expertise is national and international security, decision making and foreign policy, international political economy, and Middle Eastern, Russian, and

European political systems. His research interests relate to terrorism and security studies, with a particular focus on rebellious collective action. His PhD is from the University of Tennessee, Knoxville.

Dr Stephan Reissman focuses on continuity of operations and preparedness issues in his position with the National Oceanic and Atmospheric Administration (NOAA). He has extensive experience in emergency planning, preparedness, and response with federal (CDC, FEMA, DHS, and NOAA) and EMS agencies. He holds certifications as a Certified Emergency Manager, Master Exercise Practitioner, and Certified Business Continuity Professional. His PhD is in public affairs from the University of Colorado at Denver.

Dr Carmine Scavo is professor of political science and director of the Master of Public Administration program at East Carolina University in Greenville, NC. He teaches undergraduate courses in political science and graduate courses in public administration and security studies. His research has appeared in *Publius: The Journal of Federalism, Urban Affairs Review, and Public Administration Review* and in edited volumes. His PhD is from the University of Michigan.

Dr Alexander Siedschlag is professor of homeland security and public health sciences at Penn State (Penn State Harrisburg – School of Public Affairs, in a joint appointment with the Hershey College of Medicine). He also is chair of Penn State's intercollege Homeland Security Program. In research and teaching, he focuses on comparative homeland and civil security, security cultures, scenario foresight, and theories and methods of security studies. He has served as expert evaluator for US Department of Homeland Security and for European Union security research grant programs, as well as led security research projects in the European Union. This involved collaboration with FEMA's Strategic Foresight Initiative. Further, he has served as a senior guest lecturer at NATO School. His PhD is in political science from the University of Munich, Germany, and he in addition holds a "habilitation," or venia legendi, in political science from Humboldt University, Berlin, Germany.

Dr Jonathan Smith is professor and coordinator of the Intelligence and National Security Studies program in the Department of Politics at Coastal Carolina University in Conway, SC. He teaches courses in intelligence studies, national security strategy, and homeland security. He is also a retired naval intelligence officer who deployed in support of operations in Bosnia, Kosovo, Iraq, and Afghanistan. His PhD is in political science (national security decision making) from the University of South Carolina.

PREFACE

When the first edition of *Threats to Homeland Security* was published in 2007, there was a dearth of academic literature available on the topic to support the demand on college campuses for classes related to homeland security and terrorism after 9/11. First attempts at meeting this void were texts in traditional fields of study, such as political science or criminal justice. Terrorism studies was still a little known field in security studies programs at some colleges, such as Georgetown University, which primarily looked at the subject from a theoretical or conceptual framework. Other approaches looked at the topic in terms of policy studies, such as national security policy or foreign policy courses, which expanded to include the subject of homeland security. The consensus though was for most writers to take an exclusive view of homeland security, focusing on terrorism as the primary threat.

After Hurricanes Katrina and Rita struck the Gulf Coast in August and September 2005, causing catastrophic damage and loss of life, similar to a terrorist attack, there was shift in homeland security toward a more inclusive view, which looked at threats from an all-hazards perspective. As a result there was a new emphasis placed on producing academic literature that emphasized natural disaster response and planning, primarily in the field of emergency management. New college curricula also developed in areas of "applied sciences" that now placed greater emphasis on studying the role of first responders, as well as state and federal government agencies in responding to natural disasters, as opposed to terrorist attacks. Community colleges, four-year undergraduate institutions, and even graduate schools began to develop degree programs related to emergency management and planning in order to build on the next inclusive view of homeland security.

It was in this context that the first edition of the text was named *Threats to Homeland Security: An All-Hazards Perspective*. In other words, the goal in writing such a text was to provide students in a variety of academic disciplines and fields of study an integrated approach toward security studies and the continuing nature of security challenges to the nation through both a theoretical and practical lens. In the text, students and practitioners gained a comprehensive understanding of threats to the United States from an interdisciplinary perspective. By emphasizing the "all-hazards perspective," readers of the first edition gained a better understanding of a more inclusive view of the threats the nation faced at the time, with an expectation that these would be also be the types of "all-hazard" threats homeland security studies would need to address in the future.

Since that time, homeland security, as both an area of academic study and professional practice, has evolved considerably. Today, according to the University and Agency Partnership Initiative of the Center for

Homeland Defense and Security, there are more than 400 programs of study related to homeland security, from associate to doctoral degrees. There has been increased engagement between law enforcement agencies at the local, state, and federal levels to approach threats to public safety in new ways, to include the development of fusion centers and joint task forces. The federal government has increased the role of the Department of Homeland Security (DHS) in confronting threats, both domestically and internationally. The Department of Defense, with the development of US Northern Command, has increased its homeland defense role to coordinate military support to other federal and state agencies to confront threats that are both naturogenic and anthropogenic. And, most recently, revelations about US intelligence agencies collecting data on US citizens have expanded the dialogue on the nature of terrorist threats, breaking down traditional barriers between domestic and foreign intelligence activities.

Furthermore, in the 10 years since publication of the first edition, there has been a sea change in domestic politics and international relations, which has shaken the foundations of states and societies globally. From the international economic crisis of 2008 and the Arab Spring of 2010 to the global emergence of the Islamic State (IS) in 2014, the world has become more, rather than less, dangerous. The former director of National Intelligence, James Clapper (2014), noted, "Looking back over my more than half a century in intelligence, I've not experienced a time when we've been beset by more crises and threats around the globe."

So, what's changed in the text? With 10 years having elapsed since the publication of the first edition, all the original chapters have been revised and in some cases completely rewritten. New chapters have been added to address threats to critical infrastructure, the role of intelligence in homeland security, and homeland security planning and resources. Each chapter also addresses the overall theme of the text in reassessing whether the all-hazards perspective should continue to guide homeland security studies from an academic viewpoint, as well as homeland security policy from a practitioner's viewpoint.

In Chapter 1, Richard J. Kilroy Jr. provides an historical overview of the development of national security policies and strategies based on the threats the United States has faced since its beginning. From its early foundations focused on isolationism and nonintervention to the evolution of geopolitics that moved the United States to becoming a global superpower during the Cold War, the nature of the threats to the country has influenced the high politics of security. In the previous edition, this chapter ended with a discussion of the new Global War on Terrorism, focused primarily on al-Qaeda. Since that time, the United States has withdrawn from Iraq, is drawing down in Afghanistan, and yet continues to face an expanding terrorist threat from new groups, such as the Islamic State in Iraq and Syria (IS). This chapter has been updated to reflect the changes in national security and homeland security policies and strategy that occurred since the Obama administration came into office and changed the focus of national security away from fighting a Global War on Terrorism to focus on specific threats under the title of Overseas Contingency Operations, specifically using drone warfare to target terrorist leaders. It also touches on the early direction of the new Trump administration on national security in 2017.

In Chapter 2, Richard J. Kilroy Jr. explains the evolution from an "exclusive" view of homeland security, focused only on terrorist threats, to the "inclusive" view, which assessed all potential hazards as threats to the homeland. More recently there has been a some discussion about moving away from looking at homeland security from an all-hazards perspective, since it has tended to "water down" the threat of terrorism, as federal, state, and local agencies put every possible threat under the homeland security umbrella. From an emergency management perspective, local communities had to prepare for every possible contingency, which taxed resources and budgets. Federal homeland security funding began to dry up due to the budget crisis in 2008–2009. As a result, there was less of an all-hazards perspective to one of prioritizing the types of threats communities faced and to place their resources there. As a result, this chapter addresses these changes and the impact that moving away from an all-hazards perspective may have on the types of threats the United States faces today and in the future.

In Chapter 3, Chad S. Foster explores meanings and perspectives associated with homeland security. Questions addressed include: What are the historical traditions and prevailing theories associated with homeland security? What context is important for gaining an understanding of homeland security problems and approaches? What constitutes the homeland security enterprise, including the roles of federal, state, and local agencies? The revision to this chapter from the previous edition looks at the emergence of homeland security institutions and interests at all levels of government.

In Chapter 4, Alexander Siedschlag explores the all-hazards perspective to threat assessment, focused on management within the National Preparedness System. The chapter's focus was traditionally on prevention, protection, mitigation, response, and recovery and the "disaster impact process," as well as risk and vulnerability assessments. In the revision to the chapter, Siedschlag focuses on threat assessments and how the United States assesses threats to national security, as well as homeland security. Understanding the threat assessment process is critical to influencing intelligence collection and also how federal, state, and local agencies can better allocate resources when focused on specific threats. Siedschlag explains how threat assessment aids the decision-making process and how it can be helpful in reducing costs to local communities by allowing first responders and emergency managers to focus on the mitigation, risk reduction, and preparedness programs their communities need most.

In Chapter 5, Steven Kuhr offers a new chapter focusing specifically on critical infrastructure protection. New technologies and the increased use of "systems of systems" approaches create new efficiencies and availability of basic services such as power generation, transportation, water, and communications. However, the very nature of these technical matrices and integration of systems create new vulnerabilities and risks to homeland security. The "Internet of things" is just one example of how technology is changing even the most mundane everyday functions of people and society. Kuhr explains that as critical infrastructures expand and become more connected, our dependency on the Internet and information systems to carry the codes, programs, and instructions to make it all work grows as well, increasing the need for communities to plan for disruptions to those systems, whether that comes from a naturogenic or anthropogenic threat.

In Chapter 6, Jonathan M. Acuff provides a discussion on state-sponsored terrorism, to include a historical perspective as well as definitions of terrorism, identifying terrorists, and acts of terrorism. He also looks at the role of states and international organizations (like the United Nations) to confront terrorism, further addressing the United States and its view of state sponsors of terrorism. In the revision to this chapter, he also discusses how states can use terrorism as a means to advance their foreign policies through the use of terrorist organizations in other countries (e.g., state sponsors) but also domestically to keep dissident groups in check and prevent a possible loss of power, as occurred in Turkey in 2016. Other examples provided in the chapter include the breakup of Syria and the rise of IS, as well as Russia's intervention in Ukraine and its support for separatist/terrorist movements in that country.

In Chapter 7, Joseph Fitsanakis builds on the previous chapter, focusing on the different types of terrorist groups or organizations that function as violent non-state actors. He describes the motivations, ideologies, identities, and other factors that have given rise to terrorist movements in the past, in the present, and possibly in the future. He also discusses the various tools, tactics, and techniques that terrorist groups have used throughout the ages. He further addresses efforts by states to counter terrorist threats and the different methods employed, such as suicide terrorism. When the last text was written, the focus was on al-Qaeda as a non-state violent actor and the various offshoots of this organization. Since then, IS has emerged as a significant terrorist threat, seeking to establish itself throughout the Middle East, as well as commit acts of terrorism in states outside the region.

In Chapter 8, Richard J. Kilroy Jr. explores the pervasiveness of the Internet and its impact on just about every aspect of one's personal and public life and the threats in cyberspace coming from a number of sources, to include criminals, terrorists, and even states. In the first edition of the text, this chapter focused specifically on cyber-terrorism and cyber-warfare and addressed the US response to these types of threats provided by the government sector, to include the military. Since the first edition, there has been an exponential increase in the number and types of threats in cyberspace. Criminals, in particular, are growing in sophistication in their ability to hack into computer systems and steal personal and corporate information that threatens not only individuals but also national wealth and commerce. Revelations of China's growing cyber-warfare capability has also increased the threat of asymmetric warfare being waged in cyberspace, where a county's economic collapse would pre-stage a military attack (if even necessary). Kilroy provides a detailed look at the new dimension of threats in cyberspace with updated examples of recent cyber activity.

In Chapter 9, Christopher J. Ferrero describes the threat from Weapons of Mass Destruction (WMD), including chemical weapons, biological weapons, nuclear weapons, and radiological devices, and the potential terrorist targeting of critical infrastructure such as nuclear facilities and transportation hubs to achieve WMD-like effects. He covers the continuing threat of chemical weapons, as seen in the Syrian Civil War, and the increasing risk of biological weapons attacks by non-state actors who could use new do-it-yourself bioengineering tools to harm millions. He also addresses nuclear weapons, including the location and disposition of nuclear material and stockpiles, information on states' arms control commitments, and the terms of the Iran Nuclear Deal. He further provides information on how terrorist groups could create a WMD-like effect through the combination of nuclear or radiological substances with conventional explosives in what is known as a dirty bomb. The revised version of this chapter explores the concept of weapons of mass disruption, which suggests that terrorists can, through target analysis and selection, create a major crisis not by causing widespread death or physical destruction but by using these weapons and substances to contaminate or sabotage key infrastructure nodes, instill panic, and disrupt the flow of global commerce and public services.

In Chapter 10, Daniel Masters explores domestic terrorism in light of the new threat posed by both organized groups and individuals. Recent terrorist attacks in Europe and the United States by "lone-wolf" or self-radicalized individuals have further invigorated the debate. This significantly revised chapter not only addresses the threat posed by the different types of domestic terrorism but also expands that focus to look at the changing role of law enforcement agencies at the local, state, and federal levels to confront threats from domestic terrorism. Masters looks at the nexus between crime and terrorism as terrorist groups turn to crime to finance their operations, and criminal groups adopt terrorist tactics to spread violence and fear in order to dissuade governments from confronting them. Masters also explores the topic of mass shootings and the psychological impact these acts of hate can have as acts of terror.

In Chapter 11, Carmine Scavo focuses on how the information age, with the rise of the Internet and the media, has facilitated communication, leading both to better responses to natural disasters and to the spread of terrorist messages domestically and internationally. He explores the role of ideas and values in shaping culture and impacting societal responses to all hazards. These all serve as enablers of mass effects, meaning they can be used both by governments to increase the effectiveness of disaster response and by terrorist organizations for recruitment, fundraising, and support. In recent years, the rise of IS and the sophistication of its use of the Internet and social media, in particular, have presented a new challenge to states in countering terrorism and radical ideologies. Through these social networks, IS has been able to attract a large number of international fighters to its cause in Syria and Iraq. Since many of them hold passports and citizenship in Western countries, governments are concerned about what happens when these mercenaries return home. Scavo assesses the impact that the Internet and social media have had in contributing to the spreading of terrorist ideas and the radicalization of domestic terrorists.

In Chapter 12, Jonathan Smith adds a new chapter addressing the role of domestic intelligence in homeland security. Responding to the revelations about domestic intelligence collection on US citizens by the NSA, as a result of Edward Snowden's actions in 2013, Smith focuses on the relationship between intelligence collection and homeland security. The United States does not have a domestic intelligence organization, like the British MI-5. There was some discussion in 2002 that with the formation of the Department of Homeland Security (DHS), both the FBI and CIA be brought under the control of the new DHS; however, that was quickly dismissed due to the autonomy of these agencies and the different focus of each—one international and the other domestic. Yet, as Smith notes, that distinction has been based on the nature of the threats the nation faced with the CIA focused on external threats to national security, and the FBI focused on internal threats to homeland security (mostly being criminal threats). The nature of intelligence collection today and the use of new technologies and the Internet make those distinctions much more difficult, particularly with information technology. Smith also discusses the question that as the threats to homeland security evolve, should intelligence capabilities and resources as well? And if so, what are the threats to civil liberties and protections in democratic societies?

In Chapter 13, Stephan Reissman adds a new chapter focused on homeland security planning and resources. As a final chapter to the text, Reissman provides an important discussion on the future of homeland security, as both a function of government planning, resourcing, and direction and of educational programs that have emerged related to teaching about homeland security. In 2018, some might have thought that homeland security would no longer be in vogue, the Department of

Homeland Security would dissolve, and agencies, such as the US Coast Guard, would return to the Department of Transportation. Terrorism would no longer be the focus of US security policies abroad, and the focus at home would be to treat terrorism, as in much of the rest of the world, as criminal acts rather than national security threats. Yet, today, the world seems less secure, terrorism has not gone away, and the loss of personal freedoms and civil liberties continues to be debated. The growth in educational programs alone, related to teaching homeland security, is a testimony that reports of its death are premature.

ACKNOWLEDGMENTS

A work like this would not be possible without the collaborative efforts of all those contributors involved. Their timely submissions and quick responses to editorial comments allowed this work to come together in a relatively short period of time.

A special thanks goes out to Bob Esposito at John Wiley & Sons for approaching me about offering a second edition of the text. After 10 years, I had not expected to be revising the book after such a long period of time. I appreciate his encouragement and support to take on this project. I also appreciate Michael Leventhal's support in the contractual matters of the book, as well as his willingness to work with me on the cover design. I also want to recognize Stan Supinski and Steve Recca at the Naval Postgraduate School's Center for Homeland Defense Studies and Security. It was through their University and Agency Partnership Initiative and the Homeland Security Workshop they conducted in June 2015 that I was able to make contact with some of the new contributors to this text.

I also would like to thank the reviewers of the text for their comments and suggestions, which made this text much more readable and more thorough in its analytical and contextual basis.

Finally, I wish to thank the many editors and project managers at John Wiley & Sons, including Beryl Mesiadhas and Grace Paulin, who were involved in the production process. I appreciate their support, direction, and guidance throughout this effort from start to finish. Their constant attention to detail and editorial expertise truly made this work a success and I have learned much from their efforts.

RJK, Jr.
Conway, SC

ABOUT THE COMPANION WEBSITE

This book is accompanied by a companion website:

www.wiley.com/go/Kilroy/Threats_to_Homeland_Security

The instructor's website includes PPT slides for all chapters of the book, solutions to the Self-Check questions at the end of each major section of each chapter, and solutions to the Summary Questions at the end of each chapter.

In the student's website, I would recommend just including the Self-Check question solutions and the Summary Question solutions. I have used texts that have too much information for students who then use the "school solutions" rather than doing their own analysis.

1

THE CHANGING NATURE OF NATIONAL SECURITY
Understanding the Nature of Threats to Homeland Security and the US Response

Richard J. Kilroy, Jr.
Department of Politics, Coastal Carolina University, Conway, SC, USA

Starting Point

Go to www.wiley.com/go/Kilroy/Threats_to_Homeland_Security to assess your knowledge of the basics of national security and homeland security.
Determine where you need to concentrate your effort.

What You'll Learn in This Chapter

▲ The definitions of national security and homeland security
▲ The key players who formulate national and homeland security policy
▲ How changing international and domestic security environments affect national and homeland security policies
▲ The threats in a post-9/11 world that impact national security policy issues
▲ Contemporary challenges to national and homeland security

After Studying This Chapter, You'll Be Able To

▲ Analyze security environments and assess national and homeland security policy choices during specific historical periods
▲ Distinguish between national and homeland security policy players within government and outside government
▲ Appraise the threat situation in the post-9/11 security environment
▲ Examine US national and homeland security and policy as a response to the changing security environment and threat perceptions

Threats to Homeland Security: Reassessing the All-Hazards Perspective, Second Edition.
Edited by Richard J. Kilroy, Jr.
© 2018 John Wiley & Sons, Inc. Published 2018 by John Wiley & Sons, Inc.
Companion website: www.wiley.com/go/Kilroy/Threats_to_Homeland_Security

INTRODUCTION

Within the disciplines of political science and international relations, the study of war and conflict has been traditionally included under the umbrella of international security since the primary threats to states have been viewed as other states. The rise of non-state actors, such as terrorist groups or criminal gangs, has broadened the concept of threats to a nation's security to include both domestic and international dimension. For example, the United States, throughout the nation's history, has faced a variety of **threats or adversaries** (foreign and domestic) possessing both capability and intent to do the nation harm. To counter these threats, various policy choices emerged, each reflecting the nation's security interests at different periods of time. As a result, the nation's political leaders developed **national security** policies, which are those policies that served to protect the United States, its citizens, and its interests through the threatened and actual use of all elements of national power.

During the first half of the twentieth century, the United States changed from a nation with the seventeenth largest military in the world to one of two military superpowers. It was the leader of the free world against a physical and ideological threat in the Soviet Union and communism. This change was not preordained, however, as strong domestic political challenges also shaped foreign policy outcomes. Fifty years after the end of World War II, the United States again found itself in a new kind of security environment with both domestic and international security implications. At the turn of the twenty-first century, the nation was faced with the new threat of terrorism at home. This led to the development of **homeland security** policies, which emerged following the terrorist attacks of September 11, 2001 (9/11), to encompass the collective efforts of local, state, and federal agencies to keep the country safe, initially against terrorism, but later expanded to include an all-hazards perspective. Sixteen years later, the threats to homeland security have further evolved, and the United States faces a prolonged conflict against the particular threat of terrorism, domestically and internationally.

In this chapter, you will analyze security environments and assess national and homeland security policy choices during specific historical periods. You'll also learn to distinguish between the various national and homeland security policy players both within and outside government. Finally, you'll appraise the threat situation in the contemporary security environment, as well as examine US national and homeland security policy as a response to the changing security environment and threat perceptions.

1.1 Foundations of American Security Policy

When the nation's founders were crafting a new system of government based on a republic (vs. a monarchy), they struggled over the concept of security. How much power should be vested in the central government versus the state governments? Should the United States have a standing army or rely on the state militias alone for the nation's security? The **Federalist Papers** (authored by Alexander Hamilton, James Madison, and John Jay) argued the need for a central government strong enough to protect the nation against the threats it faced at the time while also protecting states' rights and individual liberties. As James Madison noted in

Federalist No. 41, "The means of security can only be regulated by the means and danger of attack... They will in fact be ever determined by these rules and no others" (Hamilton et al. 1961, 257).

Upon achieving its independence from Great Britain, the United States faced the possibility of British reinvasion, attacks by other European colonial powers in the region, and challenges to commerce. Its national security policy reflected George Washington's admonition in his Farewell Address to avoid entangling alliances with European powers, which would draw the United States into Europe's sectarian wars. Thus, for over a century and a half, **isolationism**, a foreign policy based on avoiding alliances with other countries, produced an American national security policy of limited military power, depending instead on the ocean boundaries, diplomacy, and commerce to keep the country safe.

Prior to its entrance into World War I, US security interests were primarily focused regionally rather than globally. An example of a security policy reflecting this regional focus was the **Monroe Doctrine** of 1823. Although the United States did not have the military power to back up such a policy, the Monroe Doctrine reflected the principle that the United States should support the desire of the new democratic nations of the Americas to break from their colonial past and exist as free nations, secure from overt European influence. This principle was tested throughout the nineteenth century by various European powers, such as the French occupation of Mexico and the continuing Spanish and British presence, primarily in the Caribbean region. With the US defeat of Spain in 1898, however, the United States displayed the capacity to live up to its principles.

Why did the United States enter these new domains? For most of America's early history, security meant maintaining territorial integrity, but it also involved protecting American trade overseas. As the United States grew economically, so did other countries, so American traders found themselves clashing more frequently with foreign interests over resources and markets. The clashes could be simply commercial competition, but violence could break out with local populations, with other commercial enterprises, or with governments. Trade was not only enriching the country but also redefining the government's duty to protect American citizens to include events that were increasing in both scope and frequency.

1.1.1 Geopolitics at the Beginning of the Twentieth Century

The emergence of American military power (primarily sea power) at the beginning of the twentieth century expanded US national security interests in the Western Hemisphere and beyond. Whereas the original Monroe Doctrine was a statement of principle, the **Roosevelt Corollary** (Figure 1-1) to the Monroe Doctrine under President Theodore Roosevelt signaled a more aggressive US security policy to exert its **hegemony** over the Western Hemisphere. The ability of the United States to project military power to other regions further increased our nation's ability to leverage other elements of national power, including the use of diplomacy, economic power, and informational power. The threat of military force therefore broadened the expression of national security interests, leading to a more expansionist role for the United States. Broadening the context of national security further affected US foreign policy interests toward Europe and European affairs. Whereas in the past the United States was comfortable in its isolationist role, in the early 1900s,

Figure 1-1

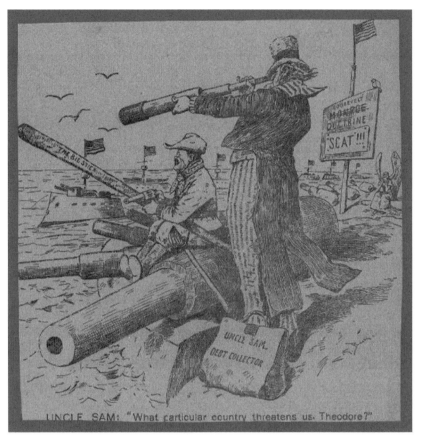

The Roosevelt Corollary to the Monroe Doctrine in the Western Hemisphere (Charles Green Bush, 1842–1909). Uncle Sam—"What Particular Country Threatens Us, Theodore?," March 12, 1905, *New York World*. Source: Reproduced with permission of MS Am 3056 (489) Houghton Library, Harvard University.

the changes in the geopolitical makeup of Europe were directly affecting America's security at home.

The causes for World War I were complex, reflecting imperial competition, the rise of industrial economies and military-industrial complexes, the decline of the aristocracy, and the rise of nationalism, anarchism, and communism. Powerful political ideas and movements swept across the European continent, creating conditions for conflict and war. Although Woodrow Wilson ran for reelection in 1916 on the campaign slogan "He kept us out of war," in 1917, he came to the realization that national security required the United States to join with the **Entente Powers** (mainly France, Russia, Britain, and Italy) against the **Central Powers** (Germany, Austria-Hungary, the Ottoman Empire, and Bulgaria). A German submarine's sinking of the *Lusitania*, an American ship loaded with supplies for Britain, underscored America's inability to cut itself off from countries at war. As Wilson noted, "I made every effort to keep my country out of war, until it came to my conscience, as it came to yours, that after all it was our war a well as Europe's war, that the ambition of these central empires was directed against nothing less than the liberty of the world" (Foley 1969, 12).

World War I revolutionized the geopolitical landscape of Europe as empires were dissolved and new nation-states emerged. Wilson pressured the European powers to accept his famous 14 points, which called for **collective security** based on concerted international response to aggression. This laid the foundation for the League of Nations, the precursor to the United Nations (UN). In effect, Wilson redefined national security policy from one based on neutrality to one based on continuing international cooperation. The US Senate refused to ratify the resulting treaty, however, and America retreated back to a period of isolationism and avoidance of European affairs. In addition, partly because of American reluctance but also because of the difficulty of constraining major powers, the League of Nations ultimately failed.

Also after World War I, the United States used naval disarmament as a means to increase international security, without having to enter into a collective security arrangement. Navies allowed the projection of power at that time, so limiting naval power also limited military potential. Proposed as an alternative to the League of Nations, Republicans in the US Senate promoted the Washington Naval Conference (1921–1922), limiting the size and growth of the world's major naval powers: the United States, Great Britain, France, Japan, and Italy. The treaty, however, delayed rather than ended such arms races.

Later, in the 1930s, Congress engaged in another effort to promote isolationism by way of the **Neutrality Acts**, laws forbidding American support for or involvement with countries at war. Under these laws, the *Lusitania* might never have been sunk, as it could not have carried supplies to Britain or even entered British ports. As a security issue, the laws represented a major challenge to presidential power, as they restricted the flexibility the president enjoys as commander-in-chief and as the chief architect of US foreign policy.

Between wars, ocean barriers and relatively secure borders continued to provide security for the United States. Canada to the north was a proven ally, requiring a minimal security presence. To the south, however, Mexico was emerging from a bitter civil war and internal revolution. In fact, before the US entry into World War I, the Mexican revolutionary leader Pancho Villa staged a series of attacks into the United States, the most famous being the Columbus, New Mexico, raid of March 19, 1916. This led to the legendary General Pershing expedition into Mexico in pursuit of Villa, and it also included a mobilization of a number of National Guard units to the border to provide security. The expedition ended in 1917 with US entry into World War I and diplomatic efforts between the American and Mexican governments to avoid further conflict. By the end of World War I, the Mexican revolution had moved toward stabilization under a new regime, which would eventually emerge as Mexico's dominant political party for the next 70 years.

Immediately prior to the start of World War II, the United States began aggressively developing its air and naval capabilities, allowing it to be able to project power where and when necessary. The United States also expanded its military overseas presence in places like the Philippines, Cuba, Panama, Puerto Rico, the Midway Islands, and the Hawaiian Islands. Set up as strategic coaling stations, naval bases at these locations provided the US forward presence in areas it deemed to have strategic interests. At the same time, Britain and France, still suffering "war weariness," were attempting to pull back from some of their overseas commitments and colonial holdings, leaving power vacuums that were quickly filled by Japan, Italy, and Germany, the countries that would be known as the **Axis Powers** during World War II.

1.1.2 National Security and World War II

World War II began in 1939 with the German invasion of Poland, followed by declarations of war by Britain and France. The United States did not officially enter the conflict until 1941, following Japan's surprise attack on Pearl Harbor. By its end in 1945, World War II had inflicted over 62 million casualties from at least 50 countries. Major operational campaigns occurred in the Atlantic and Pacific theaters, as well as throughout Europe, Eastern Europe and Russia, Asia, China, Africa, and the Middle East. British and German vessels even fought near the tip of South America. The sheer magnitude of the conflict impacted people and nations throughout the world such that security took on new meaning for different nations. For the United States, it meant that the nation would never again be able to return to an isolationist foreign policy and its national security would be directly linked to that of Europe, Asia, and other regions of the world.

From 1939 to 1941, the United States maintained its neutrality with regard to World War II, despite Winston Churchill's pleas for a formal alliance with Britain. America demonstrated this neutrality by avoiding direct conflict, preferring to support the Allies through other means. For example, Franklin Roosevelt's lend/lease program provided Britain with essential war materials to continue military operations against Germany, even though this policy contravened the Neutrality Acts. This security strategy further provided for **prepositioning** or establishing bases and supplies in foreign countries to prepare a rapid response to future crises, anticipating the time when the United States would eventually join the conflict. For Roosevelt, the United States was the "arsenal of democracy," and it was only a matter of time before the United States would become directly involved in another land war in Europe, given the expanding German threat. However, domestic public opinion was mixed, as was that of Congress, given the large numbers of German and Italian immigrants in the United States. In fact, until the attack on Pearl Harbor, 64% of the American public still thought peace was possible without US intervention. Some revisionist historians argue that knowing this, Roosevelt provoked a Japanese attack to force Congress to declare war against Japan and the Axis powers (e.g., see Williams 1978). According to this argument, Roosevelt could then support Winston Churchill's "Germany first" strategy to save Europe before opposing the Japanese in Asia. These views are clearly in the minority, however, as most recognized military historians clearly place the blame on Japan for its preemptive strike on the US Pacific fleet in order to reduce resistance to Japan's imperial strategy to conquer Southeast Asia. Roosevelt and his top military advisor, General George C. Marshall, both supported the "Germany first" war plans, recognizing the immediate need for American military intervention in the European theater of operations. Roosevelt, exercising his prerogative as commander-in-chief, set the nation's strategic policies, ordering the military to begin combat operations in North Africa rather than plan for a direct attack on France. Codenamed Operation Torch, this campaign began in November 1942, signaling the beginning of American offensive efforts in the war (Brower 2002).

During World War II, Roosevelt and his successor Harry Truman left the operational wartime decision making to their military commanders. In the European theater, General Dwight D. Eisenhower commanded US and Allied military forces in North Africa, the Italian peninsula campaigns, and the crossing of the English Channel on D-Day (June 6, 1944) and forward to Berlin. Eisenhower, as the Supreme Allied Commander, determined security policy during the war in Europe, as did General Douglas MacArthur and Admiral Chester Nimitz in the Pacific. The Army Chief of Staff, General George Marshall, served as the Chairman of the Joint Chiefs of Staff and was the President's principal military advisor at the time. He did not command forces, nor did he set operational policy decisions. Rather, the president and the Secretaries of War and the Navy set strategic security policies, which the military leaders then executed. Only later, during Korean War in the 1950s, when MacArthur challenged Truman's authority by questioning his strategic policies, did the president exercise his role as commander-in-chief to remove MacArthur from command.

US national security policy during World War II was, first and foremost, the defeat of the Axis powers, Germany and Italy first and then Japan. America applied all elements of its national power to that end. Even domestic politics took a backseat to foreign policy, as every American accepted the sacrifices required of a nation at war, to include certain deprivations of goods and services in support of the war effort. The largest domestic economic impact was the retooling of the industrial base from a consumer-based economy to a war-based economy, as America leveraged its economic and military power to achieve its national security objectives. The American public responded by investing in their country (buying war bonds), working in the factories (women joined assembly lines in record numbers), and collecting salvageable materials (children led collection efforts for scrap iron, rubber, and other items). During World War II, whether they were fighting the war in Europe, the Pacific, or the home front, most Americans felt they were directly contributing to the security goal of defeating their enemies. However, some groups, such as Japanese Americans, were not allowed to help due to fears over their true sense of loyalty to America versus Japan, and thus they were subjected to isolation in special camps during the war.

FOR EXAMPLE

Japanese Internment Camps

During World War II, the US government took the action of interring Japanese Americans from the West Coast in War Relocation Centers located away from the coastal areas in the west. Over 120 000 men, women, and children were sent to the centers. Over two-thirds of them were US citizens. President Roosevelt justified the action based on the threat of Japanese spies operating in those communities. The Supreme Court (*Korematsu v. United States* 1944) upheld Roosevelt's actions, stating that ethnic groups could be interned during a state of war because "[p]ressing public necessity may sometimes justify the existence of such restrictions" (PBS n.d.) What is not as well known is that smaller groups of Italians and Germans living in the United States were also interred during the war, classified as "enemy aliens" (Siasoco and Ross 2006).

World War II ended in 1945 with the surrender of Germany, followed by Japan's surrender after the dropping of nuclear bombs on Hiroshima and Nagasaki. The decision to use nuclear weapons for the first time was made by President Truman, knowing that short of a US invasion of the Japanese mainland, the war in the Pacific could drag out for years. Rather than accept the larger loss of American and Japanese lives from such a protracted conflict, Truman's use of this new technology was as much psychological as it was physical. Due to the magnitude of the destruction caused by nuclear weapons, the world was about to enter a new stage of both security and insecurity, as other nations sought to come under the nuclear umbrella and avoid conflict for fear it would escalate into global nuclear warfare.

SELF-CHECK

- Define national security.
- Which of the following was not one of the Central Powers during World War I?

  a. Germany

  b. Austria-Hungary

  c. Russia

  d. Bulgaria

- Italy was not one of the Axis Powers during World War II. True or false?
- The League of Nations would have replaced a collective security policy with one based on neutrality. True or false?

1.2 Security in the Cold War Era

At the end of World War II, the United States emerged as the strongest military and economic power in the world by virtue of having avoided the direct impact of the war, with the exception of the attack on Pearl Harbor. Most of Europe lay in ruins, however, as did much of Japan. Working with Great Britain and other countries, the United States created the **United Nations (UN)** and, through the **Bretton Woods Agreements**, key economic institutions that were intended to promote political and economic stability throughout the international system, including Europe and Japan. Believing the causes of World War II lay in political, economic, and social instability created by World War I, planners in 1945 sought to prevent the recurrence of those conditions.

Despite agreements made at Yalta between Stalin, Roosevelt, and Churchill, the Soviets moved quickly to fill the geopolitical vacuum of German defeat by occupying those countries they "liberated" during the war. The United States countered the Soviets by seeking to restore a balance of power to Europe through the combination of a continued US military presence in the region, as well as a large amount of direct economic aid to rebuild Europe. Conceived by US Secretary of State George C. Marshall, the **Marshall Plan** provided funds supplied by the United

States to help rebuild non-Communist countries after World War II. The Plan provided means for West Germany, in particular, to recover from the devastation of World War II and emerge later as an ally in the Cold War.

Initially, President Truman assumed that Stalin, like most political leaders, was a pragmatist and that Soviet security policy would be motivated by a quid pro quo. Truman expected that Stalin would be willing to negotiate (horse trading, as Truman called it), assuming that Soviet behavior could be modified. However, George Kennan, a US government official stationed in Moscow, published works explaining the source of Soviet behavior toward the West and challenging Truman's perception. Kennan argued that the Soviets were not willing to work with the United States and other Western nations to share power. Rather, the Soviet goal was to destroy the West, and the only rational US security policy was one that stood up to Soviet aggression, willing to match force with force if necessary (History Guide n.d.). Whether it liked it or not, America would take on a leadership role in setting the international security agenda, as well as committing the resources necessary to serve as global guarantor of a new world order. Thus began the period that would come to be known as the Cold War.

FOR EXAMPLE

Mr X and Containment

George F. Kennan was a US Department of State official who was convinced that the Soviets viewed accommodation with the United States and other Western powers as a weakness and contradictory to their goal of expanding international communism. Kennan sought to communicate his views about the true nature of Soviet ambitions through what became known as his "long telegram" back to the State Department. In this official document, Kennan laid out the reasons why the United States needed to take a hard-line strategy toward Moscow and Soviet expansionism.

This official document become public in 1947, when it was published in an article titled "The Sources of Soviet Conduct" in *Foreign Affairs*. The author was called "Mr X," but experts knew it to be the work of George Kennan. In this article, Kennan explained the motivations behind Soviet behavior in foreign affairs. He argued that the Soviet state was totalitarian in its political structures as well as its ruling ideology, communism. Kennan believed communism to be antithetical to the West and a direct challenge to our nation's democratic principles, free-market capitalist economy, and cultural and spiritual beliefs. He warned that the United States should not regard the Soviets as partners in managing international security, but rather as competitors, always seeking an advantage on the world stage. As Kennan stated, "In these circumstances, it is clear that the main element of any United States policy toward the Soviet Union must be that of long-term, patient but firm and vigilant containment of Russian expansive tendencies." The key word **containment** signified the principal national security policy pursued during the Cold War to prevent the spread of communism and Soviet influence throughout the world (History Guide n.d.).

1.2.1 Bipolarity Versus Multipolarity

Prior to World War II, the international security environment could be character-ized as a **multipolar system**, a relationship among countries in the international system where no country dominated, with a number of nation-states (primarily European) possessing military power and capable of acting independently. Hans Morgenthau (1948) popularized the use of the term **balance of power**, where no one state had a monopoly of power and nations sought to maximize security either through alliances to compensate for weaknesses or through unilateral means when they perceived it be in their national interest to do so. Morgenthau believed that a multipolar system allowed for greater flexibility for nations, who could change alliances as necessary to maximize their power and security.

After World War II, the old vestiges of the European balance of power, based on a multipolar system, disappeared, as two new spheres of military power and influence emerged: the United States and the Union of Soviet Socialist Republics (USSR). Since both powers emerged as victors after World War II, each sought to consolidate its influence over parts of Europe, as well as former European colonial interests. The new security environment that developed was therefore character-ized as a **bipolar system**, with other nation-states tending to align themselves with either the United States or the USSR. Those supporting the United States were primarily Western European nations, while Eastern European countries came under the influence of the USSR, mostly by force. Those in the US camp came to be called the First World or Free World nations, while those in the USSR camp came to be called the Second World or Communist bloc states.

George Kennan's notion of containment was a national security strategy for handling the bipolar system. Other possible strategies ranged from returning to isolation to initiating total war, where all national resources would be employed to destroy the Soviets. Containing Soviet expansion would be a long-term policy and would be very expensive, but it seemed the best way of pressuring the Soviets while minimizing costs at home. The array of threats included conventional and nuclear war in Europe, direct attacks with nuclear weapons on the United States and the USSR, proxy wars where the two major powers supported competing sides in wars of national liberation, and also espionage and subversion in the two countries.

To manage this bewildering array of threats, Congress passed the **National Security Act of 1947**. This act turned the Army Air Corps into the US Air Force and merged the War Department and Navy Department, creating the Department of Defense. The act also created a civilian organization, the Central Intelligence Agency (CIA), to manage overseas intelligence gathering and conduct **clandestine and covert operations** against foreign governments. The Department of Justice's Federal Bureau of Investigation (FBI) received responsibility for domestic counter-intelligence. Several influences drove the effort: the new Soviet threat, the intelli-gence failure that had permitted the attack on Pearl Harbor, and concerns about Communist groups operating inside the United States. Finally, some argue that the act was created to reduce turf wars between the Army and Navy.

The primary international security structures that emerged after World War II reflected the interests of these two power blocs representing the bipolar system. To counter the overwhelming conventional military force buildup by the Soviets in Eastern Europe, the United States led the development of the **North Atlantic**

Treaty Organization (NATO) in 1949. This collective defense organization was established as a political and military alliance, with each member nation pledging that an attack on any one of them would be regarded as an attack against all and bring the collective response of all member nations. The original 12 members of NATO were Belgium, Canada, Denmark, France, Iceland, Italy, Luxembourg, the Netherlands, Norway, Portugal, the United Kingdom, and the United States. Between 1949 and the end of the Cold War in 1991, four other nations were also admitted to NATO: Greece, Turkey, West Germany, and Spain. These 16 nations, led by the United States, comprised the "West" and its military response to the "East," which was led by the USSR. In response to the formation of NATO, the Soviets sought to counter the collective military powers of the West by forming the **Warsaw Pact** in 1955, composed of Albania, Bulgaria, Czechoslovakia, East Germany, Hungary, Poland, Romania, and the Soviet Union (Figure 1-2).

Figure 1-2

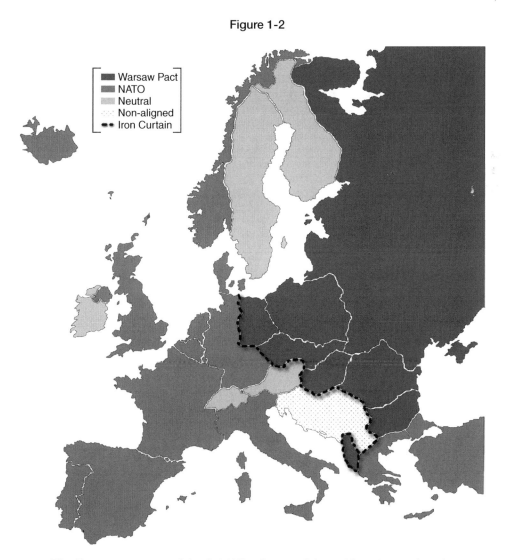

The European context of the Cold War. Source: Adapted from Rumer (2016).

Besides NATO and the Warsaw Pact, other regional security alliances also formed during the Cold War, including the Australia, New Zealand, United States Security Treaty (ANZUS), the Southeast Asia Treaty Organization (SEATO), and Organization of American States (OAS). Other Communist countries, such as Cuba, North Korea, and the People's Republic of China (PRC), were also considered to be in the Soviet sphere of influence, but they did not enter into formal alliances such as occurred with those nations under the US sphere of influence. Most Third World countries were faced with a stark choice of association with one or the other super-power, dividing most of the world into two competing camps.

This change from multipolarity to bipolarity was a significant shift in the way international politics worked. The balance of power system described by Morgenthau, where countries would make alliances in order to prevent any one country from gaining too much power, had broken down during World War I. Woodrow Wilson's idea of collective security would have had every country unite against aggression, replacing the balance of power system. Without this system, however, bipolarity arose in the absence of multipolarity. Bipolarity was based on two competing groups of countries, or "blocs." Competition became what the Soviets called managing the **correlation of forces**, a measure of comparative military power of member nations (see Table 1-1), where the two blocs were locked in combat like two wrestlers grappling for an advantage over each other. Over time, some countries might move from one bloc to the other, changing relative power, until one side had a clear advantage. Throughout this period of Cold War competition, the United States and USSR spent lavishly on weapons and political influence to ensure their own success.

Eventually, the bipolar system broke down, not from the direct tensions between the superpowers, but from the internal fragmentation of the two power blocs. The most important changes emerged in the 1960s, when France left NATO and the Peoples' Republic of China (PRC) quarreled with the Soviets. In the latter instance, the two nations fought a low-level border war in the early 1970s. President Nixon visited the PRC around that time, and the resulting relationships moved closer to the shifting patterns of the earlier multipolar system.

1.2.2 Containing Communism

During the Cold War era, Kennan's view of the Soviet Union was essentially correct, but managing the threats posed by the USSR proved difficult. This section examines the different threats mentioned previously and subsequent responses. Keep in mind that the choices were highly politicized, reflecting concerns about the desirability of peace and war and also how best to allocate defense dollars.

1.2.2.1 Conventional and Nuclear War in Europe

When tensions with the Soviets began, defense planners presumed that war would be fought in Germany and surrounding areas. Some planners wanted American forces to be limited, acting as a trigger for nuclear war, while others wanted NATO forces to be adequate for defeating a Soviet invasion. Compromises led to forward-basing substantial amounts of supplies, along with over one million American personnel. Included in this force was a substantial collection of short- and medium-range

Table 1-1: Approximations of NATO versus Warsaw Pact Military Power—Contrasting Views

	Warsaw Pact count	NATO count
Tanks		
Warsaw Pact	59 000	52 000
NATO	31 000	16 000
Armored personnel carriers		
Warsaw Pact	70 000	55 000
NATO	47 000	23 000
Artillery systems		
Warsaw Pact	72 000	43 000
NATO	57 000	14 000
Combat aircraft		
Warsaw Pact	7 900	8 200
NATO	7 100	4 000
Helicopters		
Warsaw Pact	2 800	3 700
NATO	5 300	2 400
Ground forces		
Warsaw Pact	3 600 000	3 100 000
NATO	3 700 000	2 200 000

Source: Department of Defense (1989).

nuclear weapons, and the order of battle was reorganized for fighting on a nuclear battlefield.

An important part of planning for national security was that if America should be fighting a war in Europe, it might be seen by other opponents as an opportunity to attack elsewhere. Just as World War II was fought in several theaters simultaneously, America needed to prepare for similar conditions in the future.

Some of these forces remain in Europe today, available for assignment elsewhere. Their numbers were drawn down over time, and their equipment and munitions were redirected for conflicts elsewhere, including Vietnam and Iraq. In one of the last major threats of the Cold War, the Soviets began basing intermediate-range (1000 miles) missiles in the early 1980s. American intentions to counter with similar missiles produced a treaty to eliminate these weapons from Europe. This part of the Cold War was finally winding down.

1.2.2.2 Nuclear Threats to the United States and USSR

In 1945, the United States was the only country with nuclear weapons, but Soviet spies managed to steal the technology. Thus, by the middle of the 1950s, both countries had hydrogen bombs, also known as thermonuclear weapons. The only long-range delivery platforms, though, were bomber aircraft. Suddenly, however, in 1957, the Soviets orbited a satellite, Sputnik, meaning that they had missile technology that would allow an attack on the United States without the use of airplanes. The United States thus developed a nuclear triad, composed of long-range strategic bombers, intercontinental ballistic missiles, and submarines, all of which were capable of delivering nuclear warheads. The US nuclear strategy leveraged technology, increasing its nuclear weapons capability with improved accuracy in striking targets (referred to as the **circular error probability (CEP)**) and also the use of **multiple independently targetable reentry vehicles (MIRVs)**, which allowed missiles to have more than one warhead. The Soviets relied more on "throw weight," using a brute force strategy—in other words, the more warheads the better, with accuracy not being as important.

Throughout the Cold War, there was always concern on both sides over how accurate each nation's intelligence assessments were with regard to actual nuclear weapons counts and capabilities. As a result, on two occasions, the two **superpowers**, the United States and USSR, came close to actual nuclear war. In the first instance, during the Cuban missile crisis in October 1962, the Soviets tried to base short-range missiles in Cuba. For many years, it was thought that the United States had forced the Soviets to back down. It was later discovered that the crisis was resolved by a quid pro quo of American missiles being removed from Turkey. The second occasion was during the Arab–Israeli War of 1973.

It's important to note that the possibility of nuclear war was the first major direct threat to the continental United States in decades. Further, it augmented the civil defense planning at home that began during World War II, which required the creation of shelters and food stocks for emergencies. Further, the arms race and consequent intelligence-gathering efforts produced dramatic technological advances, changing perceptions about war and war fighting by adding satellite imagery, computer analysis, and advanced communications to the mix.

The possibility of nuclear war, however, was a divisive issue for many people. Americans became divided over whether the country's leaders could, in good conscience, use such weapons, and they pressed for actions through the United Nations (UN) instead of relying on domestic politics. Others argued with equal fervor that as long as other nations had such weapons, the United States must have them as well. Such fears among the five countries that had nuclear weapons in the 1960s produced treaties to limit **proliferation**, or the supplying of other countries with the technology to build their own nuclear weapons. Eventually, using a policy called **détente** (a relaxation of tensions), the Nixon administration in the 1970s began negotiating treaties that would slow the arms race and subsequent administrations would negotiate actual reductions in nuclear weapons. President Reagan in the 1980s achieved great success in negotiation through a two-track approach. On one side, he negotiated aggressively, calling for dramatic reductions in stockpiles of nuclear weapons. On the other, he pressed for advanced technology, including the Strategic Defense Initiative (SDI). Also known as Star Wars, the SDI relied on the use of ground- and space-based systems to protect the United States from attack by nuclear missiles. In light of these actions, the Soviets could either negotiate or face economic failure by trying to keep up with American efforts.

1.2.2.3 Proxy Wars

The United States and the Soviet Union never actually fought each other during the 45 years of the Cold War. Military advisors, money, and equipment were delivered far and wide, however. For instance, the Soviets and the Peoples' Republic of China supported North Korea's invasion of South Korea, and Cuban advisors operated in Angola and Central and South America. For a time, Americans were in Ethiopia and Russians were in Somalia, until civil wars in those countries caused the two to switch sides. The last major anti-communist operation was in the island of Grenada in 1983, which was being used as a staging area for supplies for insurgents in the Western Hemisphere.

During the Cold War era, the largest commitment of American forces was in Vietnam, where the conflict dragged on for over 10 years, from the Kennedy administration into the second Nixon administration. Eventually, domestic opposition forced American withdrawal. The Soviets ran into similar problems in the late 1970s when they invaded Afghanistan, encouraging the rise of radical Islamic groups, such as al-Qaeda and the Taliban. In fact, when the Soviet Union collapsed in 1991, a contributing factor was the money spent on such foreign adventures. Such proxy wars also had profound effects on US domestic politics, forcing the end of the draft and the move to an all-volunteer military and additionally contributing to reluctance among some Americans to engage in overseas operations. Despite this tendency, both Republican and Democratic presidents continued to commit troops overseas.

The proxy wars added a new layer of responsibility for military planners. Not only did they need to plan for conventional and nuclear wars, but they were also required to create doctrine to manage low-intensity conflict, counterinsurgency, and circumstances calling for rapid troop deployments. The Green Berets, for example, were created not simply to fight an unconventional war, but to organize local populations against a common enemy.

1.2.2.4 Espionage and Subversion during the Cold War

The Cold War created difficult times for managing domestic security, as political and normative goals clashed with the needs of security. The Soviet Union operated an active program of spying and subversion in the United States, and the FBI replied with an intense counterespionage program. In the late 1940s and early 1950s, Alger Hiss and other government officials were convicted of spying for the Soviets. Senator Joseph McCarthy held hearings to investigate how Soviet spies were able to penetrate so deeply into government during the 1950s, and he also pursued subversives in the media and government. Eventually, important political actors concluded that McCarthy was going too far and was ignoring constitutionally guaranteed rights for the accused, and they forced McCarthy to back down. This debate between individual rights and national security remains a hotly contested topic to this day.

As the Cold War continued, the CIA and the Defense Intelligence Agency (DIA) were joined by additional specialized agencies, such as the National Security Agency, which monitors radio and other communications. During the 1960s, these agencies had a fairly free hand in pursuing intelligence problems. In the 1970s, however, Congress set up the Church Commission to draw up rules restraining the intelligence community. According to this commission, clandestine and covert operations would require written presidential approval in the future. Although some people use these terms interchangeably, clandestine operations are secret efforts to gather information, while covert operations are intended to influence how governments behave. Covert operations would include bribes, subversion and psychological operations, and support for insurgent forces, with the intent not to reveal the source of the operation.

Finally, while the United States was dealing with spies, Europe was struggling with bands of terrorists, such as the Baader-Meinhof Gang and the Red Brigades, operating independently of the Soviet Union. The Weathermen, Symbionese Liberation Army (SLA), Black Panthers, and other extremist groups began plotting terrorist activities in the United States as well. Cooperation between American and European intelligence and police forces became a critical effort for addressing these threats.

1.2.3 Non-Communist Threats

International communism presented the greatest, but by no means the only, threat to the United States during the Cold War. The US government preferred, however, to focus on the major threat, hoping that the others would remain minor problems. Nonetheless, wars of national liberation and revolutions in the developing world drew resources away from the main problem, as did frequent conflicts about religion and territory in the Middle East. Conflicts between Arabs and Israelis broke out four times between 1948 and 1973; these conflicts were as much about who controlled Palestine as what religion should be followed. The Carter administration withdrew support for the Shah of Iran in 1978, a move that resulted in Iran being taken over by religious extremists. A group of students seized the US Embassy in that country late in 1979, creating the famous Iran hostage crisis. American efforts at negotiation and at rescue failed, though the hostages were released at the beginning of the Reagan administration. These problems caused the government to again rethink how to manage special operations and rapid deployment.

During the 1980s, efforts at projecting power met with mixed success. American intervention in Lebanon failed after the bombing of the US Marine barracks in Beirut in 1983. A terrorist attack on a nightclub in Berlin in 1986 was found to have been planned by Libya; President Reagan retaliated by bombing many targets in Libya (called Operation El Dorado Canyon), eliminating Libya's military potential (but not its support for terrorism) for years to come. These and other attacks reflected state-sponsored terrorism (see Chapter 6), where governments encouraged extremists. An increasing problem, however, was the radical Islamists, consisting of the Muslim Brotherhood in Egypt and the Wahhabists in Saudi Arabia, both of which were factions from the majority Sunni sect of Islam, as well as the followers of the Ayatollah Khomeini in Iran, who are part of the Shiite minority. Osama bin Laden and al-Qaeda come from the Wahhabist movement. They supported efforts to drive Western influences from the Middle East and to replace existing Middle Eastern governments with newer, more radical ones.

Two points are important here. First, although many problems occurred in the Middle East during this time, they were not specifically problems with Islam.

Second, while the cases listed here involved conflict, there were also extensive efforts to encourage peaceful resolution to problems. For example, the Camp David Accords of 1979 settled conflict between Israel and Egypt and established a long-term relationship between the United States and Egypt. Although problems with groups and governments in the Middle East were present, those groups and governments did not represent a monolithic threat. However, the Islamic Revolution in Iran in 1979, and the subsequent rise of the Ayatollah Khomeini, did usher in a new era of state sponsorship of terrorism, with the rise of Hezbollah, Islamic Jihad, and other groups espousing radical Islamic ideologies that have both regional and global impact today.

SELF-CHECK

- Define balance of power.
- The principal national security policy pursued during the Cold War was called:
  a. Containment
  b. Isolationism
  c. Expansionism
  d. Unilateralism
- Covert operations seek to cover their sources. True or false?
- Terrorism is a product only of religious extremism. True or false?

1.3 Security in the Post-Cold War Era: Pre-9/11

The government of the Soviet Union collapsed in 1991 when a coup by communist hard-liners failed. The Soviet economic relationship with Eastern Europe had already been abandoned, and the leader of the new democratic government, Boris Yeltsin, moved quickly to turn the old USSR into the Commonwealth of Independent States (CIS), relieving the Russian Republic of responsibility for governing the Ukraine, Belarus, and other parts of the federal (Soviet) union. The Cold War was over, and for a brief moment, some scholars argued that the world had become a **unipolar system** characterized by one superpower—in this case, the United States.

This milestone in history complicated, rather than reduced, the national security debate. Some people foresaw an end to conflict and a "peace dividend" from the reduced need for major weapons systems and a large standing army. Americans could come home. Others argued that the UN would take on a greater role in sustaining world peace, and it would need American and NATO support. Some of these people suggested that NATO's mission, the defense of Europe, should be redefined to engage in worldwide humanitarian assistance. Still others argued that economic globalization would bind together the commercial interests of the entire world, so that the United States would still be heavily involved in world affairs, but not as a military power.

1.3.1 Changing Threats

During the 1990s, most of the old threats from superpower tensions were dramatically reduced or eliminated. New regional organizations had been established to settle conventional disputes in Europe, and NATO was negotiating with former Soviet bloc countries about joining the organization. The United States and the Soviet Union had signed agreements that dramatically reduced their nuclear arsenals. The proxy wars were now simply local and regional conflicts rather than extensions of Soviet and American policy. Espionage remained an issue, but it was the Peoples' Republic of China, rather than the Russia, that was to attract the most frequent complaints.

Non-Communist threats remained, however, and were growing in scope. A number of minor powers sought **weapons of mass destruction (WMDs)**, which included **chemical, biological, radiological, nuclear, and explosive (CBRNE) weapons**. Such weapons would give them an advantage in regional power struggles and could possibly deter the United States and other powers from threatening them. The availability of these weapons could also make terrorist groups more dangerous, so monitoring was enhanced. In 1998, for example, India and Pakistan both tested nuclear devices, attracting severe criticism from the rest of the world. Likewise, intelligence gathered by several countries indicated that during the 1990s, Iraq, Iran, and North Korea were producing an array of WMDs as well as developing missiles to carry them.

During this period, the intelligence community suffered from certain organizational shortcomings that undermined broad cooperation, so it was fortunate that terrorist groups were unable to acquire WMDs. However, terrorist attacks using conventional explosives and methods on the World Trade Center in 1993, the attacks on American embassies in Tanzania and in Kenya in 1998, the Khobar Towers apartment complex bombing in Saudi Arabia in 1998, and the attack on the USS Cole in 2000 were indications of a growing terrorist threat. An attack by homegrown terrorists on a federal office building in Oklahoma and the use of poison gas on the Tokyo subway by Aum Shinrikyo both in 1995 further indicated that it was not just Islam that was the source of extremist threats.

1.3.2 New Conflicts, New Responses

There were many competing perceptions of the proper foundations for American national security planning during the post-Cold War, pre-9/11 era. These included joint efforts with the UN and other international organizations, a general reduction of American involvement overseas, and ad hoc coalitions to address specific problems. In choosing a national security strategy, the US government needed to consider domestic concerns, the interests of its allies, and the perspectives of its opponents. Thus, security planners needed to consider how a given action might affect voters in Illinois, government officials in Beijing and London, Muslims in Cairo, dictators in Iraq, and insurgents in Colombia. The end of the Cold War made these opinions loom in importance, as the Soviet threat had previously provided an excuse for setting many of these issues aside.

The first test of this new security situation occurred in 1990, when Iraq invaded Kuwait. Through the UN Security Council, President George H. W. Bush organized an international coalition to drive the Iraqis out of Kuwait. This intervention became only the second instance of the UN using its enforcement powers against an aggressor, the first having been the response to North Korea in the 1950s.

From this point onward, the performance of international coalitions became more erratic. In 1992, American forces joined a UN effort to provide emergency food relief in Somalia. In 1994, a civil war in Rwanda turned into genocide, or widespread politically motivated murder, but the United States refused to become involved in or to push for UN intervention in what it thought to be no more than a domestic conflict. Despite increasing evidence of genocide, which would eventually leave over 800 000 people dead, governments and key UN officials including Secretary General Kofi Annan sided with the US position. Stung by criticisms of this inaction, in 1995, the United States participated in a UN intervention to stop violence in the breakaway Republic of Bosnia, where Muslims and ethnic Croatians fought Bosnian Serbs who were being supported by the army of the Former Republic of Yugoslavia (now Serbia). American efforts produced the Dayton Accords, a compromise between competing sides that at least stabilized circumstances. Interventions in a political crisis in Haiti in 1995 and against ethnic cleansing in the Serbian province of Kosovo in 1999 were added to the array of interventions. The last began as a UN response to the crisis, but it eventually became a NATO operation.

FOR EXAMPLE

US Intervention in Somalia

As a result of civil war in the early 1990s, over 350 000 Somalis died and over 1.5 million faced starvation. In December 1992, at the end of his administration, President George H. W. Bush committed 28 000 US military forces to the humanitarian mission to "stop the dying" in Somalia by aiding in relief efforts. However, as a result of the security environment in the country and attacks by armed militia groups, which impeded the mission, the US military took more offensive actions against Somali warlords by attempting to disarm them and capture key leaders, such as Mohamed Farrah Aıdıd.

In one military operation, made famous by the book (Bowden 1999) and movie *Black Hawk Down*, US military forces were caught in a firefight with the Somalia militias, resulting in the deaths of 18 US Rangers and other Special Operations Forces flying support missions. French television crews showed one dead US Ranger being dragged naked through the streets of Mogadishu. The impact of those images on the American public eventually caused the Clinton administration to pull US military forces out of Somalia and turn over the mission to a United Nations force. It also contributed to the reluctance of the United States to respond with a military intervention to the genocide that occurred in Rwanda in 1994.

On a positive note, some problems were dramatically reduced during this time. The United States negotiated a trade deal with Mexico, and Canada called the North American Free Trade Agreement (NAFTA). Other Central and South American countries began promoting free trade and democratic government as well. Countries were adopting American practices to promote mutually beneficial exchange and general prosperity. Instead of shipping weapons, countries were shipping automobile components. While drug trafficking and internal violence remained problems in some countries, the future in the Americas looked promising.

1.3.3 Reorganization of National Security Policy

The reorganization of American national security policy that took place during the 1990s actually began in the closing days of the Cold War. Many important changes sprang from the legal reviews required by the Senate Church Commission and also from the **Defense Reorganization Act of 1986**, also known as the Goldwater–Nichols Act after its two congressional sponsors. The earlier **National Security Act of 1947** had not ended the political competition between the branches of the military, which became evident during the failed hostage rescue attempt in Iran in 1980 as well as military operations against Grenada in 1983. The Defense Reorganization Act required systematic joint planning efforts, including a Joint Strategic Planning System, to augment existing defense planning and contingency planning programs. It also required a quadrennial defense review process and eventually led to the establishment of the US Special Operations Command.

A more important change was the requirement for the administration to produce a National Security Strategy (NSS) that would describe strategic concerns in order to reconcile planning for current and future threats. When the Cold War ended, Congress wanted to know what threats remained and what the priorities were. The Reagan, Bush, and Clinton administrations provided these documents every other year on average. The 1997 NSS gave a good sense of the transformation in how the nation's leaders perceived security, with a strong focus on the need for interagency integration (e.g., between the CIA and Defense Intelligence Agency) to combat problems like terrorism, drug trafficking, and international organized crime. Thus, the NSS discussed the importance of **non-state actors**, or people or organizations that exercise political influence, either domestically or internationally, even though they do not represent sovereign governments. Promoting democracy, trade, arms control, and the information infrastructure were seen as essential for sustaining peace and stability in the world at large. The security provided by tanks and missiles in the past had become part of a much broader security effort.

Finally, during this period, the government began to move away from security planning based on world war-level thinking. A commission was set up to study which military facilities were still needed, withdrawing resources from communities throughout the country. The usefulness of new weapon and support systems also came under scrutiny. These matters became political footballs: the B-2 bomber looked too expensive, but then it was noted that parts were manufactured in over 400 congressional districts. The Marine Corps' Osprey aircraft was cancelled repeatedly as a technical failure, only to be resurrected by Congress. As these examples show, many of the players involved in security planning may have had different concerns at heart when policy was created.

SELF-CHECK

- Define unipolar system.
- Which of the following terrorist incidents against US interests did not occur between 1990 and 2000?
  a. Khobar Towers bombing
  b. First World Trade Center bombing
  c. US embassy bombings in Kenya and Tanzania
  d. Marine barracks bombing in Lebanon
- Al-Qaeda is an example of a non-state actor. True or false?
- Crimes against humanity always result in US intervention. True or false?

1.4 National Security and Terrorism: Post-9/11

On 9/11, terrorists seized control of passenger aircraft and flew two of them into the two towers of the World Trade Center and a third into the Pentagon. A fourth aircraft crashed in rural southern Pennsylvania as passengers fought to overwhelm the hijackers. Close to three thousand people died in the attacks, making 9/11 the worst loss of life in a single day in the United States since the Battle of Antietam in 1862 (Civil War Trust n.d.). For a brief time, most Americans as well as people from other countries were unified by the horror of the attack. How had it happened? Who was responsible? What should be done to prevent similar attacks in the future? The warnings of many specialists in terrorism had come to pass, and Americans needed to rethink national security yet again.

The "how had it happened?" component of the 9/11 attacks proved straight-forward. A group of well-financed terrorists had come to America, taken some flying lessons, then, at an agreed-upon time, boarded aircraft and seized control. The terrorists were identified with a loose association of Muslim extremists called al-Qaeda. Operating under the direction of Osama bin Laden, a Saudi Arabian, al-Qaeda's stated goal was to restore the purity of Islam. This goal required at the very least driving Americans out of the Middle East and then overthrowing governments sympathetic to the West in the region. To this end, it was believed that al-Qaeda was responsible for many terrorist incidents in the 1990s as well.

Intelligence community analyses from the 1990s indicated that al-Qaeda had substantial financial resources and enjoyed support from several countries. Muslim fundamentalists called the Taliban had seized power in Afghanistan and were providing a safe haven for al-Qaeda. Iraq, though it was under UN sanctions, was sponsoring terror attacks in Israel and was also believed to be linked to al-Qaeda. Thus, terrorism reflected more than one group of people, and it presented a variety of targets and dangers.

Other chapters in this book present distinctions among these threats as well as specific responses. The remainder of this chapter, however, discusses some key considerations regarding understanding threats in the context of national and homeland security and preparing responses to those threats that will be presented in greater detail later.

1.4.1 Globalization and Geopolitics

In the late 1990s and early 2000s, **globalization**, the increasing economic and social interdependence among countries, created many opportunities for mutually beneficial exchange. Many argued that this change would increase stability and peace in the world through the development of complex interdependencies. Yet, interdependence also creates vulnerabilities, opening countries to short- and long-term risks. For example, if a country has a civil war, any investments from outside may be lost. Further, each country has its own form of government and its own interests. Will interdependence bind a potential adversary to peaceful behavior, or just make it stronger and create more damage when it turns on us? Scholars differ significantly on this question. One issue that they do agree on is that globalization can present a challenge to cultural integrity and national identity, creating a backlash. Terrorism by radical Islamists and other forms of extremism represent this backlash. Finding an appropriate response becomes a matter of building a coalition among seemingly competing views.

First, let's consider the threats. Terrorism problems are part of a much larger set of challenges that the United States faces, reflecting the "preventing similar attacks" issue. As trade and other forms of international cooperation increase, the importance of specific circumstances also grows. In addition, given the interconnectedness of global economies, trade, politics, and security issues, the ability of a non-state actor to use **asymmetric warfare**, or non-conventional warfare tactics and techniques

---

FOR EXAMPLE

Asymmetric Warfare Isn't New

Asymmetric warfare includes the use of terrorism and could involve the use of various WMDs (or technologies capable of producing a WMD effect). Yet, as Thomas Barnett (2005) and others have argued, asymmetric warfare is not completely new. These tactics and techniques have existed for millennia—remember the Trojan horse? For the most part, they reflect Eastern rather than Western military thought. What has changed, though, is the belief that we are now entering into a new historical phase of conflict, called fourth-generation warfare (Hammes 2004), in which **asymmetrical warfare** can be understood as "evolved irregular warfare" with a new emphasis on factors other than military power, such as moral force and sociological factors.

Terrorist groups, like al-Qaeda and now IS, apply asymmetrical tactics when they use non-conventional means to attack Western interests (car bombs, suicide bombers, truck drivers, etc.). The "tools" available to terrorists are described in detail in Chapters 8 and 9, with a special focus on those tools that can cause the most damage.

employed by a less powerful force against a more powerful nation like the United States, continues to grow as technology creates vulnerabilities.

Second, **geopolitics**, the political impact of geographical relationships, plays a key role in globalization's interdependence. Oceans protected the United States in its early history, but expanding trade links mean many American interests are far from the center of American power. For example, China is far away and still has a Communist government overseeing the capitalist aspects of its economy. If China decided to cut off or dramatically alter its economic relations with the United States, what could the United States do about it? Further, China sees some of its near neighbors, such as Taiwan and Japan (which are some of America's closest allies in the region), as rivals. An incident early in 2001 underscored this problem: a Chinese fighter aircraft collided with an American reconnaissance aircraft, killing the Chinese pilot and forcing the American plane to land on Chinese territory. The airplane and crew were returned after intense negotiations, but many felt the United States had been forced to concede too much. However, the fact that the event occurred far from the United States and close to China made other alternatives short of war unlikely. In the South China Sea in 2016, China challenged US interests and allies by increasing its naval presence throughout the region.

Domestic and international coalitions form around different interpretations surrounding this interplay of geopolitics and globalization. For example, in what was called the Bush Doctrine, national security was based on an aggressive response to perceived threats. First, certain repressive regimes, which former President George W. Bush referred to as "the axis of evil," present significant dangers to the rest of the world. These countries—Iran, Iraq, and North Korea—were suspected of developing WMDs, and they are also located in places where they can harm American interests. North Korea, for example, has been developing missiles capable of delivering nuclear warheads that can hit Japan and Taiwan and have the potential to hit the West Coast of the United States. Iran and Iraq are both in a position to disrupt the flow of oil from the Middle East and to threaten Israel. One of the more substantial concerns was that WMDs would find their way into the hands of terrorists. Finally, all three countries are geographically close to China and Russia, both of which are potential sources of materials for WMDs.

A second principle of the Bush Doctrine was **preemption**, which is taking action against a state or non-state actor *before* it becomes too dangerous a threat. As always, experts disagree as to when preemption becomes necessary. Third, under this doctrine, moral values had a stronger place in evaluating the actions of others. Finally, according to this belief system, the linchpin to world peace is creating peace between the Israelis and Palestinians, something that will require substantial political change among the latter.

The Bush Doctrine enjoyed support at first, but the coalition necessary for successful policy was weakened by a number of circumstances. First, notions like preemption were questioned by people who see terrorism as a crime to be dealt with by legal processes rather than a security matter to be dealt with by military force. Second, many observers feared that the doctrine might lead to unilateral actions in which the United States ignores the voices of its friends overseas, undermining the gains in cooperation from globalization. Although President Bush used a multilateral approach with North Korea, critics fear that the nation's efforts in dealing with Iraq and Iran will leave the United States isolated from its allies. Third, the absence of WMDs in Iraq seriously undermined the credibility of American efforts there, breaking the domestic coalition that supported the Second Gulf War. Although geopolitical concerns about oil and moral concerns about Saddam Hussein's repressiveness were important, the presence of WMDs made the threat to the United States from Iraq both greater and more direct.

The domestic political debate surrounding these issues continues. If the interdependence of globalization governs national policies, these concerns will ultimately be reduced. If Morgenthau's balance of power is the norm, however, then these remain significant problems for the United States in defining national security interests.

1.4.2 The Bush Administration's Global War on Terrorism

The 9/11 attacks on the World Trade Center and the Pentagon produced significant changes in the way agencies monitored and responded to potential and actual threats. The 2002 NSS provided direction for responding to terror as an issue, laying the foundation for increased coordination among agencies responsible for security. Later, the 2006 NSS added support for pursuing preemptive war.

In the immediate aftermath of 9/11, the United States planned and executed the campaigns in what has since become called the **Global War on Terrorism (GWOT)**. The main target was Afghanistan, the home of the Taliban regime and the base of operations for al-Qaeda. It was also believed to be the last known location of al-Qaeda's leader, Osama bin Laden, at the time. The GWOT began in earnest with the start of **Operation Enduring Freedom (OEF)** in October 2001, in which military operations commenced against the Taliban regime in Afghanistan. Initially proposed as Operation Infinite Justice, Operation Enduring Freedom actually comprised military operations in Afghanistan, the Philippines, and the Horn of Africa, with the target being terrorist groups believed to be associated with al-Qaeda. OEF also involved actions taken domestically by the Department of Defense in support of the new homeland defense mission. One example was the formation of Joint Task Force–Olympics, the military's contribution to providing security against a possible terrorist threat to the Olympic Games held in Salt Lake City, Utah, in January 2002.

After helping establish a non-militant Islamic government in Afghanistan, the United States turned its sights on Iraq and its leader, Saddam Hussein. The Second Gulf War (Operation Iraqi Freedom) commenced in April 2003, but the goal this time was not simply removing Iraqi troops from Kuwait (as it was during the First Gulf War in 1990), but rather regime change and the overthrow of Hussein. The US invasion of Iraq was an example of preemptive war, aimed at neutralizing Hussein's regime and its suspected ties to terrorist organizations, including as a potential source of WMDs for terrorist organizations. Despite the failure of the invasion to produce any hard evidence of stockpiling of WMDs or further evidence of Iraq's ties to al-Qaeda or other terrorist organizations, the Bush administration supported the war by promoting the liberation of Iraq as a key foreign policy goal in the Middle East, which would lead to further success in the GWOT. US forces remained in Iraq and Afghanistan throughout the George W. Bush administration (Figure 1-3).

Figure 1-3

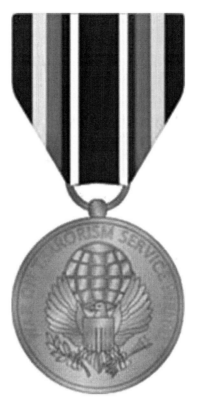

Global War on terrorism medal. Source: Department of Defense (2015).

Global War on Terrorism Service (GWOT-S) Medal: Approved Operations

Operation	Inclusive dates
Airport Security Operations	September 27, 2001–May 31, 2002
Noble Eagle	September 11, 2001–TBD
Enduring Freedom	September 11, 2001–TBD
Iraqi Freedom	March 19, 2003–Aug 31, 2010
New Dawn	September 1, 2010–Dec 31, 2011
Inherent Resolve	June 15, 2014–TBD
Freedom's Sentinel	January 1, 2015–TBD

Source: Department of Defense (2015).

1.4.3 The Obama Administration's New National Security Strategy

Once Barack Obama came into office in January 2009, he made it a priority to set a deadline for withdrawal of US forces from Iraq and Afghanistan. The United States would no longer fight a "Global War on Terror." Instead, the focus would be confronting the specific terrorist threat posed by a**l-Qaeda and its affiliated movements (AQAM)**. The 2010 National Security Strategy reflected President Obama's new focus on confronting the terrorist threat abroad through the use of military forces conducing **Overseas Contingency Operations (OCO)** rather than large military force deployments and occupations (NSS 2010). The United States completed its military withdrawal from Iraq in December 2011, with President Obama stating that "we're leaving behind a sovereign, stable, and self-reliant Iraq" (Salam 2014). Yet, the Iraqi government and military would prove incapable of dealing with the new threat posed by Sunni extremists who emerged from Abu Musab al-Zarqawi's al-Qaeda in Iraq after his death in 2006. Within three years of the US military withdrawal, Iraq, as well as Syria, would be confronted by a new threat called the Islamic State in Iraq and Syria (ISIS), the Islamic State in Iraq and the Levant (ISIL), or, more simply, the **Islamic State (IS)**.

The Obama administration initially refused to use drones to confront IS in Iraq, after the US withdrawal. Only when IS began to capture cities, such as Fallujah, which US forces fought to control during the Iraq War, did the United States respond with military support to the Iraqis to include the use of Special Operations Forces as advisers to the Iraqi military and the direct use of US-controlled drones. As IS continued to capture and hold territory in Iraq and Syria, the United States and coalition partners would begin direct airstrikes in both countries to attack IS forces.

As a result of events in Iraq, President Obama decided to delay the withdrawal of US forces in Afghanistan and even increased the US military presence in that country, as al-Qaeda and the Taliban's resurgence threatened to overturn the US-supported Afghan government and military. Despite a pledge to end the war in Afghanistan during his two terms in office, in 2016, after 15 years of conflict, the United States still maintains about 10 000 military personnel in the country. In his 2015 National Security Strategy, President Obama further stated that the United States, along with its NATO partners, will continue "a limited counterterrorism mission against the remnants of core al-Qaeda and maintain our support to the Afghan National Security Forces (ANSF)" (NSS 2015, 10).

In 2016, President Obama expanded military operations against IS to include Libya, authorizing the deployment of Special Operations Forces advisors and later direct combat aircraft strikes against IS targets. The direct involvement of US military personnel in Libya was significant in expanding US support for the Libyan Government of National Accord (GNA), which was still not a recognized government by many states (Walsh 2016). The Obama administration had previously approved a direct role for the US military in Syria, limited to flying combat aircraft missions against IS targets in that country. As of this date, no US ground forces were operating in Syria. These actions were a significant departure from President Obama's early policies of reducing the US military presence in the Middle East to combat terrorist groups, relying primarily on the use of armed drone aircraft to target suspected terrorists.

FOR EXAMPLE

Use of Drones by the Obama Administration

The use of armed drones to conduct targeted killings of suspected terrorists was started under President George W. Bush, as part of the Global War on Terror. When Barack Obama came into office, drones became the weapon of choice in his administration's counterterrorism policy. In the first three years of his administration, the use of drones by both the CIA and the US military's Joint Special Operations Command (JSCOC) increased significantly (44–240), expanding to multiple countries, to include Pakistan, Yemen, and Iraq, as well as increasing the targeting of low-level terrorists and not just key leaders. A drone strike authorized by President Obama killed Anwar al-Awlaki in Yemen in 2011. Al-Awlaki was an Islamic cleric (and US citizen) credited with radicalizing a number of terrorists, to include Major Nidal Hasan, a US Army officer who killed 13 at Ft. Hood, Texas, in 2009, and Umar Farouk Abdulmutallab, the Nigerian who tried to blow up a Detroit-bound international flight with an underwear bomb on Christmas Day 2009 (Miller 2011).

In 2016, the Obama administration released part of its secret "playbook" for drone warfare, which listed 473 total drone strikes authorized by President Obama from 2009 to 2015. In those strikes, the report stated that 2581 enemy combatants had been killed. The report also admitted that 64–116 civilians had also been killed in those strikes (Hennigan 2016).

1.4.4 Homeland Security and National Security

It is unlikely that the 9/11 attacks could have been prevented. Although some clues were available, an analysis of policies and procedures indicates that government agencies were unable to share key information, despite the intentions established in the 1997 NSS. For example, considerations of legal due process and civil liberties kept the FBI and CIA from sharing information. The FBI could gather information only with proper warrants and only about domestic lawbreaking, with the goal of presenting evidence in a court of law. The CIA's attention was on foreign matters, and it wanted to keep materials and the methods for getting them secret.

The Department of Homeland Security (DHS) was created in response to the demands of Congress, the concerns of the American people due to the threat of terrorism, and the 2002 NSS, which committed the United States to fight a "Global War on Terrorism" at home and abroad. DHS merged 22 federal agencies with over 170 000 employees under one cabinet-level office. The FBI and CIA remain outside of the Department of Homeland Security, but greater levels of information sharing have been established. In 2016, DHS had grown to over 240 000 with an equal number of contracted employees supporting the Department (Lipowicz 2010). Given President Obama's reference in the 2015 NSS to the "persistent threat posed by terrorism today," (7) it appears that Homeland Security is here to stay.

The Bush administration produced a National Strategy for Homeland Security in May 2002, before it produced its first National Security Strategy in September

2002. The National Strategy for Homeland Security was updated in 2007, listing the following four goals (NSHS 2007):

1. Prevent and disrupt terrorist attacks.
2. Protect the American people, our critical infrastructure, and key resources.
3. Respond to and recover from incidents that do occur.
4. Continue to strengthen the foundation to ensure our long-term success.

President Obama chose not to issue a separate Homeland Security Strategy when he came into office in 2009. Instead he chose to include Homeland Security within his National Security Strategy, initially released in 2010 and updated in 2015. He produced a National Strategy for Counterterrorism (2011), as a continuation of President Bush's National Strategy for Combating Terrorism (2003). Obama also supported and expanded organizations created after 9/11, such as the Department of Homeland Security, the Office of the Director of National Intelligence (ODNI), and the National Counterterrorism Center (NCTC).

With the election of President Donald Trump in November 2016, the United States entered into a new period of uncertainty in its national and homeland security policy. Domestically, the Trump campaign rhetoric focused on immigration policies and "building a wall" between the United States and Mexico to keep illegal immigrants out of the country (McCaskill 2016). It also questioned the NATO alliance and trade policies, which indicated the United States might be entering into a new isolationism. Once taking office in January 2017, President Trump found implementing such campaign promises much more difficult. Besides not being able to get Mexico to "build a wall," his other efforts to control immigration and limit travel to the United States from seven Muslim countries ran afoul of US courts. In his first trip to Europe in May, he failed to reassure NATO leaders that the United States was still a supporter of Article 5 and the concept of collective defense (Glasser 2017). As of July 2017, the Trump administration had yet to articulate a new National Security or Homeland Security Strategy.

SELF-CHECK

- Define asymmetric warfare.
- One example of a US government response, organizationally, after the 9/11 attacks, was the formation of the Department of National Security. True or false?
- Which of the following countries was not identified by President Bush as part of the "axis of evil"?

  a. Iraq

  b. Libya

  c. Iran

  d. North Korea

- The use of drones in the targeted killing of suspected terrorists declined during the Obama administration. True or false?

SUMMARY

Maintaining American national security blends several important questions, basically asking who, why, when, and how. The "who" reflects the balance among political opinions. We can speak of this as the domestic audience: when the government develops a policy, how do people feel about it? Conservatives and liberals alike may press for peace or demand war, though for different reasons. Much depends on the "why." If a problem arises in the international system, does the response involve getting American citizens to safety, or does it demand cooperation or involvement in the affairs of other countries?

The "when" is not simply the time in history during which a problem occurs. A critical "when" issue for policymaking involves whether a problem is temporary or long term. The Cold War lasted from 1946 to 1991. Was containment a good idea? When containment policy was established, it was by no means clear when the Cold War would end. Finally, the "how" reflects how the response will be managed. When America fought World War II, it was probably the largest organizational problem in our history, yet it was managed by competing government departments acting on extraordinary powers only granted to them for the duration of the crisis. It is only later that interdepartmental and interagency coordination become routine. The success of any program, however, is its ability to address the crisis at hand. Whatever the who, why, when, and how, government must adapt so as to bring appropriate organization to the problem at hand.

During the course of the last 70 years, America's security environment has undergone several key transformations. First, the creation of international institutions such as the United Nations has increased interdependence among nations. Second, the means of attack and defense have changed from rifles and battleships to WMDs, making even small groups potentially very dangerous. Third, new threats have arisen in the place of old threats, such as that once posed by the USSR. The circumstances of these new threats reflect long-standing concerns and analytical frameworks, such as geopolitics and power relationships. Fourth, as various threats have grown more complex, it's become necessary to develop new organizations, processes, policies, and strategies to manage the threats, as well as to increase the coordination among these elements. Of course, there are currently a number of competing perspectives within the American political system about what constitutes a threat and what the appropriate responses to these threats should be. The waxing and waning of these perspectives means managing national and homeland security will be a source of controversy for years to come.

In this chapter, we addressed all of these issues by taking a detailed look at the changing nature of national security throughout US history. More specifically, we analyzed various security environments and national security policy choices during specific historical periods. We also learned to distinguish between national security policy players within and outside of government and appraised the threat situation in post-9/11 America. In addition, we examined US national security strategy and homeland security policy as a response to today's changing environment and threat perceptions.

KEY TERMS

Al-Qaeda and its affiliated movements (AQAM)	Term used by the Obama administration to specifically target the terrorist threat posed by those groups connected to al-Qaeda, such as al-Qaeda in Iraq, al-Qaeda in the Islamic Maghreb (AQIM), and al-Qaeda in the Arabian Peninsula (AQAP).
Asymmetrical warfare	The use of unconventional tactics by weak states against stronger states. These tactics are often difficult for the stronger state to counter because of legal, moral, or other restrictions on what kind of violence the state may use in response to such tactics.
Axis Powers	The alliance among Germany, Japan, and Italy during World War II.
Balance of power	International relations theory where no one state has a monopoly of power and nations seek to maximize security either through alliances to compensate for weaknesses or through unilateral means when they perceive it be in their national interest to do so.
Bipolar system	A relationship among countries in the international system in which two countries dominate and other nation-states tend to align themselves with either of the two, such as the United States and the USSR during the Cold War.
Bretton Woods Agreements	Series of post-World War II agreements that created key economic institutions intended to promote international economic stability and trade, such as the International Monetary Fund (IMF), the International Bank for Reconstruction and Development (IBRD or World Bank), and the General Agreement on Tariffs and Trade (GATT).
CBRNE	Abbreviation for chemical, biological, radiological, nuclear, and explosive weapons.
Central Powers	The alliance between Germany, Austria-Hungary, the Ottoman Empire, and Bulgaria in World War I.
Circular error probability (CEP)	Term that describes the accuracy with which nuclear weapons strike their targets.

Clandestine and covert operations	Clandestine operations are secret efforts to gather information, while covert operations are intended to influence how governments behave. Covert operations could include bribes, subversion and psychological operations, and support for insurgent forces.
Collective security	An agreement among countries to unite against any aggressor.
Containment	Principal national security policy pursued during the Cold War to prevent the spread of communism and Soviet influence.
Correlation of forces	A measure of comparative military power between the United States and the USSR during the Cold War based on the combined resources of the nations that were aligned with each superpower.
Defense Reorganization Act of 1986	Also known as the Goldwater–Nichols Act, it required systematic joint planning efforts, including a Joint Strategic Planning System, to augment existing defense planning and contingency planning programs. It also required a quadrennial defense review process and eventually led to the establishment of the US Special Operations Command.
Détente	Literally, a "relaxation of tensions"; refers to the efforts of the Nixon administration to promote diplomatic compromise with the USSR.
Entente Powers	The alliance between the United States, Britain, France, Russia, and Italy in World War I.
Federalist Papers	Essays authored by James Madison, Alexander Hamilton, and John Jay in 1787–1788 that argued the need for a US federal government strong enough to provide for national security while also protecting states' rights and individual liberties.
Geopolitics	The political impact of geographical relationships.
Globalization	The increasing economic and social interdependence among countries.

Global War on Terrorism (GWOT)	Military campaign launched after 9/11 that targets terrorist groups in multiple countries.
Hegemony	A term used to express the political, economic, or military predominance or control of one state over others.
Homeland security	A term used after 9/11 to encompass the collective efforts of local, state, and federal agencies to ensure the United States is safe, secure, and resilient against terrorism and other hazards.
Islamic State (IS)	The term used to identify the Sunni extremist group that emerged initially in Iraq after the death of Abu Musab al-Zarqawi, the leader of al-Qaeda in Iraq. It is also referred to as the Islamic State in Iraq and Syria (ISIS) and the Islamic State in Iraq and the Levant (ISIL).
Isolationism	A foreign policy based on avoiding alliances with other countries.
Marshall Plan	Plan that provided US funds to help rebuild non-Communist countries after World War II.
Monroe Doctrine	A regional security policy proposed by President James Monroe in 1823 that sought to limit European influence in the Americas.
Multiple independently targetable reentry vehicle (MIRV)	Device that allows a missile to carry more than one nuclear warhead.
Multipolar system	A relationship among countries in the international system in which no country dominates, with a number of nation-states possessing military power and capable of acting independently.
National security	Protecting the United States, its citizens, and its interests through the threatened and actual use of all elements of national power.
National Security Act of 1947	A law that created the Central Intelligence Agency, the US Air Force, and the Department of Defense in order to face threats during the Cold War.
Neutrality Acts	Laws passed by Congress in the 1930s forbidding American support for or involvement with countries at war.

Non-state actors	People or organizations that exercise political influence, either domestically or internationally, even though they do not represent sovereign governments.
North Atlantic Treaty Organization (NATO)	A military alliance formed in 1949 with each member nation pledging that an attack on any one of them would bring the collective response of all member nations.
Operation Enduring Freedom (OEF)	Military operations in Afghanistan, the Philippines, and the Horn of Africa against terrorist groups believed to be associated with al-Qaeda from 2001 to 2014.
Overseas Contingency Operations (OCO)	President Obama's use of military forces to specifically confront al-Qaeda and its affiliated movements overseas rather than conducing a Global War on Terror. Emphasis was placed on the use of Special Forces and drones rather than large military deployments and occupations.
Preemption	Taking action against a state or non-state actor before it becomes too dangerous a threat.
Prepositioning	Establishing bases and supplies in foreign countries to prepare a rapid response to future crises.
Proliferation	The supplying of other countries with the technology to build their own nuclear weapons.
Roosevelt Corollary	Security policy of President Theodore Roosevelt to use military power to back up the claims of the Monroe Doctrine toward US hegemony in the Western Hemisphere.
Superpowers	The dominant military powers during the Cold War: the United States and USSR. After the demise of communism, the United States remained the world's lone superpower.
Threats or adversaries	Traditionally understood as states that possess both capability and intent to do a nation harm. That has been expanded to also include non-state actors, such as terrorist groups and criminal gangs.

Unipolar system

An international system characterized by one superpower.

United Nations (UN)

International organization established after World War II to resolve disputes and stop aggression through collective security.

Warsaw Pact

A military alliance formed in 1955 by the Soviet Union, which sought to counter the collective military powers of the West (NATO) by uniting countries of Eastern Europe under Soviet control and influence.

Weapons of mass destruction (WMD)

Device such as a chemical, biological, radiological, nuclear, or explosive weapon that can inflict widespread damage when used.

ASSESS YOUR UNDERSTANDING

Go to www.wiley.com/go/Kilroy/Threats_to_Homeland_Security to assess your knowledge of the basics of national security and homeland security.

Summary Questions

1. During its first 150 years of existence, the United States pursued an isolationist foreign policy. True or false?

2. NATO was created after the Warsaw Pact. True or false?

3. The international security environment that emerged after World War II can best be described as bipolar, with the United States and the USSR establishing spheres of influence over other nations. True or false?

4. After September 11, 2001, the United States returned to a policy of isolationism in foreign affairs, attempting to avoid conflict in other nations that would increase the possibility of terrorist incidents in the United States itself. True or false?

5. Which of the following was not an author of the Federalist Papers?
   (a) John Jay
   (b) Alexander Hamilton
   (c) Thomas Jefferson
   (d) James Madison

6. Which of the following military campaigns was not part of the Global War on Terrorism?
   (a) Operation Provide Comfort
   (b) Operation Enduring Freedom
   (c) Operation Iraqi Freedom
   (d) Operation Noble Eagle

7. Which of the following countries was an original member of NATO in 1949?
   (a) Austria
   (b) Australia
   (c) Canada
   (d) Spain

8. Which of the following organizations was created after 9/11?
   (a) DHS
   (b) NCTC
   (c) ODNI
   (d) All of the above

Applying This Chapter

1. In a classroom discussion, a fellow student argues that based on James Madison's statement that security can only be measured by the "means and danger" of attack, the greatest threat the United States faces today is a terrorist obtaining a nuclear weapon. Do you agree or disagree? Why or why not? What would you recommend for a national security strategy focused on protecting the homeland against such a threat?

2. You are a member of the president's National Security Council. North Korea continues to defy international condemnation of its nuclear development program and continues test-firing long-range missiles, which could threaten the United States. What course of action do you recommend for national security policy: containment and deterrence, preemption, or multilateral policy options? What would be some of your specific points supporting one option over the others?

3. If you were to teach a course on national security policymaking, what subjects would you include? What type of model would you employ in explaining how national security decisions are made? Who would you identify as the key players? Would you treat homeland security as a separate policy area or include it under the broader national security policy umbrella?

4. The Islamic State (IS) continues to expand its operations in Syria and Iraq and is now threatening to move into southern Turkey. After an attempted military coup in Turkey in 2016, where many military leaders were purged from the armed forces, the Turkish military is not capable of conducing sustained military operations against IS. The only effective fighting forces are the Kurds and the PKK, which is considered a terrorist organization by the United States and Turkey. Given that Turkey is a NATO ally, should the United States commit ground forces to defend Turkey against IS? Or should the United States arm and support the Kurds, despite Turkish government opposition?

YOU TRY IT

Asymmetrical Warfare

Analyze the topic of asymmetrical warfare. Look for specific examples in history where a weaker power has used asymmetrical means to defeat a more powerful adversary.

National Security Policies

Research national security policies under the Bush I, Clinton, Bush II, and Obama administrations in the post-Cold War era. Analyze the security policies or "doctrines" that emerged during each administration. How did each administration identify terrorist threats to the homeland? What policy choices were made with regard to counterterrorism both domestically and internationally?

2

REASSESSING THE ALL-HAZARDS PERSPECTIVE

Understanding the Nature of Threats Due to Natural, Accidental, and Man-Made Disasters and Their Relationship to Homeland Security

Richard J. Kilroy, Jr.

Department of Politics, Coastal Carolina University, Conway, SC, USA

Starting Point

Go to www.wiley.com/go/Kilroy/Threats_to_Homeland_Security to assess your knowledge of the basics of the all-hazards perspective.
Determine where you need to concentrate your effort.

What You'll Learn in This Chapter

▲ The difference between natural, accidental, and man-made disasters

▲ The history of the types and sources of disasters in the United States

▲ The consequences and management of natural, accidental, and man-made disasters in a post-9/11 world

▲ The definition of all hazards and the implications of the all-hazards perspective on homeland security

After Studying This Chapter, You'll Be Able To

▲ Evaluate the types of natural, accidental, and man-made disasters that can and do occur in the United States today

▲ Assess the nature of our response to natural, accidental, and man-made disasters in the United States

▲ Judge how disasters can have catastrophic effects on and implications for our nation's response in the war on terrorism

▲ Assess whether the all-hazards perspective is the best approach toward managing threats to homeland security in the future

Threats to Homeland Security: Reassessing the All-Hazards Perspective, Second Edition.
Edited by Richard J. Kilroy, Jr.
© 2018 John Wiley & Sons, Inc. Published 2018 by John Wiley & Sons, Inc.
Companion website: www.wiley.com/go/Kilroy/Threats_to_Homeland_Security

INTRODUCTION

After the terrorist attacks against America on 9/11, the national response was to elevate terrorism to the highest category of current and potential threats to the US homeland. In other words, the view within federal government toward homeland security was to take an "exclusive" view, focused primarily on terrorist threats, rather than an "inclusive" view that assessed **all hazards** as threats to the homeland.

This was the prevailing view when Hurricane Katrina hit the Gulf Coast in August 2005, followed by Hurricane Rita, less than 30 days later. The federal government, particularly the Federal Emergency Management Agency (FEMA), was criticized for its slow response to the humanitarian crisis that emerged in the city of New Orleans, where over 1800 people died as a result of the hurricane and the subsequent flooding that occurred when the city's levee system failed (Schleifstein 2009). As a result, homeland security took on a more inclusive view incorporating an **all-hazards approach** toward threats to the homeland from natural, accidental, and man-made sources.

In recent years, given the increasing incidence of terrorist attacks in the United States, the all-hazards perspective has come under increased scrutiny. Concerns have been raised, particularly within the emergency management community, that in trying to protect against every possible threat to the homeland, federal, state, and local government agency resources are stretched too thin to respond to major crises when they occur (Canton 2013; Gregory 2015). Some have even argued that by focusing on the all-hazards perspective, the United States is neglecting the main threat of domestic terrorism, which created the expansive federal bureaucracy focused on homeland security after 9/11 (Homeland Security 2015; U.S. Senate 2012).

In this chapter, you will reassess the all-hazards perspective with regard to threats to homeland security. You will evaluate the types of natural, accidental, and man-made disasters that can and do occur in the United States, as well as assess the nature of our response to these disasters. You will also judge how today's disasters can have catastrophic effects and implications for our nation's response in the war on terrorism (e.g., **cascading effects** or **secondary and tertiary effects**). Much like an act of terrorism, a disaster of any type can have devastating consequences for our nation's critical infrastructures, as well as effects on commerce and our way of life. How the United States has responded to such occurrences in the past, both organizationally and operationally, has been impacted by the events of 9/11, as well as other types of disasters. The current approach has been to take an all-hazards approach to managing disasters. Yet, as the Prussian military strategist Frederick the Great noted, "in trying to defend everything he defended nothing" (Qotlr n.d.).

2.1 Natural Disasters: Things We Can Expect to Happen

Prior to 9/11, terrorism was a relatively rare occurrence within the United States. Most of the nation's response capability at the local, state, and federal levels was focused on threats of nature, or **natural disasters**, such as hurricanes, tornadoes, floods, and forest fires. While there was concern for attacks in the form of a potential nuclear exchange with the former Soviet Union during the Cold War, most of the emphasis on **civil defense**, or the protection of the nation against threats within the United States, was focused on our nation's ability to respond to acts of nature. Various government agencies charged with civil defense and response missions, such as the Federal Emergency Management Agency (FEMA) and the National Guard, were primarily organized to respond to the consequences of natural disasters, such as occurred in New Orleans in September 2005 with Hurricane Katrina.

It seems that regardless of where you live in the United States, you are bound to be subject to the extremes of nature. On the East and Gulf Coasts, you can experience the effects of hurricanes, which occur seasonally from June to November. On the West Coast, you are more likely to be subject to earthquakes and devastating forest fires. In the heartland of America, you tend to be prone to experience the consequences of tornadoes, floods, and severe winter storms. Lest we forget about Alaska and Hawaii, they too have unique environmental problems due to hazards such as tidal waves and volcanoes.

Given the certainty that natural disasters will occur, our nation has a long history of preparation for such disasters and the ability to respond in a crisis. Local communities have developed emergency response capabilities, often tailored to the threats their communities face. For example, in Greenville, North Carolina, there is not a robust supply of road salt and sand to respond to winter storms. Thus, when such storms hit in 2004, the community was not prepared and quickly exhausted local resources. However, due to the flooding experienced in eastern North Carolina during Hurricane Floyd in 1999, the local community was much better prepared for the impact of Hurricane Michael in 2016, due to a well-rehearsed community response plan in place to deal with such a disaster (Breeden 2016).

2.1.1 The History of Natural Disasters in the United States

One of the earliest disasters recorded in history was the "Great Fire of London" in September 1666, which destroyed much of the city and caused over £10 million (British pounds sterling) in damage. Yet, ironically, there was little loss of life. In the United States, the best-known fire occurred in Chicago in 1872, destroying over 17 000 buildings and killing over 250 people. However, the most devastating fire in our nation's history occurred in Peshtigo, Wisconsin, in October 1871, where over 3.8 billion acres were destroyed and 1500 lives were lost (Infoplease n.d.).

Despite these examples, the most devastating natural disaster in our nation's history remains the hurricane that hit Galveston, Texas, in September 1900, destroying over 3500 buildings and killing over 6000 inhabitants of the island. The hurricane was estimated to have winds clocking 140 miles per hour, making it a category 5 storm by today's standards. Most of the damage, however, was not caused by winds but by the tidal surge, estimated at over 15 ft, which swamped the island, destroying a town of 37 000 people. Estimated damage was placed at $20 million ($700 million in today's dollars) (1900 Storm n.d.).

When people think of earthquakes, they naturally think of California, the San Andreas Fault, and the April 1906 San Francisco earthquake. This event was the worst earthquake recorded in American history, killing over 3000 people (Epic Disasters n.d.). Although California has the most deadly recorded earthquakes in the United States, major earthquakes have also hit Alaska, Hawaii, and South Carolina. Furthermore, the most deadly earthquakes ever in the United States could yet occur in the nation's midsection, impacting major population centers along the Mississippi Valley. For this reason, FEMA continues to consider this region, located along the New Madrid Fault Line, as one of a number of potential disaster areas due to the scale of the damage that could occur, the breadth of area impacted (eight states, four FEMA regions), and the potential for significant secondary effects due to extreme weather and climate conditions depending on the time of year such an event might occur (Lowder 2006).

FOR EXAMPLE

The New Madrid Fault Line

In 1811 and 1812, three major earthquakes occurred in the midsection of the United States along the New Madrid Fault Line. The earthquakes were huge, believed to be of a magnitude of 8.0 on the Richter scale, and were felt even along the East Coast. New lakes were formed, and the Mississippi River was reported to have flowed backward. However, harm to buildings and people was limited due to the sparse populations that existed around the quakes' epicenters at that time. If such an event were to occur today, the major population centers of St. Louis, Missouri; Cairo, Illinois; and Memphis, Tennessee, would be severely impacted. "It is the most seismically active area of the United States east of the Rockies" (Williams 2009) (Figure 2-1).

2.1.2 Natural Disaster Response

The United States has a long history of preparing for and responding to natural disasters. For instance, Benjamin Franklin helped form the Union Fire Company in Philadelphia, Pennsylvania, in 1736 as a voluntary firefighting society in which members pledged their support to protect each other's property. Later, Franklin went on to organize the nation's first fire insurance company in 1752, based on the economic threat from a fire disaster.

For most of our nation's history, response to natural disasters was dependent on grassroots, citizen-based volunteer organizations, where members of the community came together to meet the needs of others when a disaster struck. There was little expectation that the federal government would provide relief other than financial recourse, as occurred in 1803, when Congress authorized funds to support a New Hampshire town devastated by fire. Even then, and for the next 100 years, federal assistance was limited to public infrastructure, mostly roads, bridges, and so on (Federal Emergency Management Agency n.d.).

In the 1930s, during the presidency of Franklin D. Roosevelt, increased federalization impacted disaster relief through organizations like the Reconstruction Finance Corporation and Bureau of Public Roads. The federal government also made more federal support available to local communities through the assistance of organizations like the Army Corps of Engineers, which performed much of the

Figure 2-1

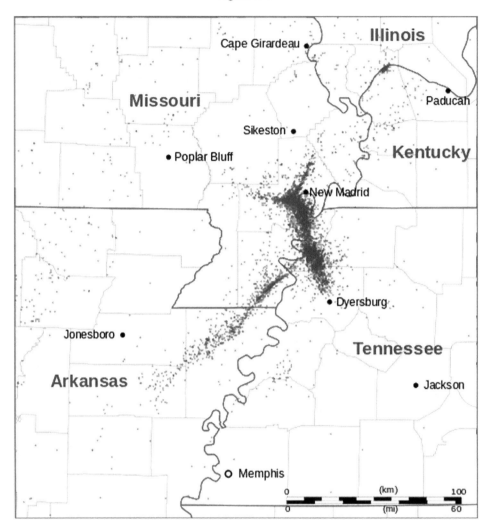

New Madrid Fault Line and major population centers (Williams 2009).

work on the nation's transportation infrastructure, including roads, bridges, dams, and waterways for flood control projects. It wasn't until 1968 and the passage of the National Flood Insurance Act, however, that the federal government made a commitment to provide financial support to private property damaged in a natural disaster.

Throughout this time, the primary organizational response to a disaster remained at the local community level, and the state was only impacted when local remedies were exhausted by the scale of the disaster. Furthermore, it wasn't until 1974 and the passage of the Disaster Relief Act that the president established the authority to declare a **state of emergency** due to a disaster, making the affected area of the country eligible for increased federal support and funding.

In 1979, the US government created a national agency to provide a coordinated federal response to local community's disaster needs. Established under the Carter administration, the Federal Emergency Management Agency (FEMA) consolidated most of nation's fragmented disaster response mechanisms, including those of the Department of Defense under its civil defense responsibilities, into one federal agency. The first director of FEMA, John Macy, "emphasized the similarities between natural hazards preparedness and the civil defense activities. FEMA began development of an Integrated Emergency Management System with an all-hazards approach that included 'direction, control, and warning systems which are common to the full range of emergencies from small isolated events to the ultimate emergency—war'" (Federal Emergency Management Agency n.d.).

Later, during the Clinton administration, under the leadership of James Lee Witt (the first professional emergency manager), FEMA became a cabinet-level agency, recognized as the **lead federal agency** for coordinating the efforts of all other federal agencies in disaster response. However, FEMA was still under the auspices of the Robert T. Stafford Disaster Relief and Emergency Assistance Act (Stafford Act), originally passed by Congress in 1985, providing the means by which the president can declare a state of emergency and thus authorize federal funds for disaster relief to both public agencies and private persons. Since its passage, the Stafford Act has been amended a number of times, with the most comprehensive changes occurring in 2000. The Stafford Act designated state governors as the lead officials for determining the need for federal assistance based on the scope of the disaster and the exhaustion of local remedies. Under the original intent of this act, the president was limited to a reactionary role, responding to a stated need rather than being proactive in anticipating a need. FEMA also operated primarily in a response mode, only showing up at the scene of a disaster once local authorities determined the need for federal assistance (Miskel 2006, 103).

During the late 1980s and early 1990s, however, FEMA came under sharp rebuke by the public and state and local governments for its slow response to disasters, even though the Stafford Act remained in effect. Also, changes to legislation during the 1980s expanded the categories of eligibility for federal disaster assistance to both individuals and organizations. Thus, between 1984 and 1988, there were only 26 disaster declarations, yet from 1989 to 1993, that number jumped to 42, and from 1994 to 1997, it rose to 97 (England-Joseph 1998).

To get a better idea of some of the events precipitating the changes to federal disaster response during this period, consider the example of Hurricane Andrew. In 1992, this devastating storm slammed into South Florida, with winds in excess of 170 miles per hour. Over 23 people were killed in the storm, and the region suffered over $26 billion in property damage. The Florida National Guard was quickly overwhelmed with the state of the disaster, prompting the president to send in active-duty service members from the Tenth Mountain Division, stationed in Ft. Drum, New York. FEMA was the lead federal agency for organizing the federal response effort. However, due to the slow response and lack of coordinated effort, FEMA was heavily criticized, prompting President Clinton to fire its director, replacing him with James Lee Witt in 1993, the first professional emergency manager to serve in this position (Glasser and White 2005; National Oceanic and Atmospheric administration 2002).

2.1.3 Natural Disasters in a Post-9/11 World

After the terrorist attacks on the US homeland on September 11, 2001, the federal government established the Department of Homeland Security (DHS) to respond to the threat of terrorism on American soil. As part of the reorganization of the federal government, FEMA was brought under the control of the new DHS structure, losing its status as an independent federal agency. The initial proposal, in theory, to consolidate all federal agencies with responsibility for responding to domestic threats (whether from terrorism or natural disasters) appeared to make sense operationally. Because terrorist incidents involved the potential for catastrophic events on par with natural disasters or with even greater consequences, FEMA would be a key player in coordinating the federal response to any incident of this scale.

One of the first significant tests of the DHS structure came in August 2005, when Hurricane Katrina, a category 3 storm, hit the Gulf Coast city of New Orleans head on with winds in excess of 125 miles per hour. Initially, the damage to the city and neighboring community of Gulfport, Mississippi, was extensive, but not catastrophic. Three days later, however, the levees broke in New Orleans, causing extensive flooding. The failure of the city government or state to exercise an effective evacuation plan left people stranded on rooftops or sheltered in places like the Superdome. The city devolved into chaos as law enforcement officers failed to show up for work and lawlessness ensued. The federal government eventually called in active-duty military forces to patrol the streets and restore order and basic services. In the aftermath, there was much finger pointing by city, state, and federal officials as to whose fault it was for the poor response. FEMA's director, Michael Brown, was fired, but he later appeared somewhat vindicated on the talk show circuit, offering evidence as to how FEMA was neglected and how his advice was ignored by senior Bush officials. In the end, over 1300 people died in Katrina's aftermath, and more than 1 million people were evacuated to other locations, such as Houston, Texas, where many remain to this day. In addition, over $44 billion in property damage occurred to New Orleans and the coastal towns of Mississippi (Gannon 2005; Lowder 2006).

Unfortunately, within 30 days after Katrina, a second barrel blast occurred with Hurricane Rita hitting the coast of Texas. Although the human tragedy of this storm was much less, the economic impact was great, with major oil refineries in Port Arthur, Texas, extensively damaged. It took months for these facilities to recover, causing fuel shortages all along the East Coast and spikes in gas prices.

After 9/11, the primary threat focus of the federal government was (and still is) terrorism. Although DHS leaders, like Michael Chertoff, stated publicly that the DHS maintained an all-hazards perspective, even before these catastrophic hurricanes hit, it was evident that with regard to funding and organizational status under the DHS, FEMA was being marginalized and its leadership ignored. On the organizational chart, the Director of FEMA at the time of Hurricanes Katrina and Rita, Michael Brown, was considered Under-Secretary for Emergency Response, a position that afforded him direct access to the Director of DHS. Yet, operationally, it made the Director of FEMA one of five undersecretaries in the organization. As for resources, FEMA saw its operational budget reduced in the years prior to 2005 as well, further indicating its loss of status within the DHS hierarchy (Glasser and White 2005).

What made the situation in the Gulf States particularly egregious was the public perception that the federal government did not care. The lack of initial concern, and slow response in the aftermath of the devastating floods, led to charges of racism against the Bush administration, since most of the victims were African American and poor, despite the fact that most of the violence and human misery was caused by victims taking advantage of other victims. Television images of looting, homeless people massed in the squalor of the Superdome, and even reports of murders and rapes made New Orleans look like a city in war-torn Somalia rather than Louisiana. US Coast Guard (USCG) and National Guard helicopters rescuing victims off rooftops further lent to charges of government incompetence at best and dereliction of duty at worst. The Bush administration did its best at damage control, trying to deflect criticism on the poor performance of New Orleans Mayor Ray Nagin and Louisiana Governor Kathleen Blanco for not doing what they should have done at the local and state level. Such attempts only proved counterproductive, however, as the public communicated their belief that in a post-9/11 world, they expected the federal government to be more proactive, whether the threat be a natural disaster or a terrorist incident.

Responding to such criticism, President Bush took proactive measures prior to Hurricane Rita, appointing then US Coast Guard (USCG) Commandant, Admiral Thad Allen (then Vice Admiral and USCG Chief of Staff), as the **Principal Federal Official (PFO)** and **Federal Coordinating Officer (FCO)** in charge of coordinating all post-Katrina federal agency support on behalf of the US government. President Bush also gave the active-duty military a more prominent role in preparation for Hurricane Rita by positioning himself in the command center at the US Northern Command headquarters in Colorado Springs, Colorado, as the hurricane made landfall. These actions were intended to communicate to the American public that the federal government was engaged and would no longer react to natural disasters in the same way again.

As a result of Hurricanes Katrina and Rita, there was some discussion by members of Congress and others that FEMA should be restored to its status as an independent federal agency, out from under DHS control. Secretary of Homeland Security Michael Chertoff argued the need to keep FEMA under DHS control in order to maintain a unified federal response to any catastrophic event, whether a terrorist incident or a natural disaster. Secretary Chertoff did make some organizational changes within FEMA, however, replacing political appointee Michael Brown with a professional emergency responder, R. David Paulison. FEMA also underwent significant internal leadership changes to deal with other post-Katrina failings with regard to the lack of accountability over federal payouts to victims and charges of waste, fraud, and abuse of the compensation programs.

In October 2006, President Bush signed the DHS appropriations bill for 2007, which made changes to the Stafford Act under Title VI, the "Post-Katrina Emergency Management Reform Act of 2006." The act gave FEMA a quasi-independent status but kept it under DHS, restoring some of its original authorities and correcting some of the weaknesses that Congress perceived in the Stafford Act. The end result of all these changes will likely be an expanding federal mandate, at the expense of local and state authorities, when it comes to homeland security policies.

SELF-CHECK

- Since 9/11, FEMA has been returned to its status as an independent federal agency, out from under control of the Department of Homeland Security. True or false?
- According to the Stafford Act, which official has responsibility for recognizing the need for a federal declaration of a state of emergency and requesting federal support?
  a. The president
  b. The Secretary of the DHS
  c. The local mayor
  d. The state governor
- Define PFO.
- James Lee Witt was the first professional emergency manager to lead FEMA. True or false?

2.2 Accidental Hazards: Things We Can Try to Prevent

When considering security from an all-hazards perspective, one area of concern that is often neglected is protection from accidental hazards. Many times, after a personal accident occurs, we ask ourselves, "What could I have done to prevent this?" The same holds true for public and private organizations, which can suffer catastrophic losses from accidental hazards. For this reason, most businesses and individuals carry accident protection insurance for both natural and accidental hazards, such as broken water pipes in our homes or traffic accidents while driving our cars.

But what is the difference between a disaster and an accident? A **disaster** that is not natural can best be understood as "an unintentional event that causes extensive damage, injury, and loss of life" (Pocock n.d.). The difference between a disaster and an **accident** is based on the scale of the accident and the impact.

From a national security perspective, what may first appear to be an accident may also be intentional and not accidental, such as the reports of the first plane crash into the World Trade Center on 9/11. The second, third, and fourth crash, of course, dispelled the belief that the first was an accident. In a post-9/11 world, with the heightened threat of terrorism occurring in the United States, any incident that may at first appear accidental requires local, state, and federal officials to conduct full investigations to determine probable cause.

2.2.1 History of Accidental Hazards in the United States

In the previous section we discussed natural disasters, highlighting some of the most significant incidents in our nation's history. Most accidental disasters, by comparison, are often much smaller in scope, but not necessarily less deadly. Accidents involving hazardous materials (HAZMAT), such as toxic chemicals, fuels, and explosives, can have devastating effects on local population groups.

For example, the worst industrial accident in the world occurred in Bhopal, India, in 1984, when a faulty vault caused a leak of methyl isocyanate (MIC) gas, eventually leading to an explosion that sent toxic cyanide gas into the atmosphere. Over 3800 people died in the immediate blast and from toxic effects of the gas. It is also estimated that as many as 20 000 people have died since as a result of health issues caused by breathing the toxic fumes (Broughton 2005).

In contrast, when a chemical fire occurred in Apex, North Carolina, in October 2006, releasing toxic fumes into the atmosphere impacting a community of 30 000, local fire departments and first responders reacted quickly in evacuating over 17 000 residents from the immediate area, resulting in no loss of life. The US Fire Administration/Technical Report cited the successful response to the chemical fire was due to the preparation of police, fire, and rescue personnel in the greater Raleigh area having intensive training in the National Incident Management System (NIMS), to include implementing the Incident Command System (ICS) and National Response Plan (NRP) protocols (Sensenig and Simpson 2008).

In the United States, one of the greatest concerns has been the potential damage caused by an accident involving a nuclear weapon. There have been numerous "incidents" since the advent of nuclear weapons technology, but to date, there is no documented nuclear "accident" that has resulted in catastrophic loss of life or property due to a nuclear explosion or emission of radiological material. Examples of nuclear weapons incidents typically include improper storage or movement of weapons, or crashes of vehicles, mostly aircraft, carrying such weapons. Most of these incidents occurred during the height of the Cold War in the 1950s and 1960s, when operational deployments involving nuclear weapons were at their height. For example, the US Air Force experienced a number of incidents of jettisoned nuclear weapons or crashes of airplanes carrying these weapons. The US Navy also experienced incidents involving nuclear weapons. As late as 1984, the Navy was involved in an accident at sea between the USS Kitty Hawk (an aircraft carrier) and a Soviet Victor-class nuclear submarine. The Kitty Hawk was carrying nuclear weapons, and it can be assumed that the Soviet sub was also carrying nuclear torpedoes (Tiwari and Gray n.d.).

FOR EXAMPLE

Nuclear Weapons Disaster

A near catastrophe occurred in eastern North Carolina on January 24, 1961, when a B-52 bomber experienced a midair implosion, causing two nuclear weapons to be jettisoned in flight. While one of the bombs deployed safety, the other did not, breaking apart as it made ground contact. Fortunately, one of six fail-safe mechanisms survived the impact, preventing the nuclear warhead from detonating. Yet, the bomb's uranium core was never found. President John F. Kennedy was informed of the accident, only to find out that there had been "more than 60 accidents involving nuclear weapons" to include "two cases in which nuclear-tipped anti-aircraft missiles were actually launched by inadvertence." The Goldsboro incident led the United States to increase the safety devices on its nuclear weapons. The Soviets were also encouraged to take similar precautions to prevent a nuclear accident (Tiwari and Gray n.d.).

2.2.2 Accidental Hazard Prevention and Response

The key to accidental hazard mitigation is to take precautionary steps intended to keep an accident from happening in the first place and, if it does occur, to keep the accident from becoming a disaster. For example, building codes today require commercial properties to have smoke detectors, alarm systems, and, in some cases, sprinkler systems. In new residential construction, homes are required to have smoke detectors pre-wired into the electrical system (with battery backups). Even though these codes may not be able to prevent property damage from occurring, they can help people escape a fire and thus prevent an accident from becoming a personal disaster. In other words, such measures can't stop accidents from happening, but they do intend to lessen the impact once an accident occurs.

In the United States, accidents involving hazardous wastes and chemicals have also occurred, promoting the federal government to develop strict safety and security guidelines for industries involving chemicals and other hazardous materials. The **Environmental Protection Agency (EPA)** is the lead US government agency for assuring compliance with US codes and statutes related to industrial plant safety and security.

The United States also belongs to the **Organization for Economic Cooperation and Development (OECD)**. The OECD's Chemical Accidents Program helps member countries in "developing common principles and policy guidance on prevention of, preparedness for, and response to chemical accidents; analyzing issues of concern and making recommendations concerning best practices; and facilitating the sharing of information and experience between both OECD and non-member countries. It is carried out in co-operation with other international organizations" (Organization for Economic Cooperation and Development n.d.).

Chemical engineers in the United States also belong to organizations that share information and educational resources on chemical safety. For example, the American Institute for Chemical Engineers (AIChE) runs the Center for Chemical Process Safety, whose goal is to "identify and addresses process safety needs within the chemical, pharmaceutical, and petroleum industries. CCPS brings together manufacturers, government agencies, consultants, academia, and insurers to lead the way in improving industrial process safety" (Center for Chemical Process Safety n.d.).

Techniques routinely employed today to prevent accidents from happening include the use of technology, particularly sensors, to monitor storage facilities, transportation conditions of hazardous material, and other dangerous areas in the production of those chemicals or materials. Examples include pressure values, closed-circuit television monitors, automated switching centers, and so on, but the key is always the "human monitor" who has to observe and respond to the technological warning signs.

However, such mechanisms are by no means foolproof. For instance, in the case of an industrial accident in Apex, North Carolina, in October 2006, a series of safety inspections that noted unsafe storage procedures went unheeded by company officials until it was too late. The facility routinely contained a number of hazardous materials, including paints, solvents, and pesticides, although exactly what was in the warehouse the night of the explosion will never be known as the company did not keep records outside of the plant. The company had been cited for numerous storage violations due to improper storage of combustible materials. There had also been concern over the location of the warehouse near residential units, churches, and schools. Although no one was killed in the explosion, 30 people did seek medical help due to inhalation of toxic fumes. In addition, some 17 000 residents, over half the town's population, were required to evacuate the area until **hazardous materials (HAZMAT)** teams could assess the damage and determine it was safe for residents to return. The explosion was a reminder of the dangers of toxic materials being handled and stored in close proximity to populated areas (CNN 2006).

When an accident occurs involving hazardous materials, most local communities have the services of trained HAZMAT teams, who are equipped to respond to accidents involving such materials. Fire departments or emergency medical service providers are most likely to have this capability. With the establishment of the Army and Air National Guard **Weapons of Mass Destruction Civil Support Teams (WMD-CSTs)** in all states within the United States, these units also have personnel trained to operate in contaminated areas due to potential terrorist acts involving hazardous materials. The creation of WMD-CSTs was authorized by President Clinton in 1988. These teams began to operate in 2000, and as of September 2006, there were 42 certified teams, with the goal of eventually fielding 55 units. Thus, every state and territory will eventually have a dedicated team. The teams are normally located in a part of the state near an airport, which allows them access to the most vulnerable areas and enables them to deploy rapidly in a crisis. The mission of the WMD-CSTs is to "support local and state authorities at domestic [WMD] incident sites by identifying agents and substances, assessing current and projected consequences, advising on response measures, and assisting with requests for additional military support" (Global Security n.d) (Figure 2-2).

Figure 2-2

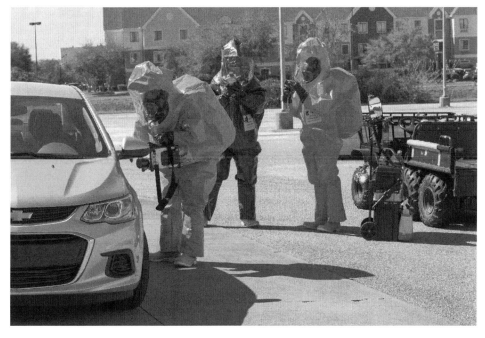

Forty-third Civil Support Team conducting HAZMAT training in March 2017 in Myrtle Beach, SC. Source: Photo courtesy of Staff Sergeant Kevin Pickering, U.S. Army (2017).

2.2.3 Accidental Hazards in a Post-9/11 World

Because accidental hazards can be understood as those events caused by technological mishap, in a post-9/11 world, the concern is that when such events occur, it may not be immediately known whether they are, in fact, accidental and not caused by deliberate, malevolent tactics by terrorists, or even simple human error. A potential train derailment carrying chemicals such as molten sulfur, benzene, or other toxic materials near a school or football stadium, where there is a large concentration of people on any given day, could give local security officials and emergency managers ulcers as they try to think through all the possible "what if" scenarios in their communities and whether such events are truly accidental or not.

For that reason, the focus today in security education with regard to all-hazard threats is on risk management. Chapter 4 explains this process in much greater detail, but an example is the insurance industry, which applies risk management strategies in its attempts to understand an individual's or corporation's tolerance for risk and loss. These companies base their cost estimates on the location of the home or business, as well as the threats (or dangers) associated with either location or type of business based primarily on three factors: vulnerability, probability, and criticality:

1. **Vulnerability** means exposure to risk, such as by living or working in or near a high-crime area.
2. **Probability** refers to the likelihood of a home or business suffering loss due to an all-hazard assessment; for example, an oceanfront vacation home in Miami, as opposed to a brick ranch house outside of Cincinnati, has greater likelihood to suffer loss due to the history of hurricanes in South Florida.
3. **Criticality** relates to the impact of loss on an individual or company; for instance, there would be a high degree of criticality if you had all your corporate assets in one location, rather than dispersed, and this location was destroyed.

The method used in the process for identifying and evaluating risks is called **risk assessment**, "an objective analysis of an organization's entire protective system" (Ortmeier 2005).

In December 2006, the DHS issued new guidelines for the "high-risk" chemical industries, in particular requiring them to perform comprehensive risk assessments that documented measures taken to prevent or mitigate the effects of a terrorist attack or other hazards. The new guidelines require these chemical plants to make their assessments and subsequent security plans to address those areas of vulnerability available to the DHS, which will then audit compliance through their own surveys and audits. Companies failing to implement required changes to their security posture will be subject to heavy fines, up to $25 000 per day for noncompliance (Department of Homeland Security 2006).

Due to the potential damage from a terrorist attack against any production, storage, or transfer facility involved with hazardous materials, there is increased sensitivity and awareness on the part of security managers and corporate leaders to the nature of the threats they face and the consequences of such actions. This increased terrorist threat awareness to inherent vulnerabilities that could be exploited by terrorist groups also has the effect of making those facilities safer from accidental hazards through increased vigilance and awareness. Reducing vulnerability to terrorist threats also can reduce vulnerability to accidental hazards through the implementation of better control and accountability practices, better physical and personnel security procedures, and better technical control procedures. Thus, a potential by-product of living in a post-9/11 world may be a decrease in both the frequency and severity of all-hazard accidents, preventing them from escalating into potential disasters.

SELF-CHECK

- Risk management involves which of the following areas of analysis?
  a. Criticality
  b. Vulnerability
  c. Probability
  d. All of the above
- What is HAZMAT?
- While there have been incidents involving nuclear weapons, to date there has not been an accident whereby a nuclear weapon has detonated, causing a nuclear explosion. True or false?
- Army and Air National Weapons of Mass Destruction-Guard Civil Support Teams came into existence after 9/11. True or false?

2.3 Man-Made Hazards: Things We Hope Don't Happen

As part of the responsibilities of any security manager or emergency planner, one must look across the full spectrum of hazards to include those that are either intentional or malevolent acts, such as a terrorism, as well as those that are created as a result of unintended consequences, such as human error. In other words, while a hazard may not exist initially, through a series of actions (or inactions), an accident or even a disaster may occur by virtue of man-made efforts, done without foresight of the consequences of those actions. Sometimes it can be a simple design flaw in a construction project, which later causes destruction, or it can be the result of demographic changes in a community that place citizens at risk, based on planning decisions made years or even decades earlier. Such scenarios tend to play out only after the fact, once an accident or disaster occurs. But in today's post-9/11 world, serious thought needs to be placed in recognizing potential hazards based on man-made actions, both now and in the future. As other chapters in the text focus specifically on terrorist acts, this section will focus on those man-made disasters caused by human error.

2.3.1 History of Man-Made Disasters Caused by Human Error in the United States

There may be a fine line drawn between many accidental disasters and man-made disasters caused by human error. In other words, an accidental disaster may be exacerbated by environmental conditions created by man, often as a process of development and modernization. This is true for natural disasters as well. One of our nation's greatest disasters caused by flooding was an example of both.

In 1889, the town of Johnstown, Pennsylvania, was destroyed in a devastating flood, which occurred after a dam broke upriver. Over 2200 people perished in the flood. While it was natural weather conditions that triggered the high water levels and placed stress on the dam structure holding back the man-made reservoir, it was a known problem at the time due to the increased development of the area and growth of vacation homes and recreational facilities upriver. Warnings to shore up the dam went unheeded. Only after the disaster occurred were engineers brought in to repair the dam to specifications that would prevent another catastrophe (JAHA n.d.).

To a certain extent, the destruction caused by the collapse of the Twin Towers in New York City on 9/11 is believed to have been a result of the unique structural design that did not allow the buildings to withstand the stress caused by the high heat and structural damage created by the impact of the jetliners. The engineers, to their credit, did not foresee a scenario such as large passenger planes crashing into these buildings, and therefore they did not plan for such a threat to the structural integrity of the Towers. However, in one of his tapes released after the attacks, Osama bin Laden is reported as saying that he knew such an event would occur based on his knowledge of the building's design. If that is true, then the potential for future terrorist attacks against targets in America, exploiting known potential man-made disasters, is extremely great and worrisome.

On the flip side, the terrorist attack on the Pentagon on 9/11, while significant in loss of life and damage, could have been much worse if not for new construction that had occurred to the building in recent years. The renovations to the Pentagon were done in "slices," meaning portions of the building were evacuated and offices relocated to other sites around Washington, until the construction had been completed. Also, the way the building collapsed around the impact site served to isolate other parts of the building from damage and physical harm to its occupants.

A recent example of a natural disaster exacerbated by man-made engineering problems was the collapse of the levee system in New Orleans during Hurricane Katrina. Part of the failure of the federal government to respond quickly was due to the initial report that the levees had held and widespread flooding had been averted. Yet that scenario quickly ended as the levees were breached and floodwaters engulfed the city, trapping people on rooftops and devastating entire neighborhoods. The levee system in New Orleans was created by the Army Corps of Engineers in 1889 and was later shored up in 1927 after flooding of the Mississippi River. Yet, as New Orleans grew and more residential housing went into areas below sea level, the risk of a catastrophic disaster increased. The levees were believed to have been designed to withstand a category 3 hurricane, although there was some doubt of that evaluation due to uneven repairs, primarily those areas that were supposed to have been repaired by the City of New Orleans and not the Corps of Engineers (Carrns and McKay 2005).

Hurricane Katrina made landfall in Louisiana on August 29, 2005, rated as a category 3 hurricane with sustained winds of 125 miles per hour. FEMA had placed such a scenario as one of its "worst-case" disasters, although their planning scenario in this case was South Florida and floodwaters coming from Lake Okeechobee as a result of a hurricane (the other "worst-case" planning scenarios were a terrorist attack on New York City and the New Madrid earthquakes) (Lowder 2006). However, even with the expectation that there would be major damage and destruction and loss of life, most planners thought the levees would hold (or at least, hoped they would).

2.3.2 Man-Made Disaster Mitigation and Response

It is virtually impossible to anticipate all potential man-made disasters that could occur on any given day. Only after the event, many times, will we learn of structural faults in construction design, or poor maintenance records, or any other combination of factors that could contribute to unintended consequences. In other words, who would have known that a disaster could result?

For this reason, the adage that "an ounce of prevention is worth a pound of cure" holds true when considering the potential for man-made disasters and the focus on mitigation over response. For example, homes can now be built with special construction techniques that enable them to better withstand the effects of high winds associated with hurricanes. High-rise buildings in earthquake-prone areas are designed with "flexible" foundations capable of withstanding the stress of ground tremors. Beachfront areas of the East Coast require elevated or "stilt housing" to raise them above coastal floodwaters. Yet, despite these known hazards, developers continue to build in floodplains or along coastlines, and homeowners continue to accept risk due to their desire to live in such areas.

FOR EXAMPLE

St. Francis Dam Failure

Around midnight on March 12, 1928, the St. Francis Dam, a 200 foot tall concrete wall, located 50 miles north of Los Angeles, California, collapsed, spilling 12 billion gallons of water. The deluge traveled 18 miles an hour down San Francisquito Canyon, reaching a height of 140 ft and a width of 3000 ft. With no warning, those small farms and towns in the flood path suffered catastrophic damage and loss of life, with 500 perishing in the disaster. The dam was only two years old when it failed. At the time of its construction, it served as a major engineering project designed to bring water and power to the growing City of Los Angeles. The chief engineer, William Mulholland, was credited with creating an engineering marvel in the construction of the aqueduct system that would bring water from the Sierra Mountains to the coast. Yet, Mulholland failed to take adequate precautions in constructing the St. Francis Dam and Reservoir, as well as ignoring faults and leaks that developed in the dam face (Wilkman 2016) (Figure 2-3).

Figure 2-3

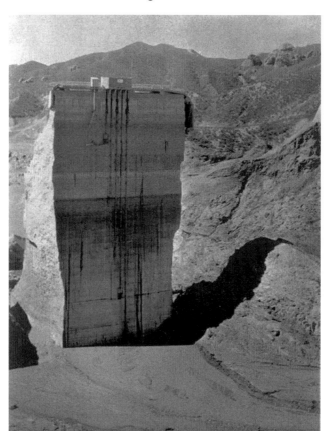

St. Francis Dam disaster 1928. Source: Historical Photo Collection of the Department of Water and Power (1928). City of Los Angeles.

To mitigate the potential damage from future man-made disasters, the EPA requires new businesses or other developers to file **environmental impact statements**, noting the hazards posed by such building projects to local communities. For the most part, these tend to focus on issues such as toxic wastes and damage to local water supplies, watersheds, and/or natural habitats from things like chemical effluents or sewage. Yet, the EPA also considers the broader impact of locating new residential construction or schools near sites that could pose potential disasters, such as chemical storage facilities or transit sites. This is due to the fact that as communities grow, what used to be located on the "outskirts" of town, such an oil refinery or commercial railroad switching center, is now located in town and could pose potential dangers to local communities.

The responses to man-made disasters caused by human error are much the same as for other disasters, but with a focus on identifying the causes and effects of the accidents. A good example is that of the Federal Aviation Administration (FAA) and its investigation process after an airline accident occurs. The investigators seek

> ## FOR EXAMPLE
>
> ### EPA-Sponsored Drill to Test Emergency Responders
>
> In September 2006, the EPA and Marathon Petroleum Company LLC cosponsored a drill to test local, state, and federal emergency response agencies' plans for managing a gasoline spill along the Kanawha River in Charleston, West Virginia. In addition to Marathon, other participants included West Virginia's Department of Environmental Protection, the City of Charleston, emergency responders from two surrounding counties, and the US Coast Guard.
>
> No actual oil spill occurred. Rather, the exercise focused on what would happen if a storage tank were to collapse and oil was spilled into the river. Participants also rehearsed how they would conduct residential evacuations, as well as road closures and other required procedures necessary to test their local emergency response plans (United States Environmental Protection Agency 2006).

to identify the cause of the accident, whether technological mishap, human error, or terrorist attack. For instance, the crash of EgyptAir Flight 990 off the coast of Massachusetts in October 1999 is one example where, to this day, the FAA does not know what caused the crash. There appeared to be no mechanical failure, no explosion, and no other suspected terrorist incident. The result of the investigation was inconclusive, not knowing whether the crash was caused by pilot error or an intentional act to crash the plane by one or more of the flight crew.

If an investigation determines that human errors caused a disaster, such as an airline crash or the meltdown of a nuclear reactor (like occurred at Chernobyl, Ukraine, in 1986), then the remediation is to offer better training or education. If the disaster is caused by design flaws or failure to follow procedures (if there were even procedures to be followed), then the response is usually organizational, with the intent to correct the error and prevent such a situation from arising in the future. However, due to the sheer volume of potential disasters caused by human error, mitigation still remains the best "response."

2.3.3 Man-Made Disasters in a Post-9/11 World

As a result of 9/11 and the attacks on buildings in New York and Washington with large concentrations of workers, new designs for buildings with high occupancy were considered, including One World Trade Center the replacement building for the destroyed World Trade Center buildings. Structural changes in building design can lessen the impact of a potential terrorist attack in the future. Simple changes include new locations for air filtration systems and return vents, keeping them from street-level access where they could become contaminated by chemical or biological agents. Also, collective protection systems, such as those designed into military vehicles, can be helpful in reducing the impact of a dirty bomb and preventing the spread of radiological contamination. Water treatment plants, food processing centers, and other potential terrorist targets can also be "hardened" against the effects of a terrorist attack by the reducing vulnerabilities inherent in these types of facilities due to man-made errors in both handling procedures and technological shortcomings of current systems.

Furthermore, recognizing the potential for **secondary and tertiary effects**, or consequences that are compounded during a natural or accidental disaster due to man-made errors, will only help emergency planners and security managers better prepare their communities for future disasters. Preventing accidents and deterring attacks is obviously the best course of action, but mitigating the effects of an accident or terrorist attack due to measures taken to correct or counter man-made hazards is equally important.

SELF-CHECK

- Due to the sheer volume of potential disasters caused by human error, what remains the best "response?"
  - a. Comprehensive recovery plans
  - b. Education of first responders
  - c. Increased funding for civil defense
  - d. Mitigation efforts to reduce vulnerability
- What is an environmental impact statement?
- Osama bin Laden believed that the collapse of the Twin Towers was ultimately caused by an "act of God." True or false?
- Secondary and tertiary effects are consequences that are compounded during a natural or accidental disaster due to man-made errors. True or false?

2.4 Reassessing the All-Hazards Perspective and Disasters

Since emergency managers and first responders face threats from both man-made and natural disasters, an all-hazards perspective of homeland security still appears to be a practical response to the challenges communities face throughout the country. Thus, for local and state-level agencies, trying to manage limited resources, personnel, and expanding mission areas and responsibilities, focusing on threats to homeland security from an all-hazards perspective has been the preferred method of operation, supporting an inclusive versus an exclusive view of homeland security. And, as Peter Gregory (2015) points out, "The same organizational structure, action plans, and command system that allows organizations to coordinate and lower operation costs prior to the occurrence of emergency events also enables them to respond to emergencies sooner and in a more unified and effective fashion, thus indirectly reducing losses and decreasing the time and resources necessary for recovery."

These same sentiments have been voiced by local and state emergency managers, who still employ an all-hazards approach toward disaster planning. For example, in South Carolina, the South Carolina Emergency Management Division (SCEMD) issued its South Carolina Hazard Mitigation Plan in 2013, which identifies "all the hazards" the state faces and assesses the risks based on probability of occurrence and consequence. The result, however, is an emphasis on disaster planning for those hazards identified as having a high probability of occurrence with the most significant consequence or impact (e.g., hurricanes and tropical storms, drought, floods, tornadoes, etc.) (SCEMD 2013). Local emergency managers also use the Threat and Hazard Identification and Risk Assessment (THIRA) process discussed further in Chapter 4 for identifying the most likely and most serious threats faced in their communities, particularly when required by FEMA to meet Emergency Management Accreditation Program (EMAP) standards.

The "one-size-fits-all" approach toward disaster planning inferred in the all-hazards perspective has actually focused on the "common operational functions" advocated by FEMA to aid local and state emergency managers in their quest to develop plans that can be applicable to a number of disaster situations. This alleviates the need to create response plans for every possible contingency. However, given the diversity of the types of threats that communities face and the unique impact of each, disaster management (vs. emergency management) with its emphasis on risk, threat, and hazard assessment is becoming a more common approach to identifying and managing threats. Disasters also have both societal impacts and environmental consequences that can extend beyond the traditional approach of emergency management, particularly for local and state governments.

At the federal level, given the changing nature of terrorism and the increase in homegrown and lone-wolf terrorist attacks, it appears that an all-hazards perspective to homeland security may not provide the necessary focus for responding to these types of threats. To increase public awareness of these types of threats, programs such as the Joint Counterterrorism Assessment Team (JCAT) at the National Counterterrorism Center (NCTC) were established by the Director of National Intelligence (DNI) to provide a means of communication and information sharing between federal and state and local agencies to help local communities better plan for these types of threats. The JCAT helps develop programs that focus on educating local communities on the threats associated with countering violent extremism (CVE) and identifying at-risk youth may prove more successful in preventing terrorist attacks in the future rather than focusing on responding to the consequences later. Interestingly those involved in the JCAT program do not consider the all-hazards perspective to be detrimental to their efforts. In fact, they feel that the all-hazards approach even facilitates the communication process to address these types of threats due to the organizations and structures brought about by the development of the common operational functions of the NIMS and ICS.

For communities facing new threats from man-made disasters as a result of terrorism, such as cyber-attacks on critical infrastructure, the all-hazards approach may be inadequate to prepare for and respond to these challenges to homeland security. Training programs, such as those offered by FEMA's Emergency Management Institute (EMI), which focus on specific threats in specific communities, help to bridge the gap between the common language and common operating procedures inherent in the all-hazards perspective and the new threats these communities face today.

Threats to homeland security from an all-hazards perspective have included natural disasters, accidental disasters, and man-made disasters. Even in a post-9/11 world, the most prevalent scenarios the nation will face continue to be threats from natural or accidental disasters rather than man-made disasters caused by terrorism. Thus emergency managers and first responders at local and state levels have employed an all-hazards approach to homeland security, trying to manage limited resources. The challenge they face is that when conducting risk assessments in response to these different kinds of threats, low probability risks (like terrorism) can have a high impact. Throughout history, incidents of domestic terrorism within the United States have been rare, yet they have had potentially catastrophic effects. On the other hand, natural, accidental, and man-made hazards may be more of the norm, but their effects are rarely catastrophic (except, of course, for those people whose lives are directly impacted by such events).

As a result of the events of 9/11, the implications for managing risks and assessing consequences from non-terrorist threats can have far-reaching implications for how well the nation is prepared to respond to a new catastrophic terrorist event. Lessons learned from Hurricane Katrina alone caused a shake-up in the Department of Homeland Security and contributed to further discussions at all levels of government on whether the new models of federal response are adequate to the task. If anything, the implication is for an ever-increasing federal mandate to deal with all kinds of threats at all levels, whether states want assistance or not. An example of the tensions that can occur with such a broadened federal response happened in Florida in October 2005, when Governor Jeb Bush did not want federal help to respond to Hurricane Wilma. Due to the poor federal response to Hurricane Katrina, the US military sought to be "proactive" by prepositioning forces in Florida under the authority of the US Northern Command. The Adjutant General of the Florida National Guard responded that the state did not need active-duty military assistance and that the local "incident commander" would be Governor Bush rather than a uniformed federal official (Sylves 2006). However, when Hurricane Matthew produced significant inland flooding in small communities in North and South Carolina in 2016, which were unprepared for such catastrophic damage, state governors were quick to request (and expect) federal support (Wilks 2016).

Preparing for and responding to threats today from an all-hazards perspective remains an important function of local, state, and federal governments. It is also a concern of the private sector. The all-hazards approach is still mentioned in the 2016 version of the National Fire Protection Association (NFPA) 1600 *Standard on Disaster/Emergency Management* publication, which is used by the private and business sector (NFPA 2016). Also, public health communities are governed by accreditation standards set by the Joint Commission, which still advocates an all-hazards approach to emergency management: "The approach calls for an organization to work toward hazard prevention while simultaneously preparing for the unexpected emergencies and unforeseen situations that inevitably occur" (Weden 2016). Communication, using a common language and common terms and procedures, is necessary for security managers at all levels of government, as well as the private and nonprofit sectors. This allows first responders, state, and federal agencies (and private sector organizations) to have a thorough knowledge and understanding of the capabilities of each other's organizations to know what each brings to the fight against threats to homeland security, from a variety of sources. However, as these threats evolve, providing new challenges for homeland security professionals, the all-hazards perspective may not be as effective as developing more tailored responses to specific threats, particularly those posed by lone-wolf terrorists or threats in cyberspace.

SELF-CHECK

- The threat of man-made hazards today is not as significant as it was in the past due to required design changes in the construction industry, an example being the levees in New Orleans, which stood up to Hurricane Katrina. True or false?

- The Joint Counterterrorism Assessment Team (JCAT) at the National Counterterrorism Center (NCTC) was established by the Director of FBI. True or false?

- Which of the following would be a secondary or tertiary effect due to a man-made hazard?

    a. A farm destroyed by flooding due to a river overflowing its banks

    b. A fire in a warehouse caused by lightning

    c. A 12-car accident on an interstate due to an ice storm

    d. A bridge collapsing during a hurricane due to structural faults during construction

- Man-made disasters can be caused by either a malevolent act (such as terrorism) or by human error. True or false?

SUMMARY

In this chapter, you learned about threats to homeland security from an all-hazards perspective, focusing on natural disasters, accidental disasters, and man-made disasters. Even in a post-9/11 world, the most prevalent scenarios we face as a nation will continue to be threats from disasters other than terrorism. Thus emergency managers and first responders at local and state levels have employed an all-hazards approach to homeland security, trying to manage limited resources. The challenge they face is that when conducting risk assessments in response to these different kinds of threats, low probability risks (like terrorism) can have a high impact. As subsequent chapters in the text note, throughout history, incidents of domestic terrorism within the United States have been rare, yet they have had potentially catastrophic effects. On the other hand, natural, accidental, and man-made hazards may be more of the norm, but their effects are rarely catastrophic (except, of course, for those people whose lives are directly impacted by such events).

Understanding the nature of threats today from an all-hazards perspective requires security managers at all levels of government, as well as the private and nonprofit sectors, to have a thorough knowledge and understanding of the capabilities of each other's organizations to know what each brings to the fight. A common saying still today among homeland security officials is that during a crisis, whether caused by a natural hazard, accidental hazard, man-made hazard, or terrorist event, it is no time to be exchanging business cards!

In this chapter, you further evaluated the types of natural, accidental, and man-made disasters that can and do occur today. You also assessed the nature of our response to natural, accidental, and man-made disasters in the United States. As a result of reading this chapter, you can now judge how disasters today can have catastrophic effects and implications for our nation's response in the war on terrorism.

KEY TERMS

Accident	An unintentional incident that causes damage, injury, or loss of life, but on a lower scale than a disaster.
All hazards	A threat or an incident, natural or man-made, that warrants action to protect life, property, the environment, and public health or safety and to minimize disruptions of government, social, or economic activities. It includes natural disasters, cyber incidents, industrial accidents, pandemics, acts of terrorism, sabotage, and destructive criminal activity targeting critical infrastructure. This also includes the effects climate change has on the threats and hazards.
All-hazards approach	An inclusive perspective toward homeland security that takes into consideration all possible threat types in a threat or risk assessment.
Cascading effects	The cumulative effects of a disaster beyond the immediate impact in terms of public safety, such as the longer-term impacts on physical, natural, economic, political, and social environments.
Civil defense	The protection of the nation against threats within the United States.
Criticality	The impact of loss on an individual or company.
Disaster	An unintentional event that causes extensive damage, injury, and loss of life.
Environmental impact statement	Statement of the hazards posed by a building project to the local community. Such statements are required under the National

	Environmental Protection Act for all major building projects or legislation that will impact the environment both positively and negatively.
Environmental Protection Agency (EPA)	The lead federal agency for assuring compliance with US codes and statutes related to industrial plant safety and security.
Federal Coordinating Officer (FCO)	The single individual, usually the head of the lead federal agency, designated to work under the PFO for coordinating the federal response to a domestic situation.
HAZMAT	Abbreviation for hazardous materials.
Lead federal agency	A single federal agency designated as having overall responsibility for coordinating federal response to a domestic situation, such as a natural disaster or terrorist incident.
Natural disaster	The effect of a naturally occurring phenomenon, usually referred to by the insurance industry as an "act of God." Examples of natural disasters include hurricanes, tornadoes, floods, and forest fires due to natural causes.
Organization for Economic Cooperation and Development (OECD)	International economic organization whose goals include developing common principles and policy guidance on prevention of, preparedness for, and response to chemical accidents.
Principal Federal Official (PFO)	The single lead federal representative with overall responsibility for the federal response to a domestic situation, such as a natural disaster or terrorist incident. This individual may or may not be the head of the lead federal agency.
Probability	The likelihood of suffering loss due to potential risks.
Risk assessment	Identifying and evaluating risks based on an objective analysis of an organization's entire protective system.
Secondary and tertiary effects	Consequences that are compounded during a natural or accidental disaster due to man-made errors.

State of emergency	A declaration by the president in response to a disaster, making the affected area of the country eligible for increased federal support and funding.
Vulnerability	Exposure to risk in general.
Weapons of Mass Destruction Civil Support Teams (WMD-CSTs)	Teams within the Army and Air National Guard that have personnel trained to operate in contaminated areas due to potential terrorist attacks involving hazardous materials.

ASSESS YOUR UNDERSTANDING

Go to www.wiley.com/go/Kilroy/Threats_to_Homeland_Security to assess your knowledge of the basics of the all-hazards perspective.

Summary Questions

1. An "inclusive" view toward homeland security would take an all-hazards perspective to threat assessments, looking beyond just terrorism. True or false?

2. As a result of 9/11 and the creation of the Department of Homeland Security, FEMA was elevated to a stand-alone cabinet-level agency, focused only on non-terrorist threats. True or false?

3. To date, in the United States, there has been no documented nuclear "accident" that resulted in catastrophic loss of life or property due to a nuclear explosion or emission of radiological material. True or false?

4. South Carolina is the only state without a dedicated Army and Air National Guard WMD-CST. True or false?

5. Man-made disasters can be caused by malevolent acts (such as terrorism) and by human error. True or false?

6. Since 1979, the lead federal agency for disaster response has been which of the following?
   (a) FEMA
   (b) DHS
   (c) US Coast Guard
   (d) EPA

7. Which federal agency is responsible for evaluating environmental impact statements?
   (a) FBI
   (b) Department of the Interior
   (c) DHS
   (d) EPA

8. Which of the following organizations possesses special teams called WMD-CSTs, who are trained in providing civil support through the ability to operate in contaminated environments?
   (a) Army and Air National Guard
   (b) FEMA
   (c) EPA
   (d) OECD

9. FEMA was established under which US president's administration?
   (a) Gerald Ford
   (b) Jimmy Carter
   (c) Bill Clinton
   (d) George H.W. Bush

10. Which event caused a change in the federal government's approach toward homeland security to focus on threats from an all-hazards perspective?
    (a) Hurricane Katrina
    (b) Superstorm Sandy
    (c) The Boston Marathon bombing
    (d) 9/11 terrorist attacks

Applying This Chapter

1. You are serving as a local emergency manager responsible for coordinating your community's response to an accidental hazard, such as a train derailment with toxic chemicals involved. What resources would you have available at your disposal? What could you count upon from the state and federal levels? How would your response have been different if this had been a terrorist attack, causing the train to derail?

2. You are an urban planner in a large metropolitan area and are considering building designs and construction. What factors would you consider in new buildings to prevent man-made disasters or secondary or tertiary effects of terrorist attacks from occurring?

3. Your local community is planning a training exercise to prepare for a possible natural disaster, such as a hurricane. What planning considerations would you recommend including in such an exercise? What local agencies and individuals would you involve in the exercise? Why?

4. Research a recent natural disaster. Consider the cascading effects: those cumulative effects of a disaster beyond the immediate impact in terms of public safety, such as the longer-term impacts on physical, natural, economic, political, and social environments in the community.

All-Hazards Perspective

Provide a study of accidents that have occurred in your state and/or local community. Determine the cause of each. Identify, if possible, whether any of these accidents could be attributed to either natural or man-made hazards. Analyze any secondary or tertiary effects that could have been caused by man-made hazards. Evaluate the remediation efforts put into place after the accident occurred.

Natural Disaster Case Study

Write a case study of the federal response to a natural disaster, such as a hurricane or flooding. Determine the roles played by local, state, and federal agencies. Assess the type of assistance provided by FEMA and evaluate the appropriateness of the aid, based on the situation. Explain what might have been different if that disaster had occurred in a post-9/11 world, yet before Hurricane Katrina. Would an all-hazards perspective have better prepared local, state, and federal agencies to respond to the disaster, or not?

3

US HOMELAND SECURITY INTERESTS
Understanding What Constitutes Homeland Security

Chad S. Foster

College of Justice and Safety, Eastern Kentucky University, Richmond, KY, USA

Starting Point

Go to www.wiley.com/go/Kilroy/Threats_to_Homeland_Security to assess your knowledge of US homeland security interests.
Determine where you need to concentrate your effort.

What You'll Learn in This Chapter

▲ Meanings and perspectives associated with homeland security
▲ Homeland security supporting traditions and theories
▲ Historical and social context for homeland security
▲ The partners involved in the homeland security enterprise

After Studying This Chapter, You'll Be Able To

▲ Assess various meanings and perspectives associated with homeland security
▲ Relate historical and social context to contemporary homeland security problems and approaches
▲ Evaluate the different roles of federal, state, and local agencies and whole community partners
▲ Evaluate the all-hazards concept in relation to homeland security

Threats to Homeland Security: Reassessing the All-Hazards Perspective, Second Edition.
Edited by Richard J. Kilroy, Jr.
© 2018 John Wiley & Sons, Inc. Published 2018 by John Wiley & Sons, Inc.
Companion website: www.wiley.com/go/Kilroy/Threats_to_Homeland_Security

INTRODUCTION

On June 12, 2016, a gunman sympathetic to international terrorist causes assaulted a nightclub in Orlando, Florida, and killed 48 individuals before being shot by local police (Alvarez and Perez-Pena 2016). Nearly 2 weeks later, a weather system halted over West Virginia resulting in rainfall that exceeded 1000-year flood levels in some areas, 23 deaths, and federal disaster declarations for 3 counties (Rice 2016). The following month, the Zika virus surfaced in the greater Miami-Dade County area leading to unprecedented travel advisories to that region by the Centers for Disease Control and Prevention (CDC) (LaMotte 2016). And the Federal Bureau of Investigation (FBI) continued to issue reports about increasing cases of ransomware—a type of malware that locks files on computers in exchange for payment—targeting individuals, businesses, and government agencies (Weisman 2016). Which of these news stories from the summer months of 2016 reflect homeland security concerns?

In this chapter, you will assess various meanings and perspectives associated with homeland security. You'll also relate historical and social context to contemporary homeland security problems and approaches as well as evaluate the different roles of federal, state, and local agencies and whole community partners. Finally you will evaluate the all-hazards perspective in relation to homeland security today.

3.1 What Is Homeland Security?

In a written testimony to the Senate Committee on Homeland Security and Governmental Affairs in September 2016, the US Department of Homeland Security (DHS) Secretary Jeh Johnson (2016) said, "[a]long with counterterrorism, cybersecurity remains a cornerstone of our Department's mission. Making tangible improvements to our Nation's cybersecurity is a top priority…." In fact, Congress passed and the president signed the Cybersecurity Act of 2015 the previous year providing a "voluntary framework for the sharing of cybersecurity threat information between and among the federal government, state governments, and private entities" (Bender 2015). And proposals for restructuring DHS to create a single Cybersecurity and Infrastructure Protection Agency were being contemplated at the time of writing.

Even before the creation of DHS via the Homeland Security Act of 2002, securing cyberspace began as a major homeland security initiative under the broader category of protecting critical infrastructures and key assets. However, addressing the threat of terrorism dwarfed other national priorities. That year, the *National Strategy for Homeland Security* defined homeland security as "a concerted national effort to prevent terrorist attacks within the United States, reduce America's vulnerability to terrorism, and minimize the damage and recover from attacks that do occur" (The White House Office of Homeland Security 2002, 2). Nearly 10 years later in the first *Quadrennial Homeland Security Review Report*, **homeland security** was defined as "a concerted national effort to ensure a homeland that is safe, secure, and resilient against terrorism and other hazards where American interests, aspirations, and way of life can thrive" (US DHS 2010, 13). This conception of the term homeland security remains consistent today.

As pointed out in Chapter 1, the threat of terrorism remains a priority for national homeland security policies, programs, and resources, but cybersecurity is now viewed as a "cornerstone" as evidenced by the aforementioned statement and newly enacted laws. This stands in contrast to the all-hazards approach to building capabilities, which is promoted by DHS doctrine and various programs. According to the latest version of the National Preparedness Goal, the term all hazards means the following:

> A threat or an incident, natural or manmade, that warrants action to protect life, property, the environment, and public health or safety, and to minimize disruptions of government, social, or economic activities. It includes natural disasters, cyber incidents, industrial accidents, pandemics, acts of terrorism, sabotage, and destructive criminal activity targeting critical infrastructure. This also includes the effects climate change has on the threats and hazards. (US DHS 2015)

For example, the Emergency Management Performance Grant (EMPG) program aims to "provide federal funds to states to assist state, local, territorial, and tribal governments in preparing for all hazards" (US DHS 2016a, 2).

Is it possible to remain focused on the threat of terrorism and cyber-attacks while also building national capabilities to respond to pandemics, earthquakes, and climate change? Does this constitute a paradox or repudiate the proverb "have your cake and eat it too?" Exploring these questions requires critical thinking on what constitutes homeland security in the United States, including the supporting traditions that comprise the homeland security profession and discipline.

3.1.1 The Merging of Traditions

To many Americans, the concept of homeland security is relatively new, a part of the national dialog only since the 2001 terrorist attacks. Though the term homeland security may be novel, is the meaning associated with the term unique, and is homeland security a new discipline? Chapter 1 presents historical context on one tradition attached to homeland security—international security or national security—with a focus on external conflicts, adversaries, and the intentional acts of nation states, groups, and individuals. This academic discipline or tradition is consistent with many of the following definitions or "ideal types" associated with homeland security as presented by Bellavita (2008):

1. **Terrorism:** Homeland security is a concerted national effort by federal, state, and local governments, by the private sector, and by individuals to prevent terrorist attacks within the United States, reduce America's vulnerability to terrorism, and minimize the damage and recover from attacks that do occur.
2. **All Hazards:** Homeland security is a concerted national effort to prevent and disrupt terrorist attacks, protect against man-made and natural hazards, and respond to and recover from incidents that do occur.
3. **Terrorism and Catastrophes:** Homeland security is what the Department of Homeland Security—supported by other federal agencies—does to prevent, respond to, and recover from terrorist and catastrophic events that affect the security of the United States.

4. **Jurisdictional Hazards:** Homeland security means something different in each jurisdiction. It is a locally directed effort to prevent and prepare for incidents most likely to threaten the safety and security of its citizens.

5. **Meta Hazards:** Homeland security is a national effort to prevent or mitigate any social trend or threat that can disrupt the long-term stability of the American way of life.

6. **National Security:** Homeland security is an element of national security that works with the other instruments of national power to protect the sovereignty, territory, domestic population, and critical infrastructure of the United States against threats and aggression.

7. **Security Über Alles:** Homeland security is a symbol used to justify government efforts to curtail civil liberties.

Bellavita argues that varied interests, which include those of government institutions and interest groups, align with each of these types. In other words, understanding perspectives and varied context is important for determining interests and institutions. From an academic perspective, it may be argued that homeland security merges many disciplines under a common umbrella; therefore, it is not a single discipline but rather multidisciplinary in nature. The international security or national security tradition supports many facets of homeland security. A parallel, if not separate, narrative may be framed relating to border security and immigration, especially given the importance placed on border security, including airport security, by the 9/11 Commission, and that a majority of DHS agencies have some responsibility for border security and immigration.

Given the scale and scope of the 2001 terrorist attacks and the fact that the Federal Emergency Management Agency (FEMA) became part of the DHS in 2002, the disciplines of emergency management and disaster studies, which encompass disaster policy and politics, are now aligned or associated with homeland security. This may be considered a third supporting discipline as illustrated in Figure 3-1. The remaining portion of this section provides historical context on this third tradition.

Long before professional fire departments and police forces, churches, civic organizations, families, and neighbors served as first responders to natural and man-made dangers. Disaster **response**—those activities in the immediate aftermath of a disaster to protect life and property (McEntire 2015, 39)—was largely handled by victims themselves, volunteers, and secular or religious groups within communities (Sylves 2015, 4). In fact, voluntary organizations continue to fulfill critical roles and address unmet needs within communities devastated by disasters today.

Over time, common hazards and threats such as flooding, fires, and disease required the administrative and financial capacities of government (Waugh 2000, 15). For example, as cities grew, catastrophic fires presented a real threat to life and property. Thus, during the eighteenth and early nineteenth centuries, local governments issued building codes requiring residents to build with brick or stone, rather than wood, to lessen the likelihood of catastrophic fires. Public health also became a concern for policymakers during the nineteenth century. As cities became

Figure 3-1

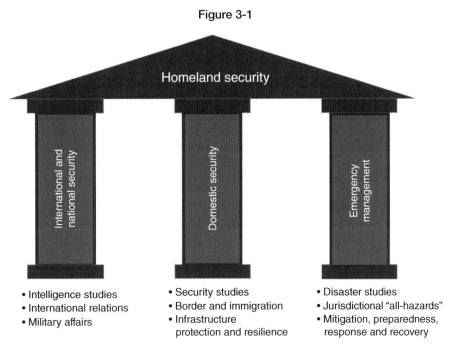

Homeland security traditions (EKU 2017).

congested and very little sanitation existed, diseases could spread easily. Frequent outbreaks of smallpox, cholera, yellow fever, and other diseases were not uncommon in American cities during the 1800s, and the 1918 influenza epidemic killed thousands in the United States. In response, local officials passed public health ordinances to regulate water use and sewage treatment (Waugh 2000, 14).

Prior to the mid-twentieth century, governmental disaster activities were generally characterized as reactive, with institutions providing relief only after disasters actually occurred (Waugh 2000, 16). This method of policymaking continued until 1950, when Congress passed the Disaster Relief Act to streamline the provision of federal disaster assistance to states by authorizing the president to approve of aid without congressional action (Sylves 2015, 60–61). Also during the period from 1930s to the 1950s and as the population grew in the United States, flooding became problematic and offering flood coverage became too costly for the private insurance market. Congress responded by authorizing studies by the US Army Corps of Engineers and eventually funding for massive structural flood control projects, mainly levees and flood walls, along the nation's river systems (Godschalk et al. 1999, 51).

Under both Presidents Truman and Eisenhower, civil defense became a national imperative beginning with the passage of the Civil Defense Act of 1950. Funding was provided to help communities prepare for nuclear war and fallout through sheltering and evacuation planning initiatives. **Preparedness**—efforts to increase readiness for a disaster response and recovery operations (McEntire 2015, 38)—entered the national lexicon. This period is important to the profession of emergency management in the United States as state civil defense agencies are considered "direct forerunners of current state and local emergency management organizations" (National Emergency Management Association [NEMA] 2011, 17).

A shift occurred in the 1960s and 1970s as the costs of flooding, hurricanes, and other natural disasters continued to rise and there was a realization that structural projects were too expensive to continue. As a result, policymakers and professionals embraced land use management practices and insurance tools; the passage of the National Flood Insurance Act of 1968 and creation of the National Flood Insurance Program (NFIP) illustrates the shift from structural projects to nonstructural projects that emphasized less costly incentives and disincentives for reducing future disaster losses.

From a natural disaster management perspective, the 1990s may be considered the era of **mitigation**—action taken to reduce or eliminate the long-term risk to human life and property from natural hazards (Godschalk et al. 1999, 5). The Robert T. Stafford Disaster Relief and Emergency Act (Stafford Act) of 1988 required that states develop post-disaster mitigation plans as a condition of receiving federal assistance and provided matching funds to states to support mitigation projects (Godschalk et al. 1999, 11–14). The passage of this act came just before some of the most costly and devastating natural disasters in the history of the United States, including Hurricanes Hugo and Andrew in 1989 and 1992, respectively, and the Loma Prieta and Northridge earthquakes in 1989 and 1994, respectively. This era was capped in 2000 by the passage of the Disaster Mitigation Act, which promoted proactive, pre-disaster mitigation planning and authorized grants to states and local subdivisions to support mitigation projects (Sylves 2015, 81).

The threat of terrorism clearly became the focus of disaster policies in 2001 and for the years following the attacks, and the era of homeland security began in earnest with emphasis on prevention and protection. **Prevention** includes those capabilities necessary to avoid, prevent, or stop a threatened or actual act of terrorism, while **protection** is oriented inward at safeguarding people, vital interests such as critical infrastructure, and the American way of life (US DHS 2015). This era witnessed a restructuring of the federal government, and many states followed suit by forming new offices of homeland security and intelligence fusion centers and adjusted to new roles and responsibilities (Foster and Cordner 2005). The mailings of letters laced with anthrax and ricin in 2001 and 2003, respectively, showed that America was vulnerable to a chemical, biological, or radiological attack (Foster and Kinsella 2004). And a sniper incident in the greater Washington, DC, region in October 2002 that resulted in 10 deaths and required the unprecedented coordination of law enforcement for 23 days kept domestic security concerns on the forefront (Murphy and Wexler 2004).

The next "jolt to the system"—a phrase commonly used by Donald Kettl (2014) in *System under Stress*—came following Hurricane Katrina in 2005 and Hurricane Sandy in 2012. Among other challenges, disaster recovery has occupied the attention of disaster policy and politics, especially given the enormous challenges and costs associated with these two disasters. **Recovery** is defined as activities to return affected communities to pre-disaster or, preferably, improved conditions (McEntire 2015, 39). Hurricanes are the costliest type of disaster based on Disaster Relief Fund historical spending data, and recovery spending for Hurricanes Katrina and Sandy accounted for approximately three-quarters of all hurricane spending since 1996 (Boccia 2016, 46). In fact, paying claims from the two aforementioned storms required FEMA to borrow billions of dollars from the US Treasury; the NFIP remains in a deficit as of December 2014, and FEMA owes approximately $23 billion

Figure 3-2

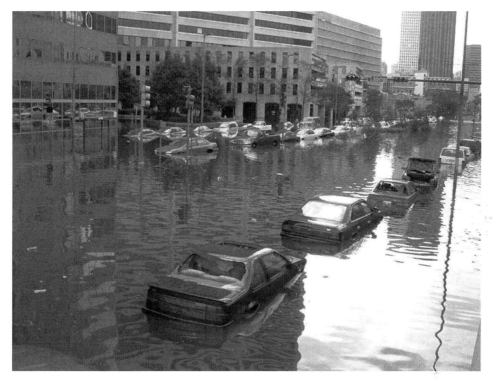

Hurricane Katrina flooding in New Orleans. Source: Photo courtesy of Marty Bahamonde, FEMA (2005).

(US Government Accountability Office [GAO] 2015, 385). For the past 10 years, significant reforms relating to disaster recovery have been underway (Figure 3-2).

Most recently, the concept of **resilience** has gained popularity within various academic disciplines. Defined by the National Academy of Sciences (2012) as "the ability to prepare and plan for, absorb, recover from, and more successfully adapt to adverse events" (1), resilience overlaps with both preparedness and mitigation and places a premium on a long-term view of hazards and their impacts, as well as community engagement. Practically speaking, resiliency is viewed as a way to reduce disaster costs, make communities more self-sufficient and less reliant on federal government support, and mitigate the impacts of climate changes.

From the viewpoint of the emergency management and disaster studies traditions, as disciplines within homeland security, this brief historical trace illustrates multiple shifts in priorities—civil defense, natural disasters, and terrorism—during the past 100 years. In fact, homeland security today, to some degree, reflects remnants of these previous eras and their long-lasting constituencies.

3.1.2 Prevailing Homeland Security Theories

Theories provide possible explanations for social phenomena and support critical thinking on both the problems themselves and the nation's political and administrative responses to the problems. This section presents a few of the more prevalent theories or explanations supported by literature.

As previously described in Chapter 1, globalization is commonly cited as a contributing factor to many homeland security problems and complexities today. It provides important context for understanding events that have occurred during the past 20–30 years, including the evolution of homeland security in the United States. It also has ramifications for security concerns outside of the United States. For example, the rapid flow of goods and social interactions has been met in many global regions by resistance to social change and clashes over cultures. The Internet and ubiquitous mobile communications have served as "force multipliers" for small radical groups intent on advancing their own narratives, especially in the absence of governmental institutions or when supported by outside nation states (McElreath et al. 2014). Even international organized crime and natural hazards such as pandemics pose a heightened global risk due to the ease of passenger travel and the shipment of cargo among nations and continents.

The "flattening of the world," as coined by book author Thomas Friedman (2005), has also resulted in the rapid industrialization of nations, the development of once forested land, and the use of natural resources. Likewise, the greater demands for energy to fuel industrialization and global transportation networks and the fierce competition for scarce resources result in companies accepting greater risks. In 2010, for example, the explosion of the Deepwater Horizon drilling rig in the Gulf of Mexico is deemed as the "largest spill of oil in the history of marine oil drilling operations" by the Environmental Protection Agency (EPA) (2016) that resulted in not only loss of life but also unprecedented damages to the environment. Likewise, recent railcar accidents and spills involving the transportation of volatile crude oil from North Dakota's Bakken oil fields to refineries along the coast has contributed to a national debate over the safest ways to transport oil—rail versus pipeline versus ship/barge—in the future.

In addition to technological hazards and threats, changing weather patterns—what many scientists and scholars now call climate change, global warming, or the climate crisis—may be linked to globalization and industrialization. **Climate change** is defined as the following:

> Changes in average weather conditions that persist over multiple decades or longer. Climate change encompasses both increases and decreases in temperature, as well as shifts in precipitation, changing risk of certain types of severe weather events, and changes to other features of the climate system. (US Global Change Research Program, n.d.)

The gradual warming of the planet is projected by experts to have serious consequences for the country.

The nation's homeland security policies and institutional framework are a result of political processes. As such, it is worth introducing a few notable public policy and management theories that help explain the evolution of homeland security. The notion that homeland security policy is driven based on events, consistent with the **issue–attention cycle** as originally advanced by the social theorists and political scientists Anthony Downs and John Kingdom, has merit (Bellavita 2008; Kettl 2014; Sylves 2015).

Essentially, a brief "window of time" opens following a significant event or large-scale disaster that gains the attention of national leaders and offers an environment

FOR EXAMPLE

Climate Change Projections by US Region

The 2014 National Climate Assessment indicates that regions of the country will experience different effects. For example, some regions such as the southeast will experience prolonged periods of excessively high temperatures or heat waves, while the severity of droughts and wildfires will increase in the southwest, and more frequent downpours and flooding occurs in the Midwest. The following provides a summary of projected climate change impacts by US region.

Northeast: Heat waves, heavy downpours, and sea level rise pose growing challenges to many aspects of life in the northeast. Infrastructure, agriculture, fisheries, and ecosystems will be increasingly compromised.

Southeast and the Caribbean: Sea level rise poses widespread and continuing threats to the region's economy and environment. Extreme heat will affect health, energy, agriculture, and more. Decreased water availability will have economic and environmental impacts.

Midwest: Extreme heat, heavy downpours, and flooding will affect infrastructure, health, agriculture, forestry, transportation, air and water quality, and more. Climate change will also exacerbate a range of risks to the Great Lakes.

Great Plains: Rising temperatures are leading to increased demand for water and energy. In parts of the region, this will constrain development, stress natural resources, and increase competition for water. New agricultural practices will be needed to cope with changing conditions.

Southwest: Increased heat, drought, and insect outbreaks, all linked to climate change, have increased wildfires. Declining water supplies, reduced agricultural yields, health impacts in cities due to heat, and flooding and erosion in coastal areas are additional concerns.

Northwest: Sea level rise, erosion, inundation, risks to infrastructure, and increasing ocean acidity pose major threats. Increasing wildfire, insect outbreaks, and tree diseases are causing widespread tree die-off.

Alaska: Alaska has warmed twice as fast as the rest of the nation, bringing widespread impacts. Sea ice is rapidly receding and glaciers are shrinking. Thawing permafrost is leading to more wildfire and affecting infrastructure and wildlife habitat. Rising ocean temperatures and acidification will alter valuable marine fisheries.

Hawaii and the US-affiliated Pacific Islands: Warmer oceans are leading to increased coral bleaching and disease outbreaks and changing distribution of tuna fisheries. Freshwater supplies will become more limited on many islands. Coastal flooding and erosion will increase. Mounting threats to food and water security, infrastructure, health, and safety are expected to lead to increasing human migration (Melillo et al. 2014).

ripe for political change. This idea may be traced back historically, but it is most clearly illustrated using recent disasters such as the September 11, 2001, terrorist attacks and Hurricanes Katrina and Sandy. This proverbial "window of time" is brief and may quickly close when the next event occurs, when the significant costs for addressing the problem are realized, or when public interest declines (Sylves 2015, 11–12). Often, new institutions are formed during this process to address the problem(s) such as the bipartisan 9/11 Commission, the Transportation Security Administration (TSA), and DHS, which were all formed in response to the 2001 terrorist attacks. Recent lone wolf terrorist attacks inspired by international groups such as the Orlando nightclub attack in 2016 may not elevate the issue of terrorism on the national agenda on par with the 2001 terrorist attacks, but they are having an impact on relevant grant and training programs, for example (Figure 3-3).

Relating to the issue–attention cycle, the political scientist Donald Kettl theorizes that **punctuated backsliding** occurs following events that stress existing systems and the status quo. Events such as the 2001 terrorist attacks and Hurricane Katrina result in neither far-reaching and significant changes nor minor incremental adjustments to policies. Rather, events result in initial significant changes to policy, and then "a subsequent slip back toward the previous equilibrium" (Kettl 2014, 159). Forces pushing back toward the previous equilibrium, among others, include bureaucracy and federalism—two national institutional factors. For example, reforms following the 2001 terrorist attacks did not result in wholesale restructuring of the nation's lead intelligence agencies—Federal Bureau

Figure 3-3

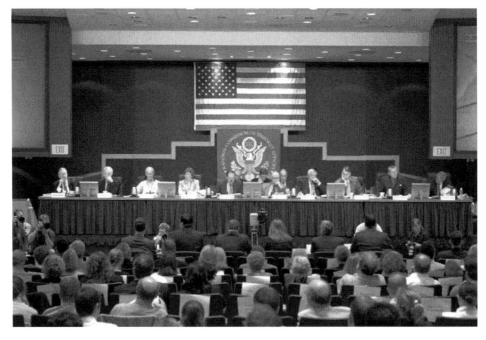

9/11 Commission presents findings in 2004 (National Commission on Terrorist Attacks Upon the United States 2004).

of Investigation (FBI), Central Intelligence Agency (CIA), and National Security Agency (NSA)—but rather laws to strengthen existing intelligence capabilities and to lessen legal–administrative constraints. The Post-Katrina Emergency Management Reform Act (PKEMRA) of 2006 consolidated preparedness programs within FEMA, among other changes, but it did not reinstate FEMA as an autonomous, independent agency as many interest groups advocated for in the years following the hurricane. Institutionalism—cultures, interest groups, oversight committees, missions, and goals—remains a strong force against change.

The second force resisting change is federalism, which relates to **intergovernmental relations** theory. Specifically, Richard Sylves (2015) applied Deil S. Wright's models for intergovernmental relations to disaster policy; it also provides a taxonomy for classifying authorities relating to homeland security.

The **coordinate-authority model** reflects clear and distinct separations of authorities and responsibilities between the federal government and states. The 10th Amendment to the US Constitution notes that "[t]he powers not delegated to the United States by the Constitution, nor prohibited by it to the States, are reserved to the States," which includes "police powers" (NEMA 2011, 14). From the perspective of disaster management, there is no reference to federal government involvement in disaster assistance in the US Constitution. Generally, states and local governments are presumed responsible for disaster management with some exceptions; for example, disasters that occur on federal lands (e.g., national parks, monuments, etc.) may be the responsibility of federal agencies such as the US Department of Interior or US Forest Service, an agency of the US Department of Agriculture. The US Coast Guard and Environmental Protection Agency (EPA) may have responsibility for management of incidents on waterways such as oil spills. However, a majority of disasters occur within the geopolitical boundaries of the 50 states, the District of Columbia, US Territories, and Commonwealths. As a result, approaches and practices may be characterized as decentralized and fragmented, which is consistent with the coordinate-authority model.

Intergovernmental relations following the 2001 terrorist attacks, what many view as the period of homeland security, has drifted toward the overlapping-authority or even inclusive-authority models. The **overlapping-authority model** accepts that responsibilities are generally shared among governments, and, likewise, no one jurisdiction retains sole jurisdiction over hazards and threats. On the other hand, the **inclusive-authority model** promotes a strong federal government with regard to homeland security decision making and power. Though some responsibilities may be shared, the main influence and authority are viewed as a hierarchy in which state and local governments are viewed as supporting the federal government and less leading in a bottom-up or unified arrangement (Sylves 2015, 42–43).

How do these models relate to the nation's approach to homeland security problems? It may be argued that the FBI will exercise broad authority for preventing and managing disasters linked to acts of terrorism. The proliferation of homeland security grant programs tied to compliance with federal mandates supports the inclusive-authority model. On the other hand, contemporary response doctrine embraces the concept of the **tiered response**; this means that incidents must be managed at the lowest possible jurisdictional level and supported by additional response capabilities when needed (US DHS 2013). This doctrine is supported by the **Stafford Act**, which was signed into law in 1988 and amended numerous times since then. This seminal law aims "to provide an orderly and continuing means of assistance by the Federal Government to State and local governments in carrying out their responsibilities to alleviate the suffering and damage which result from such disasters…" (FEMA 2007, 1). Clearly, response and recovery doctrine for most disasters supports the coordinate-authority or overlapping-authority models.

In summary, this section presented some of the more prevailing theories regarding the problems associated with homeland security and the nation's responses to the problems. Follow-on chapters describe in more depth theories relating to risk analysis, threat of terrorism, and infrastructure protection.

SELF-CHECK

- Which concept reflects the planning and drills that occurred within states and communities nationwide as a result of the Federal Civil Defense Act of 1950 and threats posed during the Cold War era?

  a. Response

  b. Preparedness

  c. Mitigation

  d. Recovery

- Prior to the mid-twentieth century, governmental disaster activities were generally characterized as reactive, with institutions providing relief only after disasters actually occurred. True or false?

- Which of the following theory(s) may be useful in understanding the extent of policy changes following significant national events?

  a. Issue–attention cycle

  b. Punctuated backsliding

  c. Both issue–attention cycle and punctuated backsliding

  d. Intergovernmental relations

- Which intergovernmental relations model may best represent authorities and systems for responding to a public health emergency such as an influenza pandemic?

  a. Coordinate-authority

  b. Overlapping-authority

  c. Inclusive-authority

  d. Exclusive-authority

3.2 Additional Context for Homeland Security

Chapter 1 and previous sections in this chapter provided both global and historical contexts for homeland security. This section provides an overview of additional context important for gaining an understanding of homeland security in the United States. This section and the next include information from the first edition in the original chapter as authored by Dr Amy Blizzard (Kilroy 2008).

3.2.1 Urban Versus Rural

Does place matter if protecting people and critical infrastructure is a core homeland security responsibility? The debate over the response to this question waged during the formative years of DHS, and it continues as DHS and states make decisions periodically regarding the allocation of federal grant funds. Urban areas are viewed, by many, as a priority for funding. In fact, 29 urban areas were the recipients of 2016 **Urban Area Security Initiative** (UASI) program funds totaling $580 million, which was approximately $180 million more than all of the states received, combined, through the State Homeland Security Program (US DHS 2016b, 31–32).

On one hand, more people live in major metropolitan areas and, thus, are vulnerable to homeland security threats and disaster events. According to the 2010 census, there are 486 urbanized areas, each with at least 50 000 people, which altogether accounted for 80.7% of the total population of the United States (US Census Bureau 2012). And growth of urban areas from 2000 to 2010 exceeded that of the entire country. Urban areas have concentrations of critical infrastructure, serve as hubs for transportation, and are considered the epicenters of economic growth and jobs across the country. Many cities such as Boston, New York City, Miami, and Los Angeles may be found in high-risk areas such as along coasts or near fault lines because of the favorable climate and availability of work in these regions. However, it also makes more people prone to hurricanes and earthquakes, for example (Figure 3-4).

On the other hand, a compelling case may also be made for investments in rural areas. Based on various government estimates, at least 75% of American land is considered nonmetropolitan or rural, including approximately two-thirds (2049) of all counties (Rural Policy Research Institute 2009; US Department of Agriculture 2016). The limited populations and tax bases often lead to shortcomings in terms of staffing, equipment, and other resources; some rural areas rely heavily on volunteers. Disaster response may be extremely challenging in rural and often remote areas that not only require traveling greater distances but also have the terrain that may consist of mountains, marshlands, and wilderness and be more difficult to traverse. Recovery in rural areas may be difficult as many areas rely on single economies. Moreover, the nation's agricultural resources and activities (e.g., supply chains and processing for animal and crop production) are highly concentrated in rural areas.

In response to these competing demands, DHS allocates funding to both states and urban areas to build capabilities across the spectrum of mission areas—prevention, protection, mitigation, response, and recovery. Furthermore, DHS and other federal departments and agencies responsible for providing grants to states

Figure 3-4

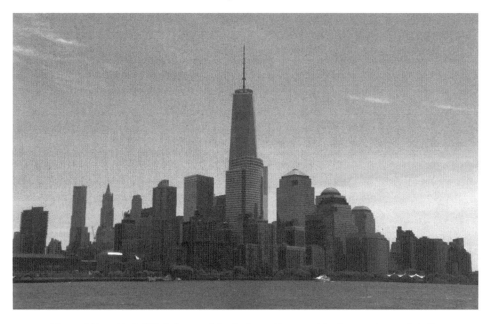

View of New York City's Lower Manhattan. Source: Photo courtesy of Jetta
Disco, DHS (2016).

and local communities have consistently used grants as financial incentives to
encourage regional approaches for a variety of reasons, such as to promote cost-
sharing and multijurisdictional planning and coordination (Foster 2006). For
example, DHS grant guidance for 2016 indicated that "Urban Areas must use UASI
funds to employ regional approaches to overall preparedness and are encouraged
to adopt regional response structures whenever appropriate" (US DHS 2016b, 45).
These approaches are viewed as one form of rescaling to address intergovernmental issues and problems presented in both urban and rural areas alike.

3.2.2 Technologies

The large-scale use of hazardous chemicals in production processes and the fact
that airplanes carry vast numbers of passengers each day are only two examples
of high-risk technologies that did not exist in prior centuries. Those on the front
line of homeland security must contend with cybersecurity such as attempted
intrusions into industrial control systems that operate and monitor critical infrastructure, biological agents found in research facilities such as anthrax, and
weaponry-like dirty bombs that can be relatively easy to make. It was well known
during the writing of the first *National Strategy for Homeland Security* (The White
House Office of Homeland Security 2002) that such technologies as information
networks enabled adversaries by providing them a platform to plan attacks, raise
funds, and spread propaganda, which continues today in the fight against adversaries like Islamic State in Iraq and Syria (IS). Technologies may also fail on
accident as was the case with the levees and flood wall system constructed in
New Orleans.

Effectively using innovation and technologies to achieve benefits, while at the same time denying and responding to those same advantages in the hands of ever-evolving and sophisticated adversaries, is an ongoing challenge for various stakeholders. Some common characteristics of newer technologies that benefit stakeholders include the following:

▲ **Enhanced awareness and intelligence:** Technologies now provide homeland security partners with enhanced situational awareness, as well as smart, intelligent systems made possible through advanced algorithms, pattern recognition software, and access to data.

▲ **Greater mobility:** Small, networked devices make it possible to monitor areas, vehicles, cargo, and so on for threats. Examples include cameras and sensors equipped to unmanned aerial surveillance (UAS) systems along the border.

▲ **Stronger predictions:** Many newer homeland security applications aim to prevent and mitigate threats and hazards by predicting their occurrence. Examples include systems that relate airline passenger information to watch lists and no-fly lists to alert authorities and modeling and simulation tools for predicting hurricanes and other natural hazards (Simpkins and Foster 2017).

3.2.3 Political and Economic Factors

Policymaking does not exist in a vacuum. Rather, government programs come to life through a policymaking process run by people. Policymakers are guided by a complex mix of values that sometimes guide decision makers and are categorized as organizational values, professional values, personal values, policy value, and ideological values (Anderson 2000, 135–137).

Organizational values involve the promotion of organizational and committee interests in the decision-making process. Professional values are professional commitments that guide decision making (e.g., first responders may tend to take a public safety perspective on issues). Personal values may involve personal ambitions, reputation, and self-interest. Policy values are those that guide decision making based on a perceived public interest or when acting in accord with beliefs about what is proper, ethical, or morally correct. Finally, ideological values legitimize actions on the basis of a political ideology or belief system. Decision makers and elected officials must balance all five categories of values during the policymaking process while setting goals for public laws and programs. This can be especially difficult when political factors enter into public debate over homeland security, especially when each person involved has a different opinion of what homeland security is and how government can best provide programs to protect society.

Likewise, the United States is a constitutional republic based on **representative democracy**, a system of government in which the ultimate political authority is vested in the people, who elect their governing officials to legislate on their behalf. Additionally, government embodies **pluralism** in that many groups or institutions share power in a complex system of interactions, which involves compromising and bargaining in the decision-making process. Under this system, majority rule must be balanced with protection of minority rights to create national policy (Plano and Greenberg 1985, 8–10). This can be difficult for policymakers, however, as the need to identify which groups are protected under homeland security policies can change from one administration to the next. Illegal immigrants, for example, may have the right to work legally and may be deported if discovered, but if an immigrant family is left homeless after a flood, will government agencies ignore their survival needs? Certainly not, but it leaves policymakers and implementers in the difficult position of trying to determine to whom homeland security applies.

FOR EXAMPLE

Immigration Policy Contentious Under President Trump

President Donald J. Trump signed two executive orders in 2017 soon after his inauguration to restrict entry into the United States and strengthen the screening procedures of individuals from select countries associated with terrorist organizations. Signed on March 6, 2017, Executive Order 13780 titled "Protecting The Nation From Foreign Terrorist Entry Into The United States" superseded a previous order that was blocked by the courts.

The order places restrictions on the issuance of visas and suspensions for 90 days on the entry of foreign nationals from three countries deemed state sponsors of terrorism—Iran, Sudan, and Syria—as well as Libya, Somalia, and Yemen. It also places a cap of 50 000 refugees entering the county via the US Refugee Admissions Program (USRAP) in 2017, as well as other provisions. In light of recent terrorist attacks in Europe and the United States, the order aims to strength the vetting and identification of individuals who "may commit, aid, or support acts of terrorism" (The White House 2017).

As of the writing of this chapter, the order was blocked by a federal judge, and this decision was affirmed by the 4th Circuit Court of Appeals on the grounds of religious freedom and tolerance; all of the countries noted in the ban are predominantly Muslim (de Vogue and Jarrett 2017).

Policymaking as it relates to homeland security is particularly challenging because of limited resources, and fears about infringing on individual liberties and the markets. While homeland security has direct benefits, it can also take away from spending for other programs that benefit public safety, such as cleaner water or safer highways. How much should be spent at the national level on low probability but high consequence and cost hazards and threats? Donald Kettl (2014) notes that homeland security is different from other government programs because there is a zero tolerance for mistakes (99). Trying to achieve perfection when conducting risk analysis and calculating trade-offs in spending, both inherently subjective processes, likely results in over-investments in some areas of security and under-investments in others. These questions regarding risks and investments confound the policymaking process.

With regard to the markets, the United States is considered a political economy—the political system is inherently linked to the economy. In other words, community stability depends in large part on economic stability. Market failures commonly lead to government intervention and programming, the provision of public goods and services; the transition of the airline's private security screeners to the Transportation Security Administration (TSA) in 2001 is an example of this phenomenon. As in other policy areas, economic factors influence homeland security policymaking and decision making.

Businesses depend on a steady cash flow, which can be disrupted if the business is forced to close by security threats. Even if the threat is short term, businesses may have difficulty remaining viable. Long-term events, like a hurricane, may force businesses to relocate to unknown markets out of their communities. In addition, marginal businesses may not be able to survive perceived threats in their communities. The ripple effect of such difficulties will be felt throughout the community in the form of short-term and long-term unemployment and inconveniences to residents who must find needed goods and services elsewhere. In addition, when their business districts are damaged by man-made or natural disasters, communities also face a host of other long-term problems, including the following:

▲ Loss of property and sales tax revenues
▲ Threats to long-term business district viability
▲ The potential loss of important businesses
▲ The need to continue to find a way to attract a client and customer base
▲ The need to undertake complex reconstruction and redevelopment projects (Waugh 2000, 6–13)

Reducing economic losses following disasters is one aim of hazard mitigation. At the local scale, building economic resiliency requires pre-disaster planning and community engagement. For example, community plans should account for major employers, interdependent industry sectors, and commercial centers or hubs and relationships between those assets and networks and supporting infrastructure. The Pacific NorthWest Economic Region (PNWER) is cited by DHS as a national model for economic resiliency (US DHS 2016c). PNWER consists of public and private sector stakeholders from US states and Canadian provinces in the Pacific northwest region who remain involved in numerous border security and disaster resiliency initiatives (e.g., planning, disaster exercises, working groups) at the regional level. They do so recognizing that agglomeration of industries and economic networks extend well beyond the political boundaries of states and follow patterns more akin to watersheds (Figure 3-5).

3.2.4 Security Versus Civil Liberties

In addition to political and economic considerations, legal context is important for gaining an understanding of homeland security. Of particular interest to the public since the 2001, terrorist attacks have been the balance between security and privacy and infringements on individual liberties as guaranteed by the US Constitution.

Figure 3-5

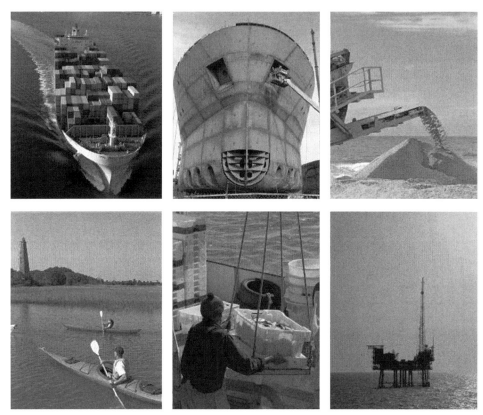

Coastal area regional economies (US Department of Commerce 2017).

Limits to personal freedoms are not a new debate. The Alien and Sedition Act of 1798 was the first law passed to limit speech that was deemed hurtful to the newly established American government. Though this was a temporary law, expiring 10 years after its passage, it sets a precedent for legal limits to personal freedoms when a national threat is perceived by government officials. Less than a century later, during the Civil War, Abraham Lincoln suspended the **writ of habeas corpus**, the constitutional guarantee that accused persons would be brought before a judge and hear the charges against them. The Supreme Court overturned Lincoln's actions, saying he had overextended his presidential powers, but by World War I, national security was once again an issue.

Thus, in 1918, Congress passed the Sedition Act. This act amended the 1917 Espionage Act and banned any language found to be "disloyal, profane, scurrilous, or abusive … and intended to cause contempt, scorn, contumely, or disrepute to the government." While many portions of the Espionage Act were repealed in 1921, major sections of that act remained part of US law, including limits to unprotected speech (see Schenck v. United States 1919). Once again, America's perceived security threat diminished somewhat, so the Supreme Court relaxed some portions of laws designed to limit personal freedoms, like the 1918 Sedition Act, but this legal stance would change again with America's entry into World War II. In 1942, for instance, the federal government authorized the forced detention of many Japanese Americans in internment camps to restrict perceived threats to national security (Dye 2005, 328; also, see Section 1.1, for additional information on Japanese internment camps).

Throughout American history, the Supreme Court has upheld limits to personal freedoms like these previous examples. Much of the debate surrounding homeland security and civil liberties stems from the passage of the Uniting and Strengthening America by Providing Appropriate Tools Required to Intercept and Obstruct Terrorism Act (USA PATRIOT Act) of 2001, which was passed to provide law enforcement agencies with greater flexibility in collecting intelligence, pursuing threats, and interrupting terrorist financing, among other provisions.

Much of the criticism against the act was directed at the provisions for surveillance and the delayed notification of a search or what many call "sneak-and-peek" searches. A **sneak-and-peak search** is a special search warrant that allows law enforcement officers to lawfully enter areas in which a reasonable expectation of privacy exists, to search for items of evidence or contraband, and to leave without making any seizures or giving concurrent notice of the search. Law enforcement has used sneak-and-peek searches for investigations involving contraband material like drugs or weapons, but the USA PATRIOT Act extends this authority to investigations involving terrorist suspects.

After passage of the USA PATRIOT Act, DHS established the Office for Civil Rights and Civil Liberties in 2003. This agency is charged with providing legal and policy advice to DHS' leadership on a wide range of civil rights and civil liberties issues.

Provisions of the USA PATRIOT Act were reauthorized in 2005, 2006, and 2011. Public outcry over the extended powers of law enforcement led to revisions in sneak-and-peak rules during the 2005 reauthorization process. Many provisions were due to expire in June 2015. As a result, Congress passed and the president signed the Uniting and Strengthening America by Fulfilling Rights and Ensuring Effective Discipline Over Monitoring Act (USA FREEDOM Act) of 2015, which continued some provisions but rescinded others such as the collection of telecommunications metadata by intelligence agencies.

Americans value their personal freedoms, and society's basic foundations include civil liberties and rights established in the US Constitution. Even though protecting the nation from threats at the expense of personal freedoms is not a new debate, the general public's views on matters of homeland security sometimes dramatically differ. This can affect politics and program implementation. Homeland security presents a new challenge to protecting personal liberties, evidenced in the debate over the USA PATRIOT Act, and many legal questions remain unanswered. The American public must continue to debate the trade-offs between personal freedoms and homeland security as federal policies and programs continue to evolve.

3.3 Homeland Security Enterprise

The policies, programs, and responsibilities for homeland security go well beyond those of a single department, most notably DHS. From the perspective of terrorism prevention, for example, only 2 of 16 members of the intelligence community—the US Coast Guard and Office of Intelligence and Analysis—reside within DHS (Office of the Director of National Intelligence, n.d.). The US Department of Defense (DoD) occupies a much greater share of intelligence capabilities used to promote national security, and the FBI and Drug Enforcement Administration (DEA) operate domestically and share in the counterterrorism mission.

In response, DHS conceived the **homeland security enterprise** concept in 2010, which consists of "the collective efforts and shared responsibilities of Federal, State, local, tribal, territorial, nongovernmental, and private sector partners—as well as individuals, families, and communities—to maintain critical homeland security capabilities" (US DHS 2010, 12). Therefore, the missions and responsibilities for homeland security are shared among both governmental and nongovernmental partners. A brief overview of select partners responsible for leading and coordinating homeland security functions are provided in the following sections.

3.3.1 Federal Partners

Bureaucracies exist at all levels of government. At the federal level, the **bureaucracy** is the sum of all departments, agencies, and offices that implement laws under the authority of the president. By definition, bureaucracies are hierarchical organizations that are highly specialized, and they operate with very formal rules (Plano and Greenberg 1985). While all departments in the federal government make up the bureaucracy, some are more involved in homeland security than others.

In 2002, 22 existing agencies were combined with new agencies to form the **Department of Homeland Security (DHS)**. The primary mission of DHS is the following: "With honor and integrity, we will safeguard the American people, our homeland, and our values" (US DHS 2016d). The supporting missions include the following:

▲ Preventing terrorism and enhancing security
▲ Securing and managing the borders
▲ Enforcing and administering the immigration laws
▲ Safeguarding and securing cyberspace
▲ Ensuring resilience to disasters (US DHS 2016d)

The supporting missions generally reflect the roles and responsibilities of the seven primary operational components of the department. It's important to comprehend the general function of these components for noting, first, how they relate to the aforementioned supporting missions and, second, what functions may be missing from DHS and coordinated by external partners.

The first agency is the **Transportation Security Administration (TSA)**, which may be the most visible to the public. Screening was largely conducted by contractors hired by the airlines before 2001. The TSA includes the Federal Air Marshal Service, and a large workforce of passenger and cargo screeners found at both commercial and private airports nationwide.

Coastal waters and inland waterways are protected by the **US Coast Guard**. In addition to serving as the lead federal agency for maritime safety and security, it has the authority to respond to oil and hazardous material spills in coordination with EPA. It also happens to be the only military organization in the United States that also has authority for enforcing laws (Figure 3-6).

Often working in close coordination with the US Coast Guard near seaports where containers and ship passengers require screening is the **US Customs and Border Protection (CBP)**. CBP is responsible for controlling all of America's land and maritime borders and ensuring that all persons and cargo entering the United States do so both legally and safely. CBP has the largest budget and workforce in DHS with about 60 000 uniformed and specialty personnel; the Border Patrol accounts for about one-third of the workforce.

Functions performed by the following two agencies were conducted by the former Immigration and Naturalization Service (INS) within the US Department of Justice: **Immigration and Customs Enforcement (ICE)** and the **US Citizenship and Immigration Services (USCIS)**. ICE is the primary law enforcement and investigative arm of DHS, which consists of agents and investigators who identify, apprehend, detain, and remove/deport criminal and other illegal aliens from the

Figure 3-6

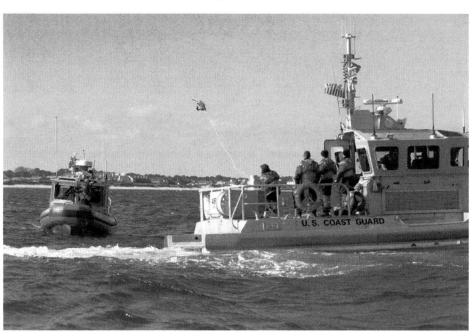

US Coast Guard response training (US Department of Homeland Security 2012).

United States. The USCIS is responsible for immigration services—facilitating legal immigration for people seeking to enter, reside, or work in the United States.

The **US Secret Service** continues to protect dignitaries and National Special Security Events (NSSEs), as well as the nation's financial infrastructure by reducing losses due to counterfeit currency, financial and electronic crimes, and identity theft.

Finally, the **Federal Emergency Management Agency (FEMA)** is responsible for coordinating the federal response and recovery efforts in support of affected states and jurisdictions included in presidentially declared disasters, among others. The 15 FEMA regional offices work closely with states on a range of preparedness, mitigation, response, and recovery initiatives for all hazards, including preparedness grants.

FOR EXAMPLE

A Glance at a Complex Security Arrangement: The Port of Los Angeles

Protecting seaports in the United States from a variety of evolving threats is a national security priority. In fact, Congress has appropriated $100 million or more for enhancing port security each year for the past 15 years.

Seaports are a critical node for transporting commercial goods and supplies. They also support the cruise ship industry, which generates a variety of business and jobs both locally and throughout the country. Both cargo and cruise ship terminals present a variety of security challenges for public and private officials by requiring unique partnerships, among other factors.

First, governance at commercial ports is provided by a variety of state and local public agencies, including port authorities, port navigation districts, or municipal port departments. The Port of Los Angeles, for example, is an example of a landlord port and operates under the direction of the City of Los Angeles. California grants local jurisdictions authority over port management and operations, which was authorized by the California Tidelands Trust Act of 1929. The port is a self-supporting department of the City of Los Angeles, California, governed by a five-member Board of Harbor Commissioners appointed by the mayor.

Second, security on the port is a shared responsibility. All companies and industries that operate terminals through a lease agreement with the port are responsible for providing security (e.g., video surveillance, access control) on their respective berths. The port police work closely with private security hired by terminal operators and protect port territory not leased to those operators.

The port police represent the local level and have authority to investigate suspicious activities and criminal actions, apprehend suspects and make arrests, conduct drug enforcement, and oversee traffic safety. The California Highway Patrol, the primary state police agency, has authority to enforce highway safety and criminal laws on and within visual sight of the interstate highways that pass through the port.

Federal security and law enforcement is largely provided at the port through three DHS agencies. The US Coast Guard is primarily responsible for safety, security, and law enforcement on the waters surrounding the ports. Additionally, it oversees the terminal operators' compliance with the Maritime Transportation Security Act of 2002 requiring review of detailed security plans and procedures as well as Coast Guard facility security regulation 33 CFR 105 (Maritime Security: Facilities). Other key federal law enforcement partners include CBP, which is responsible for screening containers entering into the port, and ICE, which enforces immigration and customs laws.

The complex security and law enforcement arrangements require close coordination among the disparate law enforcement agencies at the local, state, and federal levels of government. To this end, stakeholders at the port use the Area Maritime Security Committee (AMSC) structure as one vehicle for building consensus on the port's security-related goals and the means to achieve those goals; the MSC is comprised of a mix of law enforcement and private security stakeholders from the Port of Los Angeles (Curry and Spaulding 2006). One recent MSC product was the development of an area maritime security plan, which aims to address safety and security concerns at the Ports of Los Angeles and Long Beach (Curry and Spaulding 2006). Homeland security officials at the port ensure that their individual plans and projects such as the cargo screening system are consistent with the MSC's security initiatives.

As illustrated using the Port of Los Angeles example, seaports represent interesting cases of diverse homeland security enterprise partners working in close proximity and coordinating together toward meeting shared goals (Figure 3-7).

Figure 3-7

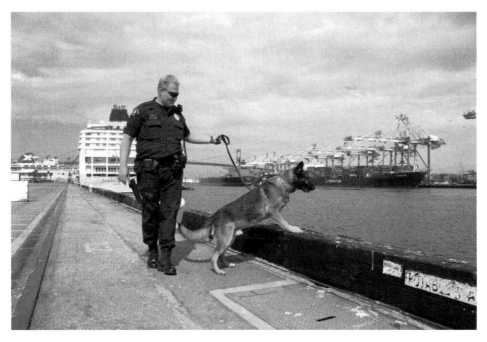

Security at the Port of Los Angeles (Port of Los Angeles 2017).

A significant number of homeland security functions are performed or coordinated by other federal departments and agencies; the following provides some examples:

▲ **Environmental Protection Agency:** Responds to spills and concerned with emergencies involving the release of oil, radioactive materials, or hazardous chemicals.

▲ **US Department of Agriculture:** Ensures the safety and security of the nation's food supply; the US Forest Service is the primary federal agency for Emergency Support Function (ESF) 4—Firefighting.

▲ **US Department of Commerce:** Responsible for regulating the export of sensitive goods and technologies and enforcing export control laws; monitors meteorological conditions, makes forecasts about storm risks, and recommends preparedness measures.

▲ **US Department of Health and Human Services:** Primary agency for Emergency Support Function 8—Public Health and Medical Services—and coordinating the federal response to potential health and medical emergencies.

▲ **US Department of Housing and Urban Development:** Primary agency for Emergency Support Function 14—Long-Term Community Recovery.

▲ **US Department of Interior:** Develops policies and procedures for all types of hazards and emergencies that impact federal lands, facilities, infrastructure, and resources.

▲ **US Department of Justice:** Responsible for criminal investigations of terrorist acts or terrorist threats by individuals or groups inside the United States.

As previously noted, the DoD works closely with DHS and other members of the intelligence community and contributes to homeland security through military missions overseas and homeland defense. In extraordinary circumstances, the DoD can conduct military missions such as combat air patrols or maritime defense operations. In fact, after September 11, 2001, a new combatant command, US Northern Command, was established specifically to coordinate military support for homeland security missions. Through US Northern Command, the DoD can, when necessary, take the lead in defending the people and territory of the country, with support from other agencies. In addition, the president can order the DoD to respond to domestic catastrophes such floods, tornadoes, and hurricanes. In these circumstances, the department may be asked to act quickly to provide capabilities that other agencies do not have.

A segue into the next section on state and local partners, the National Guard is commonly used by state governors to support civilian authorities; state governors have the authority to activate and deploy units in response to disasters or for any reason under the command of the states' adjutants general. On occasion, the federal government will approve activation under Title 32 of the United States Code, which keeps units under the control of state governors, but they are paid by the federal government. This was largely the case during the response to Hurricane Katrina. The Posse Comitatus Act of 1878 was passed to prevent the military from performing domestic law enforcement functions. However, this act doesn't apply unless the units are activated under Title 10, which commonly occurs when guard units are "federalized" for overseas missions, and it never applies to the US Coast Guard (Tussing 2012, 150–151) (Figure 3-8).

The number of Army and Air National Guard personnel fluctuates based on a number of factors; however, there are approximately 3200 units nationwide (Tussing 2012, 134). And they are often the first choice when in need of personnel and equipment (e.g., communications, air assets, transport vehicles). In addition, the National Guard has access to many specialized resources such as personal protective equipment and decontamination units for responding to chemical, biological, radiological, nuclear, and explosive (CBRNE) incidents, as well as about

Figure 3-8

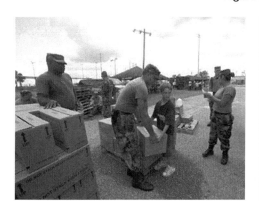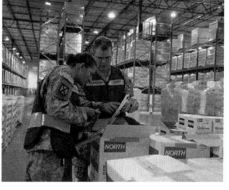

Florida Army National Guard logistical support. Source: Photos courtesy of Andrea Booher, FEMA (2005); Barry Bahler, FEMA (2008).

57 weapons of mass destruction (WMD) civil support teams (CSTs) located across the country (Tussing 2012, 152).

3.3.2 State and Local Partners

Adding to the horizontal fragmentation of the US government is the vertical division of power characteristic of the nation's **federal system**, in which the national government shares sovereignty with state and local governments as previously noted. Overall, state, county, municipal, and local governments fund and operate the emergency services that would respond in the event of a disaster. The federal government comes to the assistance of a state government when it is overwhelmed by, or incapable of addressing, a disaster. The governor asks for assistance, and a presidential disaster declaration is either granted or rejected (McEntire 2015).

When policymaking becomes fragmented between national, state, and local governments, it leads to difficulties in determining which level of government is actually in charge of homeland security functions. A compelling case may be made for states as critical partners and leaders, within the governmental framework of homeland security nationwide. States serve as linchpins between the federal government and the approximately 3141 counties and 36 000 sub-county general-purpose governments within the states and provide training and technical assistance in various professions relating to homeland security and many other services.

Consider law enforcement personnel, for example, as an indicator of resources available in the country to support terrorism prevention. According to the Bureau of Justice Statistics, there were roughly 765 000 full-time, sworn state and local law enforcement personnel in 2008, including approximately 61 000 officers employed by general-purpose state law enforcement agencies (Reaves 2011, 1–2). By comparison, the top four federal agencies with equivalent arrest and firearm authority included the CBP with 36 863, Federal Bureau of Prisons with 16 835, FBI with 12 760, and ICE with 12 446 personnel (Reaves 2012, 2). Of course state and local law enforcement perform many duties; however, the numbers cannot be overlooked.

Evidence suggests that states have experienced a significant increase in terrorism-related responsibilities following the 2001 terrorist attacks. For example, in one national survey, 75% of state law enforcement agencies reported a substantial amount of involvement in or served as their state's leader for gathering, analyzing, and sharing terrorism-related intelligence (Foster and Cordner 2005, 25).

How do state homeland security priorities compare with those of the federal government? The National Homeland Security Consortium, a group of 22 national associations that represent local, state, and private sector professionals, identified the following issues of greatest concern to them in 2016: cybersecurity, critical infrastructure fragility natural threats including climate adaptation and infectious disease, countering terrorism, and immigration reform (National Homeland Security Consortium 2016). The state of New York released a homeland security strategy for the 2014–2016 time period, which identified the following 10 goals:

▲ Strengthen CBRNE preparedness and response capabilities
▲ Protect critical infrastructure and key resources
▲ Strengthen intelligence and information sharing capabilities
▲ Strengthen counterterrorism and law enforcement capabilities

▲ Enhance emergency management and response capabilities

▲ Advance interoperable and emergency communications

▲ Promote citizen and community preparedness

▲ Build back better from disasters and become more resilient against future events

▲ Support health emergency preparedness

▲ Enhance cybersecurity capabilities (New York State Division of Homeland Security and Emergency Services 2014)

There are not only some similarities between these goals and those of DHS as noted previously, but also differences in focus (e.g., immigration vs. interoperable communications). This demonstrates the importance of perspective and context in homeland security.

Every state and many cities and counties are addressing homeland security issues either through an existing office or a newly created office. Table 3-1 shows a breakdown of state homeland security advisors and the organization that handles the day-to-day operations.

In 19 states, homeland security is operated within a combined emergency management and homeland security office, and in most of those states the designated homeland security advisor is responsible for both emergency management and homeland security. The remaining states operate homeland security from within a public safety or military affairs department or the governor's office. Interestingly, about one-third of states rely entirely on federal grants to fund their homeland security offices, and more than two-thirds receive at least 60% of their funding from the federal government (Bell 2016, 462). What does this information mean for homeland security at the state level? Quite possibly, many states may be overly dependent on federal grants to support their operations and, likewise, more influenced by the federal government than others. It may also reflect a breakdown of states that created new offices after 2001 using federal funds and those that integrated the management and coordination functions into other existing organizations such as the state police, military division, or emergency management department.

While homeland security issues can present unanticipated demands on each level and branch of government, the federal system also provides the capacity to improvise as conditions warrant. Each level of government can coordinate with other levels to minimize redundancies in homeland security actions and ensure integration of efforts. The federal government can use knowledge from states and communities to prioritize programs and address unique regional needs.

3.3.3 Whole Community Partners

In 2011, FEMA released the "**whole community**" doctrine, which is akin to the concept of the homeland security enterprise. This doctrine is based on the assumption that government-centric approaches to disaster management are insufficient in meeting all of the needs of communities impacted by disasters. According to the doctrine, this approach "include(s) a more informed, shared understanding of community risks, needs, and capabilities; an increase in resources through the

Table 3-1: State Homeland Security Structures

State	Designated homeland security advisor	Homeland security organizations
Alabama	Public safety secretary/commissioner	Public safety
Alaska	Dual title—EM/homeland security director combined EM/homeland security office	
Arizona	Homeland security director	Homeland security (stand-alone office)
Arkansas	Dual title—EM/homeland security director	Combined EM/homeland Security office
California	Dual title—EM/homeland security director	Combined EM/homeland security office
Colorado	Dual title—EM/homeland security director	Public safety
Connecticut	Deputy commissioner	Combined EM/homeland security office
Delaware	Homeland security advisor	Public safety
Florida	Florida Department of Law Enforcement commissioner	Florida Department of Law Enforcement
Georgia	Dual title—EM/homeland security director	Governor's office
Hawaii	Adjutant general	Adjutant general/military affairs
Idaho	Dual title—EM/homeland security director	Adjutant general/military affairs
Illinois	Public safety secretary/commissioner	Governor's office
Indiana	Dual title—EM/homeland security director	Combined EM/homeland security office
Iowa	Dual title—EM/homeland security director	Combined EM/homeland security office
Kansas	Adjutant general	Adjutant general/military affairs
Kentucky	Homeland security director	Governor's office

Table 3-1: (Continued)

State	Designated homeland security advisor	Homeland security organizations
Louisiana	Dual title—EM/homeland security director	Combined EM/homeland security office
Maine	Adjutant general	Combined EM/homeland security office
Maryland	Homeland security director	Governor's office
Massachusetts	Homeland security director	Public safety
Michigan	State police superintendent/director commissioner	State police
Minnesota	Public safety secretary/commissioner	Public safety
Mississippi	Homeland security director	Public safety
Missouri	Public safety secretary/commissioner	Public safety
Montana	Adjutant general	Adjutant general/military affairs
Nebraska	Lieutenant governor	Combined EM/homeland security office
Nevada	Dual title—EM/homeland security director	Combined EM/homeland security office
New Hampshire	Dual title—EM/homeland security director	Public safety
New Jersey	Homeland security director	Homeland security (stand-alone office)
New Mexico	Dual title—EM/homeland security director combined EM/homeland security office	
New York	Division of homeland security and emergency services commissioner	Combined EM/homeland security office
North Carolina	Public safety secretary/commissioner	Public safety
North Dakota	Homeland security director	Adjutant general/military affairs
Ohio	Public safety secretary/commissioner	Public safety

(Continued)

Table 3-1: (Continued)

State	Designated homeland security advisor	Homeland security organizations
Oklahoma	Homeland security director	Homeland security (stand-alone office)
Oregon	Adjutant general	Adjutant general/military affairs
Pennsylvania	Homeland security director	Governor's office
Rhode Island	State police superintendent/director/commissioner	Public safety
South Carolina	State police superintendent/director/commissioner	State police
South Dakota	Homeland security director	Public safety
Tennessee	Homeland security director	Public safety
Texas	State police superintendent/director/commissioner	Public safety
Utah	Public safety secretary/commissioner	Public safety
Vermont	State police superintendent/director/commissioner	Combined EM/homeland security office
Virginia	Public safety secretary/commissioner	Combined EM/homeland security office
Washington	Adjutant general	Combined EM/homeland security office
West Virginia	Dual title—EM/homeland security director	Combined EM/homeland security office
Wisconsin	Adjutant general	Adjutant general/military affairs
Wyoming	Dual title—EM/homeland security director	Governor's office
District of Columbia	Dual title—EM/homeland security director combined EM/homeland security office	
Guam	Homeland security director	Combined EM/homeland security office
US Virgin Islands	Dual title—EM/homeland security director	Combined EM/homeland security office

Source: Data provided by NEMA, April 2016 cited in Bell (2016).

empowerment of community members; and, in the end, more resilient communities" (FEMA 2011, 4).

This may be viewed as a significant paradigm shift in thinking about prevention, protection, mitigation, response, and recovery. In other words, first responders and emergency managers should value coordination and collaborative problem solving with a broad range of community groups and the public. Doing so may be difficult for those accustomed to top-down command and control management and decision-making models; it may run counter to existing organizational cultures. Ronald Reagan is quoted as saying that "[t]he greatest leader is not necessarily the one who does the greatest things. He is the one who gets the people to do greatest things" (McDermott 2004). Applied to the whole community concept, a successful response operation and recovery process may be defined by how well community groups and survivors care for themselves following a disaster. As such, it requires that citizens be viewed as survivors, and not victims solely reliant on government support.

San Francisco's SF72 public education campaign may be viewed as an attempt to embrace the whole community concept (San Francisco Department of Emergency Management, n.d.). Seventy-two hours or 3 days is a ballpark planning assumption for states and communities susceptible to earthquakes. People may need to fend for themselves or each other for at least 72h following a large-scale earthquake until government resources in the form of urban search and rescue, fire departments, and so on may locate and rescue them. Therefore, preparedness success may be defined in terms of the capabilities of citizens and less about the capabilities of the government agencies.

Historically important and embraced by the whole community concept are the roles of **nongovernmental organizations (NGOs)**. Technically, NGOs provide a service to a community free of charge or for a minimal cost that is required to defray the cost of the service(s) furnished. NGOs usually hold the special nonprofit federal tax exempt status—(501)(c)(3)—and financial support for voluntary agencies is generally through donations, contracts, and grants. NGOs include community service groups, church groups, and national nonprofit agencies, and they supply a range of basic necessities such as clothing, food, and household items, conduct home repairs and construct new homes, and provide for the emotional and spiritual needs of disaster survivors, for example (Phillips 2016, 220–227). Beyond the well-known disaster relief organizations such as the American Red Cross and Salvation Army, more specialized groups stand ready to assist communities following disasters. Communities in need of animal rescue and care, for example, may rely on volunteers organized by the Humane Society of the United States, the National Audubon Society, and the Association of Zoos and Aquariums (Figure 3-9).

NGOs can be important aids to state and local governments in meeting the unmet needs of survivors and very effective at communicating preparedness messages to target audiences (e.g., seniors, non-English speaking residents) before disasters occur.

In America, the private, for-profit sector provides most goods and services and owns the vast majority of America's critical infrastructure. Airlines, utilities, and agriculture production are just a few of the infrastructure and resources that are privately owned. The private sector also includes many academic, scientific,

Figure 3-9

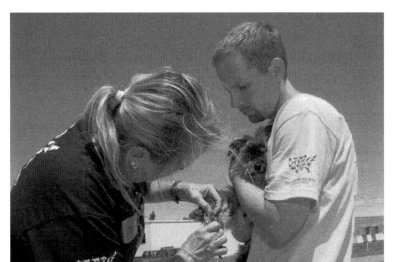

Humane Society caring for pets following disaster. Source: Photo courtesy of Patsy Lynch, FEMA (2011).

medical, engineering, and technological research facilities and institutions whose work contributes to the well-being of society as a whole. Businesses and industries have had a long relationship with the government, as both contractors for government projects and innovators whose products help government implement programs. For example, private information technology firms such as AT&T now have entire divisions dedicated to developing homeland security initiatives, and they have worked with intelligence agencies to find new ways to monitor illegal activities in publicly accessible technologies like the **Internet**.

In terms of disaster response and recovery, businesses and corporations fulfill critical roles. For example, the media disseminates alerts and warnings to the public. Hotels and motels provide temporary sheltering to displaced residents following hurricanes. Restaurants and retail establishments, which include both big "box" stores and small businesses, commonly donate needed items. Many ambulatory companies, hospitals, and healthcare organizations are privately owned and managed; they provide patient transportation and critical medical treatment. These are just a few examples of private sector partners, some literally on the front lines of disaster response and recovery.

Finally, many efforts aim to engage citizens as participants in homeland security. For example, the Citizen Corps began in January 2002 to encourage and enlist citizens across the country. The members of the Citizen Corps receive special training from the FEMA's Community Emergency Response Program to support first responders by providing immediate help to victims and by organizing volunteers at disaster sites. Citizen Corps also works with the national Neighborhood Watch Program to incorporate terrorism prevention and education into its existing crime prevention mission. It additionally includes the Volunteers in Police Service, civilian volunteers trained to support police departments, and the Medical Reserve Corps, civilian volunteers who can assist healthcare professionals during a large-scale local emergency.

Finally, DHS implemented the "If You See Something, Say Something" campaign in 2010 to "raise public awareness of the indicators of terrorism and terrorism-related crime, as well as the importance of reporting suspicious activity to state and local law enforcement" (DHS n.d.). This program relies on community-level partners such as the media and businesses to distribute information to the public about reporting suspicious activities, such as unusual items or situations.

As homeland security matures in American society, it is becoming more evident that it requires an enterprise-wide and whole community approach. The American political and social system requires coordination and cooperation between and among various levels of government, as well as among branches of government and the public as a whole, to meet the challenge of protecting citizens.

SELF-CHECK

- Define the homeland security enterprise.
- Which organization is the only military organization that also has authority for enforcing domestic laws without requiring special authority from the president or Congress?
  - a. Federal Bureau of Investigation
  - b. US Immigration and Customs Enforcement
  - c. US Coast Guard
  - d. US Northern Command
- In response to disasters, the activation of National Guard units by state governors is often preferred for the following reasons:
  - a. They have a siagnificant quantity of resources.
  - b. They are familiar with impacted areas.
  - c. They provide specialized resources such as communications equipment.
  - d. All of the above.
- Define nongovernmental organization and provide an example of one such organization with a role in homeland security.

3.4 Revisiting the All-Hazards Approach

What is the value of the all-hazards approach to homeland security from the perspective of the profession and disciplines that support homeland security? DHS clearly values the idea of all hazards as it provides flexibility to modify priorities based on changing political priorities and assessments of risks. Of course not all hazards and threats are priorities for resources, but rather those assessed as high risks, which may vary from jurisdiction to jurisdiction.

The vagueness of the approach may be viewed as a limitation. For example, ever-changing priorities influenced by elected and appointed officials and the interests of chief executives make it difficult, if not impossible, to plan long term to address problems in a strategic planning manner. Likewise, measuring progress toward meeting long-term goals is challenging when goals are constantly changed or updated. In his book titled *Managing the Climate Crisis*, Dr Robert Schneider (2016) explains why focusing on long-term problems and priorities is so problematic in today's culture of pathological shortsightedness. True for both politicians and the general public, the term temporal distortion phenomenon essentially describes how society is more focused on the current situation and what he calls the "crisis du jour"—the proverbial weather outside the window this morning—than future impacts (Schneider 2016, 94–95). The same phenomenon may partly explain why support for a range of hazard mitigation projects that only pay off in the long term is difficult to acquire.

State and local jurisdictions may have similar shortsightedness and often adjust their own strategic planning to conform to guidelines and requirements for federal grants. However, DHS' requirement that State Homeland Security Program (SHSP) and UASI funds be allocated to support individual state and urban area. Threat and Hazards Identification and Risk Assessments (THIRAs) is a policy that promotes the all-hazards approach (see Chapter 4).

On the positive end, all-hazards approaches to the preparedness function have many benefits. For example, operational communications was problematic in response to both the 2001 terrorist attacks and Hurricane Katrina. The 9/11 Commission found that "[t]he inability to communicate was a critical element at the World Trade Center, Pentagon, and Somerset County, Pennsylvania, crash sites, where multiple agencies and multiple jurisdictions responded" (National Commission on Terrorist Attacks Upon the United States 2004, 397). Likewise, Hurricane Katrina resulted in the destruction or degradation of 3 million landlines, 2000 cell towers, more than 30 Public Service Answering Points (PSAPs), 37 of 41 broadcast radio stations, and first responder land mobile radio service across the region. In fact, the New Orleans Police Department and the Mississippi National Guard were unable to establish effective communications for several days (Miller 2006; Select Bipartisan Committee to Investigate the Preparation for and Response to Hurricane Katrina 2006). Justifying the design and procurement of a costly Next Generation 9-1-1 system, interoperable land mobile radios, or a wireless network to support all-hazards response is prudent, especially in an era of scarce resources. Context is important when applying the all-hazards concept.

An approach akin to all hazards, but more applicable to acts of terrorism and other intentional acts, is the **all-crimes** approach—the model of fully integrating terrorism into other crime prevention duties. A working group sponsored by the US Department of Justice in 2005 found both benefits and challenges to this approach, especially for state and local law enforcement agencies. Of particular importance with regard to the "all-crimes" approach is the manner in which intelligence fusion centers at the state and local levels are organized and structured and the focus of intelligence analysts operating both within and external to those centers. Conceptually, the all-crimes concept and debate may be more appropriate for those solely focused on terrorism, the first of Bellavita's (2008) homeland security "ideal types."

DHS has generally adopted the all-hazards approach, but with some caveats. For example, the mission areas used to organized capabilities deemed important to the nation include prevention, protection, mitigation, response, and recovery (US

FOR EXAMPLE

The Criminal Justice System and All-Crimes Approach

State police have many competing public safety and law enforcement priorities today. As is often the case when new crimes surface, these agencies encountered challenges after the 2001 terrorist attacks with incorporating new terrorism-related demands into the existing crime-fighting framework. To this end, two views or approaches surfaced in the years following the attacks—dedicating personnel for terrorism-related duties or fully integrating terrorism into other crime prevention duties—the all-crimes approach.

The dedicated-personnel model is partly predicated on the assumption that terrorists and terrorist-related activities are not closely linked to other more traditional criminal activities such as financial crimes and drug smuggling. Proponents argue that the requirements for fighting terrorism are unlike those for dealing with other crimes. Advocates of this model also argue for a separate, specialized approach because the risks and stakes associated with terrorism are extremely high, and this approach prevents "mission creep" into other law enforcement priorities. This is a valid concern, especially given how agencies today measure performance through quantitative factors such as number of arrests and prosecutions. Unlike other crimes, three years could pass before one state-level arrest is made related to terrorism.

Other experts believe that a nexus does exist among types of criminal activity, including illegal drug operations, money laundering, fraud, identity theft, and terrorism. It is well known that some of the September 11 terrorists were cited for traffic violations prior to the attacks, while others obtained and used fraudulent driver's licenses. Proponents of this model conclude there is a high probability of identifying terrorists through their involvement in precursor or lower-level criminal activity, as was possible with the September 11 terrorists. Likewise, they argue that states should embrace an "all-crimes" approach to terrorism prevention. This strategy ensures that possible precursor crimes are screened and analyzed for linkages to larger-scale terrorist activities. Emergency management professionals use a similar approach, known as all hazards, for emergency response and preparedness (Foster and Cordner 2005, 34–35).

DHS 2015). The flow or logic of these areas is consistent with the traditional phases of emergency management. After identifying a high-risk hazard or threat, actions should be taken to prevent incidents involving those hazards and threats, protecting people, critical infrastructure, and the environment. When impossible to prevent, then the impacts of those hazards and threats should be mitigated. Finally, preparations for response and recovery should take place in case those hazards and threats result in a disaster.

According to the National Preparedness Goal, capabilities organized under prevention mission areas are solely focused on acts of terrorism, so preventing acts of terrorism remains a national priority. On the other hand, mitigation, by tradition and related policies as previously noted, is focused on natural hazards. The all-hazards approach is most broadly applicable to the protection, response, and recovery mission areas. Success of both the all-hazards and all-crimes approaches may, ultimately, depend on their applications in practice and the policies and procedures that govern their applications. For example, the all-hazards approach may be deemed favorable when applied systematically within a risk analysis framework, the topic of another chapter.

In summary, there is evidence to support each of Bellavita's (2008) "ideal types" regarding homeland security, including all hazards. What may exist today is a natural division of labor as it relates to homeland security in which each enterprise partner interprets and views homeland security differently, through their own proverbial "lens." Is this problematic or actually preferred? The general public likely associates homeland security to the threat of terrorism. If the issue–attention cycle holds true, the next national catastrophe will adjust the nation's collective views of the problem.

SELF-CHECK

- Define the all-crimes approach to criminal justice.
- DHS' requirement that State Homeland Security Program (SHSP) and UASI funds be allocated to support which of the following policy that promotes the all-hazards approach?
  - a. Whole Community Doctrine
  - b. Threat and Hazards Identification and Risk Assessments (THIRAs)
  - c. National Preparedness System
  - d. Public Service Answering Points
- According to the National Preparedness Goal, capabilities organized under prevention mission areas are solely focused on acts of terrorism, so preventing acts of terrorism remains a national priority. True or false?

SUMMARY

In this chapter, you assessed homeland security as the combination of activities that protect people, key infrastructure and assets, economic activities, and the American way of life. You also explored the fundamental questions regarding what, more precisely, constitutes homeland security. Specifically, in this chapter you delved into the traditions that support homeland security as a discipline and provided historical context on one of those traditions—emergency/disaster management.

Understanding historical context is important as homeland security today reflects remnants of these previous eras and their long-lasting constituencies. This chapter introduced a few prevailing theories both of the problems associated with homeland security and the nation's political and administrative responses to the problems. We learned that additional context in the form of social conditions, including advancements in technologies and political and economic factors, is necessary for understanding homeland security. We also explored some of the primary enterprise partners at the federal, state, and local levels of government, and other whole community partners. Finally, we learned about the benefits and limitations of the all-hazards concept.

KEY TERMS

All-crimes	A model of fully integrating terrorism into other crime prevention duties. This model or strategy ensures that possible precursor crimes are screened and analyzed for linkages to larger-scale terrorist activities.
Bureaucracy	The sum of all federal departments, agencies, and offices that implement laws under the authority of the president. By definition, bureaucracies are hierarchical organizations that are highly specialized, and they operate with very formal rules.
Climate change	Changes in average weather conditions that persist over multiple decades or longer. Climate change encompasses both increases and decreases in temperature, as well as shifts in precipitation, changing risk of certain types of severe weather events, and changes to other features of the climate system.
Coordinate-authority model	A theory of intergovernmental relations that assumes a sharp and distinct boundary between separate national and state governments. National and state governments appear to operate independently and autonomously, and they are linked only tangentially.

Department of Homeland Security (DHS)	The federal department created in 2002 with the primary missions of preventing terrorism and enhancing security, security and managing borders, enforcing and administering immigration laws, safeguarding and securing cyberspace, and ensuring resilience to disasters.
Federal Emergency Management Agency (FEMA)	Agency created in 1979 to provide a coordinated federal response to local communities' disaster needs.
Federal system	A vertical division of power found in the United States in which the national government has some exclusive powers, state and local governments have some exclusive powers, other powers are shared by all levels of government, and some powers are reserved to state and local governments.
Homeland security	A concerted national effort to ensure a homeland that is safe, secure, and resilient against terrorism and other hazards where American interests, aspirations, and way of life can thrive.
Homeland security enterprise	The collective efforts and shared responsibilities of federal, state, local, tribal, territorial, nongovernmental, and private sector partners—as well as individuals, families, and communities—to maintain critical homeland security capabilities.
Inclusive-authority model	A model of intergovernmental relations in which each level of government has a diminishing proportion of responsibilities, from the national to the state to the local government level. The federal government coordinates and shares power and responsibility; however, the authority is essentially hierarchical (top-down control).
Intergovernmental relations	The interaction and exchanges of public and private organizations across all layers of government. Intergovernmental relations reflect the growth of societal interdependence, in economic and technological terms, and have created a webbed and networked system of governance.
Internet	The global communication network that allows almost all computers worldwide to connect and exchange information. Some of the early impetus for such a network came from the US government network ARPANET, starting in the 1960s.

Issue–attention cycle	A pattern of public perception of certain domestic problems. The cycle has five stages and concerns the way major communications media interact with the public.
Mitigation	Action taken to reduce or eliminate the long-term risk to human life and property from natural hazards.
Nongovernmental organization (NGO)	An organization that provides service to a community free of charge or for a minimal cost that is required to defray the cost of the service furnished. NGOs usually hold special nonprofit federal tax exempt status and receive financial support through donations, contracts, and grants.
Overlapping-authority model	A model of intergovernmental relations in which substantial areas of governmental operations involve national, state, and local governments simultaneously. Areas of autonomy or single-jurisdiction independence and full discretion are relatively small.
Pluralism	A system of government in which many groups or institutions share power in a complex system of interactions, which involves compromising and bargaining in the decision-making process.
Preparedness	Efforts to increase readiness for a disaster response and recovery operations.
Prevention	The capabilities necessary to avoid, prevent, or stop a threatened or actual act of terrorism.
Protection	The capabilities to safeguard the homeland against acts of terrorism and man-made or natural disasters. It is oriented inward at safeguarding people, vital interests such as critical infrastructure, and the American way of life.
Punctuated backsliding	A model for how national systems and policies react to crises over time. Initially, crises result in punctuated changes to policies but then a subsequent slip back toward the previous equilibrium.
Representative democracy	A system of government in which the ultimate political authority is vested in the people, who elect their governing officials to legislate on their behalf.
Recovery	Activities to return affected communities to pre-disaster or, preferably, improved conditions.

Resilience	The ability to prepare and plan for, absorb, recover from, and more successfully adapt to adverse events.
Response	Those activities in the immediate aftermath of a disaster to protect life and property.
Sneak-and-peek search	A special search warrant that allows law enforcement officers to lawfully enter areas in which a reasonable expectation of privacy exists, to search for items of evidence or contraband and leave without making any seizures or giving concurrent notice of the search.
Stafford Act	The Robert T. Stafford Disaster Relief and Emergency Act of 1988 (Public Law 100-707) aims to provide an orderly and continuing means of assistance by the federal government to state and local governments in carrying out their responsibilities to alleviate the suffering and damage, which result from disasters. The Stafford Act is the principal legislation governing the federal response to disasters within the United States.
Tiered response	Incidents must be managed at the lowest possible jurisdictional level and supported by additional response capabilities when needed.
Urban Area Security Initiative (UASI)	A DHS program that allocates federal funds to urban areas since they have concentrations of critical infrastructure, serve as hubs for transportation, and are considered the epicenters of economic growth and jobs across the country.
Whole community	The idea that a governmental-centric approach to emergency management is not sufficient to face a catastrophic disaster. All available resources must be collectively utilized at each level of government to prepare for and respond to such an incident.
Writ of habeas corpus	The constitutional guarantee that accused persons will be brought before a judge to hear charges against them.

ASSESS YOUR UNDERSTANDING

Go to www.wiley.com/go/Kilroy/Threats_to_Homeland_Security to assess your knowledge of the basics of US homeland security interests.

Summary Questions

1. The disaster resulting from Hurricane Katrina in 2005 led many to embrace the all-hazards approach—an inclusive view of homeland security that considers all natural and man-made hazards and threats to the nation. True or False?

2. This concept is the activity in the immediate aftermath of a disaster to protect life, limit property loss, and overcome disruptions:
   (a) Mitigation
   (b) Preparedness
   (c) Response
   (d) Recovery

3. This concept is defined as the ability to prepare for, absorb, recover from, and more successfully adapt to adverse events:
   (a) Risk
   (b) Hazard
   (c) Resilience
   (d) Likelihood

4. The 1989 Exxon Valdez and 2010 Deepwater Horizon/Gulf Coast oil spills may be best labeled as the following type of hazard:
   (a) Intentional act/terrorism
   (b) Natural
   (c) Accident/technological
   (d) None of the above

5. The following theory aims to explain the brief "window of time" following significant events or large-scale disasters that is favorable to making homeland security policy and institutional changes:
   (a) Issue–attention cycle
   (b) Globalization
   (c) Decentralization
   (d) Intergovernmental relations

6. The 10th amendment of the US Constitution recognized that the basic responsibility and authority for protection and public safety rest with
   (a) Federal Emergency Management Agency (FEMA)
   (b) Federal government
   (c) States
   (d) Citizens

7. The following is considered the nation's principal legislation governing the federal response to disasters within the United States and aims to provide an orderly and continuing means of assistance by the federal government to state and local governments in carrying out their responsibilities to alleviate the suffering and damage, which result from disasters:

   (a) Civil Defense Act of 1950

   (b) Disaster Relief Act of 1950

   (c) Robert T. Stafford Disaster Relief and Emergency Assistance Act of 1988

   (d) Homeland Security Act of 2002

8. The following operational component of DHS is responsible for controlling America's land and maritime borders and has the largest budget and workforce in DHS:

   (a) Transportation Security Administration (TSA)

   (b) US Customs and Border Protection (CBP)

   (c) US Coast Guard

   (d) Immigration and Customs Enforcement (ICE)

9. The following department includes approximately half of the 16 agencies that are considered "members" of the Intelligence Community:

   (a) US Department of Defense

   (b) US Department of Justice

   (c) US Department of Homeland Security

   (d) Office of the Director of National Intelligence

10. National Guard units are commonly activated by state governors and deployed in response to disasters under the command of the following lead military official:

    (a) Attorney general

    (b) Civil affairs

    (c) Homeland security director

    (d) Adjutant general

Applying This Chapter

1. Each year, the national policymakers and administrators contemplate risks for allocating grant funds such as the UASI grant program. Assess the trade-offs between allocating funds toward major metropolitan areas and rural areas. In your response, consider social factors and infrastructure systems.

2. The monitoring or "listening" of social media among law enforcement agencies is becoming more commonplace today. For example, these monitoring strategies are deemed to be one approach to identify those who may be radicalized by foreign terrorist organizations and present a domestic threat. State and explain legal and ethical challenges that exist in implementing a social media monitoring strategy.

3. During the debate in Congress regarding funding DHS in fiscal year (FY) 2016, staffers analyzed the potential impacts of a shutdown. As an expert in homeland security, you are consulted on this question or problem. Explain homeland security functions performed by DHS that may be impacted by the shutdown and others largely performed by other homeland security enterprise partners—stakeholders external to DHS.

4. As an advisor to the new state governor, you are asked to prepare a briefing on reorganizations of state departments and agencies with a focus on homeland security. Specifically, the governor would like you to assess reorganizing the state homeland security function based on the following alternatives: (a) make it stand-alone office as a direct report to the governor, (b) assign it to the state police, (c) assign it to the military department, or (d) assign it the department of emergency management. Analyze these alternatives and prepare a briefing for the governor.

5. As a planner for a local law enforcement agency, you are tasked with updating your agency's emergency response plan. There is a chapter dedicated to responding to an influenza pandemic in the United States. Though you recognize the importance of the chapter for maintaining continuity of operations, you wonder if this chapter is a homeland security concern. Analyze an influenza pandemic through the lens of Bellavita's seven "ideal types."

Applying Homeland Security Theories

Analyze a contemporary large-scale disaster using the three public policy and management theories introduced in Section 2.1.2, which includes the issue–attention cycle, punctuated backsliding, and intergovernmental relations. Provide evidence relating to each of these theories and conclude with your own assessment of the theories.

Homeland Security Enterprise

Select any hazard or threat to your community, and then list and analyze the homeland security enterprise partners that would be involved in all of the mission areas—prevention, protection, mitigation, response, and recovery—associated with that hazard or threat. Make inferences and draw conclusions regarding the concept of the enterprise.

4

UNDERSTANDING THREAT ASSESSMENTS

A Risk Management Approach to All-Hazards Assessments

Alexander Siedschlag

Homeland Security and Public Health Sciences, Penn State Harrisburg, School of Public Affairs, Middletown, PA, USA

Starting Point

Go to www.wiley.com/go/Kilroy/Threats_to_Homeland_Security to assess your knowledge of threat assessment.
Determine where you need to concentrate your effort.

What You'll Learn in This Chapter

▲ The concept of risk management and its role in homeland security programs
▲ The different types of risk models
▲ Homeland security-specific threat assessment
▲ The role of models in risk assessment
▲ The application of models in real-life situations

After Studying This Chapter, You'll Be Able To

▲ Evaluate why risk assessment is important for homeland security programs
▲ Appraise different risk assessment models to program evaluation
▲ Assess threats to communities using risk matrices
▲ Explain why it is important to involve all stakeholders in risk management analysis
▲ Judge the usefulness of the National Preparedness System

Threats to Homeland Security: Reassessing the All-Hazards Perspective, Second Edition.
Edited by Richard J. Kilroy, Jr.
© 2018 John Wiley & Sons, Inc. Published 2018 by John Wiley & Sons, Inc.
Companion website: www.wiley.com/go/Kilroy/Threats_to_Homeland_Security

INTRODUCTION

In his statement for the record to the Senate Select Committee on Intelligence on the "Worldwide Threat Assessment of the US Intelligence Community" for 2017, Director of National Intelligence (DNI) Daniel R. Coats highlighted the need for a

> nuanced, multidisciplinary intelligence that policymakers, warfighters, and domestic law enforcement personnel need to protect American lives and America's interests anywhere in the world. (Office of the Director of National Intelligence 2017, i)

In addition to specific regional threats, the DNI's Worldwide Threat Assessment 2017 pointed out the following areas from which global threats to the United States, its allies, and partners emanate:

▲ Cyber threat
▲ Emerging and disruptive technologies
▲ Terrorism
▲ Weapons of mass destruction and proliferation
▲ Space and counterspace
▲ Counterintelligence
▲ Transnational organized crime
▲ Economics and natural resources
▲ Human security

The DNI's assessment emphasizes that on the one hand, "US and global counterterrorism (CT) partners have significantly reduced al Qaeda's ability to carry out large-scale, mass casualty attacks, particularly against the US homeland," whereas on the other hand, "US-based homegrown violent extremists (HVEs) will remain the most frequent and unpredictable Sunni violent extremist threat to the US homeland" (5). The assessment points out as the main characteristic of this particular threat that there is little to no warning possible of related attacks.

Other common threat assessments highlight a multifaceted "strategic hybrid threat" to the national and homeland security of the United States (e.g., McCreight 2015). This also shines through the DNI's Worldwide Threat Assessment. The strategic hybrid threat perspective assumes that it is necessary to reorient our perspective toward a multidimensional threat landscape that requires working across the country, in an all-of-government and whole-community approach, and around the world, with international partners, as they may exceed the single ability of the United States to confront.

In this chapter, you will learn about the Department of Homeland Security (DHS) Risk Management Doctrine and evaluate why risk assessment is important for homeland security programs. You'll also appraise different risk assessment models and learn how to assess threats to communities using risk matrices. Finally, you'll judge the usefulness of a specific set of tools known as the National Preparedness System (NPS).

4.1 Background on Threat Assessments and Risk Management

Scholars such as Arnold Wolfers (1952) had concluded early on that "national security" was a symbol leaving too much room for confusion to serve as a guiding principle for political advice or scientific analysis. He suggested that, as a first step in developing an analytical concept of the term, security should be considered, "in an objective sense, [...] the absence of threats to [a society's] acquired values, [and] in a subjective sense, the absence of fear that such values will be attacked" (483).

This already refers to the need for balanced comprehensive threat assessment that among other things involves a broad community of stakeholders, including citizens' perspectives. After the end of the Cold War, security policy continued to be understood as a normative practice, namely, as defending values (Buzan 1991). Today, defending values and the nation's heritage is an important ingredient of homeland security as seen by the US Department of Homeland Security, and reflected in the "Homeland Security Vision" put forward in the *2014 Quadrennial Homeland Security Review*:

> A homeland that is safe, secure, and resilient against terrorism and other hazards, where American interests, aspirations, and way of life can thrive. (US Department of Homeland Security 2014a, 14)

Threat assessment and responses are becoming increasingly integrated operationally and strategically. The staff of the National Security Council manages policy integration of national security and homeland security. Nevertheless, homeland security differs from national security. National security seeks to deter an attack on the country and respond to the aggressor in case an attack occurs (Dorman and Kaufman 2014). Homeland security cannot deter those who want to threaten or eliminate our way of life because they do not follow the rational and strategic purposes that national security concepts have typically seen adversaries guided by.

4.1.1 Risk Management and Threat Assessment from the All-Hazards Perspective

Homeland security therefore is about risk management in a dynamic all-hazards context that defines its evolving mission space and drives the underlying requirement for comprehensive threat assessment and response (Siedschlag 2015). The analytical approach as such is not new, and comprehensive threat assessment and preparedness across security continua and with the whole community in mind had already been the focus of classical work such as Pitrim A. Sorokin's (1942) study on *Man and Society in Calamity: The Effects of War, Revolution, Famine, Pestilence upon Human Mind, Behavior, Social Organization and Cultural Life* and George W. Baker and Dwight W. Chapman's (1962) *Man and Society in Disaster*. In awareness of such tradition, homeland security is located at the "intersection of evolving threats and hazards with traditional governmental and civic responsibilities for civil defense, emergency response, law enforcement, customs, border patrol, and immigration" (US Department of Homeland Security 2010, 14).

Homeland security's all-hazards approach though does not mean to address all and any hazards that might emerge. Rather, in order to be effective, credible, and realistic, homeland security needs to be selective, focusing on "the greatest risks" to security, within a unified national preparedness approach, which is defined in the 2015 **National Preparedness Goal** (as already addressed in Chapter 2):

> A secure and resilient Nation with the capabilities required across the whole community to prevent, protect against, mitigate, respond to, and recover from the threats and hazards that pose the greatest risk. (US Department of Homeland Security 2015a, 1)

The challenge for threat assessment in this context is threefold:

▲ First, while in need of focusing on the greatest risk, homeland security at the same time must avoid the "failure of imagination" that the *9/11 Commission Report* cited as a mistake toward failed prevention of and protection against the September 11 terrorist attacks on the United States, a mistake we cannot afford to repeat (The National Commission on Terrorist Attacks Upon the United States 2004, 336).

▲ Second, threat assessment must include anticipation of threat response, as measures to prevent, protect from, mitigate against, respond to, and recover from threats and must not infringe civil liberties, freedom, and the ultimate unifying goal of national and homeland security: protect the American societies' commonly acquired values and the American way of life.

▲ Third, national security comprising "the absence of fear that such values will be attacked" (Wolfers 1952, 483), threat assessment needs to involve the whole community. This includes two aspects:

   ▲ on the one hand, a threat assessment that takes into account citizens' perception of insecurity and fear of threats (as, e.g., identified in polls).

   ▲ on the other hand, a threat assessment that involves citizen reporting. As an example, the **National Terrorism Advisory System (NTAS)** not only increases preparedness for attacks that may occur but also includes information on protection from threats and guidance for citizens to help detect or prevent attacks before they occur.

In particular, the "If You See Something, Say Something ™" campaign across the United States encourages the public and leaders of communities to be vigilant for indicators of potential terroristic activity and to follow the guidance provided by the advisory and/or state and local officials for information about threats in specific places or for identifying specific types of suspicious activity. (US DHS n.d.)

However, whole community-based threat assessment is limited by current shortcomings of the **Suspicious Activity Reporting (SAR)** approach, as represented by the "If You See Something, Say Something ™" campaign. While "to increase the chances of having truly suspicious activities reported while safeguarding our treasured constitutional rights is no easy task," (McCreight 2015, 34), the campaign has no built-in safeguards to prevent potential freedom-infringing effects of such reporting that may turn some of its outcomes into a threat of the liberty and American way of life it seeks to defend.

Further, evidence indicates Suspicious Activity Reporting has not penetrated to the extent that it could be regarded a solid whole-community effort. For example, a Gallup poll in 2013 showed that less of half (45%) of Americans had heard the "If You See Something, Say Something ™" slogan, and only 13% correctly identified it as designed to prevent terrorism (Ander and Swift 2013). Although DHS works with different organizations to spear the campaign across the United States, 55% had never heard of it according to the Gallup poll, which also indicated the campaign does not achieve whole-community objectives; rather, considerable geographical and social gaps were apparent. Only a majority of citizens in the East (64%) were aware of it, as opposed to 44% in the Midwest, 39% in the South, and 37% in the West (Ander and Swift 2013). College graduates (55%) were found more likely to be aware of the campaign (55%) than those without an academic degree (41%); overall, campaign awareness correlated with education level.

4.1.2 Assessing Threats and Civil Liberties

Data sharing for threat assessment and how this process may lead to an oversecuritization of the American democracy that infringes its founding principles of liberty and freedom, as enshrined in the Bill of Rights (the first 10 amendments to the US Constitution), have been critically discussed since the Uniting and Strengthening America by Providing Appropriate Tools Required to Intercept and Obstruct Terrorism Act of 2001 (USA PATRIOT Act). The discussion was reignited by the Snowden case that revealed some questionable National Security Agency (NSA) collection practices, as well as by the discussion around the new Uniting And Strengthening America By Fulfilling Rights And Ensuring Effective Discipline Over Monitoring Act of 2015 (USA FREEDOM Act).

This Act renewed some expired provisions from the USA PATRIOT Act through 2019, at the same time setting limits on mass data collection by the federal government (Congressional Research Service 2015). Much about the legislative as well as public debate about the USA FREEDOM Act centered on its expected impact on domestic surveillance, specifically by the National Security Agency (NSA). The Act largely restricts domestic surveillance and the use of technology to that end to the presence of specific requests, whereas under the USA PATRIOT Act, production of domestic surveillance data would often be allowable for mere threat assessment. In particular, the Act responded to concerns about NSA surveillance of US persons without emergency authorization by putting a halt to the agency's mass phone data collection program. In addition, the Act takes steps to increase the transparency of surveillance.

Some critics continue to argue that homeland security initiatives have neither made the country safer nor protected liberty and freedom. In fact, while a majority is clearly supportive of the US Department of Homeland Security, Americans as a whole are split on the success of homeland security programs.

For instance, the latest comprehensive data available on federal agencies' public approval ratings, from a Pew Research Center survey in September 2015, indicate 64% of Americans see the US Department of Homeland Security (DHS) positively (16% of respondents had a "very favorable" opinion of DHS, and 48% had a "mostly favorable" opinion; Pew Research Center 2015). This approval rating seems to be consistent as a poll two years before had yielded that 66% of Americans had a positive view of the Department (Drake 2013).

However, a Bloomberg poll conducted right after the terrorist attacks in Paris in November 2015 found that 48% of Americans surveyed were mostly confident that the United States had done enough to protect its homeland against similar attacks, while 46% were mostly not confident, and 6% were not sure (Bloomberg 2015). Their results are similar to a Pew Research Center poll conducted after the Boston Marathon bombings in April 2013, where 45% said there is not much more the government can do to prevent such terrorist acts, and 48% believed the government could do more to thwart them (Pew Research Center 2013).

If around half of the Americans do not think homeland security is making the country safer, at least against the advanced persistent terrorist threat, around half believe the country is on the right track, and around two-thirds believe the US DHS is doing a good job altogether, which perspective is correct? Before we can even ask if programs are successful, we must first decide what the risks to our security are and what interests we need to protect. This highlights the importance of the assessment process in which we identify threats and interests in our communities. This process is necessary to implement homeland security programs more effectively, bearing in mind the whole range of threats:

> The United States homeland security environment is complex and filled with competing requirements, interests, and incentives that must be balanced and managed effectively to ensure the achievement of key national objectives. The safety, security, and resilience of the Nation are threatened by an array of hazards, including acts of terrorism, malicious activity in cyberspace, pandemics, man-made accidents, transnational crime, and natural disasters. (US Department of Homeland Security 2011, 7)

4.1.3 Homeland Security Risk Management Doctrine

Based on this fundamental assessment, the Homeland Security Risk Management Doctrine (US Department of Homeland Security 2011) sets forth an Integrated Risk Management (IRM) approach, where department efforts are integrated with federal, state, local, tribal, territorial, nongovernmental, and private sector homeland security partners. The purpose is to comprehensively manage risks emanating from major threats to the homeland. The DHS Risk Lexicon (US Department of Homeland Security Risk Steering Committee 2010) provides relevant definitions, such as the following:

- ▲ **Risk:** "the potential for an unwanted outcome resulting from an incident, event, or occurrence, as determined by its likelihood and the associated consequences."
- ▲ **Risk management:** "the process for identifying, analyzing, and communicating risk and accepting, avoiding, transferring, or controlling it to an acceptable level considering associated costs and benefits of any actions taken."
- ▲ **Hazard:** a "natural or man-made source or cause of harm or difficulty. […] A hazard differs from a threat in that a threat is directed at an entity, asset, system, network, or geographic area, while a hazard is not directed. […] A hazard can be actual or potential."
- ▲ **Threat:** a "natural or man-made occurrence, individual, entity, or action that has or indicates the potential to harm life, information, operations, the environment, and/or property." Annotation: "Threat as defined refers to an individual, entity, action, or occurrence; however, for the purpose of calculating risk, the threat of an intentional hazard is generally estimated as

the likelihood of an attack (that accounts for both the intent and capability of the adversary) being attempted by an adversary; for other hazards, threat is generally estimated as the likelihood that a hazard will manifest."

▲ **Threat assessment:** the "product or process of identifying or evaluating entities, actions, or occurrences, whether natural or man-made, that have or indicate the potential to harm life, information, operations, and/or property."

In summary, a threat is what we are trying to protect against. The effort to protect is substantially supported by analysis of vulnerability, that is, weaknesses or gaps in security programs that can be exploited by threats. Threat assessment is a part of the risk management process. Risk is the potential for loss, damage, or destruction of an asset as a result of a threat exploiting a vulnerability. Threat assessment is a precondition for risk management, as the broader "process of identifying, analyzing, assessing, and communicating risk and accepting, avoiding, transferring or controlling it to an acceptable level considering associated costs and benefits of any actions taken" (US Department of Homeland Security Risk Steering Committee 2010, 30).

While it is important to understand these US Homeland Security-specific foundations for threat assessment, it is as relevant to appreciate the state of the art context and resulting general framework for analysis, as described in the next subchapter.

FOR EXAMPLE

Awareness for Homegrown Violent Extremism

As another example, the abovementioned criticism about Suspicious Activity Reporting notwithstanding hazard assessment in the time of advanced persistent terrorist threats must be a whole-community effort:

Any successful homeland security program has to include public awareness campaigns. This would include not only educating the general public as to the threats that could affect their security, safety, and/or way of life but also how members of the public could report suspicious activity or behavior to assist in preventing a man-made incident. Consider the homegrown violent extremists (HVEs), for example. […] Violent extremist threats within the United States can come from a range of violent extremist groups and individuals, including domestic terrorists and homegrown violent extremists (HVEs). […] Contributing to the challenges associated with detecting the potential actions of HVEs is that some do not have criminal records nor have they been on the radar of law enforcement agencies. How then can we discover the plans and/or intentions of these HVEs? One very effective way is via tips from the general public. No matter in which country the HVE resides, there are generally signs that are present in and around the familial, workplace, educational, and/or social circle that would cause someone concern. These instances need to be reported to an official representing public safety and security in some capacity in order to stop the HVE before loss of life and/or damage to public property occurs. Without this type of public cooperation, the collection of this "domestic intelligence" becomes exponentially more difficult (Ryan 2015, 100).

SELF-CHECK

- National security has been defined as
  a. A whole-community approach
  b. Absence of hazards
  c. Absence of threats to a societies' acquired values
  d. Identical with homeland security
- The all-hazards approach focuses on preventing all and any hazards out of which threats may emerge to the United States. True or false?
- A threat is
  a. Potential hazard
  b. Risk × vulnerability
  c. The outcome of risk analysis
  d. None of the above

4.2 A General Framework of Analysis: What to Assess

Hazard assessment is the process by which we identify new and existing threats and assess the level of risk to a population (Lindell and Prater 2003). As an example, since 9/11, the most visible program requiring hazard assessment in the United States is airline and airport security. In 2016, exercising its dual mission of protecting the borders of the United States and facilitating legitimate trade and travel, the US Customs and Border Protection processed more travelers than ever before at air, land, and sea ports of entry, totaling to more than 390 million (of which more than 119 million travelers were processed at air ports of entry). Projections are for international air travel to increase at an annual rate of 4% over the next five years (US Customs and Border Protection 2017).

For many Americans, the airport is a prime place where federal homeland security programs may affect their lives. Consider, for example, what happened in August 2006, when American and British airports, as well as airports throughout the European Union (EU) and elsewhere in the world, adjusted carry-on luggage restrictions including a stricter ban on liquids and gels. This happened after British authorities announced an alleged terrorist plot to create explosives on board the aircraft that were capable of destroying planes. After the ban, travelers endured long security lines and dumped thousands of bottles of liquids into airport trash cans. Subsequently, the US Transportation Security Administration (TSA) relaxed the rules somewhat, but not before hearing complaints from angered passengers who threw away drinks, shampoos, baby formula, medicines, and even holy water (Pitchford 2006). Arguably, the threat assessment did not take into account the risk to which we expose airline passengers when keeping them in long lines for an extended amount of time in the departure halls, known as the least secure area of an airport. This risk had already been pointed out by the President's Commission on Aviation Security and Terrorism (1990, 33) and become tragically obvious in the Brussels Airport bombing in March 2016. When security rules create long lines and restrict people's ability to travel freely, homeland security can become a hotly debated topic with people asking, who or what is really a threat?

4.2.1 The Disaster Impact Process

When conducting any hazard assessment, you must first determine what factors to assess. At the most basic level, what you'll need to assess can be viewed in terms of interest and threats.

▲ **Interests** are the human (individual or group), environmental, political, or economic components of society we seek to protect through homeland security programs.

▲ **Threats** are generally defined as potential to harm, or more specifically, events that can destroy or damage human, environmental, political, or economic interests. Threats can be natural or anthropogenic (man-made).

Interests and threats intersect in program implementation, so it is important that we understand how disasters affect daily life. The **disaster impact process** is the way we can consider the effects a disaster will have on a community by examining the conditions before, during, and after the disaster. This process includes the following three phases:

1. The first phase of the disaster impact process is the pre-impact phase, which includes planning and mitigation efforts. Identifying pre-impact conditions can help define the characteristics and issues that make communities vulnerable to disasters. It can also identify how specific segments within a community may be affected.

2. The second phase is the actual disaster event, which includes specific hazard conditions and community response. Information about the disaster impact process can be used to identify event-specific conditions that determine the level of disaster impact within the community.

3. The third phase is the emergency management intervention phase, which includes response, recovery, and program evaluations. Understanding this phase of the disaster impact process allows planners to develop suitable emergency management responses and to determine whether their efforts are working to minimize potential threats (Lindell and Prater 2003). Whereas the first two steps of the disaster impact process are discussed in the succeeding text, this third phase is examined in a later section of the chapter.

4.2.2 Pre-Impact Conditions

As previously mentioned, the first phase of the disaster impact process is the pre-impact phase, which includes planning and mitigation efforts. Identifying pre-impact conditions can help define the characteristics and issues that make communities vulnerable to disasters. It can also identify how specific segments within a community may be affected. Pre-impact conditions are defined as hazard exposure or physical and social vulnerabilities.

Pre-impact interventions and hazard vulnerabilities will affect post-impact response and disaster effects. Additionally, individual hazards must be addressed as both individual events and multiple events. For example, hurricanes may produce tornados, flooding, and heavy winds and rain, each with different potential impacts that can also increase when they happen in combination.

Communities and states must determine to what level each type of threat may affect their population. This process involves the use of mapping, data analysis, and modeling. Models can help us define the process by which disasters produce community impacts and assess community resilience (Cutter et al. 2008; Lindell and Prater 2003). For instance, Lindell and Prater's model, as depicted in Figure 4-1, illustrates how three pre-impact conditions—hazard exposure, physical vulnerability, and social vulnerability—interact with emergency management interventions and event-specific conditions. Before we look at the model, however, let's define these three types of pre-impact conditions.

▲ **Hazard exposure** is the probability of occurrence of a given event magnitude. Hazard exposure assessment defines specific types of events, both natural and man-made, that threaten lives or property. These threats can vary in intensity and occurrence across the country. Hazard assessment can be difficult if historical data are insufficient, if the hazard is newly discovered, or if the physical and social vulnerabilities are not fully understood. Natural hazard exposure risks can be simply living in a floodplain or living on a hillside subject to landslides. Man-made hazard exposure risks can be living near places like nuclear power plants or chemical factories (Lindell and Prater 2003).

Figure 4-1

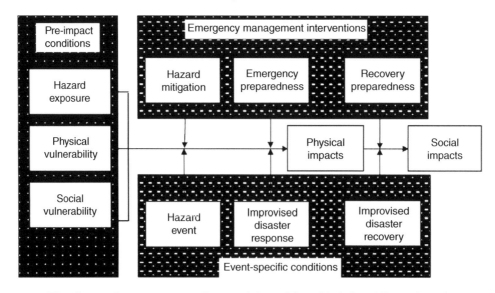

The disaster impact process. Source: Adapted from Lindell and Prater (2003).

▲ **Physical vulnerability** includes three specific categories of vulnerabilities: human, agricultural, and structural.

    a) **Human vulnerability** refers to individual vulnerabilities to environmental extremes. Extreme environments include those influenced by temperature, wind, radiation, and chemical exposure. Human vulnerabilities vary, so even when populations are exposed to a disaster, we can assume that some people will die, others will be severely injured, still others slightly injured, and the rest will survive unscathed. Typically, the people most susceptible to any environmental stressor will be the very young, the very old, and those with weakened immune systems.

    b) **Agricultural vulnerability** is agricultural plant and animal vulnerability to environmental extremes. Like humans, there are differences among individuals within each plant and animal population. Risk assessment for plants and animals is more complex than human vulnerability assessment because of the large number of species in the plant and animal kingdoms.

    c) **Structural vulnerability** describes structural limits to a building's ability to withstand extreme stresses (e.g., high wind, hydraulic pressures of water, seismic shaking) or features that allow hazardous materials to infiltrate the building.

▲ Finally, **social vulnerability** is a person's or group's ability to anticipate, prepare for, and cope with disasters.

Once a disaster actually occurs, it can have a number of impacts. These impacts may be physical, social, or both. Physical impacts include casualties (direct and indirect deaths) and damage (losses of structures, animals, and crops). Social impacts, on the other hand, are less visible than physical impacts, and they can develop over a long period of time. It is important that risk assessment includes and evens model social impacts because they can cause significant problems in the long term for individuals and communities. Types of social impacts include the following:

▲ **Psychosocial impacts** are impacts on mental health and the ability to get treatment after a disaster.

▲ **Demographic impacts** are impacts on a community's population following a disaster. One way to assess population changes after a disaster is to use the demographic balancing equation, defined as $P_a - P_b = B - D + IM - OM$, where P_a is the population size after the disaster, P_b is the population size before the disaster, B is the number of births, D is the number of deaths, IM is the number of immigrants, and OM is the number of emigrants. The magnitude of the disaster impact, $P_a - P_b$, is for the population of a specific geographical area and two specific points in time. Ideally, the geographical area would correspond to the disaster impact area, P_b would be immediately before disaster impact, and P_a would be immediately after disaster impact (Smith et al. 2013).

▲ **Economic impacts** refer to the property damage caused by disaster impact, which creates losses in asset values that can be measured by the cost of repair or replacement. Disaster losses in the United States are initially borne by the affected households, businesses, and local government agencies whose property is damaged or destroyed, but some of these losses are redistributed during the disaster recovery process.

▲ **Political impacts** are changes in the political structure of a community after a disaster. There is substantial evidence that disaster impacts can cause social activism resulting in political disruption, especially during the seemingly interminable period of disaster recovery. The disaster recovery period is a source of many victim grievances, and this creates many opportunities for community conflict, both in the United States (Bolin 1982, 1993) and abroad (Bates and Peacock 1993).

The physical impacts of a disaster combine with improvised disaster recovery to produce the disaster's social impacts (Committee on Disaster Research in the Social Sciences 2006). Thus, as you can see from Figure 4-1, it is apparent that communities should engage in two types of assessment to best plan for emergencies. First, physical impact assessment can form the basis for hazard mitigation and emergency preparedness. Second, risk assessment can direct recovery preparedness practices to reduce social impacts.

4.2.3 Event-Specific Conditions

The second phase of the disaster impact process is the actual disaster event, which includes specific hazard conditions and community response (planned and improvised). Information about the disaster impact process can be used to identify the event-specific conditions that determine the level of disaster impact within a community. However, risk assessment is difficult because of the inherent complexity of natural and man-made disasters. For example, coastal communities face a number of risks from hurricanes, including flooding, wind damage, storm surge, and rain. Thus, it can be difficult to separate the types of threats, but it is possible to characterize them in terms of six significant characteristics. These are as follows:

1. *Onset speed*: How fast the event begins
2. *Perceptual cues*: What types of cues indicate the onset of the threat, such as wind, rain, or ground movement
3. *Intensity*: How strong the threat is
4. *Scope*: The size of the area that the threat impacts
5. *Duration*: How much time the event lasts
6. *Probability*: How often the event may occur

The first two characteristics, onset speed and perceptual cues, can help determine the amount of forewarning that affected populations will have to complete emergency response actions (Lindell and Prater 2003).

We can also categorize hazard events like storms or terrorist attacks by examining the potential losses (property and lives) they may cause. For example, a tornado may cause more concentrated damage than a hurricane. Yet another way of categorizing hazard events is to examine how a hazard may expose physical, social, or structural vulnerabilities in communities. For example, floods may affect certain low-elevation neighborhoods in a community, but they may not affect neighborhoods on higher ground. Knowing the type of hazard and how it will affect an exposed community is also helpful in increasing preparedness and modeling disaster responses. For instance, a chemical attack would evoke a community response much different than a forest fire. In addition to response, an event's characteristics will affect prevention, protection, mitigation, and recovery efforts as well. Thus, a community will not respond to a hurricane in the same way that it would respond to an event such as the 9/11 attacks. At the same time, the purpose is to prepare communities to respond to an all-hazards threat environment, based on those threats that according to current assessment pose the greatest risks. The **all-hazards plus approach** (see the following "For Example" section) combines the comprehensive approach with a prevailing threats approach. It does so by fostering development of prevention, protection, mitigation, response, and recovery capabilities that are common to natural and man-made disasters while also including capabilities that are uniquely relevant to specific types of disasters.

FOR EXAMPLE

Risk Assessment and Hurricane Katrina

Hurricane Katrina, the most devastating natural disaster in US history, struck the Gulf Coast of the United States in August 2005, killing over 1300 people in Louisiana and Mississippi. This hurricane was a major natural disaster, exceeding the economic costs of Hurricane Andrew in August 1992, which had a price tag of $25 billion in storm-related damage. While models can predict the physical damage from a hurricane or even the potential flooding from failed levees, what is hard to estimate is the other social impacts of a disaster like Hurricane Katrina, such as the psychological and demographic impact on New Orleans residents in particular. The entire demographics of New Orleans has changed since the storm, with over 200 000 residents, mostly African American, relocating to other states (mainly Texas), the majority of whom will not return. Also, during the reconstruction of New Orleans, a large number of Hispanics have moved into the city, leading not only to a social impact but also to a political impact on future elections and power shifts between minority constituencies (Miskel 2006). The Post-Katrina Emergency Management Reform Act of 2006 (PKEMRA) addressed preparedness gaps that had become apparent in the disaster response. Amending the Homeland Security Act of 2002 as well as the Robert T. Stafford Disaster Relief and Emergency Assistance Act of 1988, PKEMRA among other things mandated Federal Emergency Management Agency (FEMA) to implement a risk-based, "all-hazards plus" strategy for preparedness. That means a comprehensive approach to preparedness, response, recovery, and mitigation that emphasizes the development of capabilities that are common to natural and man-made disasters while also including the development of capabilities that are uniquely relevant to specific types of disasters (Philpott 2015, 33).

4.2.4 Final Thoughts on What to Assess

To be successful in national hazard assessment, it is important that all levels of government cooperate to monitor issues and events that could lead to man-made or natural disasters. Today, the USA PATRIOT Act and the subsequent USA FREEDOM Act strengthen intergovernmental partnerships among local jurisdictions and higher governmental authorities with greater available resources, foster public–private sector partnerships, and take precautions to prevent collection of information for threat assessment to interfere with constitutional rights and liberties. The Department of Homeland Security coordinates resources for sharing information with intermediate and local jurisdictions, in part to improve risk assessment. However, as Hurricane Katrina and subsequent disasters have shown, even with new organizations and legislative initiatives, the best models and risk assessments don't always help us truly understand the long-term impact of disasters on a community or a nation. This makes the risk assessment process much more dynamic and not simply a matter of running algorithms through a computer program.

SELF-CHECK

- Which of the following is not a phase of the disaster impact process?
  a. Pre-impact phase
  b. Recovery
  c. The actual disaster event
  d. Emergency management interventions
- Hazard assessment is the process by which we identify new and existing threats and assess the level of risk to a population. True or false?
- $P_a - P_b = B - D + IM - OM$ is an example of a(n):
  a. Risk matrix
  b. Impact analysis
  c. Demographic balancing equation
  d. Recovery balancing equation
- Which is the all-hazards plus approach?
  a. A risk management approach that focuses on known plus unknown hazards
  b. A threat response plus a mitigation strategy
  c. A focus on capabilities common to natural and man-made disasters, plus disaster-specific capabilities
  d. A disaster response plus resilience approach

4.3 A Matrix Approach: How to Assess

In 2006, the US Department of Homeland Security released the first **National Infrastructure Protection Plan (NIPP)**. A revision was released in 2009, and a new NIPP followed in 2013. NIPP provides a comprehensive risk management framework, developed through a collaborative process that clearly defines critical infrastructure protection roles and responsibilities for all levels of government (federal, state, local, tribal, and territorial), private industry, nongovernmental agencies, nonprofit organizations, and academia (US Department of Homeland Security 2013a). Risk management is a systematic and analytical process to consider the likelihood that a threat will endanger an asset (e.g., a structure, individual, or function) and to identify actions that reduce the risk and mitigate the consequences. As NIPP 2013 points out,

> Managing the risks from significant threat and hazards to physical and cyber critical infrastructure requires an integrated approach across this diverse community to:
>
> ▲ Identify, deter, detect, disrupt, and prepare for threats and hazards to the Nation's critical infrastructure
> ▲ Reduce vulnerabilities of critical assets, systems, and networks
> ▲ Mitigate the potential consequences to critical infrastructure of incidents or adverse events that do occur (US DHS 2013a, 1)

An effective risk management approach includes the following types of assessments:

▲ A **threat assessment** identifies and evaluates threats based on various factors, including capability and intentions as well as the potential impact of an event. Even when such an assessment exists, however, we will never know whether we have identified every threat or event, and we may not have complete information about the threats that we have identified. Consequently, two other elements—vulnerability assessments and criticality assessments—are essential to better prepare against threats.

▲ A **vulnerability assessment** identifies weaknesses that may be exploited and suggests options to eliminate or mitigate those weaknesses.

▲ A **criticality assessment** systematically identifies and evaluates an organization's assets based on a variety of factors, including the importance of its mission or function, whether people are at risk, and/or the significance of a structure or system. Criticality assessments provide a basis for prioritizing which assets require higher or special protection.

A good risk management approach is adaptable to all levels of government and across the public and private sectors. The 2013 *National Infrastructure Protection Plan* (NIPP) uses a risk management framework that combines consequence, vulnerability, and threat information to produce a comprehensive assessment of national or sector-specific risks. The risk management framework among other things includes a call for action for more analysis: "Greater analysis of dependencies and interdependencies at international, national, regional, and local levels can inform planning and facilitate prioritization of resources to ensure the continuity of critical services and mitigate the cascading impacts of incidents that do occur" (US Department of Homeland Security 2013a, 24). The framework applies to the general threat environment, as well as to specific threats or incident situations. Further, since most critical infrastructure is privately owned or owned by local or state agencies, the 2013 NIPP stresses intergovernmental as well as whole-community cooperation to build an integrated risk assessment that all levels of government and partners in the protection of the nation's critical infrastructure can implement.

The NIPP incorporates an all-hazards approach to homeland security that addresses the direct effects of natural and man-made incidents on the nation's critical infrastructure and key assets. It is a public and private sector partnership that includes a risk assessment of America's threats and assets. The goal of risk assessment in the NIPP is to help prioritize protection activities and enable disaster responses and recovery efforts. Additionally, the NIPP requires the development and use of sophisticated analytical and modeling tools to help inform effective risk-mitigation programs in an all-hazards context.

Risk assessment can help determine the nature and extent of risk by analyzing potential hazards and evaluating existing conditions of vulnerability that could pose a potential threat to people, property, livelihoods, and the environment on which they depend (Wisner et al. 2012). Risk assessment for homeland security has two main objectives: risk reduction and hazard assessment. **Risk reduction** is an examination of the actions necessary to decrease detected or projected levels of danger and to identify the resources required for implementing those actions (Dynes et al. 1972). In other words, hazard identification and assessment are the procedures through which we can monitor environmental threats, while risk reduction is the development and implementation of activities aimed at mitigation, preparedness, response, and recovery (Mileti 1999).

4.3.1 Risk Matrices

Risk assessment is an effective tool to identify safety risks from various sources and to determine the most cost-effective means to reduce risk. One method of risk assessment is to use a matrix. A **matrix** is a tool for decision making that uses a grid design to weigh the frequency of an event against its severity to rank potential costs or damage. As shown in Figure 4-2, FEMA incorporated the risk matrix approach developed by the management consulting firm Arthur D. Little, Inc. into its practices for hazard planning and management. Construction of a risk matrix starts by first establishing how the matrix is intended to be used. Little's risk matrix approach requires the following steps (Federal Emergency Management Agency 1997, 314):

1. Identify and characterize hazards: Define and describe hazards, measures of magnitude and severity, causative factors, and interrelations with other hazards.
2. Screen risk: Rank or order the identified hazards as a function of the relative degree of risk.

Figure 4-2

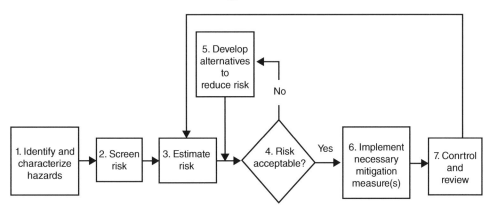

The risk matrix process. Source: Adapted from Federal Emergency Management Agency (1997, 315).

3. Estimate risk: Apply the process or methodology to evaluate risk.

4. Assess acceptability: Determine whether the risks that have been identified and estimated in the previous steps can be tolerated.

5. Develop alternatives to reduce risk: Select cost-effective actions to reduce or mitigate unacceptable risks, including technological and management controls.

6. Implement: Implement mitigation measures to control risks to acceptable levels.

7. Control and review: Periodically monitor and review risks.

The risk matrix approach assigns qualitative measures to prioritize risk by weighing the frequency of an event to its severity. For example, severity may range from minor to catastrophic impacts on lives, property, the economy, and the environment. Frequency can range from low (less than once every 1000 years) to high (more than once in 10 years). After establishing categories, a matrix can be constructed. A risk matrix can be very simple, such as a two-by-two grid, or very complex, with 10 or more categories for each factor. Different criteria for categorizing the severity and frequency of an event will vary, so using a risk matrix without clear definitions of the categories can lead to inaccurate assessments. Figure 4-3 employs categories and definitions found in the FEMA publication *Multi-Hazard Identification and Risk Assessment: A Cornerstone of the National Strategy* (1997).

As you can see, the matrix in Figure 4-3 uses the qualitative measures A, B, C, and D to prioritize action for specific hazards based on their frequency and severity. These classes are as defined follows:

▲ *Class A*: Hazards in this class are high risk and have the highest priority for mitigation and contingency planning (immediate action). Examples of potential losses include death, complete shutdown of key assets and critical infrastructure for more than 1 month, and severe damage to more than 50% of the property located in the affected area.

▲ *Class B*: Class B hazards are moderate to high-risk conditions that are addressed by mitigation and contingency planning (prompt action). Examples of potential

Figure 4-3

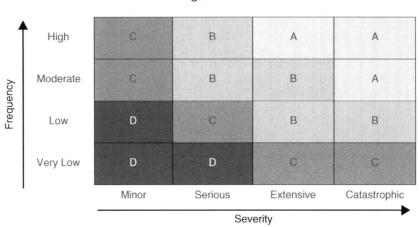

A risk matrix. Source: Adapted from Federal Emergency Management Agency (1997).

losses include permanent disability or severe injury or illness, complete shutdown of key assets and critical infrastructure for more than 2 weeks, and severe damage to more than 25% of the property in the affected area.

▲ *Class C*: These are risk conditions sufficiently high to give consideration to further mitigation and planning (planned action). Examples of potential losses include injury or illness not resulting in disability, complete shutdown of key assets and critical infrastructure for more than 1 week, and severe damage to more than 10% of the property in the affected area.

▲ *Class D*: Class D hazards are low-risk conditions that may be addressed by additional mitigation contingency planning (advisory in nature). Examples of potential losses include treatable first aid injury, complete shutdown of facilities and critical services for more than 24 h, and severe damage to no more than 1% of the property located in the affected area.

Risk matrices are effective for assessing both natural and man-made disasters. The scenarios and consequences can be adapted for any disaster, as long as they are simple to use and understand. Additionally, a good matrix design will include clear guidance on applicability and likelihood ranges that cover the full spectrum of potential scenarios and descriptions of the consequences of concern for each consequence range. A good risk matrix will also have clearly defined tolerable and intolerable risk levels and shows how scenarios that are at an intolerable risk level can be mitigated to a tolerable risk level on the matrix. Finally, a good risk matrix should provide clear guidance on what action is necessary to mitigate scenarios with intolerable risk levels. For example, a risk matrix analysis could be helpful in determining the risks associated with building a hospital in a flood zone. During Hurricane Katrina, many hospitals and medical facilities in New Orleans were flooded, requiring the evacuation of patients, supplies, equipment, and staff. It would thus appear risky to rebuild community services like hospitals in a flood zone, but decision makers must balance the risk of flooding with convenient location for the population the facility serves.

4.3.2 Composite Exposure Indicator

Another model used to determine risk is the **Composite Exposure Indicator (CEI)**. This approach ranks the potential for losses in a given region for single or multiple hazards by assigning a numeric value to the exposure potential for communities (Federal Emergency Management Agency 1997). While this method was originally designed for natural or technological disasters, it can be adapted for homeland security issues very easily.

FEMA has used this approach to quantify 14 variables in 3100 US counties, with rankings based on the amount of each variable present. This method implies that the larger a county's CEI is, the higher the county's exposure is to potential damages from natural or man-made hazards (see Figure 4-4). FEMA uses these variables to plan response levels for different regions. Based on these variables, FEMA has also drawn several conclusions about the nation's counties:

▲ The number of hospitals and the population within a county are highly correlated.

▲ Hospitals and population are moderately correlated with a county's number of bridges.

Figure 4-4

Variable	Unit of measure	Mean	Standard deviation	Minimum	Maximum
Hospitals	#/mi^2	0.005	0.028	0	1.297
Population	#persons/mi^2	213.767	1,519.663	0.053	62,245.000
Nuclear power plants	#plants/mi^2	0.000	0.001	0	0.010
Toxic release inventory	#sites/mi^2	0.059	0.228	0	4.913
Public water supplies	#/mi^2	0.005	0.077	0	4.276
Superfund sites	#sites/mi^2	0.001	0.003	0	0.056
Sewage treatment sites	#sites/mi^2	0.014	0.056	0	2.460
Utility lines	Ft/mi^2	647.161	404.752	0	2,756.591
Airports	#/mi^2	0.002	0.003	0	0.100
Roads	Ft/mi^2	665.084	443.725	0	11,633.116
Railroads	Ft/mi^2	420.221	361.616	0	4.624.799
Pipelines	Ft/mi^2	300.052	726.723	0	32,188.936
Dams	#/mi^2	0.012	0.031	0	1.246
Bridges	#/mi^2	0.270	0.591	0	13.767

A CEI analysis. Source: Adapted from Federal Emergency Management Agency (1997).

▲ The number of public water supply systems and sewage treatment sites are strongly correlated.

▲ Public water supply systems and sewage treatment plants are moderately correlated with the length of pipelines and the number of dams.

▲ The length of roads is moderately correlated with sewage treatment sites.

4.3.3 HAZUS

Another model used for risk assessment is HAZUS, which stands for **HAZ**ards **U**nited **S**tates and is a natural hazard loss estimation software package developed by the Federal Emergency Management Agency (FEMA) in 1997 (Federal Emergency Management Agency 2017a). The most recent version of the software is HAZUS-MH MR2 (MH stands for "multi-hazards"). It is available and free of charge to public and private agencies and organizations. HAZUS supports risk-informed decision making by using a geographic information system (GIS) software package that analyzes potential losses from floods, hurricane winds, and earthquakes before or after a disaster occurs. The model estimates risk in three steps. First, it calculates the exposure for a selected area. Second, it characterizes the level of intensity of the hazard affecting the exposed area. Third, it uses the exposed area and the hazard to calculate the potential losses in terms of economic losses, structural damage, or other factors determined by the user. Potential loss estimates analyzed in HAZUS-MH include the following:

▲ Physical damage to residential and commercial buildings, schools, critical facilities, and infrastructure

▲ Economic loss, including lost jobs, business interruptions, and repair and reconstruction costs

▲ Social impacts, including estimates of shelter requirements, displaced households, and population exposed to scenario floods, earthquakes, and hurricanes

HAZUS uses flexible programming that frames assessments as a series of modules. Thus, new modules, improvements, and data may be added without reworking the entire methodology. This allows for a rapid transfer of information so that decision makers have the most up-to-date data available at all times, and it saves upgrade and maintenance costs for users. The modules incorporated in HAZUS include earth science hazards, data inventories, director damage, induces damage, direct economic/social losses, and indirect losses.

4.3.4 Vulnerability Assessments

Vulnerability assessment is a technique, for example, used by the Coastal Services Center (CSC) of the National Oceanic and Atmospheric Administration (NOAA) for coastal communities facing the threat of natural hazards such as flooding and hurricanes. As depicted in Figure 4-5, vulnerability analyses include critical facilities analyses, societal analyses, environmental analyses, and economic analyses (National Oceanic and Atmospheric Administration, Office for Coastal Management 2017).

Figure 4-5

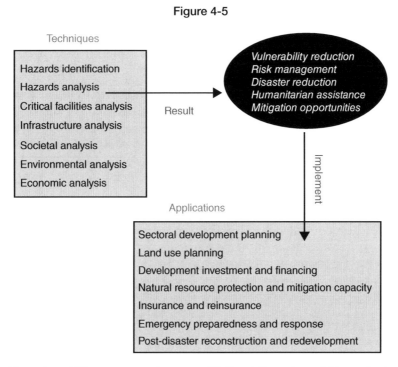

The vulnerability assessment process (National Oceanic and Atmospheric Administration 2006).

Vulnerability assessment techniques can determine the vulnerability of infra-structure networks and individual structures, as well as the economic, environmental, and societal vulnerabilities posed by natural hazards. Vulnerability assessment can be used to determine the effects of single hazards or multiple hazards, and it can address impacts on both public infrastructure and private sector interests (like tourism). These assessments can be on the macro-, micro-, and system levels.

▲ **Macro-level** *assessment*: Multinational, regional, national, or subnational level
▲ **Micro level** *assessment*: Metropolitan, urban, community, or neighborhood level
▲ **System level** *assessment*: Network, grid, area, or individual structure level (National Oceanic and Atmospheric Administration 2006)

4.3.5 Threat and Hazard Identification and Risk Assessment

Within the whole-community approach, it is important for every community to identify and understand their specific risks. Such an understanding enables well-informed decisions about how to manage risks and related resource requirements. Based on the *National Preparedness Goal*, the **Threat and Hazard Identification and Risk Assessment (THIRA)** process drives strategic priorities by helping communities determine capability targets and those resources that are required to

---

FOR EXAMPLE

Vulnerability Assessment for Indian Point Nuclear Reactor

The Indian Point power plant is located on 239 acres in Westchester County, New York, on the banks of the Hudson River 35 miles north of midtown Manhattan. The plant has two reactors that generate over 16 million megawatts of electricity every year. In 1994, the Union of Concerned Scientists used vulnerability analysis to analyze the threats to nuclear facilities throughout the United States, including Indian Point. The scientists estimated a successful attack on just one of the reactors would result in between 100 000 and 500 000 cancer deaths within 50 miles, due to non-acutely lethal radiation exposures within 7 days after the attack. The peak value corresponds to an attack timed to coincide with weather conditions that maximize radioactive fallout over New York City. Additionally, economic damages within 100 miles would exceed $1.1 trillion and could be as great as $2.1 trillion for the worst case evaluated (Lyman 2004).

---

meet them (US Department of Homeland Security 2013b). The THIRA process is a flexible and scalable four-step process designed to support the whole community—including individuals, businesses, faith-based organizations, nonprofit groups, schools and academia, and all levels of government—in understanding its specific risks and estimate the capabilities required to effectively address those risks. Figure 4-6 illustrates the four-step THIRA process. Figure 4-7 provides details on each step.

In addition to THIRA, where states, territories, tribes, and urban areas identify threats and hazards of primary concern, set capability targets to address potential impacts, and estimate the resources required to reach those targets, states and territories are mandated by the Post-Katrina Management Reform Act to use the State Preparedness Report (SPR) to assess their currently existing capabilities. Comparing current capabilities with the targets set through the THIRA process helps communities to identify specific weaknesses and prioritize resources to close them.

4.3.6 Final Thoughts on How to Assess

Risk management is a systematic and analytical process used to consider the likelihood that a threat will endanger an asset and to identify actions that reduce the risk and mitigate the consequences of an attack. An effective risk management approach includes a threat assessment, a vulnerability assessment, and a criticality assessment. Hazard assessment is the process by which we identify new and existing threats and assess the level of risk to a population. Risk reduction involves an examination of the actions necessary to decrease the detected or projected levels of danger and to identify the resources required for implementing those actions. Because the available resources are rarely equal to the threat, this process implicitly

FOR EXAMPLE

From the State of California Threat and Hazard Identification and Risk Assessment (THIRA) 2014

The THIRA as implemented in California at the state level is the first step in a more extensive process. The THIRA remains a foundational strategic document complementing the State Hazard Mitigation Plan. Additional steps include prioritizing core capabilities for development through various mechanisms such as the State Preparedness Report, training and exercise programs, operational/emergency planning, hazard mitigation efforts (pre- and post-disaster), and individual/community preparedness programs. [...] The 2014 THIRA saw good progress in a comprehensive review and update to threats and hazards. Tsunami, climate-related issues, volcanic eruption, cyber-attacks, influenza pandemic, animal disease, and attacks to mass gathering locations were added as threats/hazards and examined in 2014. [...] Several bullets were added to reflect information gathered due to the inclusion of pandemic and animal disease in the list of identified threats and hazards reviewed for 2014. In addition, the number of people affected was adjusted in several of the targets such as Public Information & Warning, Critical Transportation, Mass Search & Rescue, and Mass Care. Numbers increased in all cases except Mass Search & Rescue. The increase in numbers generally reflected the inclusion of impacts that extended beyond the initial response period in the response mission area. [...] Estimating Resource Requirements at the end of the THIRA process without a mature typology has significantly hindered the development of a common understanding of the nature and process of defining operational resource requirements. California should develop a consensus over the actual capability of NIMS [National Incident Management System] typed assets in order to better inform Resource Requirement to fulfill Capability Targets identified in the THIRA. (California Governor's Office of Emergency Services 2014, 5–7)

Figure 4-6

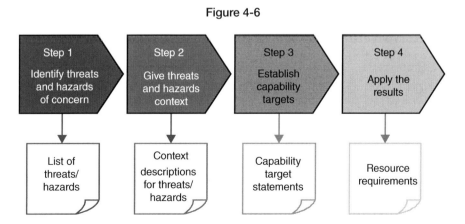

The THIRA process (US Department of Homeland Security 2013b, 2).

Figure 4-7

The THIRA process:

1. **Identify threats and hazards of concern**: Based on a combination of experience, forecasting, subject matter expertise, and other available resources, identify a list of the threats and hazard of primary concern to the community.

2. **Give the threats and hazards context**: Describe the threats and hazards of concern, showing how they may affect the community.

3. **Establish capability targets:** Assess each threat and hazard in context to develop a specific capability target for each core capability identified in the national preparedness goal. the capability target defines success for the capability.

4. **Apply the result**: for each core capability,estimate the resources required to archive the capability targets through the use of community assets and mutual aid, while also considering preparedness activities, including mitigation opportunities.

Steps in the THIRA process (Federal Emergency Management Agency 2013c).

defines the remaining level of danger considered to be acceptable. One method is to use a matrix, which is a tool for decision making that uses a grid design to weigh the frequency of an event against its severity to rank potential costs or damage. FEMA incorporated the risk matrix approach, developed by Arthur D. Little, Inc., into hazard planning and management. Other tools include the Composite Exposure Indicator, HAZUS, and vulnerability assessments. It is important to use risk assessment results in the THIRA process and SPR self-assessment to generate hazard-specific preparedness data that helps identify gaps and prioritize initiatives and resources to close those gaps.

Models can give insight into predicting damages from disasters, but decision makers need to use data appropriate to each phase. For example, if a risk assessment is used when determining the best site for critical infrastructure like a new power plant, then a model like a risk matrix would be appropriate to assess risk for different locations during the prevention phase. However, if a risk assessment is to be used for state budgets, then a CEI model would be helpful in determining fiscal considerations like rebuilding costs versus mitigation costs for different areas of the state. Thus, understanding each phase of the disaster life cycle is critical to making good decisions.

SELF-CHECK

- An effective risk management approach includes a threat assessment, a vulnerability assessment, and a criticality assessment. True or false?
- What does HAZUS stand for?
  a. Hazard Assessment Zoning Under States
  b. Hazards Under Susceptibility
  c. Hazard Zones in the United States
  d. Hazards United States
- A micro-level vulnerability assessment includes multinational, regional, national, or subnational structures. True or false?
- The Composite Exposure Indicator (CEI) ranks the potential for losses in a given region for single or multiple hazards by assigning a numeric value to the exposure potential for communities. True or false?

4.4 The Whole-Community Approach of the National Preparedness System

The *2010 Quadrennial Homeland Security Review* (US Department of Homeland Security 2010) defined the National Preparedness System based on the National Preparedness Goal (for a current description, see Federal Emergency Management Agency 2016). This goal was called for in Presidential Policy Directive 8 (2011) (US Department of Homeland Security 2015b) and expanded on regulations of the Post-Katrina Emergency Management Reform Act of 2006. As mentioned, the National Preparedness Goal is a "secure and resilient Nation with the capabilities required across the Whole Community to prevent, protect against, mitigate, respond to, and recover from the threats and hazards that pose the greatest risk" (US Department of Homeland Security 2015a, 1). By outlining 32 core capabilities, the National Preparedness Goal identifies what is necessary to foster a resilient nation based on national preparedness rooted in unified efforts across the whole community. Those core capabilities can best be thought of as significant functions that must be developed and executed across the whole community to ensure national preparedness.

The goal enables federal, state, and local agencies to better allocate resources through focusing on specific threats and those capabilities required to address them effectively and efficiently. Threat assessment based on the goal of building and sustaining national preparedness aids the decision-making process, and it can be helpful in reducing costs to local communities by allowing first responders and emergency managers to focus on the prevention, protection, mitigation, response, and recovery programs their communities need most.

The National Preparedness System provides a consistent approach to that end. Its main components include the following:

▲ **Core doctrine:** It describes the approach, resources, and tools for achieving the National Preparedness Goal.

▲ **National Planning Frameworks** and **Federal Interagency Operational Plans** for each preparedness mission (prevention, protection, mitigation, response, and recovery): They "describe how the Whole Community works together to prevent, protect against, mitigate, respond to, and recover from threats and hazards. Each framework is supported by a Federal Interagency Operational Plan, which explains how federal departments and agencies work together to deliver the core capabilities through the coordinating mechanisms outlined in the framework. [...] The frameworks are built upon scalable, flexible, and adaptable coordinating structures that align key roles and responsibilities to deliver necessary capabilities" (US Department of Homeland Security 2010, 72).

▲ **Comprehensive Preparedness Guides (CPG):** This initiative is designed to develop guidance documents on a variety of preparedness issues in support of the National Preparedness Goal. So far, FEMA has released three CPGs that are parts of the National Incident Management System (NIMS) (Federal Emergency Management Agency 2017b):

a) **CPG** 101: Developing and Maintaining Emergency Operations Plans. It encourages emergency and homeland security managers to work with the whole community in addressing all of the risks relevant to their jurisdictions.

b) **CPG** 201: Threat and Hazard Identification and Risk Assessment (THIRA) Guide. As previously discussed in this chapter.

c) **CPG** 502: Considerations for Fusion Center and Emergency Operations Center Coordination. It in centered on the critical collaboration and information exchange roles between fusion centers and Emergency Operations Centers (EOCs).

▲ **National Preparedness Report:** This annually delivered report, which includes results from integrated Threat and Hazard Identification and Risk Assessment and State Preparedness Reports, provides a comprehensive assessment of progress and challenges occurring nationwide and across all preparedness mission areas (prevent, protect, mitigate, respond, and recover) in meeting the capability targets from the National Preparedness Goal. For example, the 2016 National Preparedness Report, among other things, found (US Department of Homeland Security 2016) the following:

a) **Planning**; Public Health, Healthcare, and Emergency Medical Services; and Risk and Disaster Resilience Assessment are core capabilities at acceptable levels of performance, which however will decline if not maintained to address emerging challenges.

b) **Preparedness** of states and territories to achieve capability targets is highest in the response mission area and lowest in the recovery mission area.

▲ **Building and Sustaining Preparedness:** This is based on comprehensive campaign including public and community outreach and private sector programs. Examples include Suspicious Activity Reporting, such as known through the "If You See Something, Say Something ™" campaign.

Figure 4-8

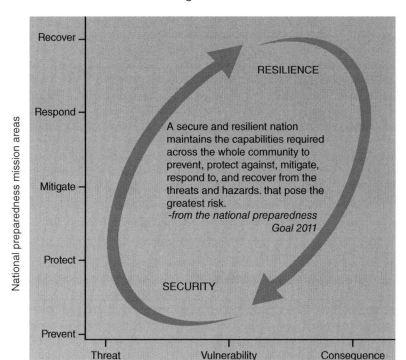

Risk elements by national preparedness mission areas (US Department of Homeland Security 2013a, 19).

When it comes to emergencies, there is a need to have an ongoing cycle that keeps planning in the forefront. The "phases" of the disaster life cycle (that is used in some variations in different countries around the world), in homeland security known as the national preparedness missions cycle—prevention, protection, mitigation, response, and recovery—also describe a model for emergency management planning. In reality, these phases might better be called functions, since they are neither discrete nor temporally sequential.

For each step of the national preparedness cycle, modeling risks can be an effective tool for decision making, but it is important to understand how a model will be used. As illustrated in Figure 4-8, listing national preparedness areas (prevent, protect, mitigate, respond, and recover) against risk elements (threat, vulnerability, and consequence) can help determine the level of resilience reached, as the National Preparedness Goal aims at a resilient nation.

The DHS Risk Management Doctrine and the National Preparedness Goal of a resilient nation are mutually reinforcing:

Risk management contributes to the achievement of resilience by identifying opportunities to build resilience into planning and resourcing to achieve risk reduction in advance of a hazard, as well as enabling the mitigation of consequences of any disasters that do occur. (US Department of Homeland Security 2011, 8)

Risk reduction is the application of appropriate techniques and management principles to reduce the likelihood of an occurrence or its consequences or both (United Nations Office for Disaster Risk Reduction 2015). Examples of risk reduction include regulations that limit construction in areas that are susceptible to hazard impacts and building construction practices that make individual structures less vulnerable to natural hazards. For example, building construction in floodplains is regulated at the federal level through the National Flood Insurance Program (NFIP), and communities participating in the NFIP must adopt minimum building standards set forth by FEMA in order for residents to be eligible for subsidized federal flood insurance. These codes set standards for various aspects of construction to protect general health and safety, including appropriate building construction practices for hazardous locations by establishing code provisions to require hazard-resistant building designs and materials. In the United States, local building codes may be based on a model code or a state code. According to a FEMA study of 2013, 22 states had building codes that prohibit further local amendment without state approval and mandated local enforcement of those statewide codes. Building codes are enforced by local governments as an exercise of police power (Federal Emergency Management Agency 2013b).

Another example of risk reduction is the Department of Homeland Security grant program to reduce risk from terrorist attacks on rail systems. The majority of mass transit systems in this country are owned and operated by state and local government and private industry, but securing these systems is a shared responsibility between federal, state, and local partners. Thus, the DHS provides grants to railways to be used for planning, training, equipment, and other security enhancements. One project funded by this program was the National Capital Region Rail Security Corridor Pilot Project, which included numerous components, including a virtual security fence that will detect moving objects, perimeter breaches, left objects, removed objects, and loitering activity. The seven-mile stretch of track was monitored continuously, and the data that is gathered was transmitted simultaneously to multiple locations, such as the US Capitol Police, the US Secret Service, CSX, and other applicable federal or local agencies (US Department of Homeland Security 2006).

4.4.1 Prevention

As defined in the National Prevention Framework, **prevention actions** are

> what the whole community—from community members to senior leaders in government—should do upon the discovery of intelligence or information regarding an imminent threat to the homeland in order to thwart an initial or follow-on terrorist attack. (US Department of Homeland Security 2014b, 2)

Those efforts are centered on seven protection core capabilities defined in the National Prevention Framework: Planning, Public Information and Warning, Operational Coordination, Forensics and Attribution, Intelligence and Information Sharing, Interdiction and Disruption, and Screening, Search, and Detection (3). Homeland security intelligence plays a specific role in prevention efforts (Steiner 2015). Intelligence, in particular threat information, can be rewritten so that the classification and controls are removed and it may be disseminated to the general public:

There are times when the general public needs to be informed about a potential threat not only to take potential action to protect themselves and their loved ones, but also to be another set of eyes and ears for those governmental agencies attempting to prevent the threat from coming to fruition. Prevention would come in the form of either stopping the potential perpetrator (via arrest or other means) or making it so the intended targets are no longer vulnerable to the planned action. (Ryan 2015, 91)

Understanding the threat assessment process further is critical to influencing intelligence collection and also how federal, state, and local agencies can better allocate resources when focused on specific threats.

4.4.2 Protection

Protection actions, according to the National Protection Framework, are those that the whole community undertakes "to safeguard against acts of terrorism, natural disasters and other threats or hazards" (US Department of Homeland Security 2014b, 3). The protective posture is increased, when required, by coordinating structures "to augment operations that take place during temporary periods of heightened alert, during periods of incident response, or in support of planned events" (4). This includes determining responsibilities and procedures for community organizations. Organizations must acquire personnel, facilities, and equipment resources to implement their plans and to remain prepared through ongoing training.

Protection thus involves **preparedness actions** or pre-impact actions that provide the human and material resources needed to support active responses at the time of hazard impact (Lindell and Perry 2000). In homeland security, this, for example, involves law enforcement task forces, critical infrastructure partnerships, state and major urban area fusion centers and other information sharing mechanisms, or health surveillance networks. Assessing threats and risks in a hazard analysis is the first step in emergency preparedness, and a hazard analysis should consist of four parts: emergency assessment, hazard operations, population protection, and incident management (Lindell and Perry 1992). Emergency assessment consists of the actions that define the potential scope of disaster impacts, such as staffing plans for first responders. Hazard operations consist of short-term actions to protect property, such as boarding up windows. Population protection actions protect people from impact; an example would be an evacuation order. Incident management actions activate and coordinate the emergency response. Incident management can be seen in communication between responders, agencies, and affected communities.

4.4.3 Mitigation

Hazard mitigation is sustained action to alleviate or eliminate risks to life and property from natural or man-made hazard events (United Nations Office for Disaster Risk Reduction 2015). Mitigation activities include land use planning, adoption of building codes, elevating structures, property acquisition, and relocation outside floodplains. Mitigation decreases the need for post-disaster response and expenditures across all levels of government and for property owners.

In homeland security, following the National Mitigation Framework, mitigation strives for a "national culture shift that embeds risk management and mitigation in all planning, decision making, and development," based on the specific core capabilities of Long-Term Vulnerability Reduction, Risk and Disaster Resilience Assessment, and Threats and Hazard Identification (US Department of Homeland Security 2014b, 5).

Mitigation is a separate phase of the disaster life cycle, but it can also take place during the planning, response, and recovery phases. In the planning phase, mitigation can include building public awareness of mitigation techniques, creating state and local hazard mitigation plans (under the Disaster Mitigation Act of 2000, also known as DMA 2000), integrating hazard mitigation criteria into local comprehensive plans and engineering public facilities to withstand the effects of an event. Mitigation during the response and recovery phases includes locating emergency equipment and supplies out of high-risk areas and permanent relocation or retrofitting.

An example of federal mitigation policy is the FEMA-administered **National Flood Insurance Program (NFIP)** comprised of three components: flood insurance, floodplain management, and flood hazard mapping. Communities participate in the NFIP by adopting and enforcing floodplain management ordinances to reduce future flood damage. In exchange, the NFIP makes federally backed flood insurance available to homeowners, renters, and business owners in these communities. Community participation in the NFIP is voluntary, but nearly 20 000 communities across the United States and its territories participate. Since the NFIP began, participating communities have saved almost $1 billion per year through implementing sound floodplain management requirements and property owners purchasing flood insurance. Additionally, buildings constructed in compliance with NFIP building standards sustain on average 80% less damage annually than those not built in compliance (Federal Emergency Management Agency 2013b).

Another federal mitigation tool is the Disaster Mitigation Act of 2000 that requires state, tribal, and local governments to conduct risk assessment though mitigation planning. DMA 2000 amended the Robert T. Stafford Disaster Relief and Emergency Assistance Act by repealing its previous mitigation planning provisions (Section 409) and replacing them with a new set of requirements. This new section emphasizes the need for state, tribal, and local entities to closely coordinate mitigation planning and implementation efforts by identifying natural and man-made threats to communities nationwide (Section 322). DMA 2000 also requires state mitigation plans as a condition of disaster assistance, and federally approved state plans can increase the amount of funding available to states and local governments through the Hazard Mitigation Grant Program (HMGP). Since the passage of DMA 2000, all 50 states have enacted laws that enforce disaster planning requirements for local governments. Under the act, local governments and states must address the following types of hazards in order for their plans to be approved:

▲ Dam failure
▲ Earthquake
▲ Fire or wildfire
▲ Flood
▲ Hazardous materials

▲ Heat
▲ Hurricane
▲ Landslide
▲ Nuclear explosion
▲ Terrorism
▲ Thunderstorm
▲ Tornado
▲ Tsunami
▲ Volcano
▲ Wildfire
▲ Winter storm

4.4.4 Response

Disaster response is the reaction individuals have when faced with the onset of a disaster. Response can be very quick, as was the case during the September 11, 2001, attacks in New York City, or it can be delayed, as was seen after Hurricane Katrina in 2005. Disaster response delays can occur because people have limited information, or they may be in denial that the disaster is actually happening to them. Disaster victims often devote considerable effort to helping their neighbors, contrary to the stereotype of selfish protection of one's self and one's property (Lindell and Prater 2003). Additionally, people in nearby areas move in to offer assistance, and when existing organizations seem incapable of meeting the needs of the emergency response, they evolve to take on new members and new tasks, or new organizations may emerge (Dynes 1970).

The National Response Framework (NRF) establishes a comprehensive all-hazards approach to enhance the ability of the United States to manage domestic incidents (natural disasters, terrorist attacks, and other catastrophic events). In addition to response from the federal government, key roles and responsibilities are aligned across tiers of government (federal, state, local, territorial, and tribal) and further include the whole community to augment government response (US Department of Homeland Security 2014b, 5–6).

The framework incorporates best practices and procedures from incident management disciplines—homeland security, emergency management, law enforcement, firefighting, public works, public health, responder and recovery worker health and safety, emergency medical services, and the private sector—and integrates them into a unified structure. It forms the basis of how the federal government coordinates with state, local, and tribal governments and the private sector during incidents. It establishes protocols to help do the following:

▲ Save lives and protect the health and safety of the public, responders, and recovery workers
▲ Ensure security of the homeland
▲ Prevent an imminent incident, including acts of terrorism, from occurring
▲ Protect and restore critical infrastructure and key resources

▲ Conduct law enforcement investigations to resolve the incident, apprehend the perpetrators, and collect and preserve evidence for prosecution and/or attribution

▲ Protect property and mitigate damages and impacts to individuals, communities, and the environment

▲ Facilitate recovery of individuals, families, businesses, governments, and the environment (US Department of Homeland Security 2008)

The NRF is built on the template of the National Incident Management System (NIMS), which provides a consistent doctrinal framework for incident management at all jurisdictional levels, regardless of the cause, size, or complexity of the incident. The purpose of the NRF is to provide an all-hazards approach to domestic incident management. The NRF provides the framework for federal interaction with state, local, and tribal governments, the private sector, and NGOs for domestic incident prevention, preparedness, response, and recovery activities. It serves as the foundation for the development of detailed supplemental plans and procedures to effectively and efficiently implement federal incident management activities and assistance in the context of specific types of incidents.

One component of the NRF is the establishment of joint field offices (JFOs), that is, temporary, federal, multi-agency coordination centers established locally following a disaster declared by the president. As shown in Figure 4-9, the JFOs provide unified coordination of national response from a centralized location close to the incident. Their primary responsibility is to serve as the primary field entity for federal response and assist with local threat response and provide incident support to state, local, tribal, and governments and the private sector. The JFO system enables the effective and efficient coordination of federal incident-related prevention by ensuring common situational awareness and providing "in the field" support for on-scene efforts and conducting broader operations that may extend beyond the incident site.

4.4.5 Recovery

Recovery is the period of time after a disaster. It can be of immediate, short-term, or protracted duration. During a disaster or immediately following, recovery often consists of providing assistance for preserving life and basic subsistence to affected populations. The recovery phase also includes damage assessment, debris clearance, and reconstruction of infrastructure and buildings. Beyond physical reconstruction, recovery should also address the social, economic, and political needs of the community. Community reconstruction can take a very long time, and after large-scale disasters, some communities never fully recover. For example, before Hurricane Katrina devastated New Orleans in 2005, the city had a population of approximately 485 000. One year later, population estimates were approximately 223 000, less than half of the pre-storm population. While New Orleans has recovered and in 2017 had an estimated population of 343 000, the city may never regain all of its lost residents (World Population Review 2017). When a portion of the population is missing, businesses lose revenue, schools lose students, and cities lose tax money. City services cannot function at optimum levels, and governments must provide services with fewer funds. Removing debris and rebuilding the physical elements of a city may be the easy part. It can be far more complex and difficult to repair the social fabric that makes a community function.

Figure 4-9

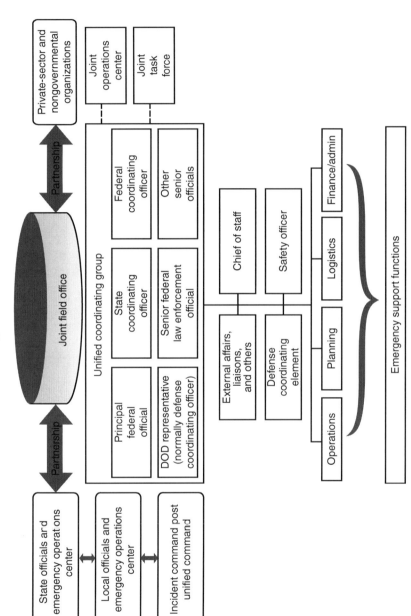

JFO structure for terrorist attacks (Federal Emergency Management Agency 2008).

For homeland security, the National Disaster Recovery Framework (NDRF)

> provides guidance that enables effective recovery support to disaster-impacted states, tribes, and local jurisdictions. It provides a flexible structure that enables disaster recovery managers to operate in a unified and collaborative manner. It also focuses on how best to restore, redevelop, and revitalize the health, social, economic, natural, and environmental fabric of the community and build a more resilient Nation. (US Department of Homeland Security 2014b, 7)

Effective recovery programs are possible only with good planning during the pre-impact phase. Communities should plan for the inevitable disaster, and pre-impact actions should include recovery planning. It is important for communities to develop the financial and material resources needed to support a prompt and effective disaster recovery. Plans should include responsibilities and assignments for impact assessment, debris management, infrastructure restoration, housing recovery, economic recovery, and linkage to hazard mitigation. Successful recovery plans should contain six components:

- ▲ First, communities should establish a recovery organization and chain of command.
- ▲ Second, recovery planning should identify temporary housing for potential evacuees.
- ▲ Third, the plan should indicate how to accomplish the essential tasks of clean up (e.g., damage assessment, debris removal and disposal, infrastructure restoration, and permit processing). This is an important step because clean up must be underway before the reconstruction can begin (Lindell and Prater 2003).
- ▲ Fourth, along with reconstruction, recovery plans should include methods to monitor contractors and retail pricing so that the population is not exploited.
- ▲ Fifth, plans also need to address historic sites that may be affected.
- ▲ Sixth, recovery plans should recognize that recovery period is a good time to enact policies for hazard mitigation projects in the community.

FOR EXAMPLE

How Much Does It Cost to Rebuild?

Hurricane Sandy, also known as Superstorm Sandy, affected the East Coast and then heavily hit the New York and New Jersey region on October 29, 2012. It was the second-largest Atlantic storm ever recorded, putting more than 8.5 million customers out of electricity, destroying thousands of homes, inflicting damage in the dimension of tens of billions of dollars, and causing at least 162 fatalities. In a large-scale preparedness effort, FEMA activated response centers and deployed over 900 personnel before the Sandy disaster struck. More than $1.2 billion in housing assistance and over $800 million for recovery such as restoration of infrastructure were delivered. FEMA used an online crisis management system to coordinate federal response, while after action it determined that, among other things, improved use of hazard-specific planning and analysis could have better driven operational decision making. This included authority issues between program staff at the Joint Field Office (JFO) and those in charge at local level, or responsible for liaison. Those shortfalls resulted in limited ability to implement a comprehensive and coordinated whole-community response (Federal Emergency Management Agency 2013a).

At state level, the Governor of New Jersey released a damage assessment according to which over 30 000 businesses and homes were destroyed or sustained structural damage, 42 000 were affected otherwise, and 233 00 persons registered for individual assistance. Total costs inflicted by Hurricane Sandy totaled $36.9 billion. This includes

- Repair, response and restoration costs (including, but by far not limited to, business; housing; water, waste, and sewer; utilities; transit, roads, and bridges.) = $29.4 billion
- Mitigation and prevention costs = $7.4 billion (State of New Jersey 2012)

SELF-CHECK

- Which of the following is not one of the phases of the disaster life cycle?
  a. Response
  b. Matrices
  c. Prevention
  d. Recovery
- Which of the following is an example of a federal mitigation program?
  a. FEMA
  b. NRF
  c. NFIP
  d. FHA
- The National Response Framework establishes a comprehensive all-hazards approach to enhance the ability of the United States to manage domestic incidents. True or false?
- The Joint Field Office system enables the effective and efficient coordination of state-run incident-related prevention only by providing "in the field" support to state and local on-scene efforts. True or false?

SUMMARY

In this chapter, you evaluated why risk assessment is important for homeland security programs, appraised different risk assessment models to program evaluation, assessed threats to communities using risk matrices, and judged the usefulness of threat and hazard identification processes and planning models.

Potential threats can be natural or man-made, and they can affect personal, economic, political, or environmental interests. Interests and threats intersect in program implementation, so it is important that we understand the "disaster impact process." Only through an assessment of threats and interests can we understand the impact disasters will have on the physical, social, economic, and political characteristics of our communities. Risk assessment aids the decision-making process, and it can be helpful in reducing costs to communities by allowing emergency managers to focus mitigation, risk reduction, and preparedness programs on those areas that need the most protection. In addition, risk assessment is an open-outcome process that should be evidence-based and data-driven and take nothing for granted. Critical thinking and continuous improvement are not signs of weakness in the process, but a natural part of the effort and ingredients of success (Harvey 2008; Kowalski 2008). Absence of critical thinking in threat identification and risk assessment can lead not only to self-serving policies but also to loss of public trust and to mass casualties (Ramsay and Kiltz 2014, 2).

KEY TERMS

Agricultural vulnerability	Agricultural plant and animal vulnerability to environmental extremes; the ability of livestock and crops to withstand disasters.
All-hazards plus approach	Comprehensive approach to prevention, protection, mitigation, response, and recovery that emphasizes the development of capabilities, which are common to natural and man-made disasters, while also including the development of capabilities that are uniquely relevant to specific types of disasters.
Composite exposure indicator (CEI)	A hazard assessment model that ranks potential for losses in a given region for single or multiple hazards by assigning a numeric value to the exposure potential for communities. FEMA has used this approach to quantify 14 variables in 3100 US counties, with rankings based on the amount of each variable present.

Criticality assessment	Process that identifies and evaluates an organization's assets based on a variety of criteria.
Demographic impacts	Effects on a community's population after a disaster.
Disaster impact process	The way to examine the effects a disaster will have on a community. The first step of the disaster impact process is the pre-impact phase, which includes planning and mitigation efforts. The second phase is the actual disaster event, which includes specific hazard conditions and community response. The third phase is the emergency management intervention phase, which includes response, recovery, and program evaluation.
Disaster response	The reaction individuals have when faced with the onset of a disaster.
Economic impacts	Changes in asset values after a disaster that are measured by the cost of repair or replacement.
Hazard assessment	The process by which we identify new and existing threats and assess the level of risk to a population.
Hazard exposure	The likelihood that specific disasters will occur; the probability of occurrence of a given event magnitude.
Hazard mitigation	Sustained action to alleviate or eliminate risks to life and property from natural or man-made hazard events.
Human vulnerability	Individual vulnerability to environmental extremes.
Interests	The human (individual or group), environmental, political, or economic components of society that we seek to protect through homeland security programs
Matrix	A tool for decision making that uses a grid design to weigh the frequency of an event against its severity to rank potential costs or damage.
National Flood Insurance Program (NFIP)	FEMA-administered program that features three major components: flood insurance, floodplain management, and flood hazard mapping.
National Infrastructure Protection Plan (NIPP)	Provides the foundation for an integrated and collaborative approach of stakeholders from all current 16 critical infrastructure sectors, all 50 states, and all levels of government and industry to manage risks and enhance resilience by reducing vulnerabilities, minimizing consequences, identifying and disrupting threats, and speeding up response and recovery.

National Planning Frameworks	Set the strategy and doctrine for building, sustaining, and delivering the core capabilities identified in the National Preparedness Goal. They describe the coordinating structures and alignment of key roles and responsibilities for the whole community and are integrated to ensure interoperability across all mission areas. There are five frameworks: National Prevention Framework, National Protection Framework, National Mitigation Framework, National Response Framework, and National Disaster Recovery Framework.
National Preparedness Goal	Defines the (currently 32) core capabilities required to achieve the goal of "a secure and resilient Nation with the capabilities required across the whole community to prevent, protect against, mitigate, respond to, and recover from the threats and hazards that pose the greatest risk."
National Preparedness System	Describes the process employed to build, sustain, and deliver core capabilities in order to achieve the goal of a secure and resilient nation.
National Terrorism Advisory System (NTAS)	Increase preparedness for attacks that may occur and includes information on protection from threats and guidance for citizens to help detect or prevent attacks before they occur.
Physical vulnerability	The ability to prepare for, cope with, and withstand disasters; this includes human vulnerability, agricultural ability, and structural vulnerability.
Political impacts	Changes in the political structure of a community after a disaster.
Preparedness actions	Pre-impact actions that provide the human and material resources needed to support active responses at the time of hazard impact.
Prevention actions	Actions performed by the whole community to counter a detected imminent threat to the homeland in the form or an impending terrorist attack.
Protection actions	Actions performed by the whole community to take precaution against terrorist threats, other man-made hazards, and natural disasters.
Psychosocial impacts	Effects on mental health and the ability to get treatment after a disaster.

Recovery	The period of time after a disaster. It can be of immediate, short-term, or protracted duration.
Risk management	The process for identifying, analyzing, and communicating risk and accepting, avoiding, transferring, or controlling it to an acceptable level considering associated costs and benefits of any actions taken.
Risk reduction	An examination of the actions necessary to decrease detected or projected levels of danger and to identify the resources required for implementing those actions.
Social vulnerability	A person's or group's ability to anticipate, prepare for, or cope with disasters.
Suspicious Activity Reporting (SAR)	Encouragement of citizens by DHS to report observed behavior reasonably indicative of pre-operational planning associated with terrorism or other criminal activity to local law enforcement in a prompt and detailed manner, to help prevent terrorist attacks or other violent crimes.
Structural vulnerability	A building's ability to withstand extreme stresses or features that allow hazardous materials to infiltrate the building.
Threat	Natural or man-made event that can destroy or damage human, environmental, political, or economic components of society.
Threat assessment	Process that identifies and evaluates threats based on various criteria
Threat and Hazard Identification and Risk Assessment (THIRA)	Process drives strategic priorities by helping communities determine capability targets and those resources that are required to meet them.
Vulnerability assessment	Process that identifies weaknesses in a structure, individual, or function.

ASSESS YOUR UNDERSTANDING

Go to www.wiley.com/go/Kilroy/Threats_to_Homeland_Security to assess your knowledge of the basics of threat assessment.

Summary Questions

1. Hazards only occur naturally. True or false?
2. The disaster impact process includes event-specific conditions. True or false?
3. CEI is a program that uses geographic information systems. True or false?
4. Effective recovery programs benefit from planning during the pre-impact phase. True or false?
5. Which of the following is not a part of the preparedness cycle?
   (a) Mitigation
   (b) Response
   (c) Recovery
   (d) Vulnerability
6. Which of the following is not a social characteristic that can be impacted by natural disasters that affect homeland security?
   (a) Demographic
   (b) Economic
   (c) Psychosocial
   (d) Ecological
7. Which of the following is not an assessment method?
   (a) Homeland Security Index
   (b) HAZUS
   (c) Composite Exposure Index
   (d) Vulnerability assessment
8. According to the Disaster Mitigation Act, which of the following is not a type of hazard that local governments and states must address in order for their plans to be approved?
   (a) Tsunami
   (b) Terrorism
   (c) Cold
   (d) Dam failure

Applying This Chapter

1. Your boss asks you to explain the processes/missions of the National Preparedness System. How would you do this? How do those missions relate to the goal of fostering a resilient nation?
2. During a community leaders meeting, someone asks how vulnerable your community is to terrorist attacks. Your initial planning assessment was that

this type of threat was low, but new information at the meeting indicates the need for a new risk assessment. Develop a risk matrix that includes terrorist threats. Explain some techniques that a community can employ to reduce the risk of this type of threat.

3. You are an analyst for an energy company that is expanding its nuclear power generation capabilities by building new nuclear power plants. You are responsible for providing a recommendation for possible sites for the new plant. Which hazard assessment method(s) would be most helpful in your analysis? What are some community characteristics you would consider when planning a new plant?

4. You are an urban planner in a major coastal city. You are responsible for making recommendations for policies that will help reduce risks from hurricanes and flooding. What threat assessment process would you use and what types of mitigation policies would you recommend? What capabilities could the town develop and what types of activities could it regulate to reduce risks?

Risk Management Models

Models are analytical tools. They are not authoritative, meaning they can help assess possible outcomes in planning efforts, but they may not be deterministic in predicting outcomes. Based on the models described in this chapter, design your own risk management model, looking at one particular man-made or natural hazard.

Vulnerability Assessment

Within your local community, perform a vulnerability assessment for various hazards, whether natural or man-made. Determine implications of your micro analysis at the macro and system analysis levels.

5

CRITICAL INFRASTRUCTURE SECURITY, EMERGENCY PREPAREDNESS, AND OPERATIONAL CONTINUITY

A Contemporary Approach to Homeland Security for the Critical Infrastructure Enterprise

Steven Kuhr

Emergency Management and Continuity, Colorado Springs Utilities, Colorado Springs, CO, USA

Starting Point

Go to www.wiley.com/go/Kilroy/Threats_to_Homeland_Security to assess your knowledge of critical infrastructure security.
Determine where you need to concentrate your effort.

What You'll Learn in This Chapter

▲ The definition of critical infrastructure

▲ The development of critical infrastructure policy

▲ The identification of the critical infrastructure sectors

▲ The application of homeland security leadership principles in managing a program to protect critical infrastructure

After Studying This Chapter, You'll Be Able To

▲ Develop an approach to critical infrastructure protection

▲ Apply a risk-based approach to protecting critical infrastructure including the use of risk assessments and homeland security intelligence

▲ Assess threats to critical infrastructure using quantitative and qualitative risk assessments

▲ Integrate a critical infrastructure protection program with state, regional, and local homeland security, emergency management, law enforcement, fire/emergency medical services (EMS) agencies, and partners within and external to the critical infrastructure sector

Threats to Homeland Security: Reassessing the All-Hazards Perspective, Second Edition.
Edited by Richard J. Kilroy, Jr.
© 2018 John Wiley & Sons, Inc. Published 2018 by John Wiley & Sons, Inc.
Companion website: www.wiley.com/go/Kilroy/Threats_to_Homeland_Security

INTRODUCTION

Critical infrastructures (CIs) provide not only the conveniences that make American life comfortable but also the lifeline services that make the American way of life possible. Lifeline services such as electric generation, transmission, and distribution provide foundational lifeline services that not only provide their base service but are also a part of a complex system-of-systems network of dependent and interdependent infrastructures that are so interactive and interconnected that they are vulnerable to failures of each of the systems at many levels. Protecting critical infrastructure (CI) therefore requires an aggressive, comprehensive, and well-planned approach to risk assessments and management, intelligence, physical security, cybersecurity, **emergency operations** and crisis management, and recovery and restoration.

> The Nation's critical infrastructure provides the essential services that underpin American society. Proactive and coordinated efforts are necessary to strengthen and maintain secure, functioning, and resilient critical infrastructure—including assets, networks, and systems—that are vital to public confidence and the Nation's safety, prosperity, and well-being. Presidential Policy Directive 21—Critical Infrastructure Security and Resilience, February 12, 2013

In this chapter, you will analyze the critical infrastructure environment and the national and homeland security implications from a threat and consequence perspective as well as critical infrastructure protection program choices. You'll also learn to distinguish between the various national and homeland security policy players both within and outside government. Finally, you'll appraise the threat–hazard risk situation in the contemporary critical infrastructure risk protection environment.

5.1 Defining Critical Infrastructure

The very essence of modern life is made possible by the things and gadgets that help us enjoy, among many conveniences, the following: safe and reliable utilities such as electricity, which in itself serves as a foundational utility for which most other conveniences are dependent on; clean drinkable water; natural gas that helps us enjoy a warm comfortable home and workplace and also allows us to prepare meals in a safe and sanitary manner; the least considered utility, wastewater systems, which help to ensure that contemporary life is sanitary and disease-free; storm water systems that ensure that our communities remain dry and safe during periods of unstable weather; transportation services that help us get around town or to work, take us on vacation, and help us shop for the food we enjoy; and communications that in themselves are vast and broad and include many modalities that we rarely consider when we make a call, send a text message, shoot an email to a friend or colleague, watch the 6 o'clock news, or catch an old movie.

The US government defines critical infrastructure as "systems and assets, whether physical or virtual, so vital to the United States that incapacity or destruction of such systems and assets would have a debilitating impact on security, national economic security, national public health or safety, or any combination of those matters" (PATRIOT Act, 130).

It is important to note that no one critical infrastructure sector can be seen as independent, suggesting that all are interdependent on another or multiple critical infrastructures. While we will examine this in greater detail, consider for a moment that all of the infrastructures mentioned are dependent on the safe and effective generation, transmission, and distribution of electricity. Let's take a quick look at drinking water, for example. Without electricity the water simply does not flow. Water transmission systems (raw water reservoirs, water tunnels, and large pipes), water treatment plants (WTPs), and water distribution systems (drinkable water storage tanks, pumps, and small pipe systems) all require electricity to operate. **Industrial control systems (ICS)**, for example, **supervisory control and data acquisition (SCADA)**, which provides an electronic means to manage and control the drinking water system from the reservoir to the tap, require electricity and safe and secure communications and hardwire and microwave communication networks. Electricity cannot be generated without water, which is part of electricity generation during a number of steps in the process, especially generator cooling systems. This chicken-and-egg scenario is hence referred to as interdependency.

5.1.1 Defining the Sectors

From a homeland security programmatic perspective, CI exists among 16 infrastructure sectors and subsectors as defined by the National Infrastructure Protection Plan (NIPP) (US DHS 2013). The NIPP, originally issued in 2009, was reissued in 2013 with the following goals:

1. Assess and analyze threats to, vulnerabilities of, and consequences to critical infrastructure to inform risk management activities (risk assessment).
2. Secure critical infrastructure against human, physical and cyber threats through sustainable efforts to reduce risk, while accounting for the costs and benefits of security investments.
3. Enhance critical infrastructure resilience by minimizing the adverse consequences of incidents through advanced planning and mitigation efforts and by employing effective responses to save lives and ensure rapid recovery of essential services.
4. Share actionable and relevant information across the critical infrastructure community to build awareness and enable risk-informed decision making.
5. Promote learning and adaptation during exercises and incidents (NIPP 2013, 5).

While the NIPP's goals are designed to provide guidance at the national level, these goals are sound and can be applied to protect CI at a local or enterprise level. For example, the director of security at a public drinking water utility must be aware of the threats and vulnerabilities that must be confronted from a security planning and operational perspective (risk assessment—goal 1); develop and provide robust security policies, plans, and procedures in order to protect the drinking water infrastructure against human-made physical and cyber threats as well as natural hazards (goals 2 and 3) as defined in goal 1, risk assessments; access and produce actionable intelligence across the homeland security and industry community so as to develop security and natural hazard protective measures based on intelligence-led security programming considering physical and cyber threat trends and natural hazard vulnerabilities (goal 4); and ensure that security and emergency operations are focused on informed decision making based on information and intelligence provided through risk assessments and an intelligence-oriented program (goal 5) (Table 5-1).

The NIPP has identified 16 critical infrastructure sectors, all of which are represented by sector-specific plans, a number of which are subdivided into subsectors, and all of which are represented by industry-specific sector coordinating councils (Figure 5-1).

5.1.2 Information Sharing and Analysis Centers

One of the greatest values provided by the NIPP is the information sharing and analysis components of the plan where information is shared by sector affiliated government agencies, the **Information Sharing and Analysis Centers (ISACs)**, and the sector/industry organizes which participate in information sharing. While we will discuss the application of intelligence, especially homeland security intelligence (HSINT) and industry-specific intelligence (ISINT), later, it is important to note that intelligence is part of a dynamic and comprehensive risk- and intelligence-driven CI protection program. In essence, we will see that risk assessments, including threat, vulnerability, consequence, and impact analyses, are not static as previously thought. Rather, risk analysis in today's high-threat/high-risk infrastructure environment is a constantly moving target, especially when we introduce intelligence into the equation.

FOR EXAMPLE

Healthcare and Public Health ISAC

The National Health (NH) ISAC, is a nonprofit organization for the nation's healthcare and public health critical infrastructure, recognized by the US Department of Health and Human Services (HHS), the HHS Health Sector Coordinating Council (SCC), the US Department of Homeland Security (DHS), the National Council of ISACs (representing all the nation's critical infrastructures ISACs), intelligence agencies, law enforcement sector, and the health sector.

NH-ISAC is a member-driven security intelligence information exchange among trusted entities for the purposes of providing members with actionable cybersecurity for intelligence situational awareness, information sharing capabilities supporting effective countermeasure solutions, and coordinated cybersecurity incident response. As a nonprofit organization, NH-ISAC represents a trusted community comprised of national healthcare and public health critical infrastructure owners and operators and the organizations supporting the health sector.

The mission of the NH-ISAC is to foster, enable, and preserve the public trust by advancing health sector cybersecurity resilience and the ability to prepare for and respond to threats and vulnerabilities (FDA 2014).

Table 5-1: Critical Infrastructure Sectors

Sector Subsectors	Sector coordinating council	Information sharing organization	Sector	Sector coordinating council	Information sharing organization
Chemical	Yes	No	Financial services	Yes	No
Commercial facilities • Entertainment and media • Gaming • Lodging • Outdoor events (amusement parks) • Public assembly (stadiums) • Real estate • Retail (shopping malls) • Sports leagues	Yes	Yes	Food and agriculture	Yes	No
Communications	Yes	Yes	Government facilities	Yes	No
Critical manufacturing	Yes	No	Healthcare and public health	Yes	No
Dams	Yes	No	Information technology	Yes	No
Defense industrial base	Yes	Yes	Nuclear reactors, materials, and waste	Yes	No

(Continued)

Table 5-1: (Continued)

Sector Subsectors	Sector coordinating council	Information sharing organization
Emergency services	Yes	Yes
Transportation systems • Aviation • Highway infrastructure and motor carrier • Maritime transportation system • Mass transit and passenger rail • Pipeline system • Freight rail • Postal and shipping	Yes	Yes
Water and wastewater systems	Yes	Yes
Energy • Electric • Oil • Natural gas	Yes	Yes

DHS, n.d.

Figure 5-1

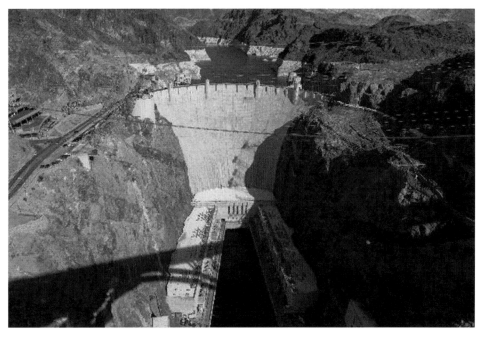

Hoover Dam, Lake Mead National Recreation Area, Nevada. Source: Photo courtesy of Alexander Stephens, US Bureau of Reclamation (2016).

SELF-CHECK

- Which of the following is not part of the transportation systems sector?

  a. Aviation

  b. Entertainment and media

  c. Pipeline systems

  d. Freight rail

- The National Infrastructure Plan defines 16 critical infrastructure sectors. True or false?

- An ISAC is an international surveillance action center. True or false?

5.2 Known Threats to Critical Infrastructure

Modern infrastructures are constantly under threats and hazards be it natural hazards, terrorism, crime, and risks inherent in the operation of particular system such as mechanical and/or technical failures. The natural hazard threat is defined by local risk assessments that determine the hazard, the likelihood of that hazard occurring, a determination of what vulnerability the hazard can have on an infrastructure, and the impact to the infrastructure, interdependent infrastructures, and ultimately the community. Take, for example, a water treatment plant (WTP) that is located in the wildland–urban interface (WUI) in a small community. A wildland fire at or near the WTP can present with a number of variables that should have been captured in a comprehensive risk assessment (CRA) and then planned for as part of the Emergency and Continuity Plan (ECP) for the facility and its dependencies. The fire, for example, can present with a threat, first and foremost, to WTP personnel. Therefore the risk assessment must ask the questions: Can the WTP operate without personnel onsite? For how long? Is there a **continuity course of action (CCOA)** such as remote plant operations? The ECP must then take into account the risk assessment, in particular the questions asked and answered, and capture this in actionable plan content. A key point here is the direct linkage between risk assessments and actionable emergency and continuity plans.

5.2.1 Natural Hazard Threats

Weather is a hazard that is constant and must be accounted for in risk assessments and ECPs based on local meteorological patterns. An emergency manager for a heavy commuter rail system on the East Coast must place great emphasis on planning for coastal storms such as hurricanes and nor'easters, whereas his or her counterpart in the Pacific Northwest must place emphasis on earthquake and tsunami planning. And while these two scenarios present with similar impacts, such as flooding, not-so-subtle differences exist that require intense focus and hazard-specific planning. While coastal storms and tsunamis, for example, both present with major flooding hazards, a coastal storm presents with high wind hazards while the tsunami may be accompanied by an earthquake. This leads to a discussion on all-hazards planning versus hazard-specific planning, which will be discussed in greater detail later in this chapter.

Severe weather, including tornadic activity, is a natural hazard that is constant throughout the nation. The term "severe weather" is often misunderstood to represent any weather scenario that can cause danger to a community. The National Weather Service (NWS) (Severe Weather Definitions n.d.) provides clarity on the definition of a number of severe weather hazards that typically refers to significant thunderstorm activity and associated storms that can produce severe lightening, large hail, rotation including tornadoes, and flash flooding. For example, a severe thunderstorm is defined in part as

A thunderstorm that can produce a tornado, winds of at least 58 mph, and/or hail at least 1″ in diameter. Structural wind damage may imply the occurrence of a severe thunderstorm. A thunderstorm wind equal to or greater than 40 mph (35 knots) and/or hail of at least 1″ is defined as approaching severe.

Likewise, the NWS defines a tornado as

a violently rotating column of air, usually pendant to a cumulonimbus, with circulation reaching the ground. It nearly always starts as a funnel cloud and may be accompanied by a loud roaring noise. On a local scale, it is the most destructive of all atmospheric phenomena.

These definitions are very specific and therefore have direct meaning to the protection of critical infrastructure when one considers how these storms can damage, destroy, and disrupt critical infrastructure services. Consider, for example, how a severe thunderstorm can impact the production of electricity. While strong winds can damage transmission and distribution lines, large hail can cause damage to various exposed components such as electric generation plants, substations, and transformers both large and small. Flash flooding can lead to damage to fuel supplies needed to generate electricity. Similarly we can point to any number of severe weather scenarios that can cause disruption of transportation services. Heavy commuter rail can be impacted by heavy rain, which can lead to flash flooding, lightning that can damage electrical components, and so forth.

Tropical/coastal weather as a category is broad and includes a variety of storm types. For our discussion we will consider hurricanes, tropical storms, and nor'easters. A hurricane is a cyclonic ocean-borne storm in the Atlantic Ocean, Caribbean Sea, Gulf of Mexico, and Eastern Pacific Ocean with sustained winds of at least 74 miles per hour. Tropical storms can be seen as "hurricane lite" storms in that they are similar in characteristics but with wind speeds from 39 to 73 miles per hour. Cyclonic ocean-borne storms in the western Pacific and Indian Oceans reaching hurricane status are called cyclones and typhoons, respectively. The National Hurricane Center (NHC) categorizes hurricanes into five different levels based on the Saffir–Simpson Hurricane Scale, which details wind speeds and destructive characteristics of a hurricane (NHC n.d.):

▲ Category 1—74–95 mph
▲ Category 2—95–110 mph
▲ Category 3—111–129 mph (major/devastating hurricane)
▲ Category 4—130–156 mph (major/catastrophic hurricane)
▲ Category 5—157 mph and higher (major/catastrophic hurricane)

(For a detailed description of the five categories, see Saffir–Simpson Scale at http://www.nhc.noaa.gov/aboutsshws.php)

The hurricane season in the United States begins on June 1 and concludes on November 30. However, micro-seasons generally exist in varying areas of the United States. For example, a hurricane requires 84° water to support convection. Emergency managers and owners and operators of critical infrastructure along the East Coast, for example, monitor water temperatures throughout the season to get a sense of the timing for the local season to become active. In the northeast, for example, August is typically the time when the hurricane season becomes active. Understanding this gives emergency managers and **critical infrastructure protection (CIP)** officials some breathing room to conduct preparedness efforts while monitoring the season and actual tropical cyclone activity.

Nor'easters differ from hurricanes in a number of ways, yet they resemble hurricanes in their impact and short- and long-term effects. The National Weather Service (NWS) defines a nor'easter, in part, as "A strong low pressure system that affects the Mid-Atlantic and New England States which can form over land or coastal waters" (NWS Glossary n.d.). While nor'easters are known to occur during the fall and spring seasons, these destructive storms are typically winter season events capable of generating winds up to and including hurricane intensity, heavy precipitation as both snow and rain, and storm surge and significant oceanic wave activity that can be a threat to life and property as well as beach erosion. Wind gusts associated with these storms can exceed hurricane force in intensity. A nor'easter gets its name from the continuously strong northeasterly winds blowing in from the ocean ahead of the storm and over the coastal areas.

Hurricane Katrina is perhaps one of the best examples of the impact hurricanes can have on critical infrastructure. Hurricane Katrina (Katrina) began life as a tropical storm on August 23, 2005, near Bermuda (Townsend 2006, 1). Over the course of the next few days, Katrina grew to catastrophic strength defined as a Category 5 hurricane on the Saffir–Simpson Hurricane Scale, with winds greater than 155 miles per hour. As the storm grew in intensity, it began a westerly path entering the Gulf of Mexico, making landfall in four Gulf Coast states. This powerful hurricane "carved a wide swath of catastrophic damage and inflicted large loss of life" (Knabb et al. 2005, 1). Katrina was the costliest and one of the deadliest hurricane disasters in the United States. Making landfall as a Category 1 storm in Florida, the storm resulted in destruction and fatalities, uncommon for a Category 1 event. As the storm traveled west, it matured in the Gulf of Mexico to a Category 5 storm. Making landfall in Louisiana and Mississippi as a Category 3 storm, the size and intensity of the storm resulted in staggering destruction and deaths in the landfall states as well as Alabama and the Florida panhandle (Knabb et al. 2005, 1). Katrina is perhaps the most significant natural disaster, in terms of loss of life, human suffering, destruction, and cost, in US history. Katrina resulted in 1833 deaths among five states, 43 tornadoes among four states, and storm surge as high as 28 ft in Mississippi and 16 ft in Louisiana (TWC 2009). The Katrina disaster resulted in $81 billion in damage of which approximately half of that was categorized as insured losses. In total, approximately 93 000 square miles of the United States was impacted by Katrina. This is roughly the size of England (Townsend 2006, 1).

The impact Hurricane Katrina had on critical infrastructure was profound. Miller (n.d.) states that the loss of infrastructure in a developed nation was the greatest since World War II and goes on to say the simultaneous failure of just about all critical infrastructure sectors presented problems for public officials in ways that had not been previously considered (192). The loss of infrastructure, communications infrastructure in particular, contributed greatly to the command and control failures. Communication systems were largely destroyed across the Katrina-impacted region. This included the loss of approximately 100 commercial radio stations, 2000 cellular telephone towers, close to 200 central office stations, approximately 40 911 call centers, and local radio towers and associated networks (193–194). The energy sector also suffered extensive damage and destruction. Mississippi Power (a Southern Company asset) is said to have been hardest impacted utility organization (Feder 2005), as it sustained damage to 65–75% of its electric transmission and distribution assets as well as the loss of more than 6000 miles of power lines (Southwire 2012). Close to 300 electric substations were also damaged. At least one electric generation plan was taken offline due to flood conditions.

Water and wastewater systems were also greatly impacted by Hurricane Katrina. The Congressional Research Service (Copeland 2005) reports that drinking water and sewerage/wastewater systems were damaged throughout the Gulf Coast with emphasis on drinking water and wastewater treatment facilities. It is estimated that over 1200 drinking water systems and more than 200 wastewater treatment facilities were affected. Iconic of the interdependent nature of utility infrastructure, many treatment facilities failed to function due to the lack of electricity and the subsequent failure to pump either raw water or raw sewerage. While a number of treatment facilities did have generators as part of their **continuity of operations** capability, fuel supplies were limited; therefore, generators and the functions they were intended to support were nonfunctional. This once again demonstrates the interdependent nature of critical infrastructures in this case the Water and Wastewater and Energy Sectors.

Wildfire is another natural hazard that can lead to destruction of critical infrastructure assets. In 2012, the Waldo Canyon Wildfire, the most destructive wildfire in Colorado history, resulted in the loss of 18 247 acres of forest, 345 homes, and two deaths (City of Colorado Springs 2012, 5). When incidents such as these occur, emphasis should be placed on the protection of life and property. This transcends to owners and operators of critical infrastructure. For example, the burn area is home or is directly adjacent to a number of critical infrastructures and national assets such as the US Air Force Academy. A number of utility assets were in the burn area and were subject to damage and destruction including a 40 000 acre foot reservoir and dam, a number of water treatment plants, water storage and distribution facilities, electric high voltage transmission and distribution lines, and community natural gas distribution. From a protection perspective, the questions that need to be asked are as follows:

▲ Is there a threat to the life safety of the asset workforce?
▲ Is evacuation needed?
▲ What is the current and forecasted impact?
▲ What is the asset disruption impact analysis?
▲ What protective measures need to be taken?
▲ What operational continuity courses of action can be applied?

The Waldo Canyon Fire provides good insight into the impact that a wildfire can have on critical infrastructure. Included in the 18 000 acres are a number of heavily populated residential communities located on the west side of Colorado Springs. These communities are served by Colorado Springs Utilities (CSU), a municipal utility organization that proudly serves as one of the nation's largest four-service utility. CSU provides electricity, natural gas, water, and wastewater services to a population of 500 000 in the city of Colorado Springs and a number of communities throughout El Paso County, Colorado, many of which were within the wildfire burn area. All services provide to the affected communities had to be aggressively monitored for potential or actual damage or wildfire destruction. At one point natural gas service to west-side communities were disrupted as a fire protective measure. This led to an ambitious gas service restoration operation when it was safe to do so.

FOR EXAMPLE

The Rim Fire, California

The Rim Fire, which began in the Stanislaus National Forest in California, progressed along the Tuolumne River Canyon and the "Rim of the World" Vista Point (SFPUC 2014, 5). The Rim Fire destroyed 257 315 acres and 112 structures. Early in the incident the fire progressed to a number of critical infrastructure assets to include two hydroelectric power houses, the Hetch Hetchy Reservoir, and surrounding watershed. As the fire progressed, it threatened the Hetch Hetchy Water and Power system, which provides electric power for San Francisco as well as water supply for most of the Bay Area (SFPUC 2014, 38). There was some damage to utility infrastructure with power outages to the burn area; however, at no point was water service disrupted to the 2.6 million customers of the Bay Area. A simple look at the impact here can help one understand the vast impact that wildfire can have on not only single critical infrastructure but also multiple dependent and interdependent infrastructures.

Earthquakes pose a significant threat to critical infrastructure by way of damage to built infrastructure, which leads to damage and disruption along lifeline- and technology-based dependent and interdependent systems. Earthquakes in densely populated centers can lead to not only direct destruction and loss of life but also degradation and even full disruption of lifeline systems such as electric and water utilities, communications, and transportation. A 2012 report by the Water Research Foundation (Eidinger and Davis 2012) provided an analysis of earthquake impact to water systems from the study of earthquakes in Chile, New Zealand, and Japan. Commonalities in damage to infrastructure included damage to buried water transmission mains (24–96″ diameter) and distribution mains (6–12″ diameter) constructed with cast iron, cement, welded steel, and high density polyethylene. Water storage tanks of various constructions were also damaged as were water treatment plants and pump stations. A picture is clearly painted here of the potential for complete collapse of water supply systems to communities resulting in a potential catastrophic loss of drinking water and water for fire suppression, critical functions needed for mass human care, and community protection in times of any disaster, especially earthquakes.

5.2.2 Terrorism and Human Threats

The threat of terrorist activity against critical infrastructure is evident through the lens of many recent terrorist attacks. While the bulk of these attacks were targeted at civilian populations, the corollary impact on critical infrastructure can be profound. The September 2001 attacks on the Pentagon in Northern Virginia and the World Trade Center in New York City resulted in not only catastrophic loss of life but also catastrophic damage to critical infrastructure systems. The attack on the World Trade Center in New York led to significant degradation to landline and cellular communication systems through the loss of telephone system equipment located near "ground zero." In addition to that was the loss of transportation infrastructure. Significant damage occurred in both the New York City Subway and Port Authority Trans-Hudson Subway systems. Attacks on transportation infrastructure can also be seen through the September 11 attacks followed by the 2004 Madrid, Spain, railway bombing and the 2005 coordinated attacks on public transportation infrastructure on the London Underground and surface busses.

The threat to lifeline utilities is of both a physical nature and of a cyber nature. In April 2013, perhaps the most notable physical attack on utility infrastructure occurred when gunmen attacked the Pacific, Gas, and Electric (PG&E) Metcalf substation that provides electric power to parts of Silicon Valley, California. At about 1:00 a.m. on April 16, 2013, an actor or actors entered a communications vault and severed telephone cables. Shortly after, actor(s) opened fire with high-powered weapons on electric substation infrastructure, firing rounds for 19 min. This attack resulted in the loss of 17 transformer units and large spill of transformer oil. Power outages were avoided by rerouting electricity through the distribution network around the site and by having regional power plants temporarily increasing generation capacity.

FOR EXAMPLE

Ukraine Power Grid Attacks

On December 23, 2015, a long-feared event occurred when cyber-attackers seized control of the electric power system in Ukraine. This attack resulted in the disruption of power to approximately 225 000 customers for as long as six hours. More than 50 electric substations were directly impacted by this attack. Concurrently a cyber-attack (denial of service) occurred on the utility telephone system rendering it useless for interaction with customers (E-ISAC 2016). At 3:35 p.m. local time, the electric distribution company Ukrainian *Kyivoblenergo* reported customer outages, which were later attributed to unauthorized access to the company's supervisory control and data acquisition (SCADA) system. Through the access into the SCADA system, seven 110 kV and twenty-three 35 kV electric substations were simply disconnected from the distribution network. It was later determined that in addition to Ukrainian *Kyivoblenergo*, two additional electric distribution companies were attacked in a coordinated cyber assault, resulting in the large number of customer outages (E-ISAC 2016). This incident, the first known or at the very least publicly acknowledged cyber-attack on the power grid, took the electric utility industry by storm as industry leaders, security professionals, and emergency managers scurried to learn about the incident and ways to prevent such an incident from occurring domestically. For a period of time, preceding the Ukraine attack, the industry was monitoring information and intelligence on BlackEnergy malware long known to be a threat to the electric grid. This incident resulted from weaponization of Microsoft Office documents with the BlackEnergy3 malware variant (E-ISAC 2016).

5.2.2.1 Insider Threat/Workplace Violence

Today's operators of critical infrastructure must be sensitive to a vast threat ecosystem that they must confront. This includes physical security and cyber security threats as well as natural hazards germane to the geolocation of the infrastructure. From a security perspective, the external threat is great. Today's CI operators must deal with potential and actual sabotage from a physical and cyber security perspective by individuals and organizations outside the organization from single actor trespass incidents to transnational terrorist and cyber threats. That said, it is important to understand that the insider threat brings with it risks on both physical and cyber security perspectives. The National Infrastructure Advisory Council (NIAC) in its 2008 report on the insider threat (Noonan and Archuleta 2008) states that any organization can be confronted with insiders, essentially employees who are otherwise entrusted to not only be a part of the service provided by an organization but also help secure it. Insiders can not only cause disruption to operations through sabotage but also remove trade and other corporate secrets through theft of both physical and electronic properties as well as espionage and cause tremendous damage to computer systems through the malicious placement of malware. On the extreme end of the threat spectrum, insiders are also in a position to conduct workplace violence against other members of the workforce as well as contractors, customers, and visitors. Today's active shooter phenomenon is a threat that organizations must confront head on, especially when one considers the access that most employees have to both secure and unsecure areas of an organization's physical infrastructure and facilities. The NIAC report (2008) actually defines an insider threat to critical infrastructure as

> one or more individuals with the access and/or inside knowledge of a company, organization, or enterprise that would allow them to exploit the vulnerabilities of that entity's security, systems, services, products, or facilities with the intent to cause harm. (5)

This definition is broad enough to cover the spectrum of threats discussed herein.

As an example, Sergey Aleynikov, a Wall Street computer programmer downloaded 32 megabytes of proprietary corporate computer code during his 2007–2009 employment. Aleynikov intended to sell the code to another organization, which could have cost the original employer millions of dollars. However, his crime was detected and he was convicted of corporate theft and transportation of stolen property (FBI n.d.). With regard to hostile and violent acts in the workplace, between 2006 and 2010 an average of 551 workplace homicides occurred annually with 518 occurring in 2010. Seventy-eight percent of the homicides in 2010 were caused by firearm incidents, 83% of which occurred in the private sector (ISC 2013), which are the primary owners and operators of America's critical infrastructure. Further, when one considers workplace violence, we must remember that the February 1993 bombing of the World Trade Center in New York, the April 1995 bombing of the Alfred P. Murrah Federal Building in Oklahoma City, and the September 2001 attacks on the World Trade Center in New York City and Pentagon in Northern Virginia were attacks on places where people work; hence these incidents must be viewed in an extreme context as attacks on the workplace.

5.2.2.2 Active Shooter and Violent Encounters

On April 20, 1999, high school students Eric Harris and Dylan Klebold shot and killed 12 students and a teacher and injured 21 others in what would be, to many, the watershed event that would spark a national phenomenon of mass violence through the use of firearms and edged weapons such as knives and axes. Owners and operators of critical infrastructure are not immune from the threat of an active shooter or violent encounter incident. Active shooter incidents have become commonplace in the United States and abroad as a means to commit mass homicide associated with various motivations including terrorism and hate. Two iconic terrorist attacks employing active shooter tactics are the November 13, 2015, attacks in Paris, France, where throughout the course a few hours terrorists shot and killed over 130 and injuring countless others; and, the December 2, 2015, firearms attacks at a holiday party that resulted in the death of 14 and injuries to 22 others. Tragically, and recently, a terrorist armed with firearms shot and killed 49 at a nightclub, which is favored by the American gay community, in Orlando, Florida. The Federal Bureau of Investigation identified 160 active shooter incidents between 2000 and 2013 (FBI 2014) in the United States with 11.4 incidents occurring annually.

Many active shooter incidents have occurred in educational facilities such as the April 2007 massacre at Virginia Polytechnic Institute where 32 were killed and the December 2012 Newtown, Connecticut, school shooting where 26 were shot and killed. Keeping in mind that education facilities are considered critical infrastructure, the National Infrastructure Protection Plan identifies education facilities as a subsector of the government sector. Another critical infrastructure sector that has experienced a number of active shooter incidents is the healthcare and public health sector. In an FBI study of active shooter incidents between 2000 and 2013 (US DOJ 2013), four active shooter incidents in healthcare facilities resulted in 10 deaths and 10 people injured including two law enforcement (LE) officers.

5.2.3 Nontraditional Aviation Technology (NTAT)

Drone aircraft commonly referred to as **unmanned aerial vehicles (UAVs)** or unmanned aircraft systems (UAS) represent an emerging threat to critical infrastructure. They are commonly observed flying near or directly above critical infrastructure such as electric generation power plants, electric transformer substations, reservoirs and dams, and military installations. The actual risk from this emerging threat is still evolving; however as drone technology improves and the capability to carry heavy payloads evolves, drone aircraft must be considered a security threat for owners and operators or critical infrastructure. Currently, surveillance of critical infrastructure, perhaps even pre-operational attack surveillance, appears the primary threat from drones along with simple nuisance drone flights from individuals who do not have nefarious goals in mind.

Drones encountered by critical infrastructure operators today are typically low altitude–low speed aircraft that weigh less than 10 pounds and are generally designed for recreational use (OCIA 2016). However, drones are growing in popularity for commercial use and are governed by FAA Part 107. Drones also have many positive operational uses (NCSL 2016). The energy industry and other utilities uses drones equipped with light detection and ranging (LIDAR) and infrared technologies to inspect communication towers, electric transmission lines, and pipelines in remote areas. Drones are also used as a cartographic tool for the creation of maps and other geographical information system (GIS) products. However, as an example of criminal, perhaps even terroristic use of drones, drone aircraft are known to have breached the airspace of 13 nuclear power plants in France (NCSL 2016). Similarly, the US Department of Energy reported at least eight known aerial intrusions over its Savannah River Nuclear Site by drone aircraft in a two-week period in early 2016. These trespass intrusion incidents were conducted primarily during the dark of night by drone aircraft described as "sophisticated." Incidents such as these once again raise the specter of aerial surveillance, perhaps pre-attack surveillance. While drones are not known to have been used in any direct terrorist attacks or other major security incidents other than surveillance and nuisance flights, as the technology matures, fear that drones could be used to conduct major and increased pre-attack reconnaissance missions and deliver explosive payloads to critical infrastructure facilities such as populated transportation hubs and utility critical infrastructure such as power plants and water treatment plants arise (NCSL 2016).

Drones are difficult if not impossible to guard against. Detection technology is not mature; therefore, security relies on effective observation and reporting. And even if drones can be detected by technology or simple observations, limited if any countermeasures exist to defend critical infrastructure from surveillance or, perhaps worse, an explosive device being delivered from above.

5.2.4 Cybersecurity Threats

While threats of physical nature including malicious manmade threats and natural threats can, and have had, catastrophic impacts on critical infrastructure, perhaps no threat is as insidious as the threat from cyber actors. Today's world is highly connected and, moreover, interconnected in ways that cause not only threats to targeted infrastructure but also cascading effects on those infrastructures that are interconnected and interdependent. While cyber threats are addressed more fully in Chapter 8, in this section we will discuss the cyber impact on our interconnected world and the primary control system, Supervisory Control and Data Acquisition (SCADA) (also known as industrial control systems) systems that help us operate critical infrastructure with efficiency. Most, if not all, of the nation's critical infrastructure is operated through SCADA systems, which "automatically monitor and adjust switching, manufacturing, and other process control activities, based on digitized feedback gathered by sensors" (Goodman 2015, 27). SCADA systems are used in transportation infrastructure as train control systems; water utilities to control drinking water treatment and distribution processes; energy utilities to generate, transmit, and distribute electricity and natural gas; critical manufacturing processes; and much more. The inherent nature of the risk associated with SCADA-oriented security threats, as mentioned earlier, is the fact that not only can a breach of a SCADA system disrupt or "take down" the target operation, but also the downstream and interdependent impacts can be quite broad. This brings us back our very basic chicken-and-egg scenario. Electricity cannot be generated without water and water cannot be produced without electricity. Take down the electric distribution system in a community by breaching the SCADA system, and you also take down the drinking water system. Water flow includes movement from reservoirs to water treatment plants through large water transmission mains as well as treatment processes that are comprehensive in and of themselves and then storage and distribution of finished drinking water. All of this requires electricity to power pump stations, treatment processes that introduce sanitizing chemicals and process water through filtration, and power to monitor treatment processes and distribution systems to include water storage tank capacity and on-demand water volumes to meet customer needs.

Unfortunately many SCADA systems are often connected to the Internet, which presents significant security implications. Many SCADA systems are aging and were designed in a time where Internet security threats were not existent or simply not common. A study in 2014 across many infrastructure organizations demonstrated that nearly 70% of these organizations had suffered at least one security breach that resulted in the loss of data or the disruption of infrastructure operations (Goodman 2015, 27).

The national electric grid (or grids as it actually is a system of interconnected power grids) is considered a target, which if impacted could have catastrophic consequences including the degradation of societal norms. The loss of utilities would be exacerbated by the loss of all things that require electric power to function: refrigerators, ATM machines, cellular phone towers, transportation systems, and police and fire department dispatch systems, just to mention a few. The American electric grid comprises system-of-systems/network-of-networks complex infrastructures that include close to 8 000 power plants—some with multiple generation units—200 000 miles of high voltage transmission lines, and hundreds of transformer substations. Adding to this complexity are community and regional electric distribution systems that bring electricity to homes and businesses. These complex interconnected and interdependent systems are connected to SCADA systems, which operate almost each and every component. Considering the enormity and vastness of this massive system of networks, one gets an understanding of the potential vulnerabilities associated with these systems and the significant burden of securing these systems. Utilities are constantly targets of hacking attempts. It is also believed that cyber actors have penetrated the US electric grid and have installed dormant software programs that can be activated on demand to disrupt the grid (Goodman 2015, 29).

The loss electric power will also lead to the loss of the Internet itself, which leads to a concept known as the **Internet of things (IoT)**. Consider for a moment that all of the devices that make American life pleasant are connected to the Internet. The IoT is defined as "a global, immersive, invisible, ambient, networked computing environment built through the continuation of smart sensors, cameras, software, databases, and massive data centers in world spanning information fabric" (Goodman 2015, 284). Lose electricity and one loses the Internet and the IoT, essentially modern conveniences that "talk" to each other and upon which so much of modern life is dependent on.

FOR EXAMPLE

Water System Vulnerability

A number of Iranian hackers successfully breached the SCADA system of a dam in the small town of Rye Brook, New York, situated 15 miles north of New York City (Berger 2016). It is unclear as to what harm the Iranians intended to cause. The dam was empty of water as it was under repair at the time of the attack. What could have happened if the dam was at capacity may never be known. Some conject that this was either simply a dry run or that the dam the Iranians intended to target was another dam with a similar name. Perhaps it was simply a probe or show of capability. Another example of a SCADA breach involved the loss of millions of liters of raw untreated waste-water in Australia when a hacker accessed the SCADA system of a sewer treatment plant. This cyber breach caused contamination of area parks and popular brand hotels (one local and one international) and destroyed local marine life.

Among the many steps in a comprehensive physical and cyber security system needed to protect SCADA systems, protecting modern systems starts with ensuring that SCADA systems are firewalled or actually air gapped and totally disconnected from the global Internet. This will help to secure SCADA systems from the security jungle that is the modern Internet. Next, SCADA systems must be isolated from enterprise computer networks through effective firewalling and security protocols. SCADA security also requires that patch management protocols are in place to ensure that the system software is constantly updated with the most current security capabilities (NSTB 2006). SCADA systems should also have multiple authentication requirements with frequent password changes for each layer of security.

SELF-CHECK

- Which of the following would be impacted by the loss of electric power?
  a. Water treatment facilities
  b. The Internet
  c. Telecommunications
  d. All of the above
- A severe thunderstorm is defined in part as a thunderstorm that can produce a tornado, winds of at least 58 mph, and/or hail at least 1″ in diameter. True or false?
- SCADA stands for Supervisory Control and Defense Actions. True or false?

5.3 Risk Identification, Analysis, and Management

Assessing risk in the homeland security domain centers on risks associated with critical infrastructure. Homeland security practitioners, especially those working in and around any critical infrastructure, must understand the risks associated with the infrastructure they are charged to protect. This leads to the discussion of risk assessments as a tool to help develop targeted protective measures including security measures (both of a physical security and cyber security nature), an emergency response and operations (crisis management) program, continuity of operations protocols, and restoration and recovery strategies. Risk assessment tools and methodologies in the homeland security domain abound and have various names depending on the goals and objectives of the risk assessment (see Chapter 4) including threat assessments that are common in the law enforcement and security industries; hazard vulnerability assessments (HVA), which is common the **emergency management** domain; security vulnerability assessments (SVAs), which is common in the corporate security environment; enterprise risk assessments, which are generally thought of as financial risk assessments in the corporate world; and so on. Regardless of what you call a risk assessment, the end result must be centered on the production of valuable and actionable information that helps provide the elements for strategies designed to compensate for the risk, overcome the risk, transfer the risk, accept the risk, or terminate the risk.

For our purposes we will discuss comprehensive risk assessments (CRAs) that are not associated with any common risk assessment tools or methodologies, but are general enough to apply to a risk assessment of a community such as a city or town, or an enterprise such as an airport, utility, or corporate environment. A risk assessment typically examines the following:

▲ Threat/Hazard—Likelihood/Probability—Vulnerability—Consequence/ Impacts
Some risk assessments use these indicators to determine a numerical value of the risk, for example, a common risk assessment model is as follows:

▲ Risk = Threat X Vulnerability X Consequence
We will examine the categories as a means of conducting a qualitative risk assessment that provides high value information to homeland security practitioners and decision makers as it is designed to provide comprehensive narrative on the risks (Threat/Hazard—Likelihood/ Probability—Vulnerability—Consequence/Impacts), not just quantitative values.

5.3.1 Inventory and Critical Assets and Functions

When conducting a risk assessment, we need to start with an inventory of **mission-critical functions (MCFs)** and **mission-critical assets (MCAs)**. If an energy sector utility generates electricity, for example, the primary mission critical function would be just that, electric generation. Electric generation would in turn have a number of dependent mission critical functions (MCFs) that would involve the activities and materials needed to generate electricity. If the electric generation facility is a coal-fueled power plant, at a high level, MCFs include the following:

▲ Operational generators/turbines
▲ A functioning control room with staff
▲ Coal on hand and an uninterrupted coal supply

At this stage in the risk assessment, it is important to also analyze dependencies and interdependencies that will help us understand what the asset needs are to ensure uninterrupted operations. This may include constant on-scene staff to ensure safe and proper operations, as well as uninterrupted supply chain for materials such as fuel and lubricants. Interdependencies would include assets provided by other critical infrastructure. For our power plant, at a minimum, that would include assets from the transportation sector, oil and natural gas subsector, and water and wastewater sector. As mentioned earlier, electricity cannot be generated without water; drinkable water cannot be produced without electricity.

5.3.1.1 Threats and Hazards

Once we catalogue all of our mission critical assets and functions, we then move on to identifying threats and hazards. Continuing with the electric generation scenario, let us define the threats and hazards that may confront a power plant. Depending on the location of the power plant, the facility may be subject to extremes of weather. A power plant in a coastal area may be subjected to strong wind and flooding from tropical storms and nor'easters. A power plant in a forested area would be subject to potential wildfires. Power plants, like all critical infrastructure across the 16 critical infrastructure sectors, are also subject to malicious human acts such as vandalism, crime, and of course acts of terrorism. We then try to identify what types of malicious acts can occur and try to remediate them by developing programmatic security policies and by constructing physical protective measures. The point is to identify the hazards so as to do directed security, emergency operations, and continuity of operations planning.

5.3.1.2 Likelihood/Probability

When conducting a risk assessment to critical infrastructure, as part of identifying risks and hazards, it is then important to try to understand the likelihood that an incident, whether it is a natural hazard or caused by a malicious act, would occur. What is the history of the facility in question? Has it been targeted before? Has it been subjected to criminal acts such as sabotage or trespass? What is the natural hazard history? Has there been a wildfire, flood, or earthquake? What about technical hazards? Has there been any incident organic to the facility such as internal flooding or incidents involving the generation facility such as fires or mechanical failures?

5.3.1.3 Vulnerability

Once we identify threats, hazards, and vulnerabilities, we then need to gain an understanding of the likelihood identified "risks." In looking at vulnerability, we determine exposure of the assets to the local hazards and threats. Is there a fire break and flood barriers around the facility? Is the facility visible and accessible by potential bad actors? Has security mitigation measures been put in place to defend against intruders? Have physical security barriers been constructed at critical access points and near mission critical assets to defend against a potential vehicle borne attack? Have security cameras been put in place?

5.3.1.4 Consequences/Impacts

Finally, once we have a clear understanding of the risks, we then need to understand the impact and consequences if the asset comes under attack, or experiences a natural hazard, and comes offline. In other words, what happens if the asset fails to function? In our scenario, if the power plant comes offline, how does that impact the community? Will there be a power outage or will other power plants in the network or overall electric grid compensate for the loss of generation? For how long? Is there a mutual aid plan in place to purchase emergency energy from nearby electric generation companies? Once we understand the impacts and consequences, we can then work with community partners such as the local and state offices of emergency management to plan for failure of the asset. We can also do internal directed planning to prepare for the loss of the asset by way of emergency operation and continuity of operations plans.

5.3.2 Intelligence Functions

The application of an intelligence function in critical infrastructure protection provides two essential avenues in which a CI protection and emergency management program can benefit. First and foremost is the use and application of actionable intelligence, and the second is general intelligence, which provides a snapshot on threat trends. Intelligence can be obtained from a number of official and unofficial sources (see Chapter 12). Official intelligence can come from a number of organizations and agencies such as state and local fusion centers, local law enforcement, and other agencies (not all intelligence is security oriented) and industry-oriented sources such as the sector coordination councils mentioned earlier in this chapter. For owners and operators of CI, one of the most common and important source of intelligence comes from the National Weather Service (NWS). As mentioned, not all intelligence is security oriented; therefore, when we consider other threats and hazards, from a CI perspective, we know that weather is a hazard that can have dramatic impact on any number of critical infrastructures. Consider the threat of winter weather to electric utilities. Blizzards with accompanying storm-force winds, ice storms with ice accretion on power lines, and accumulation of snow can result in power outages and the inability to respond effectively. Transportation agencies would also be similarly impacted by winter weather when we consider operators of highway and street infrastructure as well as public and mass transit whether it is rail or surface operations.

Having an understanding of NWS weather products, such as weather watches, advisories, and warnings and how to apply the knowledge gained from these products in the preparedness for an anticipated weather event such as a hurricane or severe winter storm, which generally provides ample advanced warning, or how to use weather intelligence during the response to no-notice weather events such as severe thunderstorms and tornado events, can prove to be highly valuable. In this regard, NWS intelligence provides both actionable and general intelligence. Typically, local NWS forecast offices (NWSFOs) have a designated phone number for emergency managers to access meteorologists for weather information. NWSFOs generally convene conference calls with area emergency managers in advance of a storm such as a hurricane and winter weather event. CI-based emergency managers should become familiar with the activities and operations of local NWSFOs and should seek out the local **warning coordination meteorologist (WCM)**, which is generally the NWS liaison to the emergency management community. Another highly invaluable source of weather intelligence is NWSChat. Most, if not all, NWSFOs operate a secure weather chat portal where weather products are posted and emergency managers, including CI-based emergency managers, can communicate directly with NWS forecasters and other emergency managers for the purpose of gaining and providing information as well as contributing to the conversation, which can be highly valuable in advance of a weather event or during weather emergency operations. NWSChat can be accessed at https://nwschat.weather.gov/

Actionable intelligence can also come from sources where the CI is operated locally. For example, many law enforcement (LE) agencies, including town and city police agencies as well as county-based sheriff's offices, operate some form of a fusion center or investigative/intelligence function. When a threat to CI becomes known to an LE agency, having a mechanism, and the relationships, in place to obtain that intelligence can prove to be invaluable in preventing or responding to a threat or security incident. Of course intelligence is a two-way street. Information regarding threats or incidents against the CI owner–operator must be transmitted to LE intelligence offices. This serves the purpose of sharing the information so that LE agencies can integrate the information to analyze it against other known investigations or to simply start a new investigation into the current threat or incident. Further, establishing a two-way communication and information sharing model establishes the CI organization as a "player" and can—and should—be seen as part of the security, intelligence, and emergency management community. While it may seem unusual for an operator of CI to operate an intelligence function, the ability to collect, analyze, and transmit actionable intelligence and intelligence trends is an invaluable undertaking in securing and protecting CI, including people and property, from known and potential threats.

Intelligence is also available from a number of agencies that support CI operators such as the US Department of Homeland Security (DHS), State Fusion Centers, and industry specific intelligence provide by Information Sharing and Analysis Centers (ISACs).

5.3.2.1 Portal-Based Intelligence

The US Department of Homeland Security (DHS) operates the Homeland Security Information Network (HSIN), which is essentially an intelligence and information sharing portal. The portal is divided into a number of "verticals" and "communities." As an example, the Critical Infrastructure Community provides documents on a daily basis, which capture happenings and trends across all 16 CI sectors. The Emergency Services portal has invaluable information targeted at the emergency services sector, which is valuable to law enforcement, fire service, emergency medical service, and emergency management agencies. Reports available might include daily DHS unclassified counterterrorism briefings, FEMA daily situation reports, and incident-specific situation reports.

Sector-specific ISACs also provide valuable intelligence through portals and email distributions. For example, the Electricity ISAC (E-ISAC) provides information that is collected from operators of electric utilities across the nation (and globally depending on the severity of the incident) on incidents such as security threats and trends, cyber security threats, and non-security incidents such as major power outages and distributes this information to subscribers via email and portal access. This source of intelligence is also complemented by a monthly webinar-based E-ISAC threat briefing. The E-ISAC is a collaborative effort among a number of agencies:

> The Electricity Information Sharing and Analysis Center (E-ISAC) establishes situational awareness, incident management, coordination, and communication capabilities within the electricity sector through timely, reliable, and secure information exchange. The E-ISAC, in collaboration with the Department of Energy and the Electricity Sector Coordinating Council (ESCC), serves as the primary security communications channel for the electricity sector and enhances the sector's ability to prepare for and respond to cyber and physical threats, vulnerabilities, and incidents. (E-ISAC 2016)

Similarly the water and wastewater sector have the Water ISAC (W-ISAC n.d.) as a source of intelligence very similar in nature to the E-ISAC for water and wastewater utilities:

> The Water Information Sharing and Analysis Center (Water ISAC) was authorized by Congress in 2002 and created and managed by the water sector. Its mission is to keep drinking water and wastewater utility managers informed about potential threat and risks to the nation's water infrastructure from all hazards, such as intentional contamination, terrorism and cyber-crime, and to provide knowledge about response, mitigation and resilience. (W-ISAC 2016)

5.3.2.2 State Homeland Security Intelligence

State fusion centers are typically a joint operation between state police and state homeland security and emergency management agencies. The US Department of Homeland Security states that

> A fusion center is a collaborative effort of two or more agencies that provide resources, expertise and information to the center with the goal of maximizing their ability to detect, prevent, investigate, and respond to criminal and terrorist activity. (Fusion Centers n.d.)

Fusion centers operate by integrating knowledge and information gained from the various participant agencies as well as from intelligence agencies at the federal level such as the DHS and FBI. Fusion centers also serve as a clearinghouse for reporting of suspicious activity and actual security incidents. Reports are then typically investigated by an appropriate agency. For example, if a state fusion center receives a report of a suspicious package at an electric transformer substation, in addition to local police and bomb squad response, the FBI and Bureau of Alcohol, Tobacco, Firearms, and Explosives (ATF) may be brought in for their expertise.

State fusion centers generate and issue intelligence reports, typically designated as Unclassified-For Official Use Only (U-FOUO). These reports contain valuable information on threats and threat trends, some general in nature and others with a specific target audience in mind such as the operator of dam or rail transportation system. As a clearinghouse, state fusion centers also redistribute U-FOUO reports such as DHS-FBI joint intelligence bulletins (known as JIBs) to individuals and agencies that have been approved for receipt of these and other similar intelligence products. In addition, state fusion centers typically convene periodic classified intelligence briefings. These briefings are typically conducted at the "Secret Level"; therefore, only those with approved security clearances that have been "passed" to the state fusion center can attend and participate in these briefings.

FOR EXAMPLE

Private Sector Security Clearances

While the possession of security clearances is typically thought to be the domain of law enforcement and other public safety agencies, the DHS Private Sector Clearance Program provides limited security clearances to CI owner–operator security and emergency management personnel.

Ensuring critical infrastructure security and resilience requires ongoing cooperation between Government and private industry. While the vast majority of information DHS shares with the private sector is at the unclassified level, some information may be classified, requiring a federal security clearance. The Private Sector Clearance Program for Critical Infrastructure (PSCP), established in 2006, ensures that critical infrastructure private sector owners, operators, and industry representatives, specifically those in positions responsible for the protection, security, and resilience of their assets, are processed for the appropriate security clearances. With clearances, these owners, operators, and representatives can access classified information to make more informed decisions. The PSCP facilitates the processing of security clearance applications for private sector partners, and is currently administered by the Department of Homeland Security (DHS), National Protection and Programs Directorate (NPPD), Office of Infrastructure Protection (IP), Sector Outreach and Programs Division (DHS 2015).

5.3.2.3 Networking and Collaboration

Unofficial and informal intelligence comes from "The Network," which is simply a collaboration among and between individuals in which relationships have been established. Owner–operators of CI and their security and emergency management personnel must seek out individuals and agencies and establish relationships and informal communication pathways. This is simply referred to as the "business card imperative" where people of importance know each other before an incident is essential in critical information sharing. As it is often said in the halls of many an emergency management office, the worst time to exchange business cards is at a command post. Using the suspicious package scenario at the electric transformer substation mentioned earlier, if the head of security for a regional utility becomes aware of this incident, by simply calling his or her counterpart at the impacted utility, informal information can be gathered and an informed decision can be made with regard to additional potential threats and impacts. Therefore, relationships should be established with area, state, and even national partners in the various CI sectors, law enforcement, fire and EMS, public works, and other utilities. Further, these relationships must be nurtured and not be allowed to become stale. Frequent phone calls, emails, and sharing of information can assist in keeping the lines of communications open during steady state and during times of emergency. Establishing and maintaining relationships with personnel from regulatory agencies can also prove to be essential especially in creating partnerships as opposed to acrimonious relationships.

SELF-CHECK

- If the electric generation facility is a coal-fueled power plant, at a high level, which of the following would not be considered a mission-critical function?
  a. General intelligence
  b. Operational generators/turbines
  c. A functioning control room with staff
  d. Coal on hand and an uninterrupted coal supply
- State fusion centers generate and issue intelligence reports, typically designated as Top Secret. True or false?
- The Warning Coordination Meteorologist (WCM) is generally the NWS liaison to the law enforcement community. True or false?

5.4 Emergency Operations and Continuity of Planning

Emergency planning for a CI organization is somewhat different than emergency planning for a community, yet there are many similarities. In planning for emergencies for CI, the approach must integrate both an all-hazards model and a risk-specific planning model that will provide for an organized approach to all emergencies and disruptions of CI operations as well as a targeted response model for emergencies and disruptions of specific infrastructure and services.

5.4.1 Critical Infrastructure Protection Planning and the All-Hazards Perspective

Using the integrated all-hazards and risk-specific model, it is imperative that emergency planning for critical infrastructure protection integrates the practices and principles of both emergency operations and continuity of operations planning.

Incorporating emergency response and recovery functions along with continuity and restoration functions into an **emergency continuity plan (ECP)** provides a holistic and comprehensive approach to managing emergencies and disruptions in a CI organization especially one that provides quality of life services for a community such as hospitals, water and electric utilities, and transportation agencies. An ECP for a CI operator can be comprehensive and detailed when one considers the complexity of operating CI and the various functions and activities that provide the service to the end user/customer.

However, an ECP for a CI organization should include at the very least the following sections:

- ▲ Alerting, Warning, and Situational Awareness
- ▲ Emergency Operations Activation and Activation Levels
- ▲ Crisis Management Team (CMT) (based on an Incident Command System (ICS)-oriented structure)
- ▲ Concept of Operations (including Crisis Management Team activities detailed by position with position-based job action sheets as an appendix)
- ▲ Continuity Courses of Action (CCAs) (detail the actions that will be taken to restore mission critical functions that were identified during the comprehensive risk assessment)
- ▲ Interagency Operations
- ▲ Public/Customer Information
- ▲ Demobilization
- ▲ After Action Review

The planning process for developing a complex plan such as an ECP requires a formal planning model as well as participation and input from many individuals representing many different functions and departments from within the CI organization as well partners from external agencies. A planning process should include the following steps:

- ▲ Identify a program lead.
- ▲ Program lead identifies preliminary planning goals (what should the plan achieve?).
- ▲ Establish a planning team (internal and external stakeholders).
- ▲ Convene and conduct formal planning meetings using a deliberative, discussion-based format (the objective here for the planning team to achieve consensus on plan activities and content).
- ▲ Develop a written plan document (socialize the plan around the planning team for review and consensus).
- ▲ Training.
- ▲ Exercises.
- ▲ Plan review cycle updates.

FOR EXAMPLE

Virginia Department of Emergency Management Continuity Planning

The Virginia Department of Emergency Management has created a template for use by state agencies and institutions of higher education in creating their individualized emergency continuity plans. These would include planning for the maintenance of critical infrastructure in an agency or institution by identifying the Mission Essential Functions (MEFs) required for continuity of operations. The template makes it easier for agencies to develop these plans by providing the basic requirements that agencies must consider during an emergency such as *loss of access to a facility or portion of a facility (as in a building fire); loss of services due to equipment or systems failure (as in telephone, electrical power, or information technology system failures); and loss of services due to a reduced workforce (as in pandemic influenza, incidents in which employees are victims or incidents that prohibit employees from reporting to the workplace)* (VDEM 2014).

5.4.2 Crisis Management Team

A **Crisis Management Team (CMT)** for a CI organization typically includes the participation of internal personnel who are trained to serve on a CMT. The Incident Command System (ICS) provides the foremost structure to manage an emergency especially one that involved complex systems. ICS training is available from many sources including state and local emergency management and homeland security offices, fire departments, and FEMA (including online ICS courses). ICS provides many capabilities to a CMT to include a structured crisis management/emergency operations organizational framework and leadership hierarchy; a framework that is common to, and recognized by, partner emergency management and public safety agencies as well other CI owner–operators; common terminology; a communications framework and linkages; an organized approach to the production of joint public information; an organized approach to response, recovery, and restoration; and, much more. An ICS organization for a CI organization would typically contain the following elements:

▲ Policy tier—Typically comprised of C-Suite Level Executives
▲ Incident management tier—Typically consisted of what is known as the command and general staff (CGS) comprising an incident commander or a unified command element; command staff consisting of safety, security, public information, and liaison functions; and general staff comprised of sections such as strategic operations, situational awareness and planning; logistics; and administration and finance.
▲ Multi-agency coordination group (MAC) that consists of representatives of external partner agencies such as local and state offices of emergency management, law enforcement, fire/EMS, public health, public works and more depending on the needs of an incident.

SELF-CHECK

- The Incident Command System for Crisis Management Team would include which of the following:

  a. A policy tier

  b. Incident management tier

  c. Multi-agency coordination group (MAC)

  d. All of the above

- An emergency continuity plan for a CI organization should include a section on Alerting, Warning, and Situational Awareness. True or false?

- The first step in the ECP planning process should include identifying a program lead. True or false?

SUMMARY

Protecting critical infrastructure requires a comprehensive approach to analyzing and preventing risk, physical and cyber security, emergency operations, and continuity of operations planning, training, and exercises, all of which requires the participation of many stakeholders both internal and external to a CI organization. Understanding the CI protection roadmap also contributes to a program that captures the threat environment and enables CI security and emergency management professionals to plan for anticipated and unanticipated emergencies and disruptions of CI operations and end-user services whether it is a customer flipping a light switch, boarding a train, or withdrawing cash from an ATM.

The path forward for critical infrastructure protection is perilous at best. As cyber criminals and terrorists refine their products and capabilities, as drone technology and payload capacity increases, and as infrastructure deteriorates and decays, critical infrastructure protection specialists must make all efforts to stay ahead of the curve. Regularly recurring threat and risk assessments coupled with rigorous physical/cyber security and emergency/continuity planning will be needed to ensure that American infrastructure continues to provide the commodities and services that society has come to enjoy and expect.

In this chapter, you analyzed the critical infrastructure environment and the national and homeland security implications from a threat and consequence perspective as well as critical infrastructure security, emergency preparedness, and operational continuity program and policy choices. You also learned to distinguish between the various national and homeland security policy players both within and outside government. Finally, you appraised the threat–hazard–risk situation in the contemporary critical infrastructure risk protection environment.

KEY TERMS

Continuity course of action	Specific pre-planned protocols and procedures designed to ensure uninterrupted operation of critical infrastructure and associated mission-critical assets.
Continuity of operations	The ability to ensure uninterrupted business operations during emergencies and disasters.
Critical infrastructure (CI)	Assets that are essential to the provision and stability and normal function of American lifestyle. CI is typically identified in 16 CI sectors designated in the National Infrastructure Protection Plan (NIPP).
Critical infrastructure protection (CIP)	Systems and procedures designed to protect CI from physical and cyber threats and to have the capability and capacity to respond to, and recover from, the said threats.
Crisis management team	A team of personnel trained to perform emergency operations functions in times of emergency.
Emergency continuity plan (ECP)	Provides a holistic and comprehensive approach to managing emergencies and disruptions in a CI organization especially one that provides quality of life services for a community such as hospitals, water and electric utilities, and transportation agencies.
Emergency management	A system of systems approach to managing threats and risks through programmatic emergency planning, emergency response, and recovery and mitigation.
Emergency operations	Activities associated with the response and recovery phases of emergency management.
Industrial control systems	Intelligent systems that are used to control business processes such as manufacturing and utility services. ICS systems are typically seen through the lens of SCADA systems.

Information sharing and analysis centers

ISACs are typically associated with NIPP sectors and are charged with developing and sharing industry-oriented intelligence.

Internet of things (IoT)

The IoT is a theory related to the broad application of Internet-connected smart devices such as home alarm systems, cellular phones, and much more, which are interconnected and in some cases not well protected, leaving them vulnerable to cyber hacking.

Mission-critical assets

Infrastructure or components thereof that are essential to safe, effective, and uninterrupted operation.

Supervisory control and data acquisition (SCADA)

SCADA systems are used to manage and mechanical industrial operations such as the transmission and distribution of electricity and the treatment and distribution of drinking water.

Unmanned aerial vehicle

An autonomous or semiautonomous airborne platform. Commonly known as a drone.

Warning coordination meteorologist (WCM)

Located within the National Weather Service Field Office, this person is generally the NWS liaison to the emergency management community.

ASSESS YOUR UNDERSTANDING

Go to www.wiley.com/go/Kilroy/Threats_to_Homeland_Security to assess your knowledge of the basics of critical infrastructure security.

Summary Questions

1. The National Infrastructure Protection Plan designates 16 infrastructure sectors. True or false?
2. ISAC stands for International Sharing and Analysis Capability. True or false?
3. A severe weather event includes large hail, high winds, and possible tornado activity. True or false?
4. The Saffir–Simpson scale is a set of metrics that measure tornado strength. True or false?
5. Electric and water utilities are an example of an interdependent system or systems. True or false?
6. An insider threat can present itself as an active shooter. True or false?
7. SCADA systems are designed to monitor tropical weather. True or false?
8. A basic risk assessment provides an understanding of threats, probabilities, and impacts. True or false?
9. Intelligence can be used to understand the threat environment near critical infrastructure. True or false?
10. The Incident Command System is the preferable organizational structure used to manage major emergencies. True or false?

Applying This Chapter

1. Critical infrastructure (CI) is rarely a linear system; rather CI is a system of networked systems. Work as a group to identify five community-based critical infrastructures and map out the dependent and interdependent systems that make the base CI operate while providing service to the dependent CI.
2. As a new member of the local Office of Emergency Management, perform a basic threat and hazard assessment of your home community by identifying threats/hazards, probability, and impact of at least six natural hazards, technical hazards, and malicious hazards and their impacts on CI.
3. As member of the state fusion center, research a recent national security or terrorist incident and provide an analysis that can be used as intelligence by local law enforcement agencies concerned about the threat to local CI.
4. As a member of a corporate security team, develop procedures to prevent and respond to an insider threat within a particular CI sector, such as power generation.

Homeland Security Information Network (HSIN)

HSIN is a secure portal operated by the US Department of Homeland Security. It contains a compendium of resources that both are near-real time and can be used for research purposes. Examples of the portal are too vast to describe here; however, it is recommended that operators of CI request access to HSIN and explore the options and communities available to them. To request access, point your web browser to https://www.dhs.gov/how-join-hsin

Basic Risk Assessment

Any good risk assessment begins with the development of an inventory of critical assets such as power plants and universities. Using the National Infrastructure Protection Plan (NIPP), identify at least one critical asset in your hometown that is associated with each of the 16 NIPP infrastructure sectors. To assess your knowledge of the NIPP, go to http://www.dhs.gov/national-infrastructure-protection-plan

6

STATE ACTORS AND TERRORISM
The Role of State-Sponsored Terrorism in International Politics

Jonathan M. Acuff

Department of Politics, Coastal Carolina University, Conway, SC, USA

Starting Point

Go to www.wiley.com/go/Kilroy/Threats_to_Homeland_Security to assess your knowledge of the basics of state actors and terrorism.
Determine where you need to concentrate your effort.

What You'll Learn in This Chapter

▲ The relationship between terrorism and other forms of collective violence

▲ Various definitions of terrorism

▲ The history of state support for terrorism

▲ Both domestic and international responses to state-sponsored terrorism

After Studying This Chapter, You'll Be Able To

▲ Analyze the similarities and differences between state violence, terrorism, and state-sponsored terrorism

▲ Evaluate how differences in definitions of terrorism are related to political interests and analytical challenges

▲ Summarize the Cold War and post-Cold War patterns of state-sponsored terrorism

▲ Analyze different approaches for dealing with state-sponsored terrorism

Threats to Homeland Security: Reassessing the All-Hazards Perspective, Second Edition.
Edited by Richard J. Kilroy, Jr.
© 2018 John Wiley & Sons, Inc. Published 2018 by John Wiley & Sons, Inc.
Companion website: www.wiley.com/go/Kilroy/Threats_to_Homeland_Security

INTRODUCTION

There are few state sponsors of terrorism left in the international system. If terrorism can be thought of as occurring in "waves," the current wave is almost devoid of state-sponsored terrorist groups (Rapoport 2004). Indeed, the two primary international terrorist threats—the Islamic State of Iraq and Syria (IS) and **al-Qaeda (AQ)**—operate using methods and seeking goals so repugnant that even states openly hostile to the United States do their utmost to keep their distance from these groups. The decline of state-sponsored terrorism suggests several questions. How are terrorism and, more specifically, state-sponsored terrorism related to other forms of collective violence? Why has state sponsorship for terrorist groups ebbed? What is the nature of the relationship between the few remaining states that sponsor terrorism and terrorist groups that are their clients? What is the nature of the threat presented by state-sponsored terrorism groups? How have governments and international organizations responded to these threats? Finally, under what conditions might we expect either a resurgence of state-sponsored terrorism or, conversely, the severing of the few remaining ties between terrorist groups and nation-states?

In this chapter we will examine the history of terrorism and state violence, as well as why states rarely sponsor terror groups in the contemporary international system. Next, we will establish current state sponsors of terror: Iran, Sudan, and Syria. We then analyze how both the international community and the United States have responded to the threats posed by the actions of the terror groups sponsored by these states. The chapter concludes with an assessment of how, despite the decline of the Cold War model of state sponsorship, the actions of Pakistan and Russia are suggestive of an enduring relationship between terror groups and states.

6.1 Defining Terrorism and Other Forms of Collective Violence

Defining terrorism is difficult, as the oft-repeated cliché "one man's terrorist is another man's freedom fighter" remains true. Even among academics, there is no widely agreed-upon definition of what constitutes terrorism (Weinberg et al. 2008). Consequently, in order to distinguish terrorism from other kinds of collective violence, as well as understand the interrelationship between terrorism and more conventional kinds of conflict, we shall examine a continuum of state and non-state violence. We begin by analyzing the origins of the modern state and the relationship between the state and violent non-state actors, such as terrorists.

The use of violence has long been a defining feature of the **territorial state**. In the archetypal definition from Max Weber (1946), states are defined as possessing a "monopoly on the legitimate use of force in a given territory" (77). Although governing organizations have been called "states" for much longer, Weber's definition describes a particular type of state that emerged at the beginning of modernity in Western Europe, roughly around the time of the Treaty of Westphalia in 1648. One of the primary differences between the modern state from its organizational predecessors is legal control over a specified territory, known as **sovereignty**.

Although ancient and medieval political organizations may have claimed the right to rule (**legitimacy**) and coercively wielded that right through a government staff, they did not see territorial borders as the "hard shells" that we do today. Prior to the advent of cartography, states simply did not recognize territorial borders as defining the limits of their authority (Branch 2014). For example, in medieval Europe, competing dukes or princes frequently claimed rights of inheritance, taxation, and authority over the same parcel of land, often located across the boundaries that existed between kingdoms and empires. These equally legitimate claims to control over a given territory were known as heteronomy. In contrast, unlike its medieval predecessor the modern state recognizes no legal competitors for legitimacy within its territorial boundaries, hence the "monopoly" component of Weber's definition.

In addition to the territorial dimension, modern states are also distinguishable from ancient and medieval states and empires in terms of their capacity for violence. There is a large literature in political science, history, sociology, and economics emphasizing the particularly violent nature of the modern state, with a superior capacity for violence characterized as crucial to its development (McNeill 1982; Tilly 1990). Although all states have been described as "protection rackets" that shake down citizens for taxes in exchange for protection (Levi 1988; North 1981; Olson 1993), modern states have frequently been viewed as much more violent (Mann 2005), with some scholars even suggesting that both world wars and the Holocaust are an unsurprising outgrowth of the nature of the modern state (Arendt 1948). Modern states have also been characterized as more violent due to their propensity to promote one dominant collective identity within their territorial borders, **nationalism**, which has led to the violent repression of other national or religious identities within the borders of the state and a drive to unite other members of the nation located within the borders of other states (Anderson 1991; Gellner 1983; Hall 1999). In light of this literature, it is worth reminding ourselves that violence in the international system is in fact declining. **Interstate wars** are historically rare and have been growing rarer (Mueller 2007). Moreover, the widely believed increase in ethnic conflict and civil wars across the globe since the end of the Cold War is largely a myth (Ayres 2000), the agony of contemporary Syria and Iraq notwithstanding.

Regardless of whether or not the modern state is more prone to violence than its historical antecedents, long before there was an international legal basis for state control over borders, there have been rules for the use of state violence. While modern conflicts are frequently interpreted based upon the deep impression made by the two world wars—all-out wars of conquest that mobilized the entire population to wage them—violence between states has historically varied considerably in terms of shared understandings between states and peoples as to the nature of war. For example, the ancient Romans and their adversaries viewed war less in terms of its modern geopolitical dimensions than as a form of status competition (Lebow 2010; Mattern 1999). In medieval Europe, the taking of members of the nobility as prisoners was widely accepted, in contrast with the equally accepted massacre of commoners who surrendered (Keegan 1983). Although the imperialist wars of conquest between Europeans and Americans and their non-Western opponents were unremittingly brutal, by the late nineteenth century new norms had emerged among Western belligerents that involved rights for all prisoners, care for the wounded, restrictions on different types of weapons systems, and rules as to who could be legally targeted in war (Finnemore 1996). The destruction wrought by the two world wars resulted in significant limitations on what kinds of force could be used legally by states, which are now codified in the **Geneva Conventions**. In addition, the use of aggressive war as state policy has been outlawed under the requirements laid out in the Charter of the United Nations, which now counts all but two states in the contemporary international system as members. Although the two non-signatories, the Vatican and the Palestinian Authority, have not been recognized as states per se, both possess a legitimate monopoly of violence within their borders.

It is not a coincidence that our modern understanding of what constitutes terrorism emerged during this same period in which norms restricting the kinds of violence had customarily used by states for millennia. One way of defining terrorism, both historical and contemporary terrorist groups, is the use of methods that explicitly violate the norms and laws of combat that emerged in the latter half of the nineteenth century, specifically the deliberate targeting of civilians to coerce the nation-state in which they reside. Yet we should be cautious using only the violation of accepted international norms as the basis of defining which groups are terrorists and which are not. First, states have often violated the laws of armed conflict, even democratic countries that have been champions of such laws. During World War II, Germany frequently ignored the distinction between combatants and noncombatants, deliberately targeting civilians in aerial bombing campaigns in Poland, the Netherlands, and the United Kingdom. But the Allies more than repaid this in kind, with bombing campaigns that killed hundreds of thousands of German civilians from 1942 to 1945, including the firebombing of the city of Dresden, a target of no military value, which killed over 25 000 people in just two nights. As the leader of British Bomber Command, Sir Arthur "Bomber" Harris put it, "the Nazis entered this war under the rather childish delusion that they were going to bomb everybody else and nobody was going to bomb them…They sowed the wind, and now they are going to reap the whirlwind" (British Pathé 1942). Although, as previously discussed, states are now significantly constrained in terms of what kinds of violence they can use, the conduct of European states in the colonial wars of the 1960s, the United States in the Vietnam War, the more recent invasion of Iraq in 2003 by the United States without the approval of the United Nations (UN) Security Council, and the annexation of Crimea by Russia in 2014 indicate compliance is not absolute.

In addition to evaluating what kind of force is being used and at whom it is directed, we must also consider the goals of the group using the illegal violence and how these activities relate to the group's overall goals or purpose. In this context, it is worth making a distinction between terrorists and organized crime. Although they often participate in the arming and financing of terrorist groups (Biersteker and Eckert 2008; Freeman 2011), organized criminal groups remain focused on the profits they derive from their illicit activities. In contrast, terrorist groups are primarily motivated by political objectives, albeit goals that are often inchoate (Abrahms 2008).

This distinction is not etched in stone, as some criminal gangs and terrorist groups are evolving to more closely resemble one another (Picarelli 2012; Scott

2013). For example, although it has recently entered into a peace agreement with the Colombian government, the Revolutionary Armed Forces of Colombia (FARC) was simultaneously an insurgent army engaged in a civil war, a terrorist group, and an organized crime syndicate that participated in narcotics trafficking, kidnapping, and extortion (see Chapter 10). Similarly, some scholars have begun using the term "**hybrid wars**" to describe conflicts involving a messy mixture of ethnic conflict, terrorism, transnational criminal activity, and foreign intervention, which have become the most common form of armed conflict over the past two decades (Schroefl and Kaufman 2014).

The matter is further complicated by the fact that all terrorist groups seek legitimacy—they want their actions to be recognized by others, particularly other states, as a justifiable means to the end of securing their right to rule (Buzan 2002). Al-Qaeda has frequently made reference to the specific tailoring of its attacks to conform with its interpretation of Islamic law, the end goal being the establishment of an Islamic empire, the caliphate (Naji 2005). Pro-government militias have often engaged in terrorism as a front for governments that don't want to be seen using such tactics against insurgents or even innocent civilians engaged in political opposition (Ahram 2016). More significantly, terrorism has also been used in state-building activities. To illustrate how these apparent polar opposites are related to terrorism, we briefly examine two cases: the use of violent non-state actors in Nazi Germany and the role of terrorism in the establishment of the state of Israel. It is worth noting in this context that analyzing these cases in no way suggests moral equivalency between them, far from it. Nazi Germany was the precipitator of a war that killed over 50 million people, including over 15 million innocent people murdered during the Holocaust. In contrast, Israel is the only democracy in the Middle East and, despite inconsistent compliance with international agreements regarding nuclear weapons proliferation and peace with the Palestinians, remains committed to the fundamental principles shared by all democracies. Indeed, that both the Nazi regime and the state of Israel were born from the use of terror should be of interest to us, as the great moral gulf between the two states illustrates one of the troubling facts about terrorism—it is not just used by "the bad guys."

FOR EXAMPLE

Terrorism and Seizure of State Control: Nazi Germany

In the 1930s, Germany was a country with democratic institutions and free elections, although both were increasingly under pressure. Many Germans had lost confidence in the ability of democracy to solve their problems. The Great Depression that began in 1929 had inflicted enormous damage on the German economy, the effects of which were much worse than even those experienced by the United States. Many Germans viewed the Weimar Republic, the regime that took power after the overthrow of the monarchy and the German defeat in World War I, as incapable of addressing the enormous challenges presented by the Depression. Moreover, some Germans believed the country's elected politicians had betrayed the country by signing the humiliating Treaty of Versailles. Although a minority, these Germans loudly proclaimed belief in the "stab in the back myth" (*Dolchstosslegende*), which also asserted an international "Jewish conspiracy" was ultimately responsible for Versailles.

In this environment, extremists were viewed more favorably than the mainstream political parties. Two of the most extreme parties were diametrically opposed to each other. The Communist Party sought to replace the Weimar Republic with a Marxist dictatorship modeled after the Soviet Union. In contrast, the goal of the National Socialist (Nazi) Party was to impose a hyper-nationalist, fascist dictatorship upon Germany, replacing its liberal institutions with uncontested rule by its party leader, Adolf Hitler. The communists and Nazis engaged in public brawls in Germany's cities, with the Nazis deploying a paramilitary army of street thugs known as the *Sturmabteilung* (SA). The SA waged a campaign of terror against opponents of Hitler, beating up communists, Jews, members of the moderate Social Democratic Party, and journalists. When the Nazis finally took power with the appointment of Hitler as Chancellor in January of 1933, the Nazi regime quickly employed members of another non-state armed group, Hitler's bodyguard, the *Schutzstaffel* (SS), to secretly set fire to the German parliament building, the *Reichstag*, and make it appear as if the communists had done it. The result was a sweeping transfer of power directly to Hitler and an orgy of violence by the SA (Evans 2003, 340–349). The Nazi leader further cemented his rule in the summer of 1934 by ordering the SS to murder dozens of political opponents of Hitler, including the previous Chancellor, Kurt Schleicher; the leader of the SA, Ernst Röhm; and other senior political figures. The Night of the Long Knives, as it became known, also resulted in the arrest and imprisonment of over a thousand others. This marked only the beginning of the use of terror by the Nazis to consolidate their power.

Terrorism and State-Building: The Lehi (Stern Gang) and Israel

For over 400 years, the historical lands of Palestine were controlled by the Ottoman Empire. During the 1870s, a new ideology, Zionism, began to emerge in Jewish communities in Europe. Zionism held that the Holy Land was the historical home of all Jews and that they could escape persecution if they emigrated to Palestine and reconstituted the state of Israel. This belief was particularly appealing to Jews in Eastern Europe, where anti-Semitism was again on the rise. A steady stream of immigrants entered Palestine, though Ottoman restrictions prevented Jews from becoming the majority. After World War I, Great Britain took control over Palestine as a mandate from the League of Nations. Although sympathetic to the plight of the Jews and formally committed to a future Jewish homeland via the secret Balfour Declaration of 1916, the British colonial authorities were concerned that a flood of Jewish immigrants would incite the native Arabs to rise up against British rule. These beliefs were confirmed when the Palestinians rose in revolt from 1936 to 1939, a conflict caused by a combination of promises broken by the British, Arab nationalism, and fear of the creation of Jewish state that would drive out the Palestinian majority. The revolt was brutally suppressed, during which the British mandate employed the Jewish paramilitary group Haganah to augment their forces. But cooperation with the British mandate authority was not a policy shared by all Jewish groups in Palestine. In the 1930s and 40s, two groups emerged among the Jewish diaspora community that argued in favor of the use of violence to found a state of Israel. Founded in 1931, the Etzel (Irgun) "regarded the use of political violence solely as a means of establishing a sovereign and democratic state of Israel" (Pedahzur and Perliger 2009, 11). In contrast, the Lehi (Stern Gang) emerged a decade later and asserted that the use of terrorism would provide a kind of catharsis—it would end forever the status of Jews as victims and targets of oppression. Before the smoke had cleared from the Arab Revolt, both terrorist groups began targeting British administrative offices.

Worldwide sympathy for the horrendous suffering inflicted on Europe's Jews during the Holocaust fundamentally changed the calculus of the British authorities. Despite the belated willingness of the mandate authorities to permit increased immigration to Palestine, the Irgun believed the British were responsible for the death of European Jews in the Holocaust (Heller 1995, 111). Consequently, both Irgun and Lehi intensified their attacks. Jewish terror cells were unraveled that had planned assassinations of the British Prime Minister and Foreign Secretary (Walton 2014, 77). In 1944, the British Minister for the Middle East, Lord Moyne, was assassinated by Lehi in Egypt, while no less than seven attempts to kill the High Commissioner of Palestine, Harold MacMichael, failed (Pedahzur and Perliger 2009, 17). Despite a significant crackdown by the British in Palestine, in 1946 the Irgun managed to bomb the King David Hotel in Jerusalem, the British mandate's chief administrative building, killing nearly a hundred people. Irgun executed attacks on the British Embassy in Rome, British transportation infrastructure in occupied Germany, a private club in London, and even the Colonial Office in the heart of the British government quarter, Whitehall (Walton 2014, 79–80). During the same time period, Lehi sent over 20 letter bombs to Great Britain, narrowly missing Sir Anthony Eden, a future Prime Minister. Additional attacks were carried out by the more formalized Jewish paramilitary group, the Haganah, though it was reluctant to use the same kinds of tactics as Irgun and Lehi, openly condemning the King David Hotel bombing (Pedahzur and Perliger 2009, 24). Despite a cease-fire between the British and Haganah in the wake of the United Nations (UN) decision to partition Palestine and form a Jewish state in 1947, Lehi and Irgun continued to attack British and Arab targets. In 1948, Lehi even went so far as to assassinate the UN Security Council representative, Count Folke Bernadotte, who had been sent to Israel to mediate the coming conflict between the newly independent Israel and the Arab states that surrounded it. Bernadotte was well known for having negotiated the release of over 30 000 prisoners from a Nazi concentration camp at the end of World War II.

> The effect of this campaign of terror was to drive the British from Palestine and enable the establishment of the state of Israel. To again reinforce the point that terrorism is not a tactic reserved only for "evil actors," the attack on the King David Hotel was carried out by Menachem Begin, who would go on to become the Prime Minister of Israel from 1977 to 1983 and win the Nobel Peace Prize with Egyptian President Anwar Sadat for forging peace between Israel and Egypt under the Camp David Accords.

As we can see from the discussion in this section, **terrorism** is a tactic used by transnational terrorist groups like AQ or IS, by insurgents against governments, by groups that combine their political objectives with transnational criminal activities like narcotics trafficking, by nation-states during wartime in the form of indiscriminate bombing and other tactics that target noncombatants, and by governments employing paramilitary militias to use tactics that the state is unwilling to use openly to oppress the population. Terrorism can take on both conventional and unconventional forms. When used by non-state actors, terrorism is often referred to as a form of asymmetric warfare, as the psychological shock induced by the terrorists' willingness to attack unarmed civilians and wreak havoc upon everyday life allows terrorists to evade and perhaps even coerce states with superior resources. In the next section, we will analyze the ways in which states and intergovernmental organizations (IGOs) like the United Nations have attempted to define terrorism in international and domestic law. In the legal context by which terrorism is defined in the contemporary international system, states also seek to draw distinctions between many of the historically employed acts of terror described earlier. Simply put, when states use their power to terrorize civilians, this is a war crime. When non-state actors do this, it is called terrorism. Yet it is not entirely clear if this distinction is useful, both analytically and legally, particularly when states cannot precisely define what constitutes an act of terrorism.

6.1.1 Legal Definitions of Terrorism

Although states have historically used tactics to induce terror in wartime populations, attacking noncombatants is illegal under the Geneva Conventions and is outlawed by a variety of instruments administered by the United Nations. A handful of states continue to administer punishments designed not just to penalize wrongdoers, but also to deter future acts through the shear brutality of the penalty. Saudi Arabia's administration of Sharia law, which includes public beheadings and mutilation, is an example of this tendency. However, violence intended to induce terror is illegal under the domestic law of most nation-states. Despite this broad consensus in the international system that terrorism is wrong, the legal definitions provided by states used to prosecute terrorists are not unproblematic.

The United States' approach to providing legally binding definitions of terrorism demonstrates the difficulty in crafting laws to combat terrorism. Multiple components of the US government have provided and continue to provide dramatically different definitions of terrorism. The specific language used in these definitions is often politicized, that is, the language is framed to appeal to a particular domestic or international political constituency from which the party in power seeks support.

For example, in the 2002 *National Security Strategy of the United States*, the George W. Bush administration defined terrorism as "premeditated, politically motivated violence perpetrated against innocents" (5). But the term "innocents" does not have the same meaning as "noncombatants." It accords a special sense of victimhood to targets of terrorism, victimhood that the US government was consciously using to mobilize support for a set of policies that its allies would not otherwise have backed, such as the invasion of Iraq and the Global War on Terrorism (GWOT). Although most countries understood and supported the US invasion of Afghanistan in the fall of 2001 to overthrow the Taliban and hunt down the members of al-Qaeda, few American allies wanted to completely militarize the struggle against transnational terrorism, which many regarded as largely a law enforcement problem, not a war. Politicized definitions of terrorism are by no means confined to the Bush administration. In the 2015 *National Security Strategy of the United States*, the Obama administration provided no definition of terrorism, preferring instead to characterize the adversary as "violent extremism and radicalization that drives increased threats" (9). At no point does the strategy define which beliefs are being "radicalized" or who or what is "extreme." This kind of language has prompted some critics to argue the administration has been unwilling to come to terms with the particularly Islamic character of the transnational terrorists targeting the United States and its allies (Bolger 2015).

Other agencies of the US government have diverged significantly from each other in how they define terrorism. As it is part of the Department of Justice (DoJ), the Federal Bureau of Investigation (FBI) employs the definition from Title 22 of the US Code, Section 2656f (d):

> premeditated, politically motivated violence perpetrated against noncombatant targets by subnational groups or clandestine agents, usually intended to influence an audience. (National Institute of Justice 2011)

However, the Department of Homeland Security (DHS), which fails to define terrorism on its website, ignores extant US code and utilizes a definition from its founding act of Congress:

> any activity that—(A) involves an act that—(i) is dangerous to human life or potentially destructive of critical infrastructure or key resources; and (ii) is a violation of the criminal laws of the United States or of any State or other subdivision of the United States; and (B) appears to be intended—(i) to intimidate or coerce a civilian population; (ii) to influence the policy of a government by intimidation or coercion; or (iii) to affect the conduct of a government by mass destruction, assassination, or kidnapping. (Congress of the United States 2002)

Finally, the Department of Defense (DoD) defines terrorism as "the unlawful use of violence or threat of violence, often motivated by religious, political, or other ideological beliefs, to instill fear and coerce governments or societies in pursuit of goals that are usually political" (Department of Defense 2014, vii).

The variance in these three definitions is significant in several important ways. First, only DoD's definition explicitly uses the expression "to instill fear," which of course is the key distinguishing feature of terrorism from other forms of coercion. Some scholars have even suggested that the purpose of terrorism is the fear itself, not the associated political objectives (Abrahms 2008). Second, DHS' definition is so broad and carries with it so many potentially included actions that almost any violation of federal, state, and even local laws could be construed to be an act of terrorism, making the definition operationally useless. Third, through its reference to "subnational groups or clandestine agents," only DoJ's definition suggests the asymmetric nature of terrorist violence, which is fundamental to distinguishing terrorists from other kinds of violence, particularly tactics used by states that are designed to terrorize. Finally, it is important to recognize that all three of these definitions are used by agencies in the Executive Branch. Although some scholars have suggested a single definition of terrorism is impossible because there are so many different kinds of terrorism (Laquer 2000), variation in definitions of terrorism leads to very different policy prescriptions. Policy drift should be avoided if said policies are to be maximally effective. And lest we assume such terminological differences are unique to US government agencies alone, it is worth noting that the United Nations (UN), European Union (EU), and North Atlantic Treaty Organization (NATO) have had similar issues with defining terrorism (Chase 2013).

On the other hand, definitional problems within the US government may have less to do with the analytical complexity of terrorism than with the missions and organizational priorities of different arms of the government. There is a research tradition in political science and international relations that suggests the specific interests of organizations tend to strongly influence how they view policy problems, which leads to policies that are not necessarily consistent with the national interest as a whole. Even knowing what constitutes the national interest itself is often not always clear. Case and point is how the US Department of State (DoS) evaluates terrorism. The everyday activity of DoS is diplomacy, and its mission is to achieve US interests through multilateral cooperation. One of the primary documents used to guide US counterterrorism strategy and transnational coordination with partner states and allies is the State Department's list of state sponsors of terrorism. Updated annually since 2004, the 2015 *Country Reports on Terrorism* (Department of State 2015) now lists only three states that currently sponsor terrorism: Iran, Sudan, and Syria. There is little doubt that each of these countries does sponsor terrorist groups, the specifics of which we will discuss in more depth in subsequent sections of this chapter.

However, several states that could easily be included as sponsors of terrorism by DoS are conspicuously absent from both current and previous reports, because their cooperation is viewed as necessary in counterterrorism efforts, their regional importance, or a combination thereof. For example, Pakistan could readily be included in this list. Although the 2015 report notes, "Pakistan has also not taken sufficient action against other externally-focused groups such as **Lashkar-e-Tayyiba** (LeT) and Jaish-e-Mohammad (JeM), which continued to operate, train, organize, and fundraise in Pakistan" (Department of State 2015), DoS continues the long-standing tradition of ignoring the fact that LeT very likely continues to receive support from the Inter-Services Intelligence (ISI), Pakistan's premier intelligence agency—LeT is best described as a proxy of the Pakistani state (Fair 2011). Ignoring Pakistan's support for LeT—a group that has killed Americans—is viewed as a necessary concession to a country the United States needs to help effect its goals in Afghanistan and maintain the status quo between the other nuclear power in the region, Pakistan's long-standing enemy India.

The omission of the Kingdom of Saudi Arabia from both current and historical lists of state sponsors of terrorism is similarly striking. Although the Kingdom has formally been a US ally in the struggle against terrorism, its historical track record is uneven at best. During the 1990s, the Saudis actively frustrated investigation of bombing of the Khobar Towers in 1996, which killed 19 Americans. Saudi Arabia was also one of only three countries that formally recognized the sovereignty of the Taliban. Finally, for over three decades Saudi Arabia has had a much closer relationship with Islamic extremism than has been publicly acknowledged by the Kingdom. Saudi Arabia has a long tradition of government funding to export its oppressive variant of Sunni Islam, Wahhabism (Hegghammer 2010). Saudi nationals have constituted the historical core of al-Qaeda; 15 of the 19 hijackers on September 11, 2001 were from Saudi Arabia. The recent release of some of the previously redacted portions of the *9/11 Report* also suggests possible collusion between the Saudis and al-Qaeda before 9/11, as there were multiple contacts between the hijackers and several people tied to the Saudi government (Congress of the United States 2016).

Certainly, the United States has strategic reasons for omitting both Pakistan and Saudi Arabia from the list of countries sponsoring terrorism. But the relationship between these two states with terrorist groups also poses several fundamental analytical questions. The spectrum of state support for terrorists has varied widely (Byman 2005). What does "sponsorship" mean? Are state-sponsored terror groups proxies in more conventional state rivalries? Are they organizations using states for their own ends? Both? What are the resultant tensions between these goals and activities? Given these tensions, how are these relationships maintained? Finally, in what sense do groups that do not necessarily consider themselves terrorists yet employ terrorism as a tactic represent a different kind of "state-sponsored" model of terrorism? In the remaining sections, we shall explore these issues.

6.1.2 The Heyday of State-Sponsored Terrorist Groups

Although the earliest identified terrorist groups can be traced to the Roman province of Judea and thus predate the territorial state, in terms of both the volume and severity of attacks, most terrorism has occurred during the last century and most terrorist groups have been sponsored by modern states. In keeping with the nature of almost all non-state actors in the modern international system, terrorist groups have lacked the necessary material resources to execute significant attacks or survive the resultant reprisals by the targets of such assaults without the backing of one or more states. Most terror campaigns are unsuccessful (Abrahms 2008; Cronin 2009), and even terrorist groups with state sponsors more often than not fail to achieve their objectives (Byman 2005, 53). Yet terrorist groups lacking such sponsors have been particularly ineffective. Even the most determined terrorist movements have often been crushed if they have not had a state sponsor to provide logistical support, training, and refuge outside the reach of the law enforcement or military assets of states targeted by such groups. For example, anarchism was a political ideology that emerged during the middle of the nineteenth century and inspired some of the most violent terrorist attacks of that century. Anarchists were responsible for dozens of political assassinations, including the killing of the Russian Czar Alexander II, French President Carnot, and US President McKinley, as well as attacks on the French parliament, the Barcelona Opera House, and the wedding of the Spanish King in 1906. Yet anarchists failed to effect any policy changes in the states they targeted and were relatively easily suppressed with the introduction of new forensic techniques and intelligence organizations in Europe (Warner 2014). By the end of the second decade of the twentieth century, anarchism had all but disappeared, replaced instead by a revolutionary belief system, Marxist–Leninism, that had a powerful state sponsor.

Although some anti-imperialist terrorist groups operated outside its influence, such as Irgun and Lehi in Israel or the National Liberation Front (FLN) in Algeria, the height of state-sponsored terrorism occurred during the Cold War under the aegis of the Union of Soviet Socialist Republics (USSR). The USSR was committed to sponsoring Marxist revolutions around the globe. Terrorism became one of several tools the Soviets used to attempt to duplicate the revolutionary experience of Russia in 1917. Consequently, as the Cold War rivalry between the United States and the USSR emerged during the late 1940s almost until the collapse of the USSR in 1991, the Soviets provided weapons, training, logistical support, safe havens, and intelligence to a wide variety of "freedom fighters" in terrorist groups. But much like the complexity of the contemporary relationship between Pakistan and LeT or Saudi Arabia and al-Qaeda, the manner in which the USSR supported terrorism varied widely from group to group, was not always based on commonly shared ideological goals, and almost never involved direct command and control. Some Soviet-sponsored groups were not even Marxists, such as the Irish Republican Army (IRA) or Carlos the Jackal's ideologically flexible group, which veered from Marxist-inspired support for the Palestinians under the leadership of Wadi Haddad in the Popular Front for the Liberation of Palestine (PFLP) to much more mercenary impulses. Another Palestinian group, the Palestine Liberation Organization (PLO), was similarly more focused on Palestinian nationalism than the finer points of Marxist–Leninist ideology. Nevertheless, under Soviet sponsorship, the PLO became one of the deadliest terrorist groups in history, responsible for hundreds of bombings, assassinations, airline hijackings, and other attacks, including the 1972 murder of nine Israeli athletes at the Münich Olympics by a PLO offshoot, Black September. Soviet sponsorship of the PLO helped "internationalize" terrorism—terrorists now attacked a much wider array of targets around the globe than their historical predecessors, executed deadlier attacks, and often struck at civilians who had no connection to the causes associated with the terrorist groups (Hoffman 2006, 63–71).

Other groups received more indirect support from Soviet client states, such as Czechoslovakia, Poland, Romania, Cuba, and East Germany, both as "cutouts" to conceal direct Soviet involvement and as sponsors of terrorism to achieve their own national political goals, which occasionally did not coincide with Moscow's wishes. For some groups, the extent of the relationship between sponsoring states and the groups remains unclear. For example, the German Red Army

Faction (RAF), French Direct Action (AD), and Italian Red Brigades all received some support from the Soviet bloc. But the RAF got most of its aid from another terrorist group, the PLO (Hoffman 2006), and endured an awkward relationship with East German Ministry for State Security (*Stasi*). Although the *Stasi* recognized the Marxist credentials of the RAF and at times provided some aid, the East German government never trusted the RAF, was concerned that its members might launch attacks in Eastern Europe, and viewed cooperation with the group cautiously, as it did not want even its tentative support for the group to damage improving relations with West Germany (Vielhaber 2013). Moreover, Czech support for the Red Brigades risked causing a serious rift between Moscow and Prague. When the Red Brigades kidnapped and assassinated former Italian Prime Minister Aldo Moro, the Soviets were concerned that should Czech sponsorship of the Red Brigades be discovered, it would undermine the Communist Party of Italy (PCI), which was heavily supported by the USSR (Andrew and Mitrokhin 1999, 298–299).

State sponsorship of terrorist groups during the Cold War was not confined to the Soviet Union and its allies. During the Vietnam War, the United States orchestrated the Phoenix Program, a covert assassination program directed by the CIA that utilized local militias to kill National Liberation Front (NLF, aka the Viet Cong) personnel and deter others from joining the NLF. Under the aegis of the School of the Americas at Ft. Benning, GA, the United States also trained and supported a variety of Latin American armed pro-government militias, some of which were tied to extrajudicial killings, including the 1980 rape and murder of four American Catholic missionaries in El Salvador (Rohter 1998). Moreover, the US government provided funding and intelligence support for the Condor system, a network of state-sponsored terrorist groups with ties to the governments of Chile, Argentina, Bolivia, Uruguay, and Paraguay. The Condor system directed a campaign of assassinations both in Latin America and in Europe of political opponents of the ruling juntas, including the murder of several Americans (Zanchetta 2016). Finally, the US government trained and supported Alpha 66, the Cuban exile group originally deployed to attempt an overthrow of the Castro regime via the Bay of Pigs landing in 1961. Following the failure of the invasion, Alpha 66 has participated in an intermittent terror campaign against the Castro regime, albeit without continued US government support, shooting down aircraft, assassinating Cuban diplomats, and bombing hotels in Havana (Korten and Nielsen 2008).

6.1.3 The End of the Cold War, Globalization, and the Decline of State Sponsorship

The end of the Cold War and the collapse of the Soviet Union in 1991 brought a sharp decline in support for the terrorist groups sponsored by the communist bloc. This reduction in material support went hand in hand with the complete delegitimization of Marxist–Leninism, depriving groups of not only the logistical support, weapons, and training formerly provided by the USSR but also the very purpose for the existence of many of these organizations. Some of the more well-known groups disbanded, including the Red Army Faction, Red Brigades, and Direct

Action (Horchem 1991; Jamieson 1990). Other groups adapted themselves to changed circumstances by eschewing violence for political solutions to their problems. In the wake of the 1998 Good Friday Accords, the IRA formally disarmed, having achieved more through negotiation in two years of multiparty talks than over 70 years of armed struggle had produced. The PLO similarly shifted to a negotiated solution to its interminable war with Israel. In 1993, the Oslo Accords created a path for a Palestinian state and fostered the transformation of the PLO into the Palestinian Authority, an organization now splintered into Fattah on the West Bank and Hamas on the Gaza Strip.

Other global trends militated against the continuance of the Cold War model of state-sponsored terrorism. First, although the collapse of the Eastern bloc ended the relationship between KGB and other communist state intelligence services with terrorist groups, other "rogue states," as they were labeled by the Clinton administration, stepped into the breach (Byman 2005). Countries such as Iran, Iraq, Libya, Syria, Sudan, Saudi Arabia, and Pakistan increased their support for terrorist groups. Second, although the resources from these new sponsors were much diminished compared with the virtual blank check provided by the USSR, other developments in the nature of terrorism would reduce the impact of such financing, making relying on a state sponsor unnecessary for many terrorist groups. Globalization has made much of what terrorists used to rely on from states far less complicated, expensive, or difficult. Terrorists have benefitted from the erosion of borders that has come about as a function of globalization (Cronin 2002; Pollard 2009). The transnational movement of people has increased in both frequency and size by so many factors that it is much easier for terrorists to hide in the sea of humanity as millions of people cross-state borders every day. Terror groups now have easier access to weapons and explosives than they did during the Cold War, as the end of that conflict has precipitated dramatic growth in the arms trade and dumped billions of dollars of surplus munitions onto the global arms market. Terrorists can now draw on a much more varied set of financial institutions and instruments to fundraise and provide support for their activities (Biersteker and Eckert 2008). Surprisingly, the global wave of democratization that spread across the planet during the 1990s may also have inadvertently made terrorist activities easier, thereby reducing the necessity of state support (Chenoweth 2010). Finally, the decline of Marxist–Leninism has partially been supplanted by the rise of Islamic, Christian, Jewish, and even Buddhist (Tamil Tigers) religious extremism (Juergensmeyer 2000), providing an ideological motivation for joining new terror groups, organizations that previously would have articulated anti-Western or anti-modern policy objectives through a Marxist or other secular ideological lens. In the Muslim world in particular, the rise of religious extremism has dramatically reduced state affiliations with terrorism, as most Muslim-majority states are not theocracies. Indeed, it is the very "apostasy" of the regimes of Egypt, Syria, and Jordan, as well as the formally Wahhabbist, yet fundamentally hypocritical Saudi royal family that funds jihad and also runs with decadent, secular Westerners in bars, hotels, and dance clubs in Europe that has motivated groups like AQ and IS.

SELF-CHECK

- Territorial states are defined in no small part by their capacity for violence. True or false?
- There is broad agreement among both scholars and policymakers as to what defines terrorism. True or false?
- A new form of conflict involving terrorism and transnational criminal activity
  a. Interstate wars
  b. Civil wars
  c. Nationalism
  d. Hybrid wars
- The US government uses one, unified definition for terrorism. True or false?

6.2 Contemporary State Sponsors of Terrorism

As recently as 2002, of the 36 terrorist groups identified by the US government, 20 had some form of state support (Byman 2005, 3). By 2016, this number has plummeted to just three states—Iran, Sudan, and Syria—and a handful of terror groups. Despite this decline in absolute numbers, the three remaining state sponsors have evinced a wide range of support for terrorist groups. In keeping with the discussion in the previous section, what constitutes "sponsorship" is not always as straightforward as direct command of the terrorist group by the state, which remains rare. The scholar Jeffrey Bale provides a useful roadmap for understanding the complex relationship between states and their associated terrorist groups worth quoting in its entirety:

1. **State-directed terrorism**—when elements of the state's security forces actually guide, supervise, or control the terrorist actions of their intermediaries
2. **State-sponsored terrorism**   when elements of the security forces provide hands-on operational assistance for acts of terrorism carried out by their intermediaries
3. **State-supported terrorism**—when elements of the security forces provide logistical support (training, specialized equipment, weapons, finances, false documents, safe houses, cover), but not operational direction or assistance, to facilitate acts of terrorism carried out by their intermediaries
4. **State-manipulated terrorism**—when elements of the security forces covertly manipulate their intermediaries into carrying out acts of terrorism, without the latter's knowledge or consent, by using informants, agents-in-place, infiltrators, or agents provocateurs

5. **State-encouraged terrorism**—when elements of the security forces incite their intermediaries to carry out acts of terrorism against mutual enemies

6. **State-exploited terrorism**—when elements of the security forces knowingly attribute terrorist actions to false perpetrators, usually declared enemies, either to protect their intermediaries or to discredit the political opposition

7. **State-sanctioned terrorism**—when elements of the security forces simply ignore or fail to punish acts of terrorism carried out independently by civilian vigilante groups against targets that are perceived to be enemies by the state (quoted in Vielhaber 2013, 533–534)

As Bale's typology of support indicates, states sponsor terrorist groups for reasons that increase the likelihood of success for the terrorist group yet are also willing to use terrorist groups to realize foreign policy objectives that may dramatically increase the risks for the terrorists themselves. States have even willingly sacrificed terror groups whose general political objectives conform with their own. For example, during the 1980s and 1990s, Egypt and Iraq provided a safe haven, logistical support, intelligence, training, and weapons to the Abu Nidal Organization. Yet following the 9/11 attacks and the United States' clearly-stated intent to make no distinction between terrorist groups and the states that harbored them, Nidal's presence in Iraq presented a potentially dangerous inconvenience for Iraqi dictator Saddam Hussein. Nidal died from gunshot wounds under mysterious circumstances in Baghdad on August 19, 2002 (Whitaker 2002).

Terrorist groups may receive support from different states that conform with different parts of Bale's model. For example, as previously discussed, the Italian terrorist group the Red Brigades received support from both the USSR and Czechoslovakia. Although the Red Brigades received more significant material support from the KGB indirectly through the Italian Communist Party (PCI), Russian support for the group more closely conformed with "state-encouraged terrorism," while Czech intelligence (StB)'s relationship with the group fits best into the "state sponsor" category. As noted earlier, the difference in the nature of support for the group by allied states in the communist bloc reflected different foreign policy goals for the USSR and Czechoslovakia, the divergence of which eventually cost the USSR its relationship with PCI.

In addition, state sponsors also shift the nature of their support over time. This change in how states assist terrorist groups may reflect changes in the political objectives of the sponsor state, the supported terror group, or both. Such shifts in support may also reflect a change in the nature of the tactics used by terrorist groups against their targets. For example, although Pakistan's ISI was a key supporter of Afghanistan's Taliban, ISI's role had to change due to the willingness of the group to continue to harbor al-Qaeda after the 9/11 attacks. Islamabad needed a better relationship with the United States on the eve of the invasion of Afghanistan to hunt down al-Qaeda and the Taliban's intransigence jeopardized that relationship.

The three remaining state sponsors of terrorism as defined by the US State Department have demonstrated different kinds of support for terrorist groups over time (Department of State 2015). It is arguable that one, Sudan, now most closely approximates "state-sanctioned terrorism" and may even be removed from the list if its cooperation with Western intelligence services continues. However, both Iran and Syria remain committed to the use of terrorism to further their respective foreign policies, which although not identical, reflect broadly shared objectives regarding Israel, the presence and role of the United States in the region, and the influence of Saudi Arabia and other Sunni-majority states.

6.2.1 Iran

In 1979, the Iranian Revolution removed the *Shah* (Emperor) from his throne, and the United States' strongest ally in the region was transformed into an Islamic republic. Yet even before the revolution had consolidated its power, US–Iranian relations had changed in a fundamental way. One of the acts accompanying the revolution was the seizure of the US Embassy in Tehran, an event almost without precedent in international politics. A group of Iranians, mostly college students, overwhelmed the weak US security force and took the embassy personnel hostage. Their objective was to compel the United States to return the *Shah* to Iran for trial for the considerable crimes he had perpetrated against the Iranian people. As the *Shah* had sought refuge in the United States for cancer treatment, President Jimmy Carter refused to return him to Iran and thus began the 444 days of the hostage crisis. During this period, the new Iranian government of Ayatollah Khomeini transitioned from tolerance of the seizure of the US hostages to overt support for the students. Even when the hostages were released in 1981, US–Iranian relations remained hostile. The United States froze all Iranian government assets held in US banks, which continued until 2015 when the bulk of the money was returned as part of Iran's agreement to halt its nuclear weapons program, a deal known as the Joint Comprehensive Plan of Action (JCPOA).

Following the revolution, the Iranian Shiite majority established a state with some democratic characteristics—the *Majles*, the Iranian parliament, and its President are elected by popular vote—as well as more authoritarian or theocratic features. The most powerful actor in Iran is the Supreme Leader, indirectly appointed by the Guardian Council, a group of 12 clerics and judges appointed by the Supreme Leader. Since the Islamic Revolution, Iran has been governed under the concept known as *Velayat e-faqih*, which holds that Iran's people and secular governmental institutions must be watched over by the country's Shiite clerical class, the *ulema*. Although the Supreme Leader has some institutional blocks on his power and is thus not a dictator strictly speaking, he appoints many of the most important civil servants, directs the country's foreign policy, and commands Iran's armed forces, including the Islamic Revolutionary Guard Corps, an organization that has been linked to terrorism since its inception and continues to sponsor terrorism through its subsidiary, the **Quds Force**.

Since 1984, the US government has listed Iran as a state sponsor of terrorism. In the years following the hostage crisis, Iran has sought to spread the Shiite Islamic revolution across the Middle East and Southwest Asia. Although Iran has never targeted US citizens outside of the region, Iranian-sponsored terror groups have killed and kidnapped US diplomatic, military, and intelligence personnel in the Middle East. During an internationally sponsored peacekeeping mission in 1983, truck bombs struck both the US Marine and French military barracks, killing nearly 300. An earlier attack that same year on the US Embassy killed nearly 20 Americans, including several prominent CIA officers. A group calling itself "Islamic Jihad" claimed responsibility for both attacks, though more recent scholarship and court findings have determined both attacks were executed by **Hezbollah** (Party of God), an Iranian-sponsored terrorist group that emerged in southern Lebanon after the Israelis invaded Lebanon in 1982 to strike at PLO staging areas and training camps. During the Israeli incursion and subsequent UN peacekeeping mission of the United States and France, Hezbollah kidnapped over 100 US citizens and other Westerners. This second hostage crisis precipitated an ill-conceived US covert attempt to buy the hostages' freedom. US Marine Lieutenant Colonel Oliver North, a staff member on the National Security Council, sold US anti-tank missiles to the government of Iran in an effort to secure the release of the hostages. This effort failed, the Iranians got the weapons, and the consequent Iran–Contra Scandal of 1987 nearly ended the presidency of Ronald Reagan. Although eight hostages were murdered, including CIA Station Chief William Buckley and UN observer Marine Corps Colonel William Higgins, through a combination of prisoner exchanges with Israel and negotiations with both UN and unaffiliated mediators Hezbollah released the remainder of the hostages in 1991.

Since the violence of the 1980s, Hezbollah has gradually evolved into a "hybrid" terrorist group (Azani 2013), with significant commitments to social welfare, education, housing construction, and economic reform. One could have made the case that during the attacks on Western targets in Lebanon, Hezbollah was performing purely as a client of Iran (Kepel 2003). Early in the group's existence, at least some of its operations "were directly controlled by Iran's Ministry of Intelligence and Security" (Rudner 2010, 227). This is hardly surprising, as the group's identity is intimately linked to the key tenets of the Islamic Revolution in Iran, chiefly *Velayat e-faqih*, and the group recognizes the clerical authority of Iran's Supreme Leader. Yet Hezbollah has also been deeply involved in the governance of Lebanon. It has openly participated in Lebanon's electoral process and become the most important political party in the country, despite its ongoing terrorist activities against the very government from which it has sought inclusion, such as the 2005 assassination of the Lebanese Prime Minister Rafic Hariri. Hezbollah continues to receive extensive weapons, training, and intelligence support from Iran, with many of its personnel trained in Iran by the Quds Force. Iran's support is so extensive that it even supplied Hezbollah with anti-ship missiles during the 2006 Lebanon War (Mazetti and Shanker 2006). Despite its ostensible evolution as a hybrid group, Hezbollah remains a terrorist group committed to striking not only in the region but also at targets as far away as Argentina, where Hezbollah executed several attacks against the Israeli Embassy and Jewish organizations during the 1990s.

Hezbollah is not the only terrorist group supported by Iran. The Palestinian group **Hamas** also receives weapons, training, and logistical support from Iran. In addition, Iran sponsors an Iraqi Shiite terrorist group, Kata'ib Hezbollah (KH), which participated in some attacks against US forces during the occupation of Iraq. More recently, Iran has been using KH to attack IS forces in Northern Iraq and

Syria. Iran continues to view its terrorist allies as one of its most important tools to menace Israel, support the Baathist regime of Syria and destroy IS, thwart Saudi Arabia's attempts to expand its influence, and supplant the US as the region's key player in power politics.

6.2.2 Sudan

Although in recent years Sudan has cooperated extensively with US intelligence agencies in the struggle against international terrorism, the country has a much longer history of support for terrorist groups. Carlos the Jackal received sanctuary from the Sudanese government for several years before they allowed the French domestic intelligence agency (DST) to apprehend him and return him to Europe for trial. In 1990, Sudanese intelligence officials actively sought out Osama bin Laden to persuade him to move his fledgling Islamic terrorist organization to Khartoum (Wright 2006, 164), where bin Laden's Egyptian ally Ayman al-Zawahiri's organization, al Jihad, was already located. Bin Laden and his core al-Qaeda followers spent over five years in Sudan, until they were expelled in 1996 following severe international sanctions against the country for sheltering al-Qaeda and al Jihad, which sponsored attacks against the World Trade Center in 1993 and an attempted assassination of Egyptian President Hosni Mubarak while they were based in Sudan. Though Sudanese officials did not cooperate as they had with DST and Carlos and allowed the CIA to seize bin Laden, Sudan ceased all support for al-Qaeda after 1996.

Despite summarily expelling bin Laden and his followers in the 1990s, Sudan did not suspend its support for terrorism. Sudan has allowed Hamas to operate in its territory, including serving as a fundraising location and weapons transshipment point (Department of State 2015, 301). However, since 2015 this support has been curtailed.

FOR EXAMPLE

Carlos the Jackal

Born the son of Marxist revolutionaries in Venezuela in 1949, Ilyich Ramirez Sanchez or "Carlos the Jackal" as he became more widely known was the world's most dangerous terrorist during the wave of terrorism following the anti-colonial insurgencies of the 1950s and 60s. Initially working under the aegis of the Marxist PFLP, Carlos eventually became involved with a variety of groups, including the Japanese Red Army (JRA) and the Baader-Meinhof Gang, before founding his own terrorist organization, the Organization for Armed Struggle, which at various times received some support from East Germany, Syria, Iraq, and Hungary. Carlos became a global figure following a daring raid on the 1975 Organization of Petroleum Exporting Countries (OPEC) meeting in Vienna. Killing three people and taking the oil ministers hostage, Carlos demanded the authorities broadcast a statement from the PFLP regarding the plight of the Palestinians, which the Austrian government agreed to, thus avoiding the summary execution of the terrorists' captives. Carlos demanded and received the use of Austrian airliner, which spirited the PFLP team away with many of the hostages. Eventually freeing all of the hostages in exchange for a large cash ransom, Carlos was subsequently kicked out of the PFLP for not killing several of the oil ministers from countries that were deemed insufficiently supportive of the Palestinian cause.

Despite his expulsion from PFLP, Carlos intensified his terrorist activities, developing and nurturing a broad network of interconnected terror teams from widely disparate countries, all operating along mission parameters determined by Carlos and his state sponsors. This kind of networked, globalized terror organization was still very new, and Carlos was regarded as an innovator in this area. He was also particularly media savvy (Hoffman 2006, 183 and 248), using print, radio, and television to his advantage, portraying his activities as heroic and the violence his affiliated groups created justified as acts of "anti-imperialist resistance." Regardless of his stated Marxist allegiance, Carlos seemed focused at least as much on cultivating his own notoriety as he was in furthering the interests of the socialist countries that sponsored him. His womanizing, relentless self-promotion, heavy drinking, and maniacal leadership style caused friction with many of his state sponsors.

Although he often had difficult relationships with his handlers, Carlos remained active in Western Europe into the 1980s. In 1982, Carlos' group exploded a bomb on a train traveling from Paris to Toulouse, killing five and wounding over two dozen, followed quickly by a bomb targeting a writer opposed to the Syrian regime (BBC 2011). In the next year, members of Carlos' organization bombed two French high-speed trains (TGV), killing four (Rault 2010, 23). Carlos and his affiliates were linked to dozens of violent attacks, including the murder of policemen, a pharmacy bombing, and an attack on a nuclear power plant in France. In the atmosphere of détente, or thawing of relations between the Eastern bloc and the West, such violence brought pressure on Carlos' state sponsors to force him to reduce his activities. His subsequent exile to Syria where his activities were frowned upon by the Baathist regime uprooted him again in 1993, this time to Sudan, where his conversion to Islam was viewed sympathetically and he was given refuge. However, Sudan's involvement with al-Qaeda and pressure by the West to reduce its support for terrorism ultimately led to his capture by French intelligence officers and repatriation to France for trial in 1994. He was subsequently convicted of killing two French policemen in 1997 and sentenced to life in prison. He has been put on trial twice since then, with a 2011 conviction for the bomb attacks in Paris during the 1980s and another in 2017 for a 1974 attack on a drugstore, marking his third life sentence.

6.2.3 Syria

Syria's involvement with international terrorism dates to at least 1979, when the country was designated a state sponsor of terrorism by the US State Department. Despite the ruling Alawite clan's Shiite faith, the Baathist regime of Syria had long viewed Iran with suspicion, due to both its close alliance with the United States (Syria was a client of the USSR) and the Shah's regional aspirations. However, following the Iranian Revolution in 1979 and the subsequent invasion of Iran by Iraq under Saddam Hussein, Syrian dictator Hafez al-Assad began to view Iran as a means of balancing against Hussein's ambition to make Iraq the dominant state in the region, as well as useful foil against the United States. Indeed, Syria immediately supported the seizure of the US Embassy by Iranian students and called on the other Arab states to do the same (Goodarzi 2006, 25). Thus, the Syria–Iran alliance was almost from the start associated with terrorism. During the US intervention in Lebanon, Hezbollah operated with Iranian support and direction from Syrian territory, activities that included the attacks on the US Embassy and Marine Barracks and the kidnapping of dozens of Western officials. Syria was implicated in these operations just as much as Iran (Goodarzi 2006, 93–94). Although Syria and Iran have been aligned in no small part due to their mutual support of Hezbollah and Hamas, Syria's historical position in the region has differed dramatically from Iran's.

Syria has enjoyed a generally lower rate of economic growth than other states in the region, lacks significant resource endowments, is composed of one of the most diverse multiethnic and multiconfessional populations in the region, and its geographic position along the borders of three states that have historically been much more powerful—Russia, Turkey, and Iran—all make Syria labor under a strategically weak position (Leverett 2005). To compensate for these weaknesses, Syria has pursued several strategies, often simultaneously, that would seem contradictory. First, in keeping with its status as a client state of the Soviet Union during the Cold War, Syria supported terrorist groups that were sponsored by other communist bloc states, including the Kurdistan Workers' Party, the Japanese Red Army, and the PLO (Leverett 2005, 10). Second, Syria has historically participated in the numerous Pan-Arab wars with Israel in 1948, 1967, 1973, and alone against Israel in 1982, thereby including Syria within the broader Arab regional community. Third, Syria used support for the PLO and Hamas as a means to further emphasize its ongoing participation in Arab efforts against Israel, while also supporting Hezbollah, thereby bolstering relations with Iran, which was increasingly viewed as a threat by the Sunni-majority states. Fourth, Syria joined the US-led international coalition against Saddam Hussein during the Gulf War. Contributing an armored division that fought alongside Egyptian and Saudi troops, Syria earned praise from the Bush administration for also "helping to restrain terrorist groups that might have targeted U.S. and other Western interests during the war with Iraq," praise forthcoming despite Syria's horrendous human rights record and support for terrorism (Moseley 1991).

In sum, under Hafez al-Assad, Syria converted a comparatively weak strategic position into one that placed Syria at the forefront of states in the region. Sponsoring terrorism was just one tool among many that made this happen, tools ranging from repeated aggression against Israel to solidifying a reputation in the West for pragmatism. With the elder Assad's death in 2000, it looked as if his son Bashar would continue his program of policy adaptability following 9/11, when Syria cooperated with the United States and provided intelligence against al-Qaeda (Leverett 2005, 16–17). Yet much like his father before him, Bashar al-Assad's pragmatism never ceased to reflect the ruthlessness that has always defined the Baathist regime. Following the US invasion of Iraq, Assad allowed large numbers of extremist Islamic fighters to cross the border with Iraq to fight coalition forces. This solved two problems for the younger Assad. First, it removed these jihadis from Syria where they would have continued to oppose his family's secular dictatorship. Second, these "foreign fighters," as they became known in the lexicon of that conflict, would harass the United States and frustrate the goals of the new Iraqi regime. If Iraq were to successfully transition to democracy under US leadership, Syria could not be far behind.

Moreover, despite his seeming cooperation in the struggle against al-Qaeda, Assad continued to support terrorism, ramping up his commitment during the early 2000s toward both Hamas and Hezbollah. This commitment was clearly on display with Syria's cooperation with Hezbollah to assassinate Lebanese Prime Minister Rafic Hariri, who had sought to sharply reduce Syrian influence in his country (United Nations Security Council 2005). The Syrian government also continued to back Hamas' opposition to efforts by its more moderate Palestinian rival organization, Fatah, to cooperate with Israel in pursuit of the "two-state solution" to the Palestinian–Israeli conflict. Yet Assad has been just as mercurial as his father, switching policy positions sharply from one extreme to another. In 2012, Syria expelled Hamas from Syria, citing the groups' support for extremist groups involved in the post-Arab Spring efforts to remove Assad from power (Cole 2015).

Despite Assad's disavowal of Hamas, Syrian support for Hezbollah remains strong. Indeed, despite the continued support of Hamas by its other sponsor, Iran, the group's fate has become even more strongly linked with the Assad regime. Several thousand Hezbollah fighters have participated in combat against Syrian opposition groups, both the Sunni extremist IS and more moderate groups supported by the West, such as the Free Syrian Army (BBC 2013). In addition to direct support for Hezbollah, the US State Department indicates that Syria's lack of interest in regulating the movement of currency in the country provides an environment for transnational terrorist group to raise money and to transfer it with impunity. Finally, Syria has commonly used terrorist tactics against the dozens of groups opposing the Assad regime, from deliberately targeting civilian hospitals to dropping "barrel bombs"—large canisters containing scrap metal and nails—in opposition neighborhoods, indiscriminately killing tens of thousands of Syrians. Syria is an incubator for all varieties of terrorist activity.

6.3 International and Domestic Responses to State-Sponsored Terror

Nation-states and Inter Governmental Organizations (IGOs) have crafted a wide variety of policy instruments to respond to the terrorist threat in general and state-sponsored terrorism specifically. These policies reflect both domestic laws creating legal instruments to restrict, sanction, and penalize the actions of states that support terrorism and multilateral international agreements to allow states to coordinate their efforts against such actors. In addition, some states have crafted bilateral agreements around specific terrorist issues or groups. Collectively, these efforts have made a significant contribution toward addressing the threats posed by international terrorism. But these laws, treaties, and agreements have occasionally made for curious partnerships. For example, although the Soviet Union was a long-standing state sponsor of terrorism and Russia has more recently used terrorist tactics to support its irredentist ambitions toward its neighbors, the United States and Russia have led efforts to establish the 86-member Global Initiative to Combat Nuclear Terrorism (GICNT 2017). GICNT is particularly important in reducing potential dangers stemming from state-sponsored terrorism, as the most likely avenue for nuclear terrorist activities remains via state support.

6.3.1 United Nations Security Council (UNSC)

On September 28, 2001, the UNSC approved Resolution 1373, which unlike most UN instruments was not presented to the General Assembly (GA) for a vote. Rather, the UNSC passed a resolution that was binding on all member states with or without their consent. UNSC 1373 is particularly important for combating state-sponsored terrorism as it provides a very specific list of activities that all states must prohibit, that states must suppress terrorist financing and access to funds, and that states must harmonize their domestic laws to make acts of terrorism criminally prosecutable. Tellingly, the resolution was passed unanimously and the meeting to vote on the resolution lasted only three minutes, suggesting a strong consensus among UNSC members toward combating terrorism and a lack of tolerance toward states that abetted their activities in the wake of the 9/11 attacks, which had occurred barely six miles away.

In 2004, the UN Security Council continued its efforts against state-sponsored terrorism by including the proliferation of chemical, biological, radiological, and nuclear explosive (CBRNE) materials to non-state actors as a proscribed activity under UNSC Resolution 1540. The Security Council also established a standing committee, the 1540 Committee, to monitor the required implementation of export control measures on CBRNE weapon materials, domestic law harmonization, and increased international cooperation to inhibit trafficking in such weapons (UNSC 1540 Committee 2017). These efforts complemented the ongoing measures to prevent access by non-state actors to radiological and nuclear material under the aegis of the International Atomic Energy Agency (IAEA).

In addition to specific resolutions undertaken by the UNSC to address international terrorism, in 2001 the UNSC established the Counterterrorism Committee (CTC), which includes all 15 Security Council member states. Subsequently, in 2004 the Counterterrorism Committee Counterterrorism Executive Directorate (CTED) was created to monitor member state implementation and compliance with UNSC 1373 around the world.

The Office of the General Secretary of the United Nations, which is the executive branch of the United Nations that oversees the UN bureaucracy, also established the Counterterrorism Implementation Task Force (CTITF) in 2005. CTITF coordinates the activities of 38 organizations around the world that are working on activities related to CTITF's strategy, which has four primary components:

1. Measures to address the conditions conducive to the spread of terrorism
2. Measures to prevent and combat terrorism
3. Measures to build states' capacity to prevent and combat terrorism and to strengthen the role of the United Nations system in that regard
4. Measures to ensure respect for human rights for all and the rule of law as the fundamental basis for the fight against terrorism (UNCTITF 2017).

6.3.2 Other Multilateral Efforts

The United Nations is not the only IGO that has served as a source of coordination in the global counterterrorism effort. As the most powerful collective security organization in history, the North Atlantic Treaty Organization (NATO) was also the first IGO to respond to terrorism with the deployment of military forces. Shortly after the 9/11 attacks, Article 5 of the North Atlantic Treaty was invoked by NATO Secretary General Lord Robertson, signaling the duty of all treaty signatories to participate in the collective defense of the United States. Within a month, the skies over the US East Coast were patrolled by aircraft from 13 countries assisting the US Air Force maintain its combat air patrol (NATO 2016a). NATO soon deployed naval forces to begin to interdict terrorist smuggling in the Mediterranean.

Although the alliance had included terrorism as part of its 1999 Strategic Concept statement, NATO had not developed a long-term strategy as to how to deal with terrorism, state-sponsored or otherwise. In May 2002, alliance members met in Reykjavik and determined that NATO would deploy forces out of its traditional area of operations to combat terrorism, thus ending one of the debates that had marked the organization since the end of the Cold War. Consequently, in 2003 NATO assumed command of the US occupation of Afghanistan, establishing the International Security Assistance Force (ISAF), which directed the coalition war effort against 29 different armed groups operating in Afghanistan and along its border with Pakistan. Although this command formally ended in December 2014, NATO forces remain in the country to continue to train and support Afghan forces. NATO has continued its commitment to counterterrorism beyond operations in Afghanistan. In a series of summits in Riga, Lisbon, Chicago, and Warsaw from 2006 to 2016, the alliance has redefined the danger of terrorism employing CBRNE as one of the greatest security threats faced by its members and further committed member states step the level of cross-national coordination to respond to terrorism (NATO 2016b).

Although not collective security organizations, several other IGOs have made significant commitments to countering terrorism. Regional governance organizations have been particularly prominent. The European Union (EU), Association of Southeast Asian Nations (ASEAN), the Organization of American States (OAS), and the African Union (AU) have all responded to the threat posed by terrorism. The EU and its predecessor the European Community (EC) have a long history of cross-border coordination against terrorism, as Europe was the site of much of the terrorist activity of the 1960s and 70s. Following the 9/11 attacks, the EU enacted the Tampere Programme, which defined specific crimes as terrorism, created a common arrest warrant for all EU members, and established a body to coordinate the efforts of member states' judiciaries. However, EU efforts to create a counter-terrorism task force that would share intelligence from security services and the police failed amidst member concerns over sovereignty and the potential violation of individual citizen's rights accompanying a broad transnational intelligence-sharing program (Coolsaet 2010, 859). ASEAN committed to a 2001 Declaration of Joint Action to Counterterrorism, which emphasized increased intelligence sharing, law enforcement coordination, and suppression of terrorist financing activities in the region (Pushpanathan 2003). OAS established the Inter-American Committee against Terrorism (CICTE) in June 2002. Though ratified by only 24 of OAS' 34 members, CICTE serves as a basis for ensuring member state compliance and coordination with UNSC counterterrorism instruments. Although the AU established the Convention on the Prevention and Combating of Terrorism in 1999 under its previous name, the Organization for African Unity (OAU), much like the other regional governance organizations, the 9/11 attacks gave new impetus for action. The AU subsequently adopted the Dakar Declaration in October of 2001 and then established a research and policy center in Algeria to aid in increasing member state capacity to combat terrorism (African Union Peace and Security 2015). The AU has deployed troops to combat terrorism in Nigeria, Chad, Cameroon, and Somalia.

Non-regional governance IGOs have also contributed to counterterrorism efforts. In 2011, the Global Counterterrorism Forum (GCTF) was established by 30 countries in New York. The GCTF partners with extant organizations like the International Institute for Justice and the Rule of Law (IIJ), the Council of Europe, and the OSCE to help build state CT capacity, reduce extremism, and improve governance, thereby reducing terrorist safe havens in weak states.

6.3.3 US International Counterterrorism Strategy

The struggle against international terrorism now spans three US administrations and has cost over \$4.79 trillion in terms of both war zone expenditures and domestic security outlays (Crawford 2016). Much like the increased coordination, information sharing, and policy harmonization demonstrated by the international community, initial US counterterrorism efforts aimed at increasing the ability of the disparate arms of the government to communicate and collaborate with each other. Although after 9/11 the United States rapidly projected power outward through the invasion and occupation of Afghanistan, Operation Enduring Freedom was undertaken with "off the shelf" military assets created long before the rise of al-Qaeda and its ilk. The US government was not ideally configured for a large counterterrorism effort, with the CIA and FBI statutorily limited in their ability to coordinate their activities and US domestic security organizations similarly unable to cooperate. The US Congress attempted to address some of these shortcomings with the controversial USA PATRIOT Act, which was hurriedly drafted in October of 2001. The USA PATRIOT Act dramatically expanded the surveillance powers of the federal government, including roving wiretaps on vehicles, authorization to search business records that might indicate support for terrorism, and even the ability to compel local libraries to release patron records to authorities. Many of the more extreme elements that probably violated the Fourth Amendment of the US Constitution were subsequently withdrawn or allowed to expire. However, the haste with which the USA PATRIOT Act was drafted and implemented indicated that a more systematic response to the threat of international terrorism was needed.

One of the key findings of Congress' bipartisan *9/11 Commission Report* was that the persistent failure of different branches of the US government to coordinate and communicate was placing considerable limitations on the ability of the government to harness its full counterterrorism capabilities (9/11 Commission 2004, 253). This was not a new claim, as both 1999's Gilmore Commission and 2000's Bremer Report had come to similar conclusions. But in what would prove to be a controversial response to the emerging consensus across these three commissions, President George W. Bush and the Congress pursued the largest reorganization of the US government since World War II. First, in 2003 the Department of Homeland Security (DHS) was established, creating a single cabinet agency responsible for domestic counterterrorism, infrastructure protection, border security, disaster response, and public health. Second, in December of 2004 the US Intelligence Community (US IC) was dramatically restructured, with the 16 agencies of the US IC placed nominally under the leadership of a Director of National Intelligence (DNI). In addition, the Office of the Director of

National Intelligence (ODNI) was created, an agency that would set common hiring and training standards across the community as well as direct the National Counterterrorism Center (NCTC).

Although the creation of DHS saw some real gains in terms of improving the speed and efficiency with which the US government could respond to terrorist attacks on the homeland, DHS also created more duplication of effort across the US IC and did not always generate increased efficiency. For example, DHS' response to Hurricane Katrina in 2005 was both lethargic and costly, marked by incompetent management and wasted resources. In contrast to the problems associated with DHS's response to Katrina, the reorganization of the US IC has improved standards across the community. However, over 80% of the US intelligence budget still remains outside the DNI's control. The ODNI's mission of increasing the integration of intelligence information has not been entirely realized, and a new layer of bureaucracy has been introduced into the national security analysis and decision-making cycle (See Chapter 12).

The major steps taken by the federal government to restructure were not directed specifically at state-sponsored terrorist threats. Indeed, al-Qaeda was viewed as the archetype of what would become the "new normal" as the Gilmore Commission characterized it. However, the US government did include counter-terrorism measures that would address the dangers posed by terrorists with state sponsors. First, the United States was at the forefront of international efforts to improve the monitoring and tracking of CBRNE, undertaken in conjunction with an ongoing intensification of US government programs to track and inter-dict the smuggling of nuclear weapons and radiological material. Chief among these efforts was the creation of the Global Threat Initiative (GTI) under the authority of the Department of Energy in 2004. GTI works alongside the Department of State's Nuclear Trafficking Response Group (NTRG) and other programs that link with the efforts of other countries to prevent terrorists from acquiring CBRNE. This work goes at the heart of one of the threats posed by state-sponsored terrorist groups. Second, in addition to preventing states from providing terrorists with CBRNE or aiding the acquisition of their precursors, the US government operates an intensified program of financial services and banking surveillance through the Treasury Department that reduces the ability of both terrorist groups and any states that support them from doing so using the global financial system.

Finally, the US government maintains a robust program of sanctions that includes

- A ban on arms-related exports and sales
- Controls over exports of dual-use items, requiring a 30-day Congressional notification for goods or services that could significantly enhance the terrorist-list country's military capability or ability to support terrorism
- Prohibitions on economic assistance
- Imposition of miscellaneous financial and other restrictions (Department of State 2015, 299).

SELF-CHECK

- The United Nations Security Council presides over a council devoted solely to combating terrorism. True or false?
- Much like the response by other countries and international institutions, the domestic response by the United States has focused on increased coordination of government agencies. True or false?
- The US government response to terrorism has concentrated primarily on the threat posed by state-sponsored terrorism. True or false?
- The Office of the Director of National Intelligence
  a. Presides over the budget of the US Intelligence Community
  b. Is responsible for making policy decisions regarding counterterrorism
  c. Failed to act to prevent the 9/11 attack
  d. Coordinates the activities of the US Intelligence Community and sets standards

FOR EXAMPLE

Coordinating US International Counterterrorism Efforts

Emblematic of post-9/11 efforts by the US government to respond to the threat posed by international terrorism is the development of a national counterterrorism strategy, or more specifically, several strategies. Both the Bush and Obama administrations formulated counterterrorism strategies. Although they both recognized the globalized, networked nature of contemporary terrorism, each outlined very different responses. Published in 2003, the *National Strategy for Combating Terrorism* noted the decline of state-sponsored terrorism and the changing nature of the threat. Despite establishing the changing nature of contemporary terrorism, the Bush administration's strategy emphasized as one of its two "fronts" denying al-Qaeda and other groups' state support (17–22). The 2003 strategy noted the importance of linking the internationally focused nature of the document to a domestic counterterrorism strategy via the new Department of Homeland Security, yet failed to do so. In contrast, the Obama administration's 2011 document *National Strategy for Counterterrorism* placed domestic security concerns at its center. Emphasizing a "whole government effort" (7), the 2011 strategy emphasized continued "hardening" of the US homeland through ongoing investment in the infrastructure of border security, immigration control, and community outreach to prevent both the infiltration of terrorists into the United States and the radicalization of potential terrorists in communities vulnerable to such recruitment efforts (11–12). In both statements of strategy, we can see the contrasting policy foci of the two presidencies, with the Bush administration much more interested in the projection of large scale US military forces overseas as counterterrorism and the Obama administration reluctant to project power after the failure of US efforts in Iraq and the stalemate in Afghanistan.

Both administrations also established separate strategies to protect the US homeland. The Bush administration produced two documents outlining the strategy to protect the domestic United States. Published in 2002, the *National Strategy for Homeland Security* made a significant effort to outline how the various parts of the federal, state, and local governments should link up to thwart terrorism and respond more effectively to terrorist attacks that did occur. Yet this strategy made no mention of the dozens of other functions of the agencies tied to the Department of Homeland Security. With its exclusive focus on counterterrorism, the 2002 strategy was out of step with the most common missions facing the various agencies it tried to coordinate. Following Hurricane Katrina in 2005 and the poor response of the federal government, 2007s *National Strategy for Homeland Security* attempted to address the prior overemphasis on counterterrorism by introducing the "all-hazards" approach (32). Choosing to emphasize his *National Security Strategy* (2015) as the primary source for homeland security strategy, President Obama never issued a stand-alone statement of homeland security strategy. Instead, DHS produced a *Department of Homeland Security Strategic Plan* (2012), which established goals and performance metrics that varied little from the previous administration's 2007 Homeland Security strategy.

Strictly speaking, none of the counterterrorism or homeland security documents outline a strategy—they fail to identify US interests and tie specific activities, both domestic and international, to protecting or furthering these interests. Although there are repeated references to American values and the nature of US democracy, both administrations repeatedly failed to establish core US interests in their attempts to define strategy. Yet with these documents, both presidencies did make significant inroads into increasing the level of coordination between all levels of government with regard to counterterrorism. Nevertheless, a recent report from the House of Representatives Homeland Security Committee found that fundamental problems in redundancy of effort, inefficient allocation of resources, and coordination with US partners overseas remain (House Homeland Security Committee 2016, 13 and 17–18).

SUMMARY

With its extraordinary violence leveled against largely defenseless civilian targets, terrorism would seem to pose a severe threat. At the height of what the Bush administration called the "Global War on Terrorism," US Army General Peter Schoomaker claimed "we're facing a national security situation that is at least as dangerous, if not more dangerous, than we faced in World War II"

(Donnelly and Waller 2005), a sentiment echoed by former Chairman of the Joint Chiefs of Staff General Martin Dempsey in 2012 (Zenko 2013). But terrorism does not pose nearly the danger that Schoomaker or others would claim. Americans are far more likely to die from car crashes or workplace accidents than from terrorism, which is more akin to "risks of using home appliances" than how it is commonly portrayed in the media or the threat it is believed to pose by a majority of the public (Mueller and Stewart 2010, 2016). Moreover, the incidence of political violence in the contemporary international system is at its lowest since the end of World War II (Human Security Report Project 2013), with overall levels of all forms of violence perhaps the lowest they've ever been in human history (Pinker 2011).

Yet state-sponsored terrorism carries with it potentially greater dangers than terrorist groups acting alone and continues to deserve our attention and vigilance. First, although globalization and technological changes have made it easier for terrorist groups to obtain financing, buy weapons, and launch attacks, terrorist groups still face enormous resource challenges if they wish to inflict mass casualty attacks against states. Groups supported by states may more readily gain access to CBRNE, something that has been almost impossible for terrorist groups lacking state support to achieve. Thus far only the Japanese doomsday terrorist group **Aum Shinrikyo** has been able to obtain WMD—sarin gas that was used in an attack on a Tokyo subway in 1995. Tellingly, Aum Shinrikyo had assets in excess of $1 billion and was skilled at recruiting Japanese government personnel with military and scientific backgrounds (Senate Government Affairs Permanent Subcommittee on Investigations 1995). Most terrorist groups seeking to inflict mass casualties on target populations lack the vast resources and pool of technical personnel of Aum Shinrikyo, making state support vital to obtain CBRNE. Some states in the international system may have incentives to use such groups as proxies against the United States and its allies, making the threat of state-sponsored terrorism potentially greater than the unaffiliated terrorism more common to the current international system.

Second, state-sponsored terrorism has historically been used and continues to be used as a means to prop up regimes during civil wars or other periods of unrest. Much as the Nazis used terror to seize and hold power, so too did the Taliban in Afghanistan during the 1990s (Coll 2004). The Taliban was the creation of Pakistan's ISI, making the Taliban a state-sponsored terrorist group, at least during this time period. The North Korean regime remains dedicated to using every form of coercion to prevent even the slightest form of opposition to its ruler, Kim Jong Un. Much of this violence has been extrajudicial in nature and employs tactics such as forced labor, public execution, torture, rape, and forced abortions (Department of State 2017). As discussed earlier, both Syria and Iran have used terrorist groups to prop up the Assad regime and combat IS.

Finally, there may be an emergent model of state-sponsored terrorism that harkens back to earlier terrorist groups. In 1914, the Serbian terrorist group the Black Hand infiltrated one of its cells across the border into a region of the Austro-Hungarian Empire that was ethnically majority Serb. Despite suffering setbacks due to the gross incompetence of its inexperienced and poorly trained operatives, the group managed to assassinate its target, Archduke Franz Ferdinand, heir to the

Austro-Hungarian throne and a moderate who had advocated a federation to address ethno-nationalist grievances, a "United States of Austria." The Black Hand was sponsored by the Serbian government and directed by the head of Serb intelligence, Colonel Dragutin Dimitrijevic (codenamed "Apis"). In achieving their aim, Apis and the Serbian government probably got more than they bargained for, as the attack understandably enraged the Austrian government and sparked World War I. Yet after four years of combat that resulted in at least 127 000 killed out of a total population of 4.5 million (Gilbert 1994, 540–541), the Serbs were nevertheless rewarded for terrorism in the name of **irredentism** with political dominance over a new multiethnic state, Yugoslavia.

Almost exactly 100 years later, dozens of so-called self-defense militias supported by Russian special forces without national or unit insignia seized Crimea from Ukraine, enabling its subsequent annexation by Russia and sparking a low-intensity insurgency in Ukraine's Donbas region that continues today. Although the backbone of the effort was the "little green men" (Schevchenko 2014) as they became known—the aforementioned Russian troops euphemistically listed as "on-leave" while they participated in the invasion—there was an indigenous anti-government movement in Crimea that did not shy away from using terror to inflict its will and pave the way for its Russian supporters. Some scholars have argued that the Russian annexation of Crimea is part of a larger plan to recover much of the territory "lost" when the Soviet Union broke apart, albeit with a more imperial than socialist tenor. Part and parcel of this campaign is the use of Russians in ethnic enclaves located in states like Ukraine, Georgia, and Estonia, groups readily converted into irregular forces (Grigas 2015). Such groups were instrumental in terrorizing loyal Ukrainian government officials and citizens in 2014.

Whether stemming from increased resources to obtain CBRNE, support regimes under pressure, or in furtherance of ethnic irredentism, state-sponsored terrorism is likely to continue, at least in the near future. Although much reduced from its height during the Cold War, terrorist groups may still find support from states at the margins of international politics. Similarly, some states may see ways in which the unconventional nature of terrorist activities may be used as an asymmetric weapon to effect real results, such as the seizure of territory and the "return" of lost members of a shared ethno-national identity or as a means to undermine the foreign policy objectives of the United States and its fellow democracies. Support for terrorism has historically allowed some regimes to "punch above their weight." Despite the sharp decrease in state-sponsored terrorism since the end of the Cold War, this remains true in the contemporary international system.

In this chapter you learned the similarities and differences between terrorism and other forms of collective violence. You established the legal bases through which nation-states wages war and the challenges this legal framework presents in both understanding terrorism and crafting strategies to combat terrorists. You studied the changing nature of terrorism, from secular, state-sponsored groups of the late twentieth century to the globalized, mostly independent groups of today. You examined the few remaining state sponsors of terror. You analyzed the various multilateral responses to terrorism in the international community, as well as the various efforts by the US government to respond to terrorism, both domestically and internationally. Finally, you noted the new pattern of irredentist terrorism pursued by ethnic Russians in Ukraine, the ongoing challenges of authoritarian regimes, and the durable incentives terrorist groups have for seeking state support.

KEY TERMS

Al-Qaeda	An international terrorist group founded in the late 1980s by Arab fighters who had supported the native Afghan resistance against the invasion of the Soviet Union. Its first leader, Osama bin Laden, was killed by US forces in 2011 and it is currently led by Ayman al-Zawahiri. Al-Qaeda has branches in dozens of countries in West Africa, the Middle East, South Asia, and Southeast Asia.
Aum Shinrikyo	Japanese terrorist group that operated primarily in the 1990s and believed the end of the world was coming. It attacked the Tokyo subway system with sarin in 1995.
Geneva Conventions	Body of international law with 196 signatory countries that defines what constitutes a legal basis to go to war and what kinds of violence may be legally used on the battlefield, and identifies specific protections enjoyed by both unarmed civilians and prisoners of war.
Hamas	Palestinian terrorist group operating primarily in the Gaza Strip, which it also governs. Formerly supported by both Syria and Iran, Syria has broken off support in protest over Hamas' support of Sunni extremists opposed to the regime of Bashar al-Assad.
Hezbollah	Shiite terrorist group based primarily in Lebanon. Sponsored by both Iran and Syria, Hezbollah is also the most important political party in Lebanon.
Hybrid wars	Conflicts that combine multiple components, both conventional and unconventional. Hybrid wars may combine narcotics trafficking and other forms of organized crime, terrorism, ethno-religious conflict, and interstate war.
Interstate wars	Armed conflict between two or more territorial states.
Irredentism	Attempts by states and non-state actors to combine groups with a shared ethno-national identity separated by international borders.
Lashkar-e-Tayyiba	Terrorist group based primarily in Pakistan-controlled Kashmir. It has links to Pakistani intelligence and is probably sponsored by the government of Pakistan.

Legitimacy	The perception of citizens that their state has the right to rule over them.
Nationalism	The most common form of collective identity in the modern era. Nationalists believe that nationalism trumps all other identities and sources of political loyalty in their state.
Quds Force	Branch of the Iranian Revolutionary Guards that supports international terrorist groups.
Sovereignty	A state's legal control over territory, including passage the movement of goods, services, and people across its borders. Sovereignty exists by virtue of its recognition by other states.
State-sponsored terrorism	When a state provides direction, logistical support, training, intelligence, safe haven, tolerance, ideological inspiration, or other forms of support for a terrorist group.
Territorial state	Defined by its legitimate monopoly over political violence in a given territory. Under international law, only the territorial state is permitted to wage war.
Terrorism	The use of violence directed at civilians to instill fear and coerce other groups that are not the immediate target of the attack.

ASSESS YOUR UNDERSTANDING

Go to www.wiley.com/go/Kilroy/Threats_to_Homeland_Security to assess your knowledge of the state actors and terrorism.

Summary Questions

1. There is general agreement among both scholars and politicians as to what defines terrorism. True or false?

2. There are now far fewer state sponsors of terrorism than there were during the Cold War. True or false?

3. Which of the following states is NOT currently considered a state sponsor of terrorism by the US government?
   (a) Iran
   (b) Syria
   (c) Cuba
   (d) Sudan

4. Which of the following states may have provided support for al-Qaeda?
   (a) Iraq
   (b) Saudi Arabia
   (c) Libya
   (d) Syria

5. The Islamic State is a state-sponsored terrorist group. True or false?

6. Which of the following have been motives for states to sponsor terrorism?
   (a) Shared ideology between the terrorist group and its sponsor
   (b) Using the terrorist group as a proxy to achieve foreign policy goals
   (c) Manipulating the terrorist group to serve as a cutout to conceal activities by the state
   (d) All of the above

7. Which of the following DOES NOT reflect the pattern of state-sponsored terrorism during the Cold War?
   (a) US support for right-wing paramilitary groups in Latin America
   (b) Support by the USSR for both Marxist and non-Marxist terrorist groups
   (c) Direct Soviet command over terrorist groups
   (d) Both US and Soviet client states providing support for terrorist groups

8. Sudan has supported which of the following organizations?
   (a) Hamas
   (b) Hezbollah
   (c) IS
   (d) Red Brigades

9. Which of the following reflect the pattern of Syria's sponsorship of terrorism?
   (a) The Baathist regime supports terrorist groups that reflect its ideology.
   (b) Syria has viewed terrorism as one among many tools of statecraft.
   (c) The Syrian government has supported terrorism primarily directed to the United States.
   (d) Syria has only supported anti-Israel terrorist groups.
10. The European Union has failed to respond to the threat of international terrorism. True or false?

Applying This Chapter

1. You meet several new people on a business trip to Europe. Over dinner, several argue that the United States has supported terrorist groups, just like Russia or Syria. How do you respond?

2. In 2015, the United States, United Kingdom, France, Russia, China, France, and Germany negotiated an agreement with Iran to halt its production of enriched uranium that could be used to build a nuclear weapon. Given what you know about Iran and its support for terrorism, how might the nuclear deal increase or decrease the likelihood that Iran will employ Hezbollah to advance its interests in the region?

3. North Korea, Zimbabwe, and Venezuela are not currently listed by the State Department as state sponsors of terror. Yet the governments of all of these countries employ techniques of repression that one could argue are a form of terrorism. Should the United States expand its definition of what constitutes state-sponsored terrorism? Would this clarify or further muddy the issue of who is a terrorist and who is a "freedom fighter?" How might this change in definition affect how the United States relates to other countries, such as Pakistan?

YOU TRY IT

Removing a State From the List

As a member of the Foreign Service, you have been tasked with evaluating whether or not Sudan should remain on the State Department's list of states that sponsor terrorism. Develop an argument supported by evidence that Sudan should in fact be removed from the list and write a short policy proposal derived from this analysis. Be prepared to respond to counterarguments for why Sudan should in fact remain on the list.

Adding a State to the List

Following the same logic as before, draft a policy proposal arguing in favor of the inclusion of a country on the State Department's list of state sponsors of terrorism that is not currently listed. Be prepared to defend your argument.

7

NON-STATE ACTORS AND TERRORISM
Understanding the Threat From Violent Non-state Actors

Joseph Fitsanakis

Department of Politics, Coastal Carolina University, Conway, SC, USA

Starting Point

Go to www.wiley.com/go/Kilroy/Threats_to_Homeland_Security to assess your knowledge of the basics of non-state actors and terrorism.
Determine where you need to concentrate your effort.

What You'll Learn in This Chapter

▲ The definition of non-state terrorism
▲ The history of terrorism and how it affects terrorist organizations' underlying rationale and continuing belief in the efficacy of violence
▲ The different types of terrorist organizations and examples of each type
▲ The methods employed by terrorist organizations
▲ What can be done to fight non-state terrorism

After Studying This Chapter, You'll Be Able To

▲ Assess the historical development of twentieth-century terrorism
▲ Evaluate the interrelated nature of all terrorism while taking note of the sociohistorical specificity of each type of terrorism
▲ Critique different types of terrorist organizations and recognize the different aims and goals they seek to achieve
▲ Manage tools for combating international terrorism

Threats to Homeland Security: Reassessing the All-Hazards Perspective, Second Edition.
Edited by Richard J. Kilroy, Jr.
© 2018 John Wiley & Sons, Inc. Published 2018 by John Wiley & Sons, Inc.
Companion website: www.wiley.com/go/Kilroy/Threats_to_Homeland_Security

INTRODUCTION

In the previous chapter, we focused on the role of states in the commission of terrorism. We examined how the interstate system is organized and how states, by their ability to employ force, also have the ability to abuse their power. When they do so (either against their own populations or against the populations and/or governments of other states), it could be considered a form of terrorism.

In this chapter, we turn our attention to terrorism conducted by non-state actors. Thus, you will learn the definition of non-state terrorism and assess the historical development of this form of terrorism throughout the twentieth century. You will evaluate the interrelated nature of all terrorism while taking note of the sociohistorical specificity of each type of terrorist act or organization. Finally, you will critique different types of terrorist organizations and recognize the different aims and goals they seek to achieve, as well as develop an understanding of the various tools used to combat international terrorism.

7.1 Explaining the Different Types of Non-state Actors

In order to acquire a detailed understanding of non-state actors and terrorism from the following text, precision is required. Therefore, before we discuss our topic, we must define two crucial terms, namely, non-state actors and terrorism. Non-state actors exist in a variety of forms and are typically of no concern to **counterterrorism** experts, unless they employ violence. Moreover, the use of violence by non-state actors does not necessarily amount to terrorism, nor does it necessarily attach the label of terrorist to the non-state perpetrator of the violence.

7.1.1 Defining Violent Non-state Actors

Non-state actors can be defined as organized entities that operate in the national and international arenas outside the realm of official state structures. Traditionally, political science literature has focused on three kinds of non-state actors, namely, intergovernmental organizations, like the United Nations or the North Atlantic Treaty Organization; nongovernmental organizations, like Doctors Without Borders or the International Committee of the Red Cross; and private corporations, many of which, like Exxon Mobil or the Vodafone Group, conduct operations in more than one country or territory (Haynes et al. 2017, 202). Historically, intergovernmental organizations have been founded and controlled by states. Some, however, like the European Union, have today developed their own distinct institutional identities and tend to operate with considerable autonomy from states.

Non-state actors that belong to one of the aforementioned categories do not operate within state structures and are therefore not usually direct agents of state power. However, they typically interact and interrelate with state structures, whether amicably or competitively. They are also at least partly visible to the public and are subjected to various forms of state regulation. But this chapter concerns a fourth category of non-state actors, that of **violent non-state actors**. The latter not only operate outside state structures but also act mostly in secret and systematically employ physical violence to achieve their **strategic goals**. Unlike violent non-state actors, violent state actors will often employ terrorist tactics. That is, they will resort to the calculated and organized use or threat of indiscriminate violence in order to attain broad political or ideological objectives.

7.1.2 Defining Non-state Terrorism

The term "terrorism" denotes one of the most elusive concepts in political science. Generations of political theorists have struggled to provide a universally agreeable definition of the term. Much of this difficulty stems from the tendency of individuals and institutions to label as "terrorism" any action that threatens their legitimacy or authority. For instance, the apartheid regime of South Africa labeled Nelson Mandela, co-founder of Umkhonto we Sizwe, the armed wing of the African National Congress, a terrorist until 1990, three years before he was awarded the Nobel Peace Prize (Cronin 2010, 394). More recently, the definition of terrorism issued in 2014 by the government of Saudi Arabia includes all actions "calling for atheist thought in any form, or calling into question the fundamentals of the Islamic religion on which this country is based" (Koch 2016, 3). To further complicate an already problematic concept, practitioners of terrorism almost never accepted their characterization of "terrorist" by their adversaries. The long list of apologists includes al-Qaeda co-founder Osama bin Laden, who described himself as a "freedom fighter" (Truman 2010, 15).

7.1.3 Terrorism and "Terrorists"

It is important to clarify here that the use of terrorism as a tactic does not make an actor inherently "terrorist." For instance, historians note that there were clearly "terrorist incidents connected with the outbreak of the American Revolution" and that the many "atrocities and massacres" that occurred as part of the American War of Independence contributed to "a campaign of political terrorism" by the insurgents (Lutz and Lutz 2005, 36) (see also Zafirovski and Rodeheaver 2013, 183). But the fact that "both the insurgent and the revolutionary will likely practice terrorism" (Herbst 2003, 151) in order to achieve their goals does not equate insurgent revolutions with terrorist campaigns. Later, when the United States gained its independence, the new nation ruthlessly targeted Native Americans with the use of what can only be described as systematic state terrorism (Smith 2005, 177). However, no serious scholar of politics or history would describe the American Revolution as a terrorist enterprise any more than he or she would describe post-revolutionary America as a terrorist state. Rather, some American revolutionaries, and later American state officials, employed terrorist tactics in the pursuit of long-term strategic objectives. The same is true for the French revolutionary experience of the late eighteenth century, which introduced the term "terror" in the **modern era of terrorism** political lexicon (Johnson 2009, 387). Undoubtedly, the French revolutionaries employed terrorism on a mass scale after 1793 as an instrument of class warfare. But this does not make the French Revolution an inherently terroristic political enterprise (Wahnich 2012).

> ### FOR EXAMPLE
>
> ### Kurdish Activism or Terrorism?
>
> The Kurdistan Communities Union (KCK) uses terrorist tactics, but is it a terrorist organization? The United States is one of a number of countries and transnational organizations that consider the Kurdistan Workers' Party (PKK)—the main member organization of the KCK—a terrorist group. There is no question that the People's Defense Forces (HPG), the armed wing of the PKK, engages in acts of terrorism against civilians, both inside and outside of its eastern Turkey stronghold (Meho 2004). But this does not mean that the HPG embodies the PKK. As an organization—indeed a movement—the PKK is far broader than its armed wing. It represents a complex set of ideological, social, and political forces that find expressions in civil rights campaigns, political activism, social work, and, occasionally, armed militancy. (Ünal 2012)

This is a crucial distinction that must also be applied to contemporary non-state militant actors. Take the example of Hamas, the Palestinian group that today controls the Gaza Strip. Few independent observers would question the statement that Hamas' military wing, the Qassam Brigades, employs terrorism in and out of the Gaza Strip (Mukhimer 2013). But this does not mean that the Qassam Brigades embodies the entirety of Hamas. Hamas is a broad political movement whose main components are ideological, social, and—after 2006, when it took control of the Gaza Strip—increasingly administrative and bureaucratic. Hamas does engage in terrorist activities through the Qassam Brigades. But it also employs school teachers, runs maternity clinics, organizes conferences, plans agricultural production, and maintains public sanitation systems (Roy 2011). To reduce Hamas to its terroristic component ignores the complexity of the organization and ultimately subverts both military and political counterterrorist efforts aimed at combating it. Similarly, one observer notes that the Shiite Lebanese group Hezbollah's "trademark of the movement" is not violent militancy but "social and humanitarian actions" that Hezbollah calls "fieldwork" (Engeland 2008, 39).

Groups like the PKK, Hamas, and Hezbollah employ a variety of terrorist acts in order to achieve broad strategic goals. Therefore their structures contain terroristic components, which they employ on a regular basis to fight wars against militarily superior adversaries. However, this does not make them principally terroristic any more than the African National Congress, which also engaged in terrorist acts from 1961 until as late as 1989, but was a principally terroristic organization. These organizations use terrorism, not for its own sake, but as a temporary tactic used in combination with other tactics (political, financial, military, and others) to achieve their long-term strategic goals. Despite its loaded undertones, therefore, the term "terrorism" refers to nothing more—and indeed nothing less—than a method of war.

SELF-CHECK

SELF-CHECK

- Define the modern era of terrorism.
- Exxon Mobil would be an example of:
  a. Intergovernmental organizations
  b. Nongovernmental organizations
  c. Private corporations
  d. Violent non-state actors
- Non-state actors typically do not use terrorism as a goal in itself. True or false?
- The American Revolution introduced the term "terror" in the modern political lexicon. True or false?

7.2 Non-state Terrorism as a Security Threat

It is often stated that "terrorism is the weapon of the weak" (Mahan and Griset 2008, 21). The phrase is taken to imply that terrorism is a method of violence resorted to by those who lack large numbers of followers or are unable to amass significant conventional military power. This statement, however, is misleading. History shows that terrorism is primarily the weapon of strong centralized governments. Indeed, when they engage in systematic terrorism, strong centralized governments tend to be far more lethal and brutal than non-state actors. The reason is evident: centralized governments are able to employ the entire machinery of the state in carrying out terrorism. The magnitude of these resources—monetary capital, material supplies, and people—tends to dwarf those of non-state actors, even when the latter have more extreme or brutal attitudes toward violence. Consequently, the terrorism employed by the Islamic State of Iraq and Syria (IS), even at the height of the group's power, cannot be compared with the magnitude of terrorism carried out by the forces of the Third Reich in Nazi Germany (Perdue 1989, 36ff).

Despite the historical truism stated previously, the lack of official legitimacy makes non-state actors more susceptible than state actors to the label of "terrorism." Thus, in the contemporary popular and scholarly literature, the term "terrorism" is far more readily associated with a non-state actor, like Hezbollah, than a state actor, like the regime of Soviet leader Joseph Stalin. In reality, the immense resources employed during the culmination of Stalinist terrorism in 1937–1938 were far more extensive in both scale and lethality than any of Hezbollah's terrorist acts (Pringle 2015, 341). It follows, therefore, that non-state actors are not as dangerous to national or international security as state violent actors. Even at the height of its power, al-Qaeda never posed an existential threat to the national security of the United States or the international security of the world. The same cannot be stated about the Soviet Union, with its 25 000 nuclear warheads at the height of the Cold War. (See Chapter 6 for a further discussion on state-sponsored terrorism.)

7.2.1 Reasons for the Prevalence of Violent Non-state Actors

If violent non-state actors are not as dangerous to states as violent state actors, then why are non-state actors so prevalent in the literature on security and terrorism? There are several reasons, not least of which is the psychological effect of non-state terrorism. The latter seeks to operate on both the tactical and emotional domains, by stressing the seeming randomness and unpredictability of indiscriminate violence. These are aimed at maximizing the emotion of terror among a population (Breckenridge and Zimbardo 2007). One expert explains that the psychological aspects of terrorism set it apart from other social phenomena, in that it "can radically distort fear perception out of proportion to the actual threat, and thus provoke extreme behavioral and emotional collective responses" (Marshall 2012, 3).

The intense psychological effect of terrorism is compounded by the fact that, unlike state actors, violent non-state actors do not usually offer their adversaries the benefit of visibility, nor do they have a clear institutional structure, or at least one that can be readily recognized by a conventional government or military. In the words of General Rupert Smith, violent non-state actors do not subscribe to conventional hierarchy, whereby a military or paramilitary force is "concentrated on achieving its singular military strategic objective, with every individual action and achievement contributing coherently towards that end" (Smith 2007, 327). Instead, violent non-state actors develop **rhizomatically**, that is, through horizontal, nonhierarchical nervous systems, consisting of semi- or entirely autonomous cells that have "no predetermined operational structure." Instead of mirroring conventional military or paramilitary structures, rhizomatic systems develop organically to suit their "surroundings and purpose in a process of natural selection" (Smith 2007, 328ff).

Moreover, violent non-state actors are rarely represented by tangible institutions. They have no recognizable international presence, no diplomats or other international envoys, nor do they recognize the—admittedly imperfect but broadly accepted—international legal system and its conventions. It is important to state here that state sponsors of terrorism also tend to operate clandestinely by interacting with non-state violent entities in secret. However, the difference is that once these activities become known, the culprits are visible and have an institutional presence.

It follows that violent non-state actors are viewed as capable of introducing a degree of instability into the international system of order that far exceeds their numerical strength or military potency. The 9/11 attacks were illustrative of the ability of a relatively small group of extremists to produce one of history's most widely televised events. As Agnieszka Stepinska (2010) has noted, the planners of the attacks carefully catered to the "timing of the newsrooms" by selecting the moment in time that would "maximize the damage" in New York and Washington and at the same time "reach audiences in all parts of the globe" (Stepinska 2010, 210). Such terrorist spectacles, whose power and effect is reinforced by the incessant news cycle of the global media, act as reminders of the fragility of daily life and the ease with which it can be disrupted by relatively small groups of determined assailants. It can be said that terrorism is the easiest form of warfare. It is precisely the ease with which it can be effectively implemented by non-state actors that elicits such strong responses from experts and the broader society alike.

7.2.2 Non-state Terrorism as a Domestic and International Threat

Broadly speaking, non-state terrorism poses a twofold national security threat for organized state structures: **domestic terrorism** and **international terrorism**. Invariably, violent non-state actors challenge the domestic authority of the state or states in whose territory they operate. They may work in small isolated cells, like Greece's Revolutionary Organization 17 November, or they may represent the violent wing of broader political movement, like the Irish National Liberation Army in the British Isles. Popular support for violent non-state actors may represent long-standing sectarian or secessionist ambitions, which may at times threaten the territorial integrity, and even the political cohesion, of a nation-state. Almost by definition, states are able to amass more power than non-state actors in such conflicts. But their efforts are not always successful. In the 1980s, the official government of Somalia was unable to curtail the secessionist campaign of the Somali National Movement, which was established as an armed rebel group by members of the Isaaq clan. The group's decade-long campaign led to the establishment of the Republic of Somaliland, an unrecognized state that today maintains control of most of northern Somalia (Bradbury 2008). A similar situation arose in Eastern Europe in 2014, with the emergence of the United Armed Forces of *Novorossiya* (new Russia). This umbrella group of armed insurrectionists took up arms against the Ukrainian state during the 2014 War in Donbass. Their campaign, which some claim was clandestinely supported by Russia (Hall 2016), eventually led to the *de facto* creation of two largely unrecognized statelets, the Luhansk People's Republic and the Donetsk People's Republic, in southeastern Ukraine.

FOR EXAMPLE

International Collaboration Against Basque Separatism

A typical case of interstate collaboration to combat terrorism was prompted by the violent campaign of *Euskadi Ta Askatasuna*. The group, which translates to Basque Fatherland and Freedom and is known as ETA, was formed in 1959 by ethnic Basque separatists living in the Pyrenees, the mountain range that forms a natural border between Spain and France. ETA has been blamed for at least 800 deaths caused by bombings, assassinations, and other terrorist acts that continue to this day. In 2000, ETA was behind the launch of a new youth organization called *Haika*, which resulted from the amalgamation of Jarrai, a militant youth group in Spain with suspected links to ETA, and *Gasteriak*, a French separatist cell operating in the French Basque Country. Soon afterward, increased attacks on French and Spanish government installations prompted Paris and Madrid to work together to combat *Haika* (Kushner 2011, 94). The group has since renamed itself to *Segi* and gone completely underground. In this case, two states that perceived their territorial integrity to be under threat by a violent non-state actor combined their efforts to combat it. In doing so, they reinstated their control over their respective populations in the Pyrenees and prevented the fragmentation of their national territories, which was *Haika*'s strategic goal.

When they transcend national borders, the activities of violent non-state actors often prompt states to work together in order to combat what they view as a common threat to their legitimacy. But even when they collaborate, states may find it difficult to respond with precision to attacks launched against them by violent non-state actors that are based abroad. International law gives a recognized state the right to respond to verified assaults by other states. But what happens when a recognized state is attacked by a violent non-state actor based abroad, which does not represent the official government of that territory? To what extent can the state on whose territory the assailants are based be held responsible for the attack? In many cases, the targets of these attacks openly accuse foreign governments of sponsoring their perpetrators. The Colombian government frequently accuses its neighboring countries of Ecuador and Venezuela of providing aid and comfort to left-wing paramilitary groups, including the Revolutionary Armed Forces of Colombia (FARC) and the National Liberation Army (ELA) (Gunaratna and Ramirez 2011, 203). In the 1980s, the government of Nicaragua regularly protested the funding by the United States of the Nicaraguan Resistance, also known as *Contras*. The *Contras* were an illegal amalgamation of right-wing paramilitary groups that took up arms against the socialist Sandinista Junta of National Reconstruction government. American support for the *Contras* continued clandestinely even after Congress officially banned it in the first half of the 1980s and culminated in the so-called Iran–Contra affair. Eventually, 14 American officials were indicted, including then Secretary of Defense Caspar Weinberger, for a number of offenses, such as violating congressional directives to refrain from providing aid to the *Contras*. Eleven of them were convicted, but all were pardoned in the concluding days of the presidency of George H.W. Bush (Kornbluh and Byrne 1993). In 1984, the Nicaraguan government filed a lawsuit against the United States at the United Nations International Court of Justice in the Netherlands. It was able to argue successfully that Washington violated international law by funding the *Contras* and mining the country's harbors. The United States refused to participate in most of the proceedings and rejected the court's ruling (Saito 2012, 207).

In the case of the *Contras*, the Nicaraguan government was able to employ international legal channels in order to identify, protest against, and eventually convict another state that assaulted it by using a non-state actor as an agent of violence. But what happens when the attacking non-state actor is not supported by a recognized state or when support is suspected but cannot be conclusively proven? For instance, in 2013 the Sunni militant group al-Shabaab attacked the Westgate shopping mall in Nairobi, Kenya, killing nearly 70 people and injuring hundreds more. The attackers were based in Somalia, but the Somali government was itself one of the group's targets. Soon after the incident, Somali President Hassan Sheikh Mohamud strongly condemned al-Shabaab's "heartless acts against defenseless civilians" and promised to "stand with Kenya" in combating al-Shabaab (Norman 2016, 148). Consequently, Kenya's gamut of responses on the interstate level were severely limited. It could only respond with increased law enforcement or intelligence activity against the assailants and only in cooperation with the government of Somalia.

The international dimension of violent non-state actors highlights yet another important aspect, namely, the potential for interstate armed conflict sparked by the actions of violent non-state actors. World War I is perhaps the most illustrative example of an interstate war that was partly sparked by the action of a violent non-state actor. In June 1914, Gavrilo Princip, a revolutionary from Austrian-occupied Bosnia and Herzegovina, assassinated Austrian Archduke Franz Ferdinand and his wife, Sophie, in Sarajevo. This action, which is widely believed by historians to have precipitated the outbreak of World War I, was carried out by a member of *Mlada Bosna* (Young Bosnia), an underground group inspired by militant **anarchism** and **revolutionary socialism** (Law 2016). Nearly 70 years later, in 1982, when Israel invaded Lebanon, it claimed that its target was not the Lebanese state. Israeli officials justified the invasion as an effort to eliminate the Palestine Liberation Organization (PLO), which Israel accused of using Lebanon as a base from which to launch attacks on Israel (Schiff and Ya'ari 1984).

FOR EXAMPLE

Russia, Turkey, and the Syrian Civil War

The bilateral relationship between Russia and Turkey suffered intensely following the outbreak of the Syrian Civil War in 2011. Both countries became involved militarily in the war—Russia on the side of the Syrian government of Bashar al-Assad and Turkey in support of several Sunni rebel groups opposed to the government. In November 2015, a Russian Su-24 attack jet was shot down by a Turkish F-16 fighter aircraft along the Syrian–Turkish border. The incident caused worldwide alarm and was condemned by Russian President Vladimir Putin as "a stab in the back by the accomplices of terrorists." The heightened tensions prompted some commentators to warn that "a further conflict between Russia and Turkey may be imminent and […] could even result in a world war" (Buhari-Gulmez 2015). Relations between the two countries were strained further in December 2016 when Russia's ambassador to Turkey was assassinated by a Turkish policeman in Ankara, apparently in protest over Russia's military involvement in Syria. According to news reports, the assassination of the ambassador occurred a day after nationwide protests in Turkey against Russia's military and diplomatic support for President al-Assad by groups sympathetic to armed rebels in Syria (BBC 2016b). It can be reasonably argued that the threat to global security posed by the Syrian Civil War is not posed by the activities of violent non-state actors; rather it is the possibility that these activities may spark an armed confrontation between major regional or international powers.

7.2.3 Assessing the Threat Posed by Violent Non-state Actors

Following our analysis, we are able to explain why non-state actors are so prevalent in the scholarly and popular literature on security and terrorism. Their actions cause an intense psychological effect on populations and leaders, which is compounded by the realization that violent non-state actors choose to wage war by their own standards, not those of their opponents. Moreover, violent non-state actors are largely invisible, refusing to be represented by tangible institutions like official seats of government, elected or appointed public administrators, or military leaders. Their lack of a recognizable international presence makes them seem elusive and threatening to the established order of states. They are thus seen as capable of introducing a degree of instability into national and international systems of order, which far exceeds their numerical strength or military capability. On the domestic front, violent non-state actors pose direct challenges to the authority of the state or states in whose territory they operate. On the international front, states find it difficult to respond with precision to attacks launched against them by violent non-state actors that are based abroad. Finally, the actions of violent non-state actors have the potential to spark interstate armed conflict between national actors.

SELF-CHECK

- Define international terrorism.
- Violent non-state actors are more prevalent than state violent actors in the literature on security and terrorism, even though violent state actors are generally more dangerous. True or false?
- The United Nations International Court of Justice in the Netherlands determined that in the 1980s the United States did not violate international law in Nicaragua by funding the Contras and mining the country's harbors. True or false?
- Which war is arguably the most illustrative example of an interstate conflict that was partly sparked by the actions of a violent non-state actor?
  a. World War I
  b. World War II
  c. The Korean War
  d. The Persian Gulf War

7.3 The Typology of Violent Non-state Actors

Aside from their conscious use of terrorism as a tactic of war, most violent non-state actors have little in common, even when they seem to be fighting for the same goals. This has been true historically and it is true today, despite persistent—and predominantly media-led—oversimplified narratives that blend such actors together. Terrorism scholars often caution that "we should be discussing terrorisms—plural—[…] rather than searching for a unified theory of explaining all terrorist behavior […]. There is not a 'one size fits all' explanation" (Club de Madrid ctd in Jones and Libicki 2008, 7). The case of the **War in Afghanistan**, which erupted following the American withdrawal in 2014, is illustrative here. In the minds of many, the war is being fought between the official Afghan military, a state actor, and the Taliban, a non-state actor. In reality, the government side includes several non-state groups that employ terrorist tactics. Among them is the National Islamic Movement of Afghanistan, with a disparate membership drawn from Uzbek Sunnis, some of whom are former communists. They are fighting alongside the Jamayat-E-Islami (Islamic Society), a predominantly Tajik and fervently anti-communist Sunni group with links to Pakistan and Saudi Arabia (Haqqani 2005, 171). The anti-government side is even more complex, consisting of the Taliban, a non-state actor with both **ethno-nationalist/separatist** and religious components, among many other groups. The latter include the very powerful Haqqani Network, which agrees with many of the Taliban's religious views, but has historically oper-ated autonomously, based on its own command structure and tactical priorities (Fitsanakis 2016). Other anti-government groups include the Khalis faction and the Mullah Dadullah Front, which at times cooperate with the Taliban but whose pri-mary allegiance is to localized insurgencies or to warlord families (Chandrasekaran 2012, 290). And of course it includes al-Qaeda-aligned insurgent groups, like the Shadow Army (Lashkar al-Zil) and the Islamic Jihad Union, whose agenda could not be more different to that of the average Taliban fighter, as will be explained later.

The microcosm of the War in Afghanistan illustrates the complexities in trying to compare or categorize violent non-state actors, even within a single conflict. This does not mean that it is impossible or pointless to devise a system of classifica-tion for non-state violent groups. On the contrary, the study of the typology of violent non-state actors can help the student of counterterrorism recognize the broad sociopolitical forces and historical trends that generate and shape terrorist activity. However, one must remain cognizant of the danger of oversimplification that is embedded in every system of typology. There is admittedly little point in attempting to classify violent non-state actors based on the tactical manifestations of their terrorism (the techniques they use to carry out terrorism), for these are markedly common. But there are arguably some shared elements in the **primary motivations**—the core reasons and motives—that prompt violent non-state actors to use terrorism as a tactic of war. To a lesser extent, we can also classify non-state actors based on commonalities in their strategic goals—that is, the ultimate ambi-tions and objectives toward which they employ terrorist tactics.

Most terrorism experts differentiate between three distinct types of violent non-state actors based on their primary motives. These are actors that are moti-vated by (i) **political/ideological** views, (ii) ethno-nationalist creeds, and (iii) religious doctrines (Forest 2012; Martin 2011; Stepanova 2008). Before we pro-ceed to examine each of these categories, two important complications must be acknowledged. First, even if a primary motivating factor behind a group's use of terrorism is readily apparent, one must not disregard the multitude of—often subterranean—factors that underline it. These can be economic, cultural, environ-mental, and even psychological in nature. Second, many violent non-state actors combine elements of more than one of these categories. It is not rare to find a non-state actor using terrorism in order to achieve a long-term vision that includes defined political, ethno-nationalist, and religious creeds. One example of such a group is the Turkistan Islamic Party (TIP), a non-state actor representing separatist Uyghurs in the western Chinese province of Xinjiang. The group, which has been active since at least 1997, operates with the stated aim of creating "East Turkestan," an independent state for Turkic-speaking Muslim Uyghurs. The TIP is motivated by a clear ethno-nationalist creed, which places it squarely in the ethno-nationalist category of violent non-state actors. However, the group also propagates a strict version of conservative Islam and has links to al-Qaeda. That doctrinal element points more toward a religious motivation for terrorist activity. Observers note that the TIP is also fervently anti-communist and actively opposes the political and economic policies of the Chinese government. That places it closer to politically motivated terrorism (Debata 2007).

FOR EXAMPLE

Vietnam: Communism or National Liberation?

The Vietminh (League for the Independence of Vietnam) fought Vietnam's Japanese and French colonialists using a variety of methods, including terrorism. Its parent organization was the Indochinese Communist Party (what eventually became the Communist Party of Vietnam), founded by Hồ Chí Minh, the future President of Vietnam. Its stated aim was to create an independent Vietnam. But its underlying motive was to establish **communism** as a means of social and political organization in the country. As its fighters made clear during the Second Indochina War (1955–1975, known in America as "the Vietnam War"), they were not prepared to concede to an independent Vietnam that was not communist. That is not to say, of course, that every last Vietminh fighter was a committed communist who had read Marx and had internalized core Marxist principles. On the contrary, its rank-and-file members were Vietnamese peasants who were primarily—indeed, often exclusively—fighting for national liberation. (Tanham 2006)

One could suggest that one of these motivating factors must be the primary reason that prompts the TIP to engage in terrorist activities. But the problem is further compounded by the fact that many violent non-state actors deliberately mask their primary motivation if they think it will be unpopular. This illustrates yet another problem of typology, namely, that the stated primary motivating force of violent non-state actors can differ depending on who is asked. In some cases, the groups themselves appear confused or uncertain about their motivations and even their goals. An illustrative example of such a group is the brutal band of guerillas who make up the Lord's Resistance Army (LRA). The group has been active in the jungles of northern Uganda, the Democratic Republic of the Congo, the Central African Republic (CAR), and South Sudan, since the late 1980s. According to specialists, it is exceedingly difficult to identify a clear agenda behind the actions of the group. Depending on the day, the latter appears to be seeking more power for the Acholi people of northern Uganda, the establishment of a multiparty democracy in Central Africa, the incorporation of the Christian Ten Commandments into the Ugandan Constitution, the abolishment of the Ugandan Constitution, or the unquestioned worship of the group's leader, Joseph Kony, who is seen as a prophet by his followers (Branch 2010; Dolnik and Butime 2016).

7.3.1 Political/Ideological Terrorism

The political ideologies of violent non-state actors can be categorized according to standard political typologies, which range from the far left to the far right. It is often the case that far-left or far-right groups use terrorism to subvert the conventions and norms of liberal democratic states. Equally often, however, these groups target each other. For instance, in the early interwar period, Germany saw the rise of the Ruhr Red Army, a paramilitary force of tens of thousands of German communists. These vigilantes fought primarily in armed street battles against the *Freikorps*, a rival paramilitary force of World War I veterans, which later acted as the underground armed wing of the National Socialist German Workers' Party, known commonly as the Nazi Party (Besier and Stokłosa 2014, 132).

The vast majority of politically motivated violent non-state actors subscribe to far-right or far-left ideologies, ranging from anarchism and communism to National Socialism (Nazism) and fascism. Many also propagate one or more variants of **nationalism**. The latter is usually underpinned by political undertones that center on a strong belief in national identity, usually combined with notions of national purity. But they can also be informed by racial undertones, in which case their adherents advocate strictly racial definitions of national identity. Nearly all such groups put forward relatively rigid and inflexible critiques of the state in whose territory they operate, whether liberal democratic or totalitarian. They typically dismiss the state's foundational principles and accuse it of failing to serve the core interests of their members—or "the people"—if they claim to speak for a silent majority. In most cases, these groups seek to bring down the existing state mechanism and replace it with an alternative administrative apparatus that propagates their political vision. In some cases, these groups have a strictly national agenda— meaning that their aspirations do not exceed the borders of the country in which they operate. In other cases, these groups are internationalist in outlook and consciously develop relations with like-minded groups abroad.

7.3.1.1 Russian Prerevolutionary Movements

For much of the twentieth century, notable examples of ideologically motivated terrorism by non-state groups originated from the anarchist and communist political spectrum. Anarchist terrorism emerged in France as a theory and in Russia as a terrorist tactic, before spreading to the rest of the world. What was interesting about the anarchist wave of terrorism of the late nineteenth and early twentieth centuries was that many of the groups that practiced it seemed to hold no concrete hope of actually changing the world. It was almost like they believed that their isolation from society and its norms was the only honest stance for a true revolutionary. That attitude was especially prominent in the nihilist movement, a subset of the anarchist movement that emerged in Russia. **Nihilism**, which became popular among middle-class Russian youth in the last two decades of the nineteenth century, derives its name from the Latin term for "nothing." In its philosophical sense, it signifies a general mood of despair felt upon the realization that existence is meaningless and that society's norms, values, and laws are equally purposeless.

In its political sense, nihilism signifies the desire to bring an end to the existing social order, sometimes through violence. What made nihilist violent groups different to other anarchists was not that they proposed to "destroy the existing order through armed conflict" but that they had "no vision for a future society" and offered "no clear alternative for the aftermath of the destruction of the existing social order" (Martin 2011, 109). As terrorism expert Gus Martin notes, nihilists defined victory "simply as the destruction of the old society" (Martin 2011, 109). In 1881, a group of Russian nihilists, all members of the outlawed revolutionary group *Narodnaya Volya* (People's Will), set up a separate radical cell called *Pervomartovtsy* (March 1), with the sole aim of assassinating Alexander II of Russia. They managed to do so on March 13 of that year, as the Czar was inspecting his troops in Petrograd. As one observer noted at the time, "their desire was not a coup, it was vengeance" (Hingley 1967, 89).

7.3.1.2 Left-Wing Movements

Throughout the twentieth century, communist violent non-state actors were considerably more ambitious than anarchists or nihilists and significantly more intentional in their use of terrorism to achieve wide-ranging political goals. Most such groups subscribed to various interpretations of revolutionary communism, including Marxist–Leninist (the official state ideology of the Soviet Union), Trotskyist (anti-Stalinist communism, named after Leon Trotsky, the founder of the Soviet Armed Forces), and Maoist (an agrarian form of militant communism developed by the founder of communist China, Mao Zedong). Together, these groups are often classified under the label "New Left" or "third wave" of terrorism that began in the 1960s and ended around 2000 (Rapoport 2001). One prime example of a communist New Left violent group was the Japanese Red Army (JRA). It was founded by Japanese revolutionary communists in Lebanon in 1971 and officially disbanded in 2001. The group's stated aims were to bring an end to the Japanese monarchy, overthrow the government, replace it with a communist provisional government, and use it to start a worldwide communist revolution (Hirai-Baun 2004, 450). The JRA achieved considerable notoriety by carrying out attacks all over the world, in places such as The Hague, Istanbul, Rome, and Kuala Lumpur. The group's most sensational operation, known as the Lod Airport Massacre, was a large-scale attack at the main international airport in Tel Aviv, Israel, which killed 26 and injured nearly 100 people. Many of the JRA's surviving members are currently in prison in a number of countries, including the United States. But several remain in Lebanon, where they have been granted political asylum and continue to enjoy a "hero's status among some in the Arab world" (Guardian 2000).

The tactics of the JRA were emulated by a host of communist revolutionary groups in 1970s Europe, most notably the Red Brigades (*Brigate Rosse*) in Italy and the German Red Army Faction (RAF) (known also as the Baader-Meinhof Gang). One common operational aspect of these groups was their **internationalization** outlook (Rapoport 2017), which favored contacts with similar groups across the world, and especially with Palestinian groups operating in the Middle East and North Africa. The United States also saw its share of New Left terrorism during that time, with groups such as the Revolutionary Armed Task Force, the May 19th Communist Organization (which bombed the US Capitol in 1983), and perhaps most notably the Weather Underground Organization (WUO). More commonly known as the Weather Underground, the WUO declared war on the US government in 1970 and proceeded to bomb the Pentagon (US Department of Defense headquarters) in 1972 and the headquarters of the Department of State in 1975 (Berger 2006, 340–347). American New Left violent groups lacked the internationalist connections of their European counterparts. Notable exceptions to that rule were Black Nationalist groups, such as the Maoist Black Panther Party for Self-Defense, which had links with China and Cuba, and maintained a branch in Algeria in the late 1960s and early 1970s (Meghelli 2009).

Assessing the effectiveness of politically/ideologically motivated terrorism is complicated for two main reasons. First, a scholar of terrorism should not necessarily take a group's stated aims as a criterion by which to judge the effectiveness of its terrorist tactics. As we have seen, violent non-state actors tend to use ambitious rhetoric in their missionary language, which often masks their actual intentions, size, and strength (Homer 1988, 223). It is difficult to believe, for instance, that the JRA's leadership truly believed at any point during the group's existence that it would be able to bring about "world revolution" (Hirai-Baun 2004, 450) with its activities. Or that the tiny, isolated leadership of the Black Liberation Army, a violent offshoot of the New York branch of the Black Panther Party, truly believed that the group would establish "a new Afrika [*sic.*] in the southern United States" and instigate "the socialist overthrow of the United States government" (Kushner 2002, 223). What is more plausible is that these groups used deliberately inflated language to "separate rhetoric from reality" (Berger 2006, 159), promote their image, and help steer broader historical forces in favor of their ideology. They were resoundingly unsuccessful in the latter part of their mission. However groups like the Weather Underground and the RAF "provoked reactions vastly disproportionate," not only to their limited size but also "to the violence they unleashed" (Varon 2004, 2).

The second reason why it is difficult to assess conclusively the effectiveness of politically/ideologically motivated terrorism is that results vary by case. Unquestionably, the New Left wave of terrorism in Western Europe and North America was short-lived (Balz 2015, 298). But some New Left violent groups in the developing world not only continue to exist today but are still formidable. They include remnants of the People's Guerrilla Army (*Ejército Guerrillero Popular*), the armed wing of the Communist Party of Peru (also known as the Shining Path, or *Sendero Luminoso*), and several armed groups in India's so-called red corridor (east India). The latter include the Communist Party of India-Maoist, whose paramilitary wing, the People's Liberation Guerrilla Army, is believed to be 100 000-strong (Shah 2015).

7.3.1.3 Right-Wing Movements

Right-wing violent non-state actors have a centuries-old history of violence, which continues unabated today. Right-wing terrorism is informed by elements of ultra-conservative beliefs that can range from single issues—such as xenophobia or hatred of homosexuals—to broad ideologies, such as Nazism or its Italian-rooted variant, fascism. In America, the historical roots of right-wing terrorism are most clearly discernible in the creation of the first Ku Klux Klan (KKK), a white supremacist and white nationalist organization that emerged in the southern United States at the conclusion of the American Civil War. The KKK operated as the underground armed **insurgency** of the defeated Confederacy during the Reconstruction Era and aimed to overthrow the pro-Union southern governments and prevent economic and civil rights reforms that threatened white supremacy (Chalmers 1987, 8ff). For over a decade, members of the KKK, who numbered in their tens of thousands, were responsible for tens of thousands of acts of terrorism throughout the United States (Parsons 2015). In its second period, which began in 1915, the KKK amassed millions of members and had branches in Canada and supporters throughout Europe. The KKK has since reemerged in at least two more waves and is today seen as one of the most powerful and enduring violent forces in modern American history.

In the postwar era, far-right terrorism has its roots in late 1970s Europe, with the emergence of violent underground groups like the neo-fascist Armed Revolutionary Nuclei (*Nuclei Armati Rivoluzionari*) in Italy. The group, which aimed to overthrow democracy in Italy and replace it with a fascist regime, is mostly known for carrying out the notorious bombing of the Bologna main train station in 1980, which killed 85 people (Anderson 2009, 48). Far-right violent groups have also been active in France, where they became especially active after France lost its Algerian territories, a development that spurred the creation of openly neo-Nazi groups. In recent times, French far-right groups have propagated the systematic use of violence against immigrants and Muslims (Mammone 2015). More recently, the German neo-Nazi group National Socialist Underground (NSU) engaged in a 13-year-long systematic campaign to murder immigrants while funding its operations through a series of bank robberies. After each murder, the group abstained from issuing political declarations and never sought to make its existence publicly known or recruit new members. Consequently, German police were left completely unaware of the political motive behind the murders. The discovery of the group's existence, and its peculiar tactics, led some observers to describe its approach as "a new kind of right-wing terrorism unlike anything Germany has seen" (Various 2011).

FOR EXAMPLE

Combat 18

An example of the connection between football hooliganism and far-right militancy is a neo-Nazi group calling itself Combat 18 (Garland and Rowe 2001, 92). The number 18 in the group's name is derived from the first and eight letters in the Latin alphabet, which are the initials of Adolf Hitler. The group formed in 1992 from football hooligans, who were members of the far-right British National Party (BNP) but opposed the party's participation in the electoral process. They engaged in attacks against left-wingers, immigrants, and nonwhite British citizens while continuing to recruit in football grounds and prisons. Since the early 2000s, former members of Combat 18 have created several violent splinter groups in Britain, including the Racial Volunteer Force and the British Freedom Fighters. There are also numerous Combat 18 groups in other European countries, such as the Czech Republic, Belgium, and Russia. (Goodrick-Clarke 2003)

Britain and the United States have arguably been the two most prolific centers of right-wing terrorism in the West in modern times. In Britain, the growth and anatomy of far-right terrorism is closely related to the culture of football hooliganism, which is in turn related to organized crime. In addition to football hooliganism, British right-wing terrorism is also closely connected with the violent politics of Northern Ireland. Northern Irish paramilitary groups like the Loyalist Volunteer Force, Red Hand Defenders, and the Real Ulster Freedom Fighters continue to oppose the 1998 Good Friday Agreement, which ended decades of sectarian violence in the region (see next section for an explanation of violent sectarianism in Northern Ireland). These groups can be categorized as ethno-nationalist, in the sense that they base their *raison d'être* on their nationalist affiliation with the United Kingdom. But they also display strong religious and political/ideological components that derive from ultraconservatism.

The United States has a long and complex history of domestic far-right terrorism by non-state actors. Aside from at least four different reincarnations of the Klan, the United States experienced terrorist attacks by Nazi, neo-Nazi, and white supremacist groups in the twentieth century. One of the most violent groups was The Order, a secret white supremacist and anti-communist group founded in 1983. The name, mission, and internal structure of the organization were inspired by *The Turner Diaries*, a novel written in 1978 by American neo-Nazi William Luther Pierce, which has inspired generations of American neo-Nazis. The main aim of the group was to establish a "homeland for white people" in North America, known among North American white supremacists as "the Northwest Territorial Imperative" (Gardell 2003, 112ff). The Order conducted a series of armed robberies and bombings in 1983 and June 1984, when it killed the nationally known Colorado-based radio host Alan Berg. The media attention generated by the case prompted an extensive counterterrorism operation by the US government, in which nearly 100 members of the secretive group were arrested and convicted for a variety of crimes (Wexler 2015). The Order influenced many contemporary and subsequent American far-right violent groups, including the Aryan Republican Army, a white supremacist organization that was found to have contacts with Timothy McVeigh (Hamm 2002). In April 1995, McVeigh, with the help of Terry Nichols, an anti-government militant, bombed the Alfred P. Murrah Federal Building in Oklahoma City, Oklahoma, killing 168 people. The incident marked the deadliest terrorist incident in the United States until the 9/11 attacks (Crenshaw and Pimlott 2015, 561).

In comparison to far-left groups, far-right non-state actors display a narrower degree of **transnationalization** in the operational field—that is, they have not historically sought to establish operational ties with ideologically comparable groups across national borders. However, this may be changing, as far-right violent actors are establishing ideological consensus within national borders and are becoming increasingly capable of joining forces abroad. This is especially visible in Europe, where the integrated area of the European Union is enabling far-right groups to "frame nationalist sentiments in [increasingly] European terms" (Fielitz and Laloire 2016, 16). Additionally, in both Europe and the United States, the contemporary emergence of far-right terrorism appears to be fueled by populist reaction to immigration from non-Western regions. For instance, Norwegian neo-Nazi Anders Behring Breivik cited nonwhite immigration as a justification for his terrorist attacks, which killed 77 and injured over 100 people on July 22, 2011. The incident was the deadliest attack on Norwegian soil since World War II. In his 1500-page manifesto, entitled *2083: A European Declaration of Independence*, Breivik rallies against **Marxism** and Islam and argues that multiculturalism must be eliminated in order to safeguard the future of a "Christian Europe" (Jackson 2014).

7.3.2 Ethno-Nationalist or Separatist Terrorism

Politically/ideologically motivated terrorism appears in waves that tend to be spectacular but relatively brief. The same cannot be said for ethno-nationalist and separatist terrorism, which can be described as one of the most permeating political forces of the twentieth century. Ethno-nationalist or separatist non-state actors are usually represented by groups that want to see the ethnic or national identity of their members reflected in the structure and makeup of the governing system. In other words, these actors view ethnicity as the basis from which to launch a project of nation-building. It must be noted that not all such groups use violence as a primary means of political expression. For instance, with the exception of the fringe and now defunct *Front de libération du Québec*, the Quebec sovereignty movement has waged a largely peaceful campaign to advocate for the province's independence from Canada (Wright-Neville 2010, 87–88). The case of the Scottish independence movement is also interesting. Over the last 40 years, a number of small violent secessionist groups have made occasional appearances, with names such as the Army of the Provisional Government of Scotland (also known as the Tartan Army), the Scottish National Liberation Army, the Army for Freeing Scotland, and the Army of the Gael. Collectively, they have been responsible for blowing up a few oil pipelines and mailing incendiary devices to British public figures, including the Queen. But these are fringe groups with no significant role in the broader secessionist movement in Scotland, whose main agent is the conscientiously nonviolent Scottish National Party (Thackrah 2004, 284). Similarly, the Non-Cooperation Movement, which was started by Mahatma Gandhi in 1920 to rid India from British rule, specifically set out to employ nonviolent means as methods of political agitation (Bakshi 1983).

But many ethno-nationalist or separatist non-state actors do use violence to pursue their goals. When they do so, these actors are often able to mobilize large numbers of members, supporters, and sympathizers. This differentiates them from anarchist groups, which are typically small in number, isolated from society, and often operate through individual mobilization using lone-actor methods (Jensen 2016).

In many cases, ethno-nationalist or separatist violent non-state actors employ a paramilitary structure that is considerably more hierarchical than those of religiously or ideologically motivated groups. Moreover, their campaigns display the characteristics of an organized—and typically protracted—insurgency. The latter can be defined as an armed struggle fought between one or more recognized states and one or more entities that have no official international recognition but exist in a *de facto* capacity. Terrorism is then used as one tactic in a broader conflict that includes many other means of fighting. Usually, however, the predominant method used by the insurgents is **guerrilla warfare**, rather than terrorism. That is frequently the case when an ethno-nationalist non-state actor fights a foreign colonizing force.

This is being practiced today by the Sahrawi People's Liberation Army (SPLA), a group of Sahrawi tribespeople fighting to end Morocco's occupation of the Western Sahara. The SPLA, which is the armed wing of the Frente POLISARIO movement, maintains a thousand-strong territorial army that includes armored vehicle and tank divisions (Zunes and Mundy 2010, 17). When an ethno-nationalist non-state actor wages a violent campaign of autonomy or independence within the borders of an existing state, it typically uses terrorism as its main mode of warfare. Sometimes these conflicts do assume features that are akin to an insurgency or isolated guerrilla battles, but such cases are rare.

FOR EXAMPLE

The Strategic Failure of the LTTE

History is replete with examples of ethno-nationalist groups that have failed to achieve their mission, despite leading mass secessionist movements. In 2009, the Liberation Tigers of Tamil Eelam, commonly known as the LTTE or the Tamil Tigers, admitted defeat after a 35-year war against the Sri Lankan state. The group had been founded in 1976 with the goal of creating Tamil Eelam, an independent state for the Tamil ethnic group in northern Sri Lanka. Despite the Tamil people being mostly Hindus, the LTTE was a socialist group that campaigned for secularism. In 1983, it launched an insurgency against the Sri Lankan state, which included the use of terrorist tactics, such as suicide bombings, assassinations, and kidnappings. Throughout that time, the LTTE enjoyed the support of India and North Korea, among other countries. At the peak of its power, the group's military included an air force and navy and its own police force, as well as separate women's units. Yet despite controlling nearly 80% of northeast Sri Lanka in 2000, in 2009 the group had been resoundingly defeated by the Sri Lankan military, which launched a brutal all-out war in the Tamil-populated regions of the country (Weiss 2012). Today, the LTTE military has been completely obliterated, and most of the group's senior leadership is either dead or has escaped to India. (Hashim 2013)

7.3.2.1 Irish Republicanism

Ethno-nationalist groups are responsible for the majority of terrorism conducted by non-state actors in the past century. The Irish Republican Army (IRA) in Ireland, and its postwar offshoot, the Provisional IRA (PIRA) in British-held Northern Ireland, are two of the earliest and most prominent examples of ethno-nationalist groups. The IRA, also known as the "Old IRA," was formed in 1917 with the aim of gaining Irish independence from Britain. After 1922, when Ireland gained its independence from Britain, IRA volunteers were amalgamated into the armed forces of the Irish Free State. But in the six counties of Northern Ireland, which remained under British rule after 1922, the IRA continued to exist as a paramilitary force. It remained mostly dormant until the summer of 1969, when Protestant groups in the North initiated a campaign of violence against Catholic civil rights activists. That prompted members of the dormant IRA to split from the organization and create the PIRA. Their stated aim was to use paramilitary tactics to defend the Catholic population from Protestant violence, as well as from the presence of the British forces, which had been ostensibly deployed by London to protect the region's Catholic population, but which the PIRA saw as an occupying army. Within two years, however, the PIRA was engaging in an offensive campaign with the goal of ending British rule in Northern Ireland (Dingley 2012, 77ff). The group used guerrilla tactics against the British Armed Forces in both rural and urban areas of the British Isles. Its gamut of methods included nonviolent agitation, such as hunger strikes, as well as sabotage, ambushes, bombings, and other violent acts. After 1973, the group carried out a protracted bombing campaign in England. Following protracted negotiations with the British government after 2005, the political wing of the IRA, Sinn Féin, shared power in Northern Ireland with Protestant loyalists. But the PIRA did not achieve its ultimate goal—secession of Northern Ireland from Britain—despite its four-decades-long armed campaign. In this, it is not alone. History is replete with examples of ethno-nationalist groups that have failed to achieve their mission, despite leading mass secessionist movements.

7.3.2.2 Jewish and Israeli Groups

Other ethno-nationalist and secessionist movements have been far more successful than the PIRA in realizing their immediate goals. One of the most notable examples in modern history was the use of terrorism by Zionist activists in Palestine between 1920 and 1948. These activists advocated the view that Jews had the right to return to what they claimed was their historical home after thousands of years of absence. The roots of Jewish terrorism in Palestine date from the early 1900s, with the formation of vigilante groups like the Bar-Giora (named for Simon Bar Giora, a Jewish leader in the First Jewish–Roman War), the Hashomer (Hebrew for "watchman"), and, most notably, the Haganah ("defense"). Founded in 1920, the Haganah's initial goal was to provide physical protection for Jewish settlements from terrorist attacks by local Arabs, who were trying to discourage more Jews from moving to what was then British-controlled Palestine. But in the late 1930s, the organization had become offensive in nature. It maintained a unit called FOSH (an acronym from the Hebrew initials for "field troops"), whose members conducted targeted killings of Arab paramilitaries (Climent 2015, 110ff). Eventually, a group of hard-line Zionists split from the Haganah to create the National Military Organization in the Land of Israel. Known simply as Irgun or Etzel, the organization openly advocated the use of terrorism in order to intimidate Palestine's British rulers and predominantly Arab population and establish a Jewish state (Climent 2015, 114). In July 1938, Irgun detonated land mines at an Arab fruit market in Haifa, killing 74 and injuring 129. In July 1946, the same organization bombed the King David Hotel in Jerusalem, killing nearly 100 and injuring dozens more. In April 1948, Irgun joined forces with Lehi, another hard-line Jewish paramilitary group, and carried out the so-called Deir Yassin massacre, an attack on an Arab village that killed over 100 civilians (Climent 2015, 115). In another notorious operation in 1948, Lehi killed Folke Bernadotte, the Swedish diplomat and United Nations mediator in the Arab–Israeli conflict, while he was in Jerusalem attempting to strike a peace treaty between the newly established Jewish state and its Arab neighbors.

One of many interesting aspects of Jewish terrorism in Palestine was the disparate ideological underpinnings of the various groups involved. The Haganah was primarily socialist in outlook, whereas the Irgun politically conservative. The Lehi (its full name was Fighters for the Freedom of Israel) is perhaps the most interesting of all of them. The roots of the group were in Revisionist Zionism, which is the ideological basis of the nonreligious right in Israeli politics. Zionism has traditionally been dominated by socialist principles, so Revisionist Zionism has been the minority ideology within the broader movement. But Lehi never aspired to be a politically homogeneous group and drew its members from a variety of ideological, religious, and cultural backgrounds. It also refused to propose a concrete vision of what an independent Israel would look like politically. Instead, it consistently portrayed itself as a practically oriented anti-imperialist organization, whose sole aim was to remove the British from Palestine and create an independent Jewish state. To that extent, Lehi went so far as to seek cooperation with fascist Italy and Nazi Germany in its war against the British. The Israeli diplomatic historian Sasson Sofer has written about two separate occasions in which Lehi's founder, Avraham Stern, attempted to "establish contact with representatives of the Third Reich, in the hope of making an alliance with Nazi Germany" (Sofer 1998, 254). In one of those, which took place in late 1940, the Zionist group presented the German diplomat Werner Otto von Hentig with a document pledging an alliance between Nazi Germany and a future Jewish state. The latter, said the document, "would be based on nationalist and totalitarian principles, and linked to the German state by an alliance" (Sofer 1998, 254). The alleged reason for the proposed alliance was that the leadership of Lehi agreed with the Nazi Party's view that Jews should leave Germany. At the same time, however, Lehi's leaders admired British liberalism and fundamentally mistrusted undemocratic political systems. And there was even a "leftist deviation" in Lehi, led by one of the group's main leaders, Nathan Friedman-Yellin-Mor, who later developed "a pro-communist and pro-Soviet stance" (Bauer 2014, 78). In the words of Israeli historian Joseph Heller, the leaders of groups like Irgun and Lehi "behaved eclectically," taking "from fascism what [they] found convenient, especially its socio-economic ideas." But at the same time, they remained "firm proponents of democracy [and] rejected the leadership principle so characteristic of fascism" (Heller 2012, 6). Ultimately, as Sofer states, "LEHI represented a unique synthesis, taking ideas from both Right and Left while seeking to separate tactical means from any normative predisposition" (Sofer 1998, 255).

The ideological variance in Jewish terrorism can also be observed in the fate of Jewish paramilitary groups following the creation of Israel in 1948. Remarkably, in 1956 some members of Lehi formed Semitic Action, an Israeli political party that advocated that Hebrew-speaking Israelis should sever their connections with the global Jewish diaspora and should instead seek to integrate into the Middle East. The party even proposed that Israel should create a confederation with its neighboring Arab states "on the basis of an anti-colonialist alliance with indigenous Arab inhabitants" (Beinin 1998, 166). On the other hand, some Lehi members refused to give up terrorism after 1948 and founded the Kingdom of Israel, a violent paramilitary group that sought to use armed violence to promote what it saw as Jewish interests. The group bombed the embassies in Israel of the Soviet Union and Czechoslovakia, which it accused of anti-Semitism. It also tried to assassinate the

Chancellor of Germany, Konrad Adenauer, in protest to what it said were Germany's insufficient financial reparations to the Jewish people after the Holocaust (Perliger 2006, 38). However, the vast majority of Haganah, Irgun, and Lehi members gradually integrated into the Israel Defense Forces, the official military of the state of Israel. In return for decommissioning their weapons and seizing their terrorist operations, the government of Israel offered the members of these groups amnesty from prosecution. Later, the Israeli government issued official service ribbons to be worn in place of medals by veteran members of Jewish paramilitary groups, including the Haganah and Lehi. In 1977, Irgun's last commander, Menachem Begin, who had ordered the bloody attack on the King David Hotel, became Israel's sixth prime minister. In 1983, Yitzhak Shamir, a former Lehi leader who had helped organize the assassination of Bernadotte in 1948, was elected prime minister of Israel. Bob Baer, an American former officer in the CIA, wrote that Shamir's transformation marked "the first instance […] where a democracy elected an assassin as a head of state" (Baer 2015, 83).

In evaluating the effectiveness of the use of terrorism by ethno-nationalist or separatist groups, we must be careful not to make broad generalizations. Clearly, Zionist paramilitary groups like Irgun and Lehi achieved their main goal, which was the creation of an independent Jewish state. At the same time, it is worth keeping in mind that Jewish terrorism against the British Mandate in Palestine took place "in the shadow of the dismantlement of the British Empire after the First World War" (Golani 2013, ix–x); the British would have eventually left Palestine even without the specter of Jewish terrorism. Thus, the extent to which terrorism in Mandatory Palestine contributed to the eventual establishment of a Jewish state is questionable. Indeed, it can be argued that the terrorism of the Jewish paramilitaries worsened ethnic divisions in Palestine and antagonized the British colonial authorities, thus delaying their departure from Palestine (Golani 2013, 40). We must also ask whether the legacy of interethnic violence, to which the Jewish paramilitary groups contributed heavily, ended up subverting Israel's internal security and damaging the prospects for a lasting peace between Jews and Arabs after 1948.

7.3.3 Religious Terrorism

For people who are not religious, it is admittedly difficult to distinguish religion from other forms of ideology, such as nationalism or communism. Some terrorism experts observe that "the assumed causal connection between religious belief and [terrorist] behavior" is not only misleading but also "inaccurate and analytically unhelpful, and in most cases serves to obscure and distort, rather than illuminate" the scientific study of terrorism (Jackson et al. 2011, 169). In terms of classification, how does one even distinguish politically or ethnically motivated violent non-state actors from groups that are motivated by religion?

Take the example of Hamas, which is an avowedly Sunni Muslim religious group and features several clerics in leading roles. Yet, despite its religious identity, the organization has tens of thousands of members and supporters who are either secular or Christian (Hroub 2006, xix), while much of its political program is secular in nature. Or take the example of the PIRA, which is officially a secular organization. However, it is no secret that most Northern Irish secessionists have a Catholic background, whereas most loyalists to the British Crown are either practicing or non-practicing Protestants. Is the clash between the British state and Irish secessionists, or between Israel and Hamas, ethnic, political, or religious in nature—or perhaps all three? And does it matter?

As always when discussing such complex topics, one must not generalize. With that in mind, it could be argued that violent actors who are motivated by religion tend to act with more fervor and a greater degree of inflexibility than those motivated by secular ideologies. This may be attributable to their belief that their way of thinking and actions are mandated by a divine being and are thus absolute and nonnegotiable. We can therefore draw an operational connection between religiously motivated terrorism and its practitioners' deep-seated belief that their violent actions are a personal testament of their commitment to an all-powerful god. This can lead them to conduct intense acts of violence and arms them with a persistent unwillingness to negotiate with their opponents. In such cases, religiously motivated violent actors view negotiating with non-believers as compromising their faith, which they see as a *sui generis* value that is inherently nonnegotiable. Additionally, the strategic mindset of religiously motivated violent actors tends to be dominated by a certain degree of **magical thinking**. The term denotes the idea that ultimate victory is granted—and often predestined—by a divine being irrespective of material factors on the ground, such as the military strength of one's adversary. Politics, therefore assumes a secondary role in the strategic outlook of religiously motivated violent actors.

Much of contemporary terrorism appears to be religiously motivated. This has led some scholars to argue that groups like al-Qaeda, which are motivated by rigid religious doctrines, represent "the emergence of a new and more dangerous form of terrorism" (Guanaratna 2010, 16). Regardless of the validity of such bold statements, it is important to stress here that the term "new" is used here within the context of modern terrorism—that is, terrorism practiced during and after the French Revolution. Prior to that monumental event in world history, it is indeed difficult to find any notable incident of terrorism that was not motivated or justified by an absolutist religious doctrine (Rapoport 2001, 7). Most subject matter experts, therefore, view the French Revolution as the beginning of the secular era in the history of terrorism, which continued throughout the nineteenth and twentieth centuries. During that era, terrorism "essentially had no religious dimension" (Chaliand and Blin 2007, 96). It follows that, if religiously motivated terrorism is indeed resurgent at the present time, it signifies a new trend in the post-1789 era; yet, when examined within the context of recorded history as a whole, it should be seen as a return to the norm, after about two centuries of secularism as the motivating force for terrorism.

7.3.3.1 Buddhist Movements

Ever since the tragic events of 9/11, the popular and scholarly narratives on terrorism have tended to concentrate on Islam as a motivating factor of organized violence. However, it is important to remember for counterterrorism purposes that no religion is immune to being used as a justification for terrorism. A characteristic example of this is Buddhism, the world's fourth largest religious tradition, which encompasses a set of teachings and practices that are attributed to Gautama Buddha. Buddhism is widely known as an intensely peaceful doctrine that places emphasis on the strict observance of moral precepts, like love, compassion, and kindness. But the religion, which has over half a billion followers, has a long history of violence in India, Japan, Sri Lanka, and—most recently—Burma. The Southeast Asian country, which is today known as Myanmar, is predominantly populated by Buddhists. But it has a sizeable minority of Muslims (about 6% of the population), who have been subjected to intense persecution for nearly five centuries. The oppression of Myanmar's Muslims originates from both state and non-state actors (Seth 2003). The so-called 969 Movement is one of the most hard-line vigilante groups that have been blamed for inciting violence against Muslims in the country. The group has been termed anti-Muslim and Islamophobic and has at times advocated the systematic boycott of businesses owned or operated by Burmese Muslims. The movement's leaders were widely blamed for helping incite the 2012 Rakhine State riots, a series of armed sectarian disputes between Buddhists and Muslims, which killed close to 200 people and caused the displacement of over 100 000 (Cruz-del Rosario and Dorsey 2016, 105).

7.3.3.2 Christian Movements

Like Buddhism, Christianity too features a long history of armed violence and non-state terrorism against Christians and non-Christians alike. We have already discussed the cases of the KKK, whose symbol is the Christian cross, and the Lord's Resistance Army, led by Joseph Kony, a self-described Christian prophet. But these are only two of many examples of Christian violent non-state actors that continue to use terrorism to promote their agenda. During the Lebanese Civil War of the 1980s, Christian Phalangists—many of whom supported the Lebanese Phalanges Party militia and the South Lebanon Army—perpetrated systematic acts of terrorism against Lebanese, Palestinian, Syrian, and Kurdish civilians. Their most notorious act was the massacres at Sabra and Shatila in 1982, when hundreds of armed Christian militia members massacred between 500 and 3500 people in the Sabra neighborhood of south Beirut and the adjacent Shatila Palestinian refugee camp (Al-Hout 2004). At around the same time, several Christian violent groups emerged in the Indian subcontinent. Among them were the National Liberation Front of Tripura and the National Socialist Council of Nagaland, which still exist today. Their goal is to establish what they call "sovereign Christian states" in northeast India, which will act like "the Kingdom of God and Jesus Christ" on Earth (Prakash 2008).

But arguably the most violent post-9/11 Christian paramilitary groups are the Anti-balaka (anti-machete) militias in the Central African Republic (CAR). Though they count secularists and animists among their members, Anti-balaka militias employ strong Christian imagery and terminology and advocate the forcible conversion of Muslims to Christianity. The militias have their roots in local-based vigilante forces set up by Christians and animists to provide security for villages during the intercommunal violence that swept the country in the 1990s. Since 2013, Anti-balaka groups, which represent the CAR's majority Christian population, have committed mass atrocities against the small and mostly nomadic Muslim minority. The violence has displaced about a quarter of the country's population and prompted the United Nations to warn that the region is "descending into complete chaos" and risks "spiraling into genocide" (Raghavan 2013).

In the United States, aside from the KKK, the oldest Christian non-state violent group is the Aryan Nations, which describes itself as a Christian separatist and white supremacist group. It has been in existence since 1974, when it was established as the political wing of the Church of Jesus Christ Christian, a white supremacist Christian denomination founded in 1946. In its history of the Aryan Nations, the Research and Development Corporation (RAND), which conducts research on behalf of the US Department of Defense, described the organization as "the first truly nationwide terrorist network" in the United States (Southers 2014, 32). In 2000, as a result of a lawsuit, the Aryan Nations went bankrupt and lost its private compound in northern Idaho. Although that development was a positive one, it prompted the geographical dispersal of the group's members and complicated counterterrorism efforts against them. The post-2000 dispersal generated a plethora of Christian violent groups. It also prompted the revival of the Creativity Movement (known initially as the World Church of the Creator), which proclaims that Christianity had been hijacked by the Jews in order to subvert the white race. The group was dissolved in 2005, after its leader, Matthew Hale, was jailed for soliciting the murder of a federal judge (Michael 2009). One of the most violent American Christian groups of recent times was The Covenant, the Sword, and the Arm of the Lord, known as CSA. With roots in the Baptist denomination, the group operated from 1971 to 1985 with the stated aim of resisting what it described as the "Zionist-occupied government" of the United States. In 1983, the group declared war on the US government and carried out a spree of bank robberies in order to raise funds for its operations. In 1985, when authorities raided the CSA compound in the state of Arkansas, they found that it had been mined by nearly 100 members of the group who lived there. Inside the compound they found weapons, including submachine guns, an antitank rocket, and plastic explosives that the group had planned to use against the government (Atkins 2011, 149ff).

7.3.3.3 Islamic Movements

If the presence of religious violent groups with backgrounds such as Buddhist or Christian is so extensively documented, why is the contemporary counterterrorist narrative focused primarily on Islamic-oriented militant organizations? First, because the attacks of 9/11, which were perpetrated by al-Qaeda, shocked Western populations. The latter were not used to seeing large-scale, spectacular terrorist attacks perpetrated on their own soil. Second, because, unlike Buddhist and Christian violent groups, which have strictly localized aspirations, some of the most notorious Sunni Islamists advocate an ambitious globalist agenda. The goal of creating a global Islamic caliphate is one of the primary distinguishing features of al-Qaeda, the Sunni Islamist organization founded in 1988 by Arab Salafists, including Osama bin Laden and Abdullah Azzam. In describing al-Qaeda, we have already used two terms that must be explained, namely, **Islamism** and **Salafism**. Islamism is a political ideology that seeks to shape society, often by force, according to conservative interpretations of Islam. Salafism is a nineteenth-century doctrine that emerged in Egypt as a reaction to the European colonialism of the Arab world. It advocates strict adherence to early Islamic doctrine, especially of the first 3 centuries of Islam's existence on Earth. It is often used synonymously with **Wahhabism**, which is a similar doctrine that emerged in Saudi Arabia, and today forms that country's state-authorized religion. Another term that is often used in relation to Sunni Muslim militants is **jihadism**. It refers to the belief that Islam is currently under attack by secularism, as well as Christianity, Judaism, and other religions, and that every Muslim has a sacred personal duty to resist by any means necessary. Consequently, al-Qaeda is a Sunni Islamist Salafist group that advocates violent *jihad*, which is Arabic for "holy war."

Al-Qaeda is one of numerous Sunni Islamist Salafist groups in the world that advocate *jihad*. However, it stands out in two major ways: First, it has historically been the best organized and best funded. To a large extent, that was because the individuals who founded it were previously involved in the Afghan Services Bureau (MAK), which provided logistical support to those fighting the Soviet Red Army during the Soviet–Afghan War of the 1980s. The MAK, which in many ways was al-Qaeda's forerunner, was supported by several states that used it to weaken the Soviet Union's military capabilities. These state supporters included Saudi Arabia, Pakistan, and, some claim, the United States, though this is disputed in the specialist literature (Plaw 2008, 106f). Second, al-Qaeda is one of very few groups of its kind that have managed to project a truly global profile, both in terms of membership and operational reach. That is in fact a major difference between al-Qaeda and almost every other Sunni militant group that is active today, including the Taliban. Unlike al-Qaeda, the Taliban's aspirations concentrate on the Afghanistan–Pakistan region, and it never had any interest in fighting Western militaries until they appeared in Afghanistan in 2001. Additionally, the vast majority of the Taliban's members are drawn from a single ethnic group, the Pashtuns. Al-Qaeda, on the other hand, draws its membership from dozens of different countries, including America. The group has a global agenda and strategy, which includes confronting the United States.

It is true that many al-Qaeda members and branches, like the Somali-based group al-Shabaab, are radicalized through local interethnic conflicts. Al-Qaeda's success has been its ability to skillfully utilize local enmities to coax localized groups and turn them into troops for its globalized agenda (Kilcullen 2009). That agenda culminates with the eventual creation of an Islamic caliphate, a Sunni Muslim empire that will use Quranic law (known as **sharia**) as its primary constitutional document. That, however, is al-Qaeda's ultimate goal. It cannot be achieved until apostate regimes in the Middle East—that is, regimes in Muslim countries that collaborate with non-believer governments—are toppled. To do that, *jihadists* must "cut off the head of the snake," namely, the United States, a "far enemy" whose political, financial, and logistical power sustains the apostates (Mendelsohn 2016, 95). That explains al-Qaeda's decision to attack the United States on 9/11. The goal was to spark an all-out war against the leading sustainer of the apostate regimes of the Middle East, primarily the Gulf States and Egypt, the Arab world's most populous country. According to al-Qaeda's plan, its forces would emerge victorious and would then proceed to topple the Muslim world's apostate regimes before uniting the "liberated" lands into a Sunni Islamic caliphate. Again, al-Qaeda is not the only group in the world with such aspirations. But the group's operational efficiency and the advanced training of its members enabled it to carry out 9/11, which made the West—and the Muslim world—pay attention.

It is safe to say that al-Qaeda's global campaign has stalled in recent years. The group's initial goal of confronting the United States has somehow morphed into a battle of "a pronounced sectarian and localized nature that has blunted al-Qaeda's emphasis in attacking the American far enemy" (Celso 2014, 2). Some claim that the change in al-Qaeda's emphasis is due to "[t]he American military retaliation after 9/11 [that] shattered al-Qaeda command and control capability and effectively fragmented the organization into a loose network of aligned groups and affiliates" (Celso 2014, 1). That opinion is highly debatable, especially when one looks at the utterly disastrous American invasion of Iraq and the subsequent **War in Iraq**. The latter actually strengthened both militant Sunni Islam and the status of the Iranian factor in a very volatile region. It is arguably far more sensible to suggest that, for a number of reasons, including the death of its founder, the spread of the Arab Spring, as well as the outbreak of the Syrian Civil War, al-Qaeda has undergone a conscious process of devolution. The latter is defined as "the erosion of an organization's central authority and the empowerment of its local branches to develop and implement policy" (Celso 2014, 2). It may be, therefore, that the various branches of the organization are today far more dangerous to international security than its center—to the extent that it even exists as anything more than an idea.

The gradual demise of al-Qaeda does not signify the demise of militant Sunni Islamism. On the contrary, it may be argued that violent Sunni fundamentalism is today more powerful than on 9/11 (Heistein 2016). To that extent, the emergence of IS should be primarily understood, not as an instigator of violent Sunni Islamism, but as its symptom. The group's lineage dates to late 1990s Jordan, where it operated as an al-Qaeda-inspired cell and referred to itself as The Organization of Monotheism and Jihad. Shortly after the 2003 invasion of Iraq by the United States, most of the group's hard-line members moved to Iraq, pledged allegiance to al-Qaeda, and participated in the Iraqi insurgency. The occupying forces responded to the insurgency with the so-called surge, a multifaceted counterinsurgency plan. It included a dramatic increase in the number of troops deployed in Iraq and a campaign of targeted killings of insurgency leaders. At the same time, the United States facilitated the creation of an anti-al-Qaeda alliance of Iraqi Sunni tribes. The loose coalition eventually gave rise to what became known as "the Anbar Awakening," an armed conflict between al-Qaeda and several Sunni tribes in western Iraq (Nance 2015, 284ff). In response to the Awakening, the leadership of al-Qaeda in Iraq reached out to several smaller jihadi groups in the region and created an anti-Awakening coalition, known as the Islamic State of Iraq (Nance 2015, 285).

By most accounts, al-Qaeda's operations in Iraq were severely impacted between 2007 and 2011, as a result of its war with rival Sunni tribes, strikes by the occupation forces and by the American-supplied Iraqi national army (Celso 2014; Silverman 2011). At that crucial moment, however, the chaos created by the outbreak of the Syrian Civil War allowed the Islamic State of Iraq to protect some of its most skilled operatives, by sending them across the border into Syria. That group called itself the Front for the Conquest of the Levant and was referred to in short as the al-Nusra Front. Between 2011 and 2013, the group managed to attract a large number of followers from Syria's Sunni-majority eastern regions, many of whom were former members of Syria's armed forces. It was also able to acquire significant quantities of weapons from looted Syrian military warehouses and storage facilities. In April of 2013, al-Nusra was more powerful than its parent group in Iraq. At that time, the leadership of the Islamic State of Iraq called for a transnational merger of the two groups under the common name IS. In addition to being a strategic move, the merger was also an attempt to disassociate the Sunni campaign in the region from al-Qaeda, which by that time was seen as a failing brand. As can be expected, al-Qaeda's central command rejected the move, which led to a split in the al-Nusra Front between pro-al-Qaeda and pro-IS factions. The pro-al-Qaeda faction continued to pledge allegiance to Osama bin Laden's successor, Ayman al-Zawahiri, which it saw as the emir (commander) of the global Islamist insurgency. But many of al-Nusra's forces sided with IS and recognized its leader, Abu Bakr al-Baghdadi, as the new emir of Sunni Islam (Steed 2016).

In early 2014, the Syrian-based wing of IS crossed the border into Iraq with thousands of well-armed fighters. The sudden appearance of this new Sunni force in western Iraq surprised the Iraqi army and its Western backers, as well as Iran, which has traditionally seen itself as a protector of Iraqi Shiites (Cockburn 2014). The IS forces were welcomed by the predominantly Sunni Arabs of western Iraq, who felt excluded and neglected in the post-2003 Shiite-dominated Iraq. By that time, the Iraqi military was almost exclusively Shiite, as a result of systematic purges of Sunni officers by the Shiite-dominated government after 2003. This contributed to the sense of marginalization among Iraqi Sunnis and made many of them see the presence of IS as a counterbalancing force against what was essentially a Shiite army. In fact, the Sunni–Shiite dispute in Iraq is the crucial context in which one must view the meteoric growth of IS in the region (Cockburn 2014). As we have already discussed, the 2003 American invasion of Iraq sparked the Iraqi insurgency. But the insurgency was not unified. There unfolded what was in essence a war within a war, an increasingly bloody sectarian violence between Iraqi Sunnis and Shiites. In the process, thousands of Iraqi Sunnis, who were seen by many Shiites as supporters of the regime of Iraqi President Saddam Hussein, were expelled from their homes and traditional strongholds in west-central Iraq (Amos 2010). Throughout that time, al-Qaeda's branch in Iraq joined the Sunni insurgency and gradually emerged as one of the protectors of Iraq's Sunni Arab minority (Hashim 2009, 13–16). By reaching out to other Sunni insurgents in Iraq, al-Qaeda gradually became an umbrella group that brought together Sunni jihadists from Iraq and Syria, secularist former members of Saddam Hussein's military and intelligence apparatus, as well as non-aligned Sunni tribes who resent the empowerment of Shiites in post-2003 Iraq (Williams 2017, 191). The same policy was practiced by militant Sunnis in Syria after 2011 (Kilcullen 2016, 77). Unquestionably, the primary identity of IS is religious, which is why the group is correctly classified as a religious violent state actor. But the presence of secularist elements in its ranks—especially in its military branch—as well as the support that it enjoys among Sunnis who fear for their future in a Shiite-dominated Iraq should not be discounted (Ayadinli 2016, 131).

Furthermore, the emergence of IS marks a crucial change of jihadist strategy that breaks with al-Qaeda's strategic trajectory. Unlike al-Qaeda, which views the creation of the caliphate as the crowning achievement of a protracted process, IS has decided to essentially reverse the process. The group began by first announcing the creation of the caliphate, thus offering Sunni jihadists tangible evidence of success. The goal is to then use the caliphate as a base from which to expand, both geographically and in terms of influence. The visible starting point of IS' break with al-Qaeda's plan was the speeches given by al-Baghdadi, the group's emir, in the Iraqi city of Mosul, shortly after it was captured by IS forces in the summer of 2014. Upon declaring himself emir and announcing the creation of the caliphate, the IS leader issued "a special call" to Muslim activists and to "people with military, administrative, and service expertise, and medical doctors and engineers of all different specializations and fields" to come to Syria and Iraq and help strengthen the Islamic State (SITE 2014).

Al-Baghdadi's call was heeded by IS sympathizers from all over the world, who descended into Syria and Iraq in their thousands to help bolster the caliphate. In the meantime, IS continued to display extraordinary professionalism in the battlefield, conquering much of northeastern Iraq and western Syria, including Raqqa, the self-styled caliphate's capital. During that time, IS affiliates emerged in several countries, including Libya, Egypt, Yemen, Algeria, Afghanistan, Pakistan, and Russia. The group's territorial acquisitions included overseas *vilayets* (administrative territorial units) in Egypt, Libya, and Afghanistan (Nance 2015, 146). While it solidified its territorial presence in Iraq and Syria, IS-affiliated militants conducted dozens of terrorist attacks in Europe, North America, South Asia, the Middle East, and Australia. But it is fair to say that the group's main preoccupation was to solidify its control over its territory and project it as a physical and symbolic epicenter of global jihad. Many observers suggest that, if and when IS loses its territorial base, the group will abandon its large-scale conventional military tactics and revert to an al-Qaeda-style, cell-based structure (Powell 2016). What is certain is that IS is a symptom of Sunni militancy, not its cause. Sunni jihadist ideology will survive IS and will continue to be a factor in regional—and possibly global—politics for many years to come.

7.3.4 Motivational Trends in Non-state Terrorism

Admittedly, violent non-state actors have little in common. However, classifying them along general characteristics can help us understand the forces that generate and shape terrorist activity. To do so, one must look at the primary motivations—the core reasons and motives—that prompt violent non-state actors to employ terrorism. Broadly speaking, most experts distinguish between three different types of violent non-state actors, namely, those that are motivated by politics and ideology, by ethno-nationalist or separatist ambitions, and by their religious views. Regardless of their particular ideological orientation, politically oriented violent actors tend to advocate strict visions about how society should be administered or governed. Ethno-nationalists and separatists wish to see the ethnic or national identity of their members reflected in the structure and makeup of a future governing system. Religiously motivated violent actors see their actions as mandated by a divine being. Although, as history shows, no religion is immune to being used as a justification for terrorism, our century has witnessed a resurgence of Sunni Islamist militancy. This is to some extent embodied by violent jihadist groups that have a globalist agenda, namely, al-Qaeda and IS. Despite common roots, these two groups represent two markedly different strategies in Salafi jihadism. Their demise should not be excluded; however, it will not terminate the wave of Sunni discontent that has generated them.

SELF-CHECK

- Define jihadism.
- Which of the following is not one of the distinct types of violent non-state actors, based on their primary motives?
  a. Ethno-nationalist or separatist
  b. Religious
  c. Political/ideological
  d. Economic
- Ethno-nationalist groups are responsible for the majority of terrorism conducted by non-state actors in the past century. True or false?
- The Oklahoma City bombing was the deadliest terrorist attack in the United States even after 9/11. True or false?

7.4 Methods of Non-state Violence

Depending on their longevity, violent non-state actors usually develop distinct techniques for carrying out terrorist attacks. These characterize their violent activities and often become "signature methods" that authorities use to identify the perpetrators of terrorist attacks. Militant groups tend to develop their *modus operandi* based on their motivations, resources, and overall strategies. Indicatively, some groups seek to maximize human fatalities. Others make it a tactical goal to cause only property damage, so as to project a public image of themselves as social radicals that respect human life. Despite such differences, it can be stated with accuracy that all violent non-state actors seek two things when dispensing violence: first, methods that are technically successful and second, methods that will enhance and even inflate their public image of strength.

Whether violent groups achieve these two goals is highly dependent on their technical sophistication and level of organization. Most violent non-state actors have limited access to financial and material resources, as well as to scientific and technical know-how. These constraints limit their ability to conduct technically sophisticated attacks, which largely accounts for the operational conservatism of most terrorist groups. Many theorists pose that violent non-state actors, much like military organizations, "are conservative in nature," which means that they "prefer to preserve tried strategies and structures rather than adopt new ones" (Dolnik 2007, 10). Consequently, the discussions about the concept of innovation in non-state terrorism begin from the premise that the technologies used by non-state actors to dispense violence "have never been completely new" (Dolnik 2007, 10).

Innovation, therefore, is rare in non-state terrorism circles and tends to be incremental rather than radical in nature. Groups tend to copy each other's techniques and change them only when their effectiveness is threatened by the evolving counterterrorist methods of state agencies. Technological progress—for example, the invention of the fully automatic, portable machine gun, or plastic explosives—is important here as a factor: violent non-state actors do tend to gradually adopt new technologies. However, just because a new technology becomes available and within technical reach does not mean that militant organizations will necessarily employ it.

7.4.1 Conventional and Unconventional Methods of Non-state Violence

Physical attacks by violent non-state actors typically aim to destroy property, inflict physical harm or death on targeted individuals (assassinations), injure or kill indiscriminately, or all of the above. Their implementation can be carried out using conventional or unconventional means. Conventional means include unarmed assaults, armed assaults using small firearms or sharp objects, armed assaults using bombs of various magnitudes, kidnappings, hijackings, and barricade/hostage incidents. Some groups use these methods in combination, so as to maximize operational unpredictability and dilute their adversary's counterterrorism resources and arsenal.

7.4.1.1 Small Firearms and Explosives

The most often used conventional method of non-state terrorist violence involves the employment of small firearms. These are preferred because they require minimal technical expertise but can have maximum effect, especially when used with frequency, thus creating "a relatively steady threat stream" (Garternstein-Ross and Trombly 2012, 6). The use of small firearms should not be confused with small-scale attacks. Small firearms used in a synchronized fashion by large assault teams can generate complex attacks that wreak havoc on a mass scale. In November 2008, a 10-member commando unit of the Pakistan-based militant group Lashkar-e-Taiba used a combination of rifles, time bombs, and grenades to carry out a series of centrally coordinated attacks on popular tourist locations in the Indian megacity of Mumbai. The series of attacks lasted 3 days, during which 166 people were killed and nearly 300 were injured, while Mumbai came to a near-complete standstill (Rabasa et al. 2009).

Bombings are used by violent non-state actors to maximize the effect of their violence without stretching their financial resources or materiel. They can be used to symbolically disrupt key targets, like international airports, without necessarily causing large numbers of casualties. They can also be used with to kill *en masse*. In 1993, a car filled with 1000 pounds of explosives blew up in the underground parking garage of the World Trade Center in New York, killing six and injuring over 1000 people. Ramzi Yousef, the al-Qaeda member who drove a car to the parking lot, told investigators that his ideal goal had been "to topple one [World Trade Center] tower on top of the other and kill 250,000 people" (Steven and Gunaratna 2004, 66). On the other side of the spectrum is Eric Rudolph, a far-right American militant who bombed the Olympic Centennial Park in Atlanta during the 1996 Olympic Games. He also bombed a gay nightclub and two family planning clinics in Georgia and Alabama. After his arrest in 2003, he told authorities that he had "nothing personal" against his dead and injured victims. His goal, he said, had been to rally public opinion against abortion and homosexuality, two behaviors that he stated "should be met with force if necessary" (Mattingly and Schuster 2005). Explosive devices planted in vehicles have been used with increasing frequency since the 1970s, when they were first regularly employed by the PIRA and by several belligerents involved in the Lebanese Civil War. A particularly brutal bombing technique involves the planned use of secondary explosions, which are timed to detonate several minutes after an earlier explosion. These kill first responders, media crews, and bystanders from the general public, who typically gather around the site of the first explosion. There have also been cases of safe-area bombings, namely, planned attacks that occur at areas where evacuees have been taken by authorities in response to a bomb threat (Purpura 2016, 482).

7.4.1.2 Kidnapping and Planned Hostage-Taking

Non-state violent groups conduct kidnappings to retaliate or exact revenge against adversaries, to attract publicity, to extract confessions from their victims, or to exchange them for their own imprisoned members (Steven and Gunaratna 2004, 70). The practice is ancient (Baumann 1973, 32ff) but was systematized mostly by left-wing violent groups in the late 1960s and early 1970s. The first notable incident took place in 1968 when the US Ambassador to Guatemala, Gordon Mein, was kidnapped by the *Fuerzas Armadas Rebeldes* (Rebel Armed Forces (FAR)), a leftist guerrilla group. He was eventually executed, becoming the first American ambassador to be assassinated while in office. In 1970, the same group kidnapped and killed the German ambassador to Guatemala. By that time, the practice had become commonplace in Latin America and had been copied by separatist groups in Canada, Spain, and Turkey (Stechel 1972, 203). History's most notorious and consequential high-profile kidnapping by a non-state group occurred in 1978 when Italy's former prime minister, Aldo Moro, was kidnapped by the Red Brigades. At the time of his kidnapping, Moro was the leader of the center-right Christian Democracy, Italy's largest political party, and was strongly favored to be the next president of Italy. After killing his five bodyguards at the scene of the abduction, the kidnappers executed Moro and dumped his body in the trunk of a car, where it was found 55 days after his disappearance. Moro's killing had an immediate and dramatic political effect: it contributed to the rise of a powerful sentiment in parliament against the Italian Communist Party (PCI), which at the time was Italy's second largest, having received 30% of the popular vote. The division quickly deepened and ended the so-called historical compromise, the governing alliance between the PCI and Christian Democracy (Engene 2004, 239), thus changing the course of Italian politics forever. Today kidnapping is practiced frequently in large parts of the Middle East and Africa, where it is such "a lucrative industry [that some] terrorist groups even subcontract kidnappings to other organizations" (Steven and Gunaratna 2004, 70).

Non-state actors regularly utilize planned barricading and hostage-taking—as opposed to unplanned hostage-taking, for instance, when a robbery goes wrong. They do so in order to attain safe passage to another location (typically a third country), attract publicity, raise funds, or exchange hostages for their own imprisoned members. Unlike kidnapping, which obscures the physical whereabouts of the victim(s), seized hostages are forcibly imprisoned at a known location. The latter method is a public act that typically results in some form of direct interaction between the hostage-taker(s) and the authorities (Mahan and Griset 2008, 140). Famous historical instances of barricading and hostage-taking include the 1979 armed seizure of the US embassy in the Iranian capital Tehran by a group calling itself the Muslim Student Followers of the Imam's Line. The seizure led to the so-called Iran hostage crisis, in which 52 Americans, most of them diplomats, were held captive for 444 days. Many, including US President Jimmy Carter himself, have suggested that the hostage crisis cost him his second term in office (Carter 2010, 526ff). Another long-lasting hostage-taking incident was the December 1996 takeover of the Japanese ambassador's residence in Lima, Peru, by 20 armed members of the Túpac Amaru Revolutionary Movement (MRTA), a Marxist–Leninist group. Over 400 were held hostage, some of them for as many as 126 days, until the residence was stormed by the Peruvian security forces in April of 1997. By all accounts, after liberating the hostages, the Peruvian security officers executed the MRTA men by shooting them in the head (Mahan and Griset 2008, 140).

Unlike these historical cases, contemporary barricading/hostage-taking operations are conducted by armed groups that "are increasingly effective in making tactical responses to barricade incidents [by the authorities] both more costly and less likely to succeed" (Dolnik and Fitzgerald 2008, 2). The hostage-takers are well read about past incidents and "know most of the standard tricks" (Dolnik and Fitzgerald 2008, 2). Additionally, they have access to wireless devices and thus maintain "direct lines of communication with colleagues and others [including media crews] beyond the location of the incident" (Dolnik and Fitzgerald 2008, 2). Most of all, contemporary hostage-takers usually appear determined to execute their victims and even die for their cause. A tragic illustration of this phenomenon was the 2004 Beslan school siege in Russia, where a group of between 50 and 70 Islamist separatists held over 1200 people, most of them children, hostage at a school. In addition to carrying heavy weapons, the hostage-takers booby-trapped the school with nearly 130 explosive devices and began executing hostages almost immediately after taking over the school. The 3-day siege ended in the death of 331 of the hostages. An estimated 176 of the dead were children. Today the Beslan school siege remains one of the three deadliest terrorist attacks in world history (Dolnik and Fitzgerald 2008, 3).

7.4.1.3 Hijackings

Many hostage-taking operations by non-state actors involve aircraft, maritime, or vehicular hijackings. One of history's most sensational maritime hijackings was the seizure of the Italian cruise ship MS *Achille Lauro*, by the members of the Syrian-backed Palestine Liberation Front, in October 1985. After holding 550 people captive for several days, the hijackers abandoned the ship without achieving their goal, which was the release of several dozen Palestinian activists held in Israeli prisons. But the incident demonstrated the sophistication of the perpetrators, who said they had planned the operation for over a year and had made several previous test runs by posing as passengers on the cruise ship (Newton 2002, 2). Aircraft hijackings are far more common than maritime hijackings by non-state groups seeking media attention, because they are more sensational. As Karen Feste (2015) states, the hijacking of commercial jets "is a special form of theater [...], a spectacle of fear and excitement and communication" that offers the news media suspense combined with unpredictability (75). Before 1960, the majority of aircraft hijackings were carried out by individuals from communist countries, who used hijacked aircraft to reach the West—primarily the United States—and seek political asylum. The latter was usually granted, despite persistent calls by communist countries for the United States to extradite the hijackers, or at least try them on American soil (McCann 2006, 101). Feste notes that during the first few decades of the Cold War, the United States "did not see these acts as terrorist or criminal behavior but [as] part of politics" (Feste 2015, 75). That changed quickly after 1960, however, when countless American sympathizers with the communist government of Cuba hijacked civilian airliners and forcibly diverted them to Caribbean island. In 1972, militant groups in Europe, the Middle East, and Africa had begun to copy the method, prompting a phenomenon of "epidemic proportions," with 325 aircraft hijackings recorded worldwide between 1968 and 1972 (McCann 2006, 101).

The phenomenon of aircraft hijacking died out due to advancements in airport security screenings but returned at the turn of the century with the 9/11 hijackings. It has been suggested that the 9/11 hijackings were operationally innovative, because they included multiple simultaneous hijackings, as well as the suicidal use of the aircraft as weapons against ground targets. But Magnus Ranstorp and Magnus Normark (2015, 1) have suggested that the 9/11 attacks may have been inspired by the 1970 Dawson's Field hijackings, which involved five attempted simultaneous takeovers of civilian airliners bound for New York and London. The hijackings were carried out by members of the left-wing Popular Front for the Liberation of Palestine (PFLP), who boarded the airliners in several European airports. Four were successful. One of the airliners was blown up after being diverted to Cairo, Egypt, thankfully after all passengers had managed to escape. The remaining three were evacuated and blown up in spectacular fashion by the PFLP hijackers before the world's media on September 12, 1970, causing "headline-grabbing, front-page coverage" (Elias 2009, 4). Ranstorp and Normark (2015, 1) have further suggested that the 9/11 attack planners may have been influenced by the so-called Bojinka plot. The term denotes a plan devised in 1994—but never implemented—by an al-Qaeda cell based in the Philippines. It centered on blowing up simultaneously 11 American civilian aircraft over the Pacific Ocean with the use of small capsules of nitroglycerine. The plot was characterized as "a new dimension of airplane hijacking" for its time, because it involved "the use of passenger aircraft as suicide bombs" (Smith 2015, 169).

The 9/11 attacks may not have been as innovative as some believe, but they did combine the use of conventional and unconventional terrorist methods by a non-state group. The unconventional aspect of the attacks was the suicide of the perpetrators, which was tactically integrated into the overall operation. As a method of dispensing violence, suicide terrorism was not alien to al-Qaeda, nor to Americans, in 2001. In fact, the 9/11 attacks were preceded by two earlier suicide attacks against American targets by al-Qaeda. These were the attacks on the US embassies in Tanzania and Kenya in 1998 and the attack on the *USS Cole* in Yemen in 2000. Thus, the 9/11 attacks marked the third instance of the use of suicide terrorism by al-Qaeda against American targets in less than three years.

7.4.1.4 Suicide Attacks

Any discussion about suicide as a method of terrorism must start by dispelling the notion that it is an irrational choice by a desperate actor. As a tactic of warfare, suicide terrorism is no more irrational than soldiers sacrificing themselves to help secure victory for their side during a battle or troops voluntarily responding to their commanders' call for a "mission of no return"—as was the case with Japanese *kamikaze* aviators in World War II. Rosemarie Skaine (2013) writes that a planned suicide mission is neither random nor mindless, but rather "a tactic of war. [As such, it] reflects the goals of the organization" that plans and executes it (xiii). Some scholars argue against the use of the biased term "suicide terrorism" to explain the phenomenon, because it carries within it cultural connotations of recklessness and even mental illness. The term may be especially unhelpful when trying to understand religiously motivated suicide terrorism, given that many of the world's religious cultures, including Christianity and Islam, tend to look down upon—or even outright forbid—suicide. Consequently, religious communities that support suicide terrorism do not refer to it as suicide, preferring instead to use the term "martyrdom." Arabs use the term *shaheed*, meaning a martyr who dies while carrying out the religious commandment of *jihad*. Even secular non-state groups that employ suicide terrorism, like the Tamil Tigers, do not refer to it as "suicide," but rather as "donating oneself to the cause" (Mahan and Griset 2008, 142).

Voluntary self-sacrifice has been employed as a tactic of regular and irregular warfare since ancient times, notably in Greek city-states like Sparta, which at times discouraged the return of defeated soldiers from the front (Rahe 2016, 33). In the modern era, non-state suicide terrorism was systematized by some nineteenth-century anarchist and nihilist groups that spearheaded the use of dynamite in terrorist campaigns (Powell 2014, 7). Despite their occasional use of suicide terrorism, there is no evidence that anarchist and nihilist groups prioritized the method as a form of commitment to principles. It is more likely that they deployed suicide bombers as a way to compensate for the rudimentary nature of their improvised explosive devices. The latter had to be detonated close to the intended targets so as to maximize casualties or to kill individuals singled out for assassination. The method faded away when the Russian school of anarchism and nihilism dissipated. But it reappeared in the early 1980s during the Lebanese Civil War when it was used by Shiite paramilitaries.

Around the same time, suicide bombings were used on a large scale by two secular Marxist groups, the Tamil Tigers in Sri Lanka and the PKK in Turkey. The Tigers used the method in a systematic fashion, even establishing a specialized suicide unit, called the Black Panthers. In 1993, when they killed Sri Lankan President Ranasinghe Premadasa, the Tigers became the world's only non-state actor to have assassinated two heads of state, in both cases with the use of suicide terrorism (Skaine 2013, 86). However, there are no examples of non-state violent groups that have used suicide terrorism as a permanent military tactic. Even in the case of the Tamil Tigers, who systematized the use of martyrdom like few other groups in history, suicide terrorism was never more than a temporary tactic and did not shape the overall strategy of the organization. The tactical aspects of the practice of suicide terrorism are crucial in the study of the phenomenon. As can be expected, dominant media narratives give overwhelming attention to the execution stage. However, the act of the so-called martyr must be understood as the culmination of "a whole set of tactical moves" (Dzikansky et al. 2012, 97) that include strategizing, indoctrination, logistical planning, reconnaissance, and operational security. Thus, the execution is "the last link of a long organizational chain that involve[s] numerous actors" (Mahan and Griset 2008, 142).

FOR EXAMPLE

Al-Qaeda's Use of Suicide Terrorism

Al-Qaeda's pioneering use of suicide terrorism was evident not only in the organization's planning of the 9/11 attack but in its assassination of Ahmed Shah Massoud, leader of Afghanistan's Northern Alliance. In the late 1990s, Massoud emerged as the most charismatic and arguably the most capable Afghan leader, a strong competitor to the Taliban's popularity. In January of 2001, al-Qaeda supplied Dahmane Abd al-Sattar, a Belgium-based member of the organization, with a forged passport and detailed "legend," a complex story that supported its cover of "journalist." Accompanied by an extensive network of al-Qaeda affiliates in Europe, al-Sattar traveled to Britain, where he was given a reference letter by a prominent Islamic cleric. From Britain, al-Sattar and several other members of the assassination team traveled to Islamabad, Pakistan, where they showed officials at the Afghan embassy the letter of reference from Britain. That convinced the officials to grant them journalistic visas to enter Afghanistan. After lengthy negotiations, the assassins managed to gain access to Massoud. They killed the charismatic Afghan leader by exploding a bomb that had been carefully built into one of their fake cameras. The killing took place on September 9, 2001, 2 days before 9/11. (Smith 2002)

In many ways, al-Qaeda pioneered aspects of modern suicide terrorism. The group professionalized the organizational chain that precedes the execution stage, especially promoting a culture of patient, long-term planning, and advanced operational security. Evidence of the use of suicide attacks by IS as a tactic of war seems to suggest that the group follows the operational principles established by al-Qaeda (Nance 2016, 329). Some added elements introduced by IS include the use of suicide attacks in the battlefield. It is believed that, in early 2017, nearly every IS battalion had in its ranks a dedicated suicide unit, whose members were typically being used as a first weapon—launching attacks or counterattacks by breaching defenses. In many cases, suicide bombers were placed inside customized armored vehicles and sent toward the enemy. This technique allowed the suicide bombers to approach enemy positions with as many as 150 tons of explosives packed inside a single vehicle (Nance 2016, 327). After an initial wave of sometimes up to

20 suicide bombers attacking the enemy in a coordinated fashion, IS would follow with an attack by conventionally armed troops in formations, who advanced with the support of armored vehicles and artillery. What we are seeing, therefore, in IS' military strategy is the systematic use on the battlefield of highly unconventional terrorist methods but in conventional ways (Coker 2015; Kilcullen 2016, 114).

SELF-CHECK

- Gordon Mein, the first American ambassador to be kidnapped and assassinated while in office, was killed by which terrorist group?
  a. Rebel Armed Forces (FAR) in Guatemala
  b. Shining Path (SL) in Peru
  c. Revolutionary Armed Forces (FARC) in Colombia
  d. Zapatistas (EZLN) in Mexico
- Evidence of the use of suicide attacks by the Islamic State as a tactic of war seems to suggest that the group follows the operational principles established by al-Qaeda. True or false?
- Aircraft hijackings far more common than other types of hijackings by non-state violent groups. True or false?
- The Iran hostage crisis, in which 52 Americans, most of them diplomats, were held captive for 444 days, led to US President George H.W. Bush not being reelected to a second term of office. True or false?

7.5 International Strategies for Countering Non-state Violence

Analysts distinguish strategies for opposing terrorism into two broad fields, namely **anti-terrorism**, which describes defensive measures taken to limit and impede terrorist activities, and counterterrorism, an offensive method that aims to prevent or even eliminate the phenomenon altogether. An example of anti-terrorism measures would be **target hardening** which are efforts to make it physically difficult for violent non-state actors to carry out attacks against targets that are generally perceived as soft, such as shopping malls or schools. Anti-terrorism has been described as "the shield" and counterterrorism as "the sword" (Johnson 2013, 67). These metaphors may be useful in helping us visualize the overall process, but they ignore the majority of measures taken to oppose terrorism, which are non-military in nature. Furthermore, to the extent that anti-terrorism and counterterrorism are indeed separate, the distinguishing lines between them are often blurry and difficult to ascertain. What is certain is that, if practiced properly, they collectively incorporate a vast array of practices, including public policy, intelligence planning, and a variety of military strategies and tactics.

To be coherent and enduring, a strategy of opposition to non-state violence must concentrate primarily on addressing the sociopolitical context in which terrorism is generated rather than on combating its violent outcome. The latter may be senseless, irrational, even unprovoked. But a serious anti- or counterterrorism strategy must always strive to understand and conceptualize the underlying motivation behind organized acts of violence (Cioffi-Revilla 2012, 152). This may not be easy to ascertain, given that, as we have already discussed, violent non-state actors are not always motivated by coherent, or even attainable, goals. There is also much research showing that the primary goal of many nonviolent state actors is not the realization of their goals, but rather the continuation of their existence (United States Army 2007, 15). Thus, violent non-state actors who realize their original aims have been known to adjust their objectives in order to justify their continued existence. They do so usually by officially disbanding one organization and forming another, with expanded aims.

FOR EXAMPLE

The Panhellenic Liberation Movement

An example of a violent non-state actor that refused to disband after achieving its stated aims was the Panhellenic Liberation Movement (PAK). The group was established in 1968 in Sweden with the aim of ending the rule of the Greek military junta and establishing a socialist government through agitation and violent means. The junta fell in 1974, and in 1981 the PAK founder, Andreas Papandreou, by then leader of the Panhellenic Socialist Movement (PASOK), became Greece's prime minister. But many members of the PAK refused to disband and set up or joined several underground paramilitary organizations, including Revolutionary Organization 17 November, the Revolutionary People's Struggle, and others. (Kassimeris 2013, 17ff)

It is not only non-state groups that pose barriers to ending conflict by their obstinacy. In some cases, elements within the state are equally recalcitrant. At times, state actors find that they have more to gain by prolonging a conflict against violent actors than by ending it. Alternatively, they may be unwilling to share power and resources with an insurgent group and its supporters. They are thus insufficiently invested in resolving a conflict and essentially contribute to its protracted nature. Critics of Israel, for example, accuse successive Israeli administrations of having consistently chosen illegal territorial expansion over the prospect of peace with the Palestinians (Deeb 2013, 31 and 71). Some Israeli historians suggest that this choice informs the basis of Israeli state policy, which is "premised on the view that Israel, the dominant military power in the Middle East, ha[s] no need to limit itself through negotiations" (Thomas 2011, xv and 111ff). This may explain why, in 2006, the Israeli government, supported by the United States and the European Union, refused to accept the outcome of the internationally monitored Palestinian legislative election. The reason was that the election had given a clear victory to Hamas, with 74 of the 132 seats in the legislature of the Palestinian National Authority. The argument of the Israeli government was that Hamas was a terrorist organization and therefore could not be allowed to represent the Palestinian people. However, the terrorism literature is replete with examples of violent non-state groups that end their violent campaigns once they entered the field of politics (Jones and Libicki 2008, xiii). There is no reason to exclude the possibility that Hamas could have been one such group. In other cases, a state involved in a conflict with a violent non-state actor may itself engage in, or sponsor, terrorism. The situation can become even more complex when third states contribute to a protracted conflict by sponsoring one or more non-state actors involved in it (see Chapter 6).

7.5.1 The Military Option

States typically enter conflicts with non-state actors with zero-sum bias, meaning that they intend to pursue the complete elimination of their opponent. In most cases, this type of thinking promotes a military approach to counterterrorism, guided by the "conviction that the conflict […] cannot be terminated short of a complete military victory" (O'Leary and Tirman 2007, 2). Thus, the state deploys the machinery of its armed forces—and sometimes those of allied states—in its effort to crush a non-state opponent. This can involve the selected use of targeted operations aiming to "decapitate" a non-state actor's senior leadership, either reactively or preemptively (Gunneflo 2016, 111). It can also involve—separately or in combination—large-scale military operations, usually in response to an actual or perceived insurgency by a non-state actor. An example of such an action is the Second Chechen War of 1999, when an estimated 80 000 Russian troops descended on the Russian Caucasus to fight against Russian and foreign Islamist fighters of the Islamic International Brigade. The war lasted approximately a year and restored Russian federal control of the region, where in 1991 Chechen secessionists had declared independence, under the name Chechen Republic of Ichkeria. As is often the case with large-scale military campaigns against non-state actors, the official end of the war was followed by a protracted counterinsurgency campaign, which lasted for nearly 10 years (Schaefer 2010). The Russian example of a large-scale military campaign launched against secessionists is not unique. It has been used repeatedly, for example, by Sri Lanka in its fight against the LTTE, by Turkey against the PKK, and by Nigeria in its fight against Boko Haram. Results have been mixed. One major problem with this approach is that it tends to display the characteristics of a total war against the civilian population and can backlash severely on the government's moral character and reputation (Gilligan 2010).

Perhaps the most pertinent modern example of employing the military option against a non-state actor is the so-called Global War on Terror (GWOT), declared by US President George W. Bush in the aftermath of the 9/11 attacks (Widmaier 2015, 104). The war, which dominated global politics in the opening years of the twenty-first century, presents terrorism experts with several controversies and problems (see Chapter 1). To begin with, the term "war on terror" poses central issues of conceptualization. Terror is an emotion, a feeling of intense fear that may be caused by an act of terrorism. Launching a war against an emotion is a nonsensical concept, which has rightly been described as "nebulous" by experts—though it is perhaps slightly less nonsensical than a "war on evil," another rhetorical device employed by President Bush at the time (Richardson 2006, 175). Presumably, the American president meant "war on terrorism," but even that term makes no logical sense, given that terrorism is simply a tactic of war. One cannot launch a war against a tactic, let alone win it. In 2006, the eminent Irish terrorism expert Louise Richardson, later vice-chancellor of the University of Oxford in England, was among many scholars who correctly pointed out that a "war on terror" was a militarily useless concept. The way it was termed by the White House, said Richardson, the "war on terror" offered no "clear matrices of success or failure by which progress could have been measured" (Richardson 2006, 175). Admittedly, sending troops to the battlefield to fight a "war on terror" or a "war on terrorism" without first defining a clear enemy—like al-Qaeda or the Taliban—is not only nonsensical but also reckless. It precludes the possibility of victory and ensures that the troops engaged in the war will either die or return home in defeat, for an emotion and a tactic can never be militarily defeated.

After 2001, it became apparent that the war launched by America in 2001 was a narrow—and certainly not global—campaign against some state and non-state actors who use terrorism and some of their supporters. Looking back, even the most ardent supporter of the war would have to admit that its course has been convoluted and at times perplexing. Although it is too early to draw broad historical conclusions, it appears that the outcome of the war has been mixed—if not counterproductive—in Afghanistan and possibly catastrophic in the Middle East. Instead of ending "terror" and "evil," the war, along with the Arab Spring and the Syrian Civil War, has arguably inflamed militant Islamism. Consequently, it can be argued that the war made America less safe than it was in the aftermath of 9/11. The Bush administration had received ample warning of the dangers involved in an over-reliance on the military as part of its global counterterrorism policy, especially in Iraq. We now know that the Intelligence Community had prepared intelligence reports warning about the negative consequences of a possible US military involvement in the Middle East. Prepared in August 2002 and January 2003, the reports suggested that the toppling of the Hussein regime would lead to a dangerous and unpredictable period of large-scale violence in Iraq. One of the reports, entitled "The perfect storm: Planning for negative consequences of invading Iraq," cautioned that an American invasion would be met by protracted guerrilla warfare. The insurgency would be led by supporters of Iraq's deposed government, said the reports, who would wage war against US forces "either by themselves or in alliance with terrorists." Moreover, the reports predicted that the removal of the Iraqi regime would fuel internal sectarianism and would lead to "a significant chance that domestic groups would engage in violent conflict with each other" (Bailey and Immerman 2015, 88). Intelligence reports by the CIA went as far as to suggest that not only would Iraq break up into ethnically based states under the weight of sectarian violence but that the ensuing anarchy would be "exploited by terrorists and extremists outside Iraq." That, warned the reports, would fuel "militant Islamism" and lead to a "surge of global terrorism" that would hurt US interests (Myers and Windrem 2007). These reports describe the primary outcome of the American invasion of Iraq with astonishing accuracy.

7.5.2 The Political Option

Research by a variety of sources, including the RAND Corporation, a defense contractor with close ties to the US Department of Defense, consistently shows that "a transition [of a non-state actor] to the political process is the most common way" to terminate its violent activities. This means that the most realistic method of ending the violent campaign of a non-state actor is through a political strategy, though the latter can be implemented in conjunction with limited military or other methods. However, "the possibility of a political solution is inversely linked to the breadth of [...] goals" advocated by the non-state actor (Jones and Libicki 2008, xiii). In other words, the narrower the goals of a violent non-state actor, the higher the possibility that it will be able to reach a politically negotiated settlement with a state actor. But even in cases when the goals of a violent non-state actor are broad mitigation of terrorism can be achieved through reaching out to the more moderate elements involved in a non-state actor's violent campaign. In 2016, after the Colombian government and the FARC agreed to bring their 52-year conflict to an end, some FARC units distanced themselves from the leadership of the group, refusing to demobilize. Some dissenters even launched a number of attacks against government targets in late 2016. But these units were isolated by the FARC, thus fragmenting the group and allowing the more moderate voices within the organization to proceed with implementing the peace agreement with the government (Brodzinsky 2016).

A political option that ends in a form of power-sharing can be especially effective when applied to conflicts involving ethno-nationalist or separatist non-state actors. In 1998, the Good Friday Agreement was signed between representatives of the British and Irish governments and the leaders of most Northern Irish political parties. The Democratic Unionist Party, which had close connections with loyalist paramilitary groups, openly opposed it. Sinn Féin, the political arm of the Irish nationalist movement, with connections to the PIRA, also expressed skepticism. However, the agreement was ratified by over 70% of voters in a referendum in the same year, leading to the power-sharing arrangement between the two opposing parties. In 2007, the British Army terminated Operation BANNER, its counterterrorism deployment that began in 1969. At the time of its termination, BANNER was the longest continuous deployment of troops in British military history and had cost the lives of nearly 1500 British soldiers (Mumford 2012, 95). Much has been written about the remarkable changes in the attitudes of many loyalist and republican activists, whose families had suffered numerous deaths as a result of the Troubles. Often neglected, however, is the change of stance by the British government, represented by the administrations of two successive British prime ministers: the Conservative Party's John Major and the Labour Party's Tony Blair. Their predecessor, Conservative Prime Minister Margaret Thatcher, was vehemently opposed to any negotiation with Irish republicans, even when 10 of them voluntarily died by going on a hunger strike in prison in 1981, demanding to be treated as political—not criminal—prisoners by the British government (McKittrick and McVea 2002, 134–149).

FOR EXAMPLE

Counterterrorism and Human Rights in Turkey

An example that illustrates the significance of striking a balance between counterterrorism and human rights, as well as civil liberties, is that of Turkey. On July 15, 2016, Turkey witnessed an attempted coup by elements of the military. The coup culminated in a dramatic armed attack on the country's parliament in Ankara. By the time it ended in failure, in the early hours of July 16, it had resulted in the deaths of over 200 people across Turkey. In response to the coup, the administration of Turkish President Recep Tayyip Erdoğan embarked on a campaign against supporters of Muslim cleric Fethullah Gülen, whom the government accused of orchestrating the coup from his home in the United States. Within 6 months, the government had arrested nearly 40 000 people and summarily dismissed or suspended 100 000 public servants across the country. Turkey, which was once hailed by the West as "a model for the Muslim world" and "an anchor of stability in the Middle East," was identified in November of 2016 as the world's leading jailer of journalists (Lowen 2016). During that same month, the World Justice Project placed Turkey in 99th place out of 113 countries on its Rule of Law Index, a primary-data-based evaluation of how the rule of law is experienced by each country's general public. (Lowen 2016)

SELF-CHECK

- Define the target hardening.
- Which US president employed a military option to defeat al-Qaeda after 9/11?

  a. Bill Clinton

  b. Barrack Obama

  c. George W. Bush

  d. Jimmy Carter

- A transition of a non-state actor to the political process is the most common way to terminate its violent activities. True or false?
- In 1998, the Good Friday Agreement was signed between representatives of the British and Irish governments and the leaders of most Northern Irish political parties. True or false?

SUMMARY

All non-state groups that use terrorism eventually cease to exist, because they are defeated, because they compromise or quit, or because they achieve their goals. However, despite the proclamations of US President George W. Bush after 9/11, it is impossible to end terror, or for that matter the phenomenon of terrorism. State actors can confront violent groups by practicing both defensive and offensive techniques that incorporate a vast array of practices, such as military and intelligence operations, policy measures, and law enforcement work. In the majority of cases, both state and non-state actors confront each other with the intention of completely dominating the conflict. But limited or large-scale military campaigns by states against violent non-state actors are rarely successful and risk becoming total in nature.

In this chapter you learned that terrorist movements are typically followed by insurgency campaigns that are protracted as they are bloody. Most non-state actors who decide to stop using violence do so after being invited to join the political arena. Many such instances lead to various forms of power-sharing that have been shown to work, especially in violent conflicts with ethno-nationalist or separatist components. You also learned that in the twenty-first century, terrorism cannot be effectively confronted without the use of intelligence and police work. Governments must exercise close surveillance of communications to guard against nonhierarchical non-state actors. They must also use human intelligence to penetrate some of the more hierarchical violent groups, like al-Qaeda. However, measures must be taken to protect human rights and civil liberties, which are as important as the physical safety of the citizenry in a democratic society.

KEY TERMS

Anarchism	A political philosophy that rejects hierarchical systems of organization and advocates the creation of self-governing social systems based on volunteerism.
Anti-terrorism	Describes defensive measures taken to limit and impede terrorist activities.
Communism	A form of radical socialism, which propagates that collective action by workers and their allies is the only effective way of halting global capitalism.
Counterterrorism	An offensive method that aims to prevent, or even eliminate, terrorist activities.
Domestic terrorism	Terrorism directed by individuals or groups at targets located within the territory of the state or states they are fighting against.
Ethno-nationalism/separatism	Espoused by individuals or groups that want to see the ethnic or national identity of their members reflected in the structure and makeup of the governing system.

Guerrilla warfare	A type of irregular warfare usually practiced by small teams of combatants, who rely primarily on hit-and-run tactics against a conventional military adversary. Guerrilla warfare is frequently employed by ethnonationalist groups fighting foreign colonizers.
Insurgency	An uprising or rebellion against a recognized government or state by a non-state actor.
International terrorism	Terrorism directed by individuals or groups at targets located beyond their adversary's territory.
Internationalization	A conscious decision to broaden the visibility of a terrorist campaign by launching attacks in, or involving targets of, third countries in order to draw global attention to the perpetrator's grievances and press for their resolution.
Islamism	A political ideology that seeks to shape society, often by force, according to conservative interpretations of Islam.
Jihadism	Refers to the belief that Islam is currently under attack and that every Muslim has a sacred personal duty to resist by any means necessary.
Magical thinking	The idea that ultimate victory is granted—and often predestined—by a divine being irrespective of material factors on the ground, such as the military strength of the adversary.
Marxism	A philosophical critique of the capitalist system, which Marxists view as inherently contradictory and unstable. Its founder, the nineteenth-century German philosopher Karl Marx, believed that the working class should engage in revolutionary activity as a way of hastening capitalism's inevitable collapse.
Modern era of terrorism	Terrorism practiced during and after the French Revolution of 1789.
Nationalism	An ideological identification with one's nation, which is usually underpinned by political undertones that center on a strong belief in national identity and sometimes combined with notions of national purity.
Nihilism	Strong skepticism and opposition to existing social order, accompanied by a rejection of conventional religious or moral principles. In some cases, nihilists call for society's destruction without offering solutions to what they perceive to be social ills.

Political/ideological terrorism	Practiced by individuals or groups that propagate strict normative visions about how society should be administered or governed. These visions are usually informed by a body of underlying ideas that form the group's ideology.
Primary motivations	The core reasons and motives that prompt violent non-state actors to use terrorism as a tactic of war.
Religious terrorism	Practiced by individuals or groups who believe that their way of thinking and actions are mandated by a divine being and that their violent actions are testaments of their commitment to their god.
Revolutionary socialism	The view that social revolution—violent or non-violent—is necessary in order to accomplish the transition from capitalism to socialism.
Rhizomatic	A model of organization that relies on horizontal, nonhierarchical systems, consisting of semi- or entirely autonomous cells that display no predetermined operational structure.
Salafism	A nineteenth-century doctrine of strict adherence to early Islamic doctrine that emerged in Egypt as a reaction to the European colonialism of the Arab world.
Separatism	The belief that a group of people—usually connected by common cultural, ethnic, religious, racial, or other characteristics—should exist separately from a larger group.
Strategic goals	The ultimate ambitions and objectives toward which non-state actors employ terrorist tactics.
Target hardening	Efforts to make it physically difficult for violent non-state actors to carry out attacks against targets that are generally perceived as soft, such as shopping malls or schools.
Transnationalization	The establishment of operational ties between ideologically comparable non-state violent groups across national borders.
Violent non-state actors	Organized entities that operate outside the realm of official state structures, act mostly in secret, and systematically employ physical violence to achieve their strategic goals.
Wahhabism	A Sunni Muslim doctrine similar to Salafism, which emerged in the eighteenth century in what is today Saudi Arabia and today forms that country's state-authorized religion.

War in Afghanistan   Armed conflict that erupted between the government of Afghanistan and various ethnic and religious factions, as well as between these factions themselves, following the withdrawal of US and NATO troops from the country in 2014.

War in Iraq   Armed conflict between an international coalition, led by the United States, and a host of insurgency groups. The war began immediately following the American-led invasion of Iraq in March of 2003 and ended in late 2011, when the last substantial numbers of American troops left the country.

ASSESS YOUR UNDERSTANDING

Go to www.wiley.com/go/Kilroy/Threats_to_Homeland_Security to assess your knowledge of the basics of national security.

Summary Questions

1. Some scholars argue that terrorism is not a derogatory moral classification, but rather a method of war. True or false?

2. Which of the following is an example of a violent non-state actor that has developed "rhizomatically?"
   (a) ETA
   (b) IRA
   (c) AQ
   (d) PLO

3. Politically motivated violent non-state actors tend to operate with more fervor and less flexibility than religiously motivated terrorist groups. True or false?

4. What was the first far-right violent group that appeared in American history?
   (a) KKK
   (b) Weather Underground
   (c) Black Panthers
   (d) Army of God

5. The most often used conventional method of non-state terrorist violence involves the employment of small firearms. True or false?

6. Which of these violent non-state actors do not constitute a distinct type?
   (a) Motivated by politics or ideology
   (b) Motivated by ethno-nationalist or separatist creeds
   (c) Motivated by religious doctrines
   (d) Motivated by Islam

7. The emergence of IS marks a crucial change of jihadist strategy that breaks with al-Qaeda's strategic trajectory. Unlike al-Qaeda, which views the creation of the caliphate as the crowning achievement of a protracted process, IS has decided to essentially reverse the process and already declared the creation of the caliphate. True or false?

8. In comparison with far-left groups, far-right non-state actors display a narrower degree of transnationalization in the operational field—that is, they have not historically sought to establish operational ties with ideologically comparable groups across national borders. True or false?

9. Which of the following is an example of terrorist group that has recently pursued the political option as an end to its decades-old conflict?
   (a) SL
   (b) IS
   (c) FARC
   (d) PKK

10. History's most notorious and consequential high-profile kidnapping by a non-state group occurred in 1978, when Germany's former chancellor Helmut Kohl was kidnapped by the Red Army Faction. True or false?

Applying This Chapter

1. The British Broadcasting Corporation (BBC) refuses to use terms such as "terrorism" or "terrorist" in its reporting. In Section 11 of its Editorial Guidelines, the BBC cautions that terms such as "terrorist" can be "a barrier rather than an aid to understanding" and that its use in reporting would essentially force the Corporation to "adopt other people's language as [its] own" (British Broadcasting Corporation 2016a, 120). According to the BBC, terrorism is too "emotive [a] subject with [too many] significant political overtones" to be of any use in serious scholarly analysis (British Broadcasting Corporation 2016a, 120). Do you agree? Why, or why not?

2. If you were the US Ambassador to Israel, how would you argue your nation's condemnation of Palestinian groups such as Hamas and their use of terrorism in support of their goal of establishing a Palestinian state in light of Israel's use of similar tactics to gain its independence?

3. Explain to a student in your class the difference between the three types of terrorist groups described in this chapter. Ask him or her to then provide examples of each type of group.

4. A newspaper headlines describes a suicide attack at a nightclub in London, where 29 people were killed, including the bomber. A classmate comments that it really should be called "homicide terrorism" rather than suicide terrorism, since the goal of the bomber was to kill as many people as possible, along with himself. Do you agree or disagree? Why or why not?

Analyzing Terrorist Organizations

You work in the State Department and are charged with researching foreign terrorist organizations and determining how to classify them based on the three primary motivations of political ideology, ethno-nationalism or separatism, and religious beliefs. Analyze the following organizations and determine their primary motivational factor. Choose one group and decide how best to craft a policy to counter its goals and objectives.

1. MRTA (Peru)
2. PKK (Turkey)
3. Palestinian Islamic Jihad (Palestine)
4. Tamil Tigers (Sri Lanka)

Transitioning from Terrorism to Politics

In the 1970s, Protestant paramilitary groups in Northern Ireland, such as the Ulster Defence Association and the Ulster Volunteer Force, had close links with the Democratic Unionist Party. But in 2017, the party joined the Conservatives to form a coalition government in London. Similarly, national leaders like Nelson Mandela and Menachem Begin began their careers as leaders of violent paramilitary groups, whose opponents described as "terrorists." Would you ever accept the political rehabilitation of a former member of a non-state violent group? If so, would you ever negotiate with people like IS leader Abu Bakr al-Baghdadi? If not, why? What is the difference between al-Baghdadi and Martin McGuinness, commander of the PIRA in the city of Londonderry, who eventually became deputy first minister of Northern Ireland?

8

CYBER-CRIME, CYBER-TERRORISM, AND CYBER-WARFARE

Understanding the Threat to Information and Information Systems

Richard J. Kilroy, Jr.

Department of Politics, Coastal Carolina University, Conway, SC, USA

Starting Point

Go to www.wiley.com/go/Kilroy/Threats_to_Homeland_Security to assess your knowledge of cyber-crime, the basics of cyber-terrorism, and cyber-warfare. *Determine where you need to concentrate your effort.*

What You'll Learn in This Chapter

▲ The definitions of cyber-crime, cyber-terrorism, and cyber-warfare

▲ The capability and intent of nations and non-state actors with regard to the threat they pose in cyberspace

▲ The consequences of a cyber-attack

▲ The defenses against cyber-terrorism and offensive cyber-warfare capabilities of the United States

After Studying This Chapter, You'll Be Able To

▲ Assess information-based threats to the nation's critical infrastructures

▲ Evaluate the difference between capability and intent with regard to cyber-terrorism threats

▲ Appraise the consequences of cyber-terrorism and its effect on our nation's critical infrastructures

▲ Judge our nation's defensive and offensive capabilities concerning cyber-warfare

Threats to Homeland Security: Reassessing the All-Hazards Perspective, Second Edition.
Edited by Richard J. Kilroy, Jr.
© 2018 John Wiley & Sons, Inc. Published 2018 by John Wiley & Sons, Inc.
Companion website: www.wiley.com/go/Kilroy/Threats_to_Homeland_Security

INTRODUCTION

The information age brought both blessings and curses as we became more enamored with technology. Nearly everyone has gone to the grocery store or bank and heard the dreaded words, "Our computer system is down. I can't help you right now." Or, much worse, imagine taking a child to the hospital for an emergency, only to find out important medical information needed to treat the child, such as blood bank data or drug interaction information, is not available due to a computer glitch. Whether we like it or not, we are citizens of a new world, called **cyberspace**—the notional environment in which digitized information is communicated over computer networks—and the ability to collect, store, retrieve, and process information is critical to our lives, as well as our nation's survival.

In this chapter, you will assess information-based threats to our nation's information-based critical infrastructures, to include cyber-crime. You will learn what cyber-terrorism is, as well as evaluate the difference between capability and intent with regard to cyber-terrorism. Next, you'll appraise the consequences of cyber-terrorism and its effect on our nation's information infrastructure. Finally, you'll learn about our nation's defensive and offensive capabilities concerning cyber-warfare.

8.1 The Cyber Threat

> There's a war out there, old friend. A world war. And it's not about who's got the most bullets. It's about who controls the information. What we see and hear, how we work, what we think… it's all about the information! Cosmo, *Sneakers* 1992 (Wikiquote n.d.)

What was a plot in a 1990s Hollywood film has now become a fact of life 25 years later: it's all about the information and who controls it. In the news today, we hear of Russian hackers and their role in influencing US presidential elections (Becker 2017; Riley and Robertson 2017); cyber criminals using ransomware, stealing millions from businesses, schools, and government agencies (Kessem 2016); and countries waging cyber-warfare against their adversaries (Greenberg 2017).

In the past, such information control remained in the hands of gatekeepers such as the media, government, and educational institutions. Today, information is more diffuse, and the means to use it, both positively and negatively, have grown considerably in the last decades. As one example, think about computers and how they are now nearly as common as television sets in American homes. Today's schools require classes to teach computer literacy. Businesses require basic computer skills for practically any conceivable job. For example, auto mechanics depend on a computer chip in a car to diagnose a problem; wait staff and merchants use computers to read credit cards, process orders, and manage inventories; soldiers use sophisticated weapons guidance programs to conduct fire-control missions; and scientists depend on high-speed computers to process mathematical formulas and determine complex algorithms in their experiments. At the end of the day, there are very few of us who can claim not to have had some interaction with computers at school, home, and/or work.

On a larger scale, consider all of the things we take for granted each day: electricity, potable water, indoor plumbing, telephones, televisions, airlines, etc. All of these comprise elements of our nation's critical infrastructures—systems and assets, whether physical or virtual—that are so vital to the United States that the incapacity or destruction of such systems and assets would have a debilitating impact on physical security, national economic security, national public health or safety, or any combination of these matters. These systems supply power generation, communications, transportation, and many other elements of daily life, and they provide us the standard of living we've come to enjoy (and expect) in this country (see Chapter 5).

Yet, all of our nation's critical infrastructures ride on information systems that are vulnerable to disruption, whether that disruption comes from natural or man-made sources. We all know the effects of a thunderstorm on television reception during the Super Bowl, or a programming error on a cellphone satellite. Most times, such disruptions are a minor inconvenience and are fixed rather quickly. Sometimes, however, the outage lasts much longer, such as during a hurricane, when we may not be able to restore power or communications for days or weeks on end.

Unfortunately, our understanding of how to manage information and protect our critical infrastructures from both accidental and intentional damages is limited at best. It usually takes some type of catastrophic failure before we realize how interconnected our world is and how complex those linkages can be. For many, it took the threat of a global computer shutdown on January 1, 2000. Called the Y2K bug (a programming technique used to save computer memory space by using two digits instead of four for the year portion of dates), it caused global panic from both government and the private sector, as millions of dollars were spent correcting the error. Many feared that major industries would be impacted by computer systems that were not "Y2K compliant," causing them to shut down. In the end, much of the concern appeared to have been for naught, as the year 2000 began with few disruptions to any of our critical infrastructures. Yet, Y2K did wake us up to the fact that we are an information-dependent society and that a major disruption, such as the one predicted for Y2K, would have catastrophic consequences for the United States and for commerce in a globalized world. If anything, the preparations for Y2K caused our leaders in government, business, the military, and law enforcement to seriously consider the consequences of such a disruption (Winerip 2013).

For this reason, the potential for a cyber-attack by a terrorist organization or a nation-state actor using cyber-warfare has the ability to create a similar effect psychologically on our society as would the use of a weapon of mass destruction (WMD). In other words, if a terrorist is able to demonstrate an ability to attack one of our nation's critical infrastructures, it would be considered akin to using a weapon of mass disruption in that it would cause more than a simple inconvenience to our everyday lives. Rather, it would evince the government's inability to protect us from future attacks, leading to a loss of trust or confidence in our nation's leadership. Such an attack could also have the effect of rendering our nation financially bankrupt and our law enforcement authorities helpless to deal with the consequences and the potential for widespread panic. For example, if such an attack on the power grid were able to effectively disable major sections of our country in winter, people's lives could be threatened directly. In fact, just such a scenario was envisioned for Y2K by the Canadian military, as it prepared for the worst in its remote northern provinces (CBC 1999).

8.1.1 Defining Cyber-Crime, Cyber-Terrorism, and Cyber-Warfare

In order to understand the threat posed by cyber-crime, cyber-terrorism, and cyber-warfare, we must first define what they are. The National Crime Prevention Council (2012) defines **cyber-crime** as "crime committed or facilitated via the Internet" or "any criminal activity involving computers and networks" (1). Types of cyber-crime involve primarily financial transactions, including nondelivery of payments/merchandise, FBI-related scams, identity theft, credit card fraud, and other illegal money transfers. However, cyber-crime can also include cyberbullying, child pornography, contraband, copyright infringement, money laundering, online gambling, and computer hacking (NCPC 2012). Cyber-crime is estimated to have cost the global economy $3 trillion in 2015 and could grow to $6 trillion by 2021 (Morgan 2016).

FOR EXAMPLE

Ransomware Attacks on Public Schools

In Horry County, South Carolina, in March 2016, cyber criminals infected the Horry County Public Schools with ransomware demanding payment of $10 000 to unlock their computer system. The county ended up paying the hackers in bitcoins, which are virtually untraceable. Although school officials stated that no student data in the 43 000 student school district was actually stolen in the hack, they admitted that their system lacked the security procedures necessary to prevent such attacks (Webb 2016).

In contrast, when Bigfork, Montana, schools were hacked with ransomware in 2016 and cyber criminals demanded payment for a key to unlock the 900 student school district's files, officials said no. Since they had backed-up their data on off-site servers, the school district was able to rebuild their network within a week (Doran 2017).

Dorothy Denning defines **cyber-terrorism** as the use of computer-based operations by terrorist organizations conducting cyber-attacks that "compromise, damage, degrade, disrupt, deny and destroy information stored on computer networks or that target network infrastructures" (Denning 2004, 91). Because computer technology has become inexpensive and the tools (basically, a computer and a modem) are readily available, practically anyone has the capability to become a cyber-terrorist today. A teenager's attempt to "hack" into a Department of Defense (DoD) website may seem innocent enough at first, but the shortcomings or "holes" in the computer system's defenses exposed by these hacks could be exploited by terrorist organizations which could then utilize cyber espionage to steal information from the computer systems while remaining undetected to the authorized users.

What makes cyber-terrorist acts difficult to detect is that, for the most part, computer attacks are anonymous, making it hard to determine the source of an attack. While most computer intrusions thus far have been attributed to self-proclaimed computer hackers or possible criminal elements, there is a possibility that some of these intrusions have been probing actions—cyber-reconnaissance conducted by terrorist organizations to detect the nation's defenses and responses. Such actions would likely be performed before a full-scale cyber-assault on our banking system, for example. Since the volume of cyber incidents grows each year, determining which could be terrorist related becomes more problematic. The DoD Joint Task Force for Computer Network Operations (JTF-CNO) reported that there were 780 cyber incidents against DoD information systems in 1997, rising to over 28 000 incidents in 2000 (Denning 2004, 92). In 2013, the Department of Defense was reporting as many as 10 million cyber attempts per day (Fung 2013). The number of these actual attacks attributed to terrorist groups is problematic. Much of that increase also has to do with better detection and awareness, but the implications are still enormous.

As compared with cyber-terrorism, the term **cyber-warfare** connotes conflict between nation-states using cyber-based weapons. For example, during both the First and Second Gulf Wars, the US military conducted cyber-warfare against the Iraqi military, using conventional electronic warfare tools (radar jamming, electronic deception, etc.), as well as computer-based tools to attack Iraqi communications and command and control infrastructure, such as air defense systems. Cyber-warfare can be used to target both military and civilian infrastructures during a military conflict, or as part of operations prior to actual hostilities. In other words, following the teachings of ancient Chinese philosopher Sun Tzu, it is better to win wars without having to fight, by convincing your adversaries of the futility of their efforts (Watson 2017). For this reason, cyber-warfare can have its greatest impact before conventional military operations, as it attempts to influence the decision making of key adversary leaders. An example of this application of cyber-warfare occurred during the NATO air campaign against Serbian forces in Kosovo in 1999. While NATO air forces used the hard power of military air strikes to destroy the Serb military, cyber-warfare efforts used "soft power" to target Serb leader Slobodan Milosevic's inner circle of advisors, business contacts, and family in an attempt to get him to capitulate to NATO's terms. Russia also conducted cyber-warfare against Estonia in 2007 and to support its invasions of Georgia in 2008 and Ukraine in 2014 (Greenberg 2017; Hollis 2011).

Based on these experiences in previous conflicts, the United States recognizes that as much as we can use cyber-warfare to our advantage in a conflict, our adversaries can also utilize it against us. In most cases, we are more vulnerable to cyber-attacks, given our military's dependency on a robust **C4I (command, control, communications, computers, and intelligence)** architecture. For this reason, the military response to cyber-warfare will be addressed in detail in a later section of this chapter.

8.1.2 What Can Cyber-Crime, Cyber-Terrorism, and Cyber-Warfare Do?

Cyber-crime, cyber-terrorism, and cyber-warfare are all focused on information systems and using the many means available—electronic, human, and otherwise—to cause both physical and psychological effects. As discussed earlier, our society is a networked society, completely dependent on information systems for processing and storing data related to practically every aspect of our daily lives. Even minor disruptions can have major consequences. When a homeowner in Indiana received a tax bill for $8 million dollars on a house worth $122 000, the "glitch" also impacted the state tax budget, reflecting a $3.1 million dollar shortfall for the year (Astahost 2006). Such glitches can also have life and death consequences, such as when one programming error left five Pacific Island nations off of a tsunami warning list (Song 2006).

One key sector of our economy that depends on information technology is the banking and finance industry. We all have bank accounts, and many of us struggle to balance our checkbooks each month. Imagine the global impact if a computer glitch (either intentional or not) suddenly caused a "bank error in your favor" and every account holder suddenly had an additional $5000 in his or her account. Hopefully, if it were your account, you would call the bank before spending it, but many people would not, leading to multiple financial problems for the bank, consumers, and merchants when those checks bounced. On a larger scale, banks and businesses do report losses every year due to computer glitches or computer hacking, and these losses have broad economic impact. In 2016, identity theft alone, a major component of cyber-crime that impacts banking and financial institutions, topped 1 billion individuals who had their personal information, including credit card or financial data, compromised due to cyber-attacks (ISTR 2017).

Could terrorists or other nations target our banking system with a cyber-attack aimed at crippling our economy and destroying public confidence in our financial institutions? The federal government thinks so, as well as the banking sector. As a result of such concerns, the Clinton administration established a system of **Information Sharing and Advisory Councils (ISACs)** in 1998 in an attempt to foster public–private partnerships in all sectors of our nation's critical infrastructures, including banking and financing. The ISACs were just one recommendation that emerged from a study of our nation's vulnerability to cyber-based threats.

For instance, in 1997, the President's Commission on Critical Infrastructure Protection (PCCIP) published its findings on the vulnerability of our nation's critical infrastructure to terrorism, primarily using cyber weapons. In the report, the commission reported that our nation was ill-prepared for cyber-terrorism or cyber-warfare, identifying the eight critical infrastructures listed in the following text. In the follow-up implementation plan, Presidential Decision Directive (PDD) 63: Critical Infrastructure Protection (May 1998), the Clinton administration assigned each infrastructure to a federal agency for oversight and coordination with the private sector through the ISACs. The eight critical infrastructures and the agencies identified in 1998 to which they were assigned are as follows:

- ▲ Information and communications: Department of Commerce
- ▲ Banking and finance: Department of Treasury
- ▲ Water supply: Environmental Protection Agency (EPA)
- ▲ Aviation, highways (including trucking and intelligent transportation systems), mass transit, pipelines, rail, and waterborne commerce: Department of Transportation
- ▲ Emergency law enforcement services: Department of Justice

▲ Emergency fire service and continuity of government services: Federal Emergency Management Agency (FEMA)

▲ Public health services, including prevention, surveillance, laboratory, and personal health services: Department of Health and Human Services

▲ Electric power, oil, and gas production and storage: Department of Energy (PDD 63 1998)

The commission report also led to the formation of the **Critical Infrastructure Assurance Office (CIAO)** under the Department of Commerce, as well as the **National Infrastructure Protection Center (NIPC)** under the Department of Justice. The CIAO became the center for coordinating the ISAC process and encouraging the private sector to cooperate with the federal government in ensuring it was protecting itself against threats from cyber-terrorism, as well as other threats from both man-made and natural disasters. In other words, cyber-terrorist threats were one of many threats to these critical infrastructures, ranging from insiders, such as disgruntled employees, to cyber-warfare by nation-states, to environmental disasters, such as floods.

The CIAO played a crucial role in coordinating the government response to the Y2K scare in 2000. Because it was located in the Department of Commerce, it provided accessibility to government agencies (local, state, and federal) as well as private sector corporations responsible for running our nation's power industries, financial centers, telecommunications systems, and transportation systems—all of which were concerned with a possible cyber shutdown due to a computer programming error. After the "end of the world as we know it" did not occur on January 1, 2000, most people returned to business as usual in both the public and private sectors. Much of the work of the CIAO was then transferred to the new National Infrastructure Protection Center (NIPC), which was housed in the J. Edgar Hoover FBI Headquarters building in Washington, D.C. Rather than simply addressing the implications of a computer programming error, the NIPC became the operations center for tracking cyber-attacks on the nation's critical infrastructures, utilizing people from the FBI, Department of Defense, intelligence community, Department of the Treasury, and Department of Energy. The component that was missing was the private sector, because most corporations in America, due to the use of proprietary information, did not want to be as open with their company's operations and possible vulnerabilities with military, law enforcement, or intelligence agencies as they were with the Department of Commerce.

Today, the functions of the NIPC have been assumed under the Department of Homeland Security's (DHS) Office of Cybersecurity and Communications, which runs the **National Cybersecurity and Communications Integration Center (NCCIC)**. It includes NCCIC Operations & Integration (NO&I), US Computer Emergency Readiness Team (US-CERT), Industrial Control Systems Cyber Emergency Response Team (ICS-CERT), and National Coordinating Center for Communications (NCC). The NCCIC expands on the previous mission of the NIPC by "working closely with federal departments and agencies and actively engages with private sector companies and institutions, along with state, local, tribal, and territorial governments, and international counterparts" (US-CERT n.d.).

SELF-CHECK

- Define cyber-warfare.
- Which of the following is not one of our nation's critical infrastructures vulnerable to a cyber-attack?

  a. Water supply systems

  b. Information and communication systems

  c. Public health services

  d. National park service
- The Department of Homeland Security runs the National Cybersecurity and Communications Integration Center. True or false?
- The functions of the CIAO, after the Y2K scare, were initially transferred to the NIPC, which was run by the Department of Defense alone. True or false?

8.2 Assessing Capability and Intent

The intelligence community determines whether a nation-state or non-state actor poses a threat to the United States based on a combination of two variables: capability and intent. Capability refers to the means to inflict harm, whereas intent relates to the broader political goals and objectives of a nation or non-state actor vis-à-vis the United States. For example, Great Britain possesses nuclear weapons (capability), but it does not show the political will (intent) to use them against the United States; thus, it is not a threat. Similarly, if a nation does not possess capability to do us harm, even though their rhetoric indicates a desire to do so, it is not a threat. During the Cold War, the US intelligence community categorized countries by level of threat (tier 1, tier 2, etc.) based on these two criteria of capability and intent.

Later, with the end of the Cold War and the demise of the former Soviet Union and its satellite states, the new threat of global terrorism emerged, including state sponsors of terrorism and non-state actors, such as al-Qaeda. Intelligence analysts continue to use a similar spectrum in assessing the level of threat based on the criteria of capability plus intent. This model also pertains to cyber-terrorism and cyber-warfare, with the greatest threat still being a nation-state that has both cyber-warfare capability and the intent to use it against the United States and its allies. Figure 8-1 displays the types of cyber threats that exist today, based on capability and intent. Here, threats are classified as ranging from hackers to professional information warriors.

8.2.1 Who Can Conduct Cyber-Crime, Cyber-Terrorism, and Cyber-Warfare?

Figure 8-1 also shows the range of threats to information systems that control our nation's critical infrastructures. The common thread throughout this figure is the damage that can be done by insiders, or trusted individuals who work at a plant,

Figure 8-1

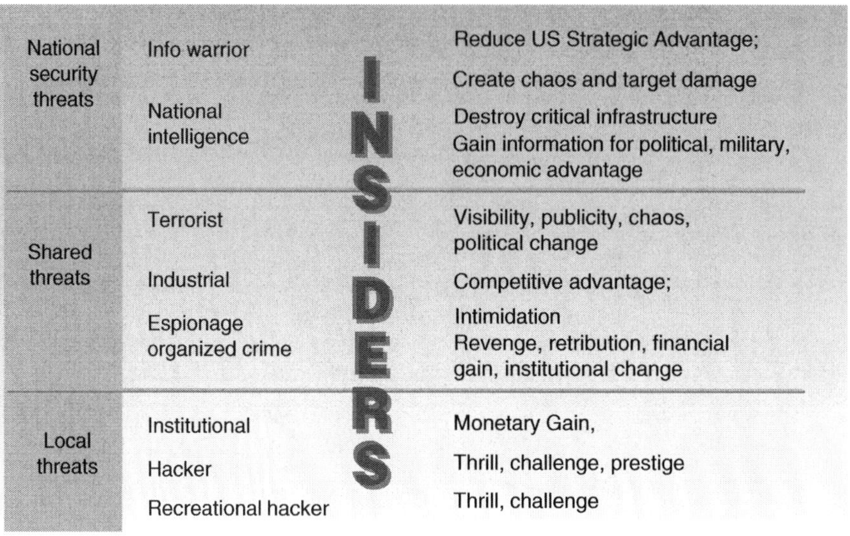

National security threats	Info warrior	Reduce US Strategic Advantage; Create chaos and target damage
	National intelligence	Destroy critical infrastructure Gain information for political, military, economic advantage
Shared threats	Terrorist	Visibility, publicity, chaos, political change
	Industrial	Competitive advantage;
	Espionage organized crime	Intimidation Revenge, retribution, financial gain, institutional change
Local threats	Institutional	Monetary Gain,
	Hacker	Thrill, challenge, prestige
	Recreational hacker	Thrill, challenge

Types of cyber threats (Kilroy 2008).

facility, organization, etc., who have access to critical information architecture, such as an information technology expert or systems administrator. Such individuals, if they are bent on causing damage or destruction (intent), clearly possess the capability to do so. However, the level of threat can vary depending on the motivation. Most insider threats are considered lower-tier threats, because they are motivated by revenge due to being fired, demoted, etc.—typically not the same threat posed by an apocalyptic terrorist with insider access, bent on greater destruction or disruption.

8.2.1.1 Criminals

In the banking and finance industries, there is more concern over institutional hackers linked to criminal activities than over terrorists. Criminals using identity theft and other cyber means to gain personal information are routinely robbing banks of millions of dollars each year. Knowing that federal law enforcement officials are not concerned with small dollar amounts (usually <$50 000), these criminals go for less conspicuous activity. They also rely on the terrorist threat to gain information, using social engineering tricks (impersonating FBI agents) to gain access to financial records (Sullivan 2005). In the summer of 2017, Europe experienced a widespread ransomware attack by cyber criminals, exploiting a malware program initially developed by the NSA that was leaked by a former NSA employee. The hackers were demanding payments or 300 bitcoins (approximately US$800 000 in 2017) by a Ukrainian media company to unlock their computer system (Thompson Reuters 2017).

The link to terrorism became clear after the post-9/11 investigations, which showed that fraudulent accounts were used by the terrorists for transferring funds to support the attacks. Bank officials also believe that terrorists are gaining financial support through criminal activity—using the vulnerabilities in the information system, rather than attacking the system—but an actual attack could be only be a matter of time (see Chapter 10).

8.2.1.2 Terrorist Groups

To date, the threat from terrorist groups, such as al-Qaeda and IS, using cyber-based weapons has yet to materialize, although the evidence exists that they are aware of the capability. We suspect that terrorist groups use the Internet for communication and cyber-reconnaissance of suspected targets. We also suspect they are familiar with the use of standard hacking tools and believe they have been probing our nation's cyber-defenses, looking for weaknesses that could be exploited. For example, in fall 2001, an FBI investigation of cyber activity turned up significant probing of critical infrastructures in the United States, such as emergency telephone systems, electrical power generation systems, water facilities, nuclear power plants, and so forth (Gellman 2002). Also, captured computers from al-Qaeda training sites in Afghanistan showed an increased level of interest by terrorists in the feasibility of conducting cyber-terrorism, possibly in conjunction with a physical WMD attack. This is one reason that Y2K caused so much concern, because it did expose many weaknesses in the information systems involved in operating our nation's critical infrastructures. In addition, recreational and institutional hackers can also expose vulnerabilities, and terrorist organizations can learn from these actions and possibly exploit the weaknesses they expose.

In his 2017 testimony before the Senate Armed Services Committee, the Commander of US Cyber Command (USCYBERCOM) (and Director of the National Security Agency (NSA)), Admiral Mike Rogers, voiced his concern that terrorist groups, like IS, use the Internet for recruitment and propaganda, which have led to the radicalization of lone-wolf terrorists inspired by extremist organizations to carry out attacks on US citizens (Rogers 2017). He also raised the prospect that terrorist groups could turn the Internet from a tool for recruitment into weapon of choice, due to the emerging Internet of things that connects so much of society today (see Chapter 5).

8.2.1.3 Nation-States

The greatest concern at the national level has been (and remains) the threat of cyber-warfare conducted by a nation-state against the United States, either as an act of war, in conjunction with military action, or conducted asymmetrically, attempting to negate America's military superiority by preventing the United States from even being able to deploy its forces overseas. By attacking our critical infrastructures using both conventional acts of sabotage and cyber-warfare, an adversary could do such harm to our nation that our military and economic power could be negated. One such series of incidents that raised these concerns occurred as the United States prepared for Operation Desert Fox in Iraq in 1998. Just prior to initiating combat operations, the DoD noticed increased cyber activity targeting DoD information systems, which appeared to be coming from a Middle-Eastern country, possibly Iraq.

> ### FOR EXAMPLE
>
> **Solar Sunrise**
>
> The incidents, termed Solar Sunrise, occurred in February 1998, indicating a pattern of behavior that could be considered a threat to DoD information systems. Probing actions by an unknown source caused the DoD to take a number of precautions to protect critical information related to the planning and execution of Operation Desert Fox. The probing incidents were widespread against Air Force, Navy, and Marine Corps information systems throughout the world. After a series of investigations, the "attackers" ended up being two teenagers living in California, who were being mentored by an Israeli, Ehud Tannenbaum, who was only suspected of being a recreational hacker. (Global Security n.d.)

Despite the results of the Solar Sunrise investigation, the cyber threat from nation-states is real. Beginning in the mid-1980s, foreign intelligence agencies, such as the former Soviet KGB and East German STASI, were conducting cyber espionage, using third parties. The first documented case occurred in 1986, when a group in West Germany, known as the Hanover Hackers, and their ring leader, Markus Hess, were arrested and charged with espionage. They had hacked into a number of DoD computer systems, stealing classified information and selling it to the KGB and STASI. They were only discovered when a University of California employee, Cliff Stoll, noticed a 75-cent billing error on their computer accounts and decided to investigate. He tracked it to an unauthorized account accessing the Lawrence Berkeley National Laboratories, which was conducting classified work for the DoD. Stoll's pioneering work in computer security and the resulting arrest of Hess was documented in a book, *The Cuckoo's Egg: Tracking a Spy Through the Maze of Computer Espionage* (Stoll 2005).

Later, an unclassified Defense Science Board report issued in 1996 identified ten countries that were developing capabilities related to information warfare, which included the use of information and computer security. These countries were Russia, China, India, Iran, Iraq, North Korea, Cuba, Libya, Syria, and Egypt. Although it mentioned varying degrees of sophistication, the study concluded that each nation recognized its own vulnerability to cyber-warfare, thus demanding an increase in defensive capabilities, as well as an interest in developing offensive capabilities (Defense Science Board 1996).

In 2017, intelligence estimates indicate that more than 30 nations are suspected of having some form of offensive cyber-warfare capability (Ranger 2017). Termed **computer network attack (CNA)**, the offensive component of Computer Network Operations (CNO), it is often a simple turning of a switch or keystroke, which changes the intelligence and espionage function, called computer network exploitation (CNE), into a hostile offensive action. CNE is considered a passive activity, since the cyber-sleuth's goal is to remain anonymous and undetected. By going offensive, the "cover" is blown, and a known vulnerability in a computer system used to gain intelligence and information now becomes the same means by which an offensive cyber-attack takes place.

Former Director of National Intelligence, James Clapper, identified Russia, China, and North Korea as countries developing more complex and sophisticated CNA capabilities as a means to offset the overwhelming military superiority of the United States (Ranger 2017). Seen as a "cheap fix," these countries will employ asymmetric tactics to defeat the United States by crippling our nation's ability to even wage war. In a book published in 1999, two Chinese colonels advocated employing such an approach, using cyber-warfare and other means to attack the United States in a future conflict (Liang and Xiangsui 1999). The tactics they advocated to undermine our support networks and digitally destroy critical infra-structure were very much in line with Eastern military philosophy as seen in Sun Tzu's classic, *The Art of War*, where the ultimate military goal is to defeat an adver-sary's will to fight without having to actually enter into military combat (Watson 2017). What is interesting in the Chinese colonels' text is the assertion that it is not a matter of *if* China goes to war with the United States, but simply *when*.

8.2.2 Tools of Cyber-Terrorism

What makes Computer Network Attacks (CNAs) so pernicious is the universality of the required weapons—in this case, simply a computer and a modem (capabil-ity). If an individual or nation-state has the intent, then becoming a threat in cyber-space is a relatively easy proposition. The question is the severity of the action and the ability to, in fact, detect where a cyber-attack comes from and how someone is doing it. Laws do not allow federal government agencies, such as the DoD, from "hacking back" on Internet service providers (ISPs), because computer attacks are still initially considered criminal activity, putting them under the purview of law enforcement agencies, such as the FBI, for investigation. In other words, if a system administrator detects a CNA occurring against his or her information system, he or she can only determine the immediate source of the intrusion (ISP), which may or may not be where the attack is originating from. In the case of the Solar Sunrise incidents mentioned earlier, the attacks against DoD computer systems appeared to be coming from university computers, such as those at Harvard and Texas A&M, because the Israeli student organizing the attacks knew that security protocols on most university computer systems were lax and easy to manipulate. Only through a thorough investigation of related ISPs did FBI investigators determine the sources of the attacks (Reed and Wilson 1998).

8.2.2.1 Denial-of-Service (DOS) Attacks

The most typical CNA is a **denial-of-service (DOS) attack**, which renders a user's computer useless, or targets an entire network. These can be done by computer viruses, such as the I LOVE YOU virus detected in 2000, which is estimated to have affected over 45 million users worldwide, causing over $10 billion in dam-age due to lost revenue, remediation, and so on (*Times of India* 2000). What made the I LOVE YOU virus so sinister is that it occurred shortly after the MELISSA virus was detected the previous year, which also caused major disruptions world-wide. It appeared that the hacker, in this case, used lessons learned from the MELISSA virus to create a more deadly virus with broader consequences. In other words, instead of just sending an e-mail with an infected file, which when opened could damage other computer files, the newer virus created self-extracting files that proliferated through an affected computer's e-mail address book, sending infected files to one's contacts—which they, in turn, thought were coming from a trusted source.

If a terrorist organization or nation-state wished to use a CNA, they would not have far to go to study the effects of and responses to such incidents in order to develop an ever deadlier "strain" of computer viruses. In October 2016, the largest scale denial of service attack to date occurred using the Mirai botnet, which attacked Dyn, a company that controls most of the Internet's domain name system (DNS) architecture. The attack brought down media sites including Twitter, The Guardian, Netflix, Reddit, and CNN. What made the attack unique was that the Mirai botnet comprised the "Internet of things" that Dyn identified as involving "100 000 malicious endpoints," with an attack strength of 1.2 Tbps (Woolf 2016).

8.2.2.2 Hacking Tools

Another means of CNA is the use of computer hacking tools that can be used to deface websites and insert false information. For example, stock market data could be manipulated to show either a loss or gain that did not occur, causing panic selling or buying. Given the volatility of oil futures and other petroleum markets, you can image what the global consequences of such an attack would be. For this reason, the Securities and Exchange Commission (SEC) is particularly watchful of unusual investor activity and market vulnerability. For example, in 2015, an SEC investigation uncovered a massive case of computer fraud that involved over 30 individuals, who took in more than $100 million in illicit profits by hacking into computer systems and stealing nonpublic information and trading stocks based on that information. Securities and Exchange Commission Chair, Mary Jo White, stated, "this international scheme is unprecedented in terms of the scope of the hacking, the number of traders, the number of securities traded and profits generated" (SEC 2015). Another example of this sort of attack would be manipulating data or generating false activity, such as fictitious e-mail, unbeknownst to the user that would cause a large financial sell-off of stock options or purchase of bogus stock funds.

8.2.2.3 Synchronized Cyber-Attacks and Physical Attacks

Returning to our previous discussion on the use of SCADA and related digital control systems (DCS) from Chapter 5, one scenario that worries cyber-defenders in the United States is the possibility of terrorists being able to conduct cyber-attacks that are synchronized with physical attacks. In other words, it's not just "digital bullets" that authorities are concerned about but rather the potential for real physical destruction that could occur from cyber-terrorism due to the linkages between information systems and physical infrastructure. An example would be manipulating a DCS that controls the floodgates for a hydroelectric dam. The fact that one al-Qaeda laptop seized in Afghanistan showed multiple visits to a website known as "the Anonymous Society," with a link to a sabotage handbook that explained how to conduct just such an attack, makes such a scenario plausible (Gellman 2002).

In 2015, IS hackers calling themselves, the "Cyber Caliphate" hacked into the US Central Command's Twitter account. They also claimed the ability to hack into a number of other sites, threatening to unleash an "electronic war" that would control America's "electronic world" (Shiloach 2015). Although no further intrusions were detected and nor did any physical attacks coincide with this hack, the US military's US Cyber Command is taking such threats seriously. Although the Commander, Admiral Mike Rodgers, considers IS capabilities as "limited," there is growing concern that terrorist groups like IS could hire cyber mercenaries who did have the expertise to conduct cyber-attacks on our critical infrastructure that may be combined with physical terrorist attacks in the United States (Browne 2016).

SELF-CHECK

- The two variables used to assess threats to our nation include capability and access. True or false?
- Which type of person can do the most damage across all threat levels?
  a. Cyber-terrorist
  b. Trusted insider
  c. Computer hacker
  d. Organized criminal
- Define Computer Network Attack (CNA).
- The most common CNA is a Denial of Service (DOS) attack, which renders a user's computer useless or targets an entire network. True or false?

8.3 Assessing Consequences

On March 23, 1996, the RAND Corporation ran an exercise in Washington, DC, with over 60 participants, using a scenario developed by David Ronfeldt and John Arquilla called "The Day After … in Cyberspace." The purpose of the exercise was to assess how our national decision makers would respond to a series of acts related to cyber-warfare coming from an unknown source. In the exercise, what began as cyber-reconnaissance soon developed into cyber-attacks on the nation's banking and financial infrastructure, leading to more targeted attacks on our defense and intelligence communities. The exercise ended with the United States launching a preemptive nuclear strike on China, the supposed source of the cyber-attacks, only to realize after that the source wasn't China at all but rather cyber-terrorists whose goal was to precipitate a global conflict (Anderson and Hearn 1996).

Since the terrorist attacks of 9/11, the US government has conducted a series of national-level exercises called **TOPOFF** or Top Officials, which involve senior leaders from federal, state, and local agencies involved in responding to a terrorist attack. The scenarios have included a bioterrorism attack in Portsmouth, New Hampshire; a chemical weapons attack in Denver, Colorado; and a radiological bomb in Phoenix, Arizona. For the first 10 years, all exercises were meant to assess the consequences of a terrorist group obtaining a weapon of mass destruction. Not until 2012 did a national-level exercise focus on a scenario that involved the simulated effects of a weapon of mass disruption, like a cyber-attack, on critical infrastructure (Public Intelligence 2012).

The US Department of Homeland Security's National Cyber Security Division (NCSD) began conducting its own exercises, called **Cyber Storm**, beginning in 2006. Cyber Storm provides participants with a "controlled environment in which to exercise a coordinated cyber incident response, including information sharing mechanisms, procedures for establishing situational awareness, public and private organizational decision making, and public communications during a cyber-related Incident of National Significance" (DHS 2006, 1). The early Cyber Storm exercises focused on federal- and state-level communication and coordination of efforts to track cyber incidents across geographical areas, through the US-CERT and Multi-State Information Sharing and Analysis Centers (MS-ISAC). The latest Cyber Strom V exercise occurred in March 2016 and included "more than 1200 participants, representing entities from the public and private sectors within the United States and abroad. Participants represented nine Cabinet-level departments, eight full player states, 12 International partners, and nearly 70 private sector companies and coordination bodies, to include: Information Technology (IT); Communications; Healthcare and Public Health (HPH); Commercial Facilities (Retail Subsector); and critical infrastructure sectors" (DHS 2016, 1).

The Department of Homeland Security has also developed exercise materials to be provided to other agencies and sectors to help them train for cyber-attacks. In 2013, DHS, working with the Department of Health and Human Services and the National Health Information Sharing and Advisory Council (NH-ISAC), produced a Table Top Exercise (TTX) specifically for the healthcare industry. The TTX provided private sector healthcare workers an opportunity to understand the implications of a cyber-attack by criminals (ransomware) or terrorists (DDOS) on local service providers by scripting a number of vignettes to include the compromise of patient information, billing system disruptions, medical equipment malfunction, and loss of health records due to system failure (DHS 2013).

One of the key lessons learned from these exercises in assessing consequences from a cyber-attack is the problem of attribution, or determining the source of any cyber-attack. Computer forensics is a new and growing discipline, leading to some intelligence agencies coining the phrase **COMPUINT**, or computer intelligence—what we can learn from analyzing computer traffic, e-mail, website hits, hard drives, etc. Yet, even though we are learning more about the technology involved, it appears the "bad guys" are also becoming more sophisticated at covering their tracks and using commercial off-the-shelf hacking tools that are readily available (one such tool is called "anonymizer," which allows you to remain anonymous), leaving less of a signature to follow.

> ### FOR EXAMPLE
>
> ### Moonlight Maze
>
> A cyber-sleuth investigation under the codename Moonlight Maze began in March 1998, after the accidental detection of a series of intrusions into computer databases at the Department of Defense, Department of Energy, NASA, and private universities and research labs doing classified government work. Documents accessed included military installation maps, military organizational information, and military-related research. The Department of Defense investigators eventually traced the activity back to Russia (PBS Frontline 2006).
>
> Although the case was eventually closed in 2008 and classified documents were obtained through the Freedom of Information Act, the source of the attacks was never identified. What Moonlight Maze, and another case, titled Titan Rain (believed to be of Chinese origin), did reveal was that cyber espionage conducted by nation-states would be an ongoing challenge for the intelligence and law enforcement community (Doman 2016).

8.3.1 Why America Is Vulnerable to Cyber-Attacks

While the openness of our democratic society is one of our nation's greatest strengths, it is also one of our greatest weaknesses when it comes to cyber-defenses and protecting ourselves from cyber-attacks, whether they be from criminals, terrorists, or nation-states. Information systems and architecture are built for efficiency, not necessarily security. Also, due to the highly competitive commercial marketplace, most companies attempt to get systems and programs out to consumers quickly, before their competition. This results in the later need for a number of software "fixes" or "patches" to correct operational problems or vulnerabilities. In addition, most companies prefer not to spend the extra time and money to enhance computer security, knowing that the average replacement cycle is three to five years anyway due to the speed at which technology develops. Ultimately, profit trumps protection.

The nature of the Internet itself also creates inherent vulnerabilities, which were not really anticipated when the technology moved from the government into the private sector. When the Internet was invented with the assistance of researchers at the Advanced Research Projects Agency (ARPA) in the 1960s, it was designed as an open architecture network operating within a closed system (e.g., the Department of Defense). It was based on a system of trust, in which those people with access also had a "need to know" the information that would be shared. The "language" designed to allow this sharing of information packets over the Internet was referred to as Transmission Control Protocol/Internet Protocol (TCP/IP). Today, this could be considered the most widely spoken "language" in the world, as the Internet is now a major means of global communication.

Because the Internet has global connectivity, it remains highly unregulated, either by individual governments or by industry. For this reason, it is considered a truly democratic entity influencing nations and individuals around the world. It is also considered a legal "wild west" in the sense that there is little in terms of legal precedent over content, access, and issues regarding privacy rights. For example, when the USA PATRIOT Act became law almost immediately after the terrorist events of 9/11, a great deal of controversy arose over the right of government to monitor Internet activity, particularly in public libraries (this provision was included as part of the USA PATRIOT Act because the FBI suspected that terrorists were using public library computers to communicate and do research).

Controversy still rages over any government attempt to either restrict Internet access or monitor the communication of private citizens. In 2006, President Bush admitted to authorizing the National Security Agency to monitor phone conversations to private citizens from suspected terrorists living overseas. Although the Attorney General's office declared such monitoring legal, there was a large public outcry over how intrusive the government was in pursuing suspected terrorist activity. There was also some disagreement as to the extent that terrorists used the Internet for communication through the use of special coding called **steganography**, or the embedding of messages or files in computer websites. Knowing that law enforcement and intelligence officials were prevented from accessing pornography sites in the workplace, terrorists were suspected of using steganography in images on such restricted sites, thereby avoiding detection (Kessler 2004).

The same openness principle applies in the use of SCADA and DCS, as previously discussed in Chapter 5. Because the computer commands used by this technology to manage controls and switches were originally meant for a closed system, safeguards were minimal. The designers did not expect someone to actually hack in and access these systems. However, cyber-terrorists, bent on attacking the United States using a computer and modem, clearly have the intent and capability to do so. Only since 9/11 have both private sector and government institutions begun to seriously look at our vulnerabilities and determine ways to better defend the nation from the threat of cyber-terrorism, in particular.

In recent years, there have been attempts to regulate cyberspace to make it more secure through legislation. In 2015, President Obama signed into law the Cybersecurity Act of 2015. At the time, this was the most significant piece of legislation created at the federal level to deal with cybersecurity issues. It focused primarily on information sharing between the public and private sectors. For companies it provided a legal "safe harbor" from liability claims for private companies, which has always been a sticking point in the past. Companies would not share their vulnerabilities in cyberspace with the federal government for fear of legal action, as well as the compromise of proprietary information. Another significant part of the legislation is that it authorizes agencies outside the federal government to monitor both government and private sector information systems and take defensive measures for cybersecurity purposes. The Act also contains provisions designed to increase cybersecurity measures at federal agencies that impact cybersecurity employees, as well as address cybersecurity preparedness of critical information systems and networks (ODNI n.d.). In 2017, President Trump signed an executive order titled "Strengthening the Cybersecurity of Federal Networks and Critical Infrastructure." Although not an act of Congress with legal authority, this executive order is aimed specifically at the executive agencies of the federal government to take actions to better protect their information system architecture against attacks in cyberspace. It concludes strengthening the security and resilience of cyberspace is an important part of the homeland security mission. The president's executive order builds upon existing capabilities and authorities while strengthening the department's ability to carry out its mission of protecting federal networks, supporting critical infrastructure owners and operators, and ensuring an open and reliable Internet for all Americans. (DHS 2017)

8.3.2 The Impact of a Cyber-Terrorist Attack

We've already discussed the types of tools available to cyber-terrorists and what they can do with them. This section deals with the consequences of cyber-terrorism and what these acts could do to us. Being able to turn off the lights in Houston may not be that big a deal, but combine a cyber-attack on the power grid with a conventional explosive attack against a benzene storage facility at the port of Houston, and there is the potential for many more casualties and a high level of confusion. Benzene is a highly toxic chemical that can release a plume cloud that would have the same effect as a chemical weapons attack on the city of Houston, due to prevailing winds. If a cyber-terrorist attack occurred at the same time, cutting off power to local hospitals bracing for casualties or water supplies feeding firefighters putting out chemical fires, you can imagine the results. In this case, cyber-terrorism would become a "casualty multiplier," increasing the effect of a conventional weapon attack.

One major consequence of a potential cyber-terrorist attack is the financial impact. For example, the airline industry today is still feeling the effects of 9/11. Immediately after the attacks, both passengers and aircrew refused to fly. Many smaller airlines went bankrupt or were forced to merge with larger carriers to survive due to fear of a follow-up attack. Insurance companies also went bankrupt due to the large number of claims, and some smaller businesses went out of business since they couldn't afford insurance against acts of terrorism. Wall Street temporarily shut down. President Bush, in an effort to ease the economic blow of 9/11 on the US economy, told the American people the best thing they could do to support their country was shop. A cyber-attack on the banking and financial sector would have an even greater financial impact, since it would have also impacted the public's perception of the safety and security of their investments, possibly causing people to hoard money, rather than spend it or place it in the bank.

Thus, another consequence of a cyber-terrorist attack is psychological. Banks today do not want to admit to the public how much money they actually lose due to computer glitches, much less criminal or terrorist cyber-robberies. Banks fear panic and the loss of public confidence. The government has similar concerns over the loss of public confidence in their ability to provide protection and basic human services after a terrorist incident. Think about the damage done by Hurricane Katrina, a natural disaster, particularly with regard to the poor response by the New Orleans city government, as well as state and federal agencies, such as the Federal Emergency Management Agency (FEMA). When the public loses confidence in the institutions established to provide basic protective services in a crisis, such as the police or their elected officials, the inability to regain that trust can have a long-term effect. Cyber-terrorists can further exploit those seams of public confidence, creating a cascading effect by playing on public fears that are already established. The concern expressed by state and local officials over the federal government's proposed response to a possible bird flu epidemic in summer 2006 reflects just such a scenario, one in which cyber-terrorism could seriously undermine the nation's ability to respond to such a crisis.

FOR EXAMPLE

Costs of a Cyber-Attack

Lloyd's of London analysts said an extreme global cyber-attack could cost as much as $121.4 billion in damages, equivalent to the cost of Hurricane Katrina in 2005, Bloomberg reported. In the hypothetical attack, the failure of a widely used cloud-based service provider would cost about $53 billion. Insurers could process claims anywhere from $620 million to $8.1 billion, Lloyd's said. But insurers would likely only cover up to $2.1 billion of the cost of an extreme event, which could cost as much as $28.7 billion. The market for cyber insurance has grown to between $3 billion and $3.5 billion and could rise to as much as $10 billion by 2020. Hacker attacks such as May's WannaCry and June's Petya have raised awareness and encouraged insurers to offer cyber-crime coverage. (Grant 2017)

SELF-CHECK

- Define COMPUINT.
- The use of a cyber-terrorism can be a casualty multiplier during a conventional or WMD attack. True or false?
- What federal agency was involved in inventing the Internet?
  a. ARPA
  b. DHS
  c. FBI
  d. CIA
- The Cybersecurity Act of 2015 was abrogated by the Trump administration's executive order on Cybersecurity in 2017. True or false?

8.4 Determining Defenses against Cyber-Crime, Cyber-Terrorism, and Cyber-Warfare

Our nation's first attempts to protect itself in cyberspace occurred during the final days of the Reagan administration in December 1988. At that time, **DARPA** (previously known as ARPA) provided the charter to the Software Engineering Institute (SEI) at Carnegie Mellon University in Pittsburgh, Pennsylvania, to establish our nation's first national **computer emergency response team (CERT)**. This was a result of a computer virus (the Morris worm incident) in November of that year, which affected 10% of the entire Internet system at that time. Even then, computer experts recognized the danger posed to information systems from the effects of viruses, although the focus at the time was not necessarily on terrorist or nation-state threats due to the nature of the technology and its connectivity. They also recognized that the task of cyber protection was beyond the scope of any one agency. For example, consider the following statement issued by DARPA:

> Because of the many network, computer, and systems architectures and their associated vulnerabilities, no single organization can be expected to maintain an in-house expertise to respond on its own to computer security threats, particularly those that arise in the research community. As with biological viruses, the solutions must come from an organized community response of experts. The role of the CERT Coordination Center at the SEI is to provide the supporting mechanisms and to coordinate the activities of experts in DARPA and associated communities. (Carnegie Mellon University 1988)

Later, under the Clinton administration, our nation first began to organize its cyber-defenses across various federal government sectors, as a result of the findings published in the President's Commission on Critical Infrastructure Protection (PCCIP) discussed earlier in the chapter. One organization created in 1997 to meet a shortcoming identified in the report was the aforementioned National Infrastructure Protection Center (NIPC), located in the FBI building. Because it was composed of FBI, intelligence community, and Department of Defense personnel, the NIPC went beyond simply cyber-defense to providing an interagency response to cyber-attacks. The NIPC served as an indications and warning (I&W) center, providing proactive alerts and advisories intended to prevent cyber incidents from spreading throughout government computer systems. The NIPC coordinated its efforts with the CERT at Carnegie Mellon and was also linked to Department of Defense cyber-defense efforts (discussed later).

On the policy side, President Clinton also took the initiative to establish the office of National Coordinator for Security, Infrastructure Protection, and Counter-Terrorism, under Richard Clarke. In this capacity, Clarke also served as the administration's "cybersecurity czar" responsible for overseeing the nation's cyber-defenses from cyber-terrorist incidents. Clarke was a holdover when the Bush administration came into office in January 2001, though his position on the National Security Council was less visible under Condoleezza Rice, the new National Security Advisor. After the terrorist attacks of 9/11, Richard Clarke testified before the 9/11 Commission and became a popular media figure due to his pointed criticism of the Bush administration and the president's lack of response to his reported warnings of imminent terrorist threats. Clarke also accused the Bush administration of pressuring him to provide evidence of Iraqi complicity in the 9/11 incidents in order to justify going to war with Iraq (PBS 2006).

In February 2003, the Bush administration issued the *National Strategy to Secure Cyberspace*. One of the first critiques of this plan came from former cybersecurity czar Richard Clarke, who claimed that the administration's plan would leave a significant gap in cyber protection. Yet, three years later, with the normal bureaucratic issues facing any massive government reorganization, the new Department of Homeland Security (DHS) assumed many of the previously disparate cybersecurity functions performed by the CIAO, NIPC, and other Clinton-era agencies under its National Cyber Security Division (NCSD).

Under President Obama, a new *Cybersecurity National Action Plan* (CNAP) was proposed in 2016, which combined both short-term goals to shore up the nation's cyber-defenses and long-term strategy to confront the growing threats in cyber-space. Some of the proposed initiatives under Obama's plan included starting a commission on enhancing national cybersecurity, creating a new Federal Chief Information Security Officer, setting up a $3.1 billion Information Technology Modernization Fund and investing over $19 billion for cybersecurity as part of the President's fiscal year (FY) 2017 budget (The White House 2016). Yet, most of the proposed initiatives became unfunded mandates as result of the 2016 presidential election.

8.4.1 The Government and Private Sector Response to Threats in Cyberspace

Not waiting for the Obama administration to develop a new *National Strategy to Secure Cyberspace*, the Department of Defense released its *Cyber Strategy* in 2015. In it the DoD proposed the following main mission areas: "defend DoD networks, systems, and information; defend the nation against cyberattacks of significant consequence; and support operational and contingency plans" (DoD 2015, 3). To accomplish these three goals, our nation's cyber-defenses can best be understood in the context of the cybersecurity framework originally proposed by the National Institute of Standards (NIST) in 2014 and reissued by the NIST under the Trump administration in 2017. The framework consists of five critical functions: identify, protect, detect, respond, and recover (Figure 8-2).

Figure 8-2

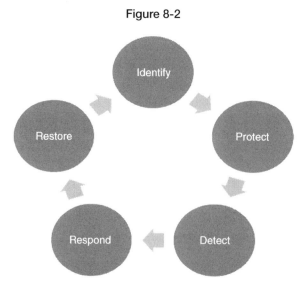

Cyber Security Framework. Source: Modified from NIST (2017).

8.4.1.1 Identify

The first function in the framework, Identify, involves understanding the threats and being able to identify their capabilities and intent. This would include cyber criminals, cyber-terrorists, and nation-states with cyber-warfare capabilities. Identify also means to "know oneself" (as stated by Sun Tzu). You also need to know your own organization's capabilities, and limitations, to include conducting risk assessments against different threats and devising risk management strategies to protect against these threats.

8.4.1.2 Protect

The second function in the framework, Protect, involves proactive measures to prevent a cyber-attack, whether that attack is from terrorists or nation-states. Protection involves mainly passive measures taken to safeguard information systems and critical infrastructures. These can be both technical means and nontechnical means. For example, a firewall is a technical means to protect an individual computer workstation, as well as a computer server. Computer passwords and antivirus and antispyware programs are other examples of technical means to protect information systems. A nontechnical means would be providing physical security around a computer workstation or server complex by locking doors, using cipher-locks for accessing mainframes, providing user education and awareness training, and so on. All these are means to prevent an attack from having negative consequences on individual users' systems. At the national level, prevention takes on larger significance with regard to safeguarding critical infrastructures and their associated information systems. In this case, preventive measures to protect information systems must be assessed within the larger context of the associated information environment. In other words, risk-based assessments must occur, because we can't protect everything.

8.4.1.3 Detect

The next function in the cybersecurity framework, Detect, is more complex in cyberspace than in a closed system, involving our nation's ability to even know it is being attacked by a terrorist, nation-state, teenage hacker, or possibly even a construction worker's backhoe! Former Deputy Secretary of Defense John Hamre was once quoted stating that in cyberspace, we may not know we are under attack until it is too late and an "electronic Pearl Harbor" has occurred (Donnelly and Crawley 1999). Detection of cyber incidents, whether they are actual cyber-attacks or not, requires 24-hour-a-day, 7-day-a-week monitoring in order to provide adequate I&W of an attack. The intelligence community maintains their I&W centers to track hostile activities by nation-states deemed to be a threat to US security interests. In addition, because the source of a cyberspace attack may not be known, both the government and the private sector have established a number of **network operations security centers (NOSCs)** to provide Indications and Warnings (I&W) capability in cyberspace.

The Department of Defense originally established their NOSC within the **Defense Information Systems Agency (DISA)** located in Arlington, Virginia. Because this center looked at the global information infrastructure, it was called the Global NOSC, or GNOSC. However, the military reorganized after 9/11 to create new command and control organizations to deal with cyber threats. This included changing the GNOSC to the **Joint Task Force–Global Network Operations (JTF-GNO)**. Each of the military service components also established NOSCs for their own operational commands in order to provide immediate I&W of an attack on that particular unit's information systems. These service NOSCs were linked to regional and larger operational NOSCs, which were eventually linked to the GNOSC as a means to quickly send information both up and down the chain of command. This structure has been replaced under the US Cyber Command to a new operational concept discussed in the next section.

The civilian NOSC counterpart was initially the NIPC. It was from this location that the various government agencies could detect cyber-attacks, both on government infrastructure and the private sector. After 9/11 and the formation of the Department of Homeland Security (DHS), the NIPC detection function became embedded in DHS's US-CERT Command Center, which is also linked to the national CERT at Carnegie Mellon University, described earlier. These public and private sector centers serve as the conduit of information to first determine whether a cyber-attack or cyber-terrorist incident has occurred. If such an incident has taken place, the centers then ascertain the nature and severity of the attack in order to determine the appropriate response. But before that occurs, remedial action may be necessary to restore basic services impacted by the incident(s).

8.4.1.4 Respond

The offensive function in defending information systems is to determine how to Respond to a cyber-attack. Once an attack is detected and determined to be a hostile action by either a nation-state or a terrorist or criminal organization, then a decision must be made on how to respond. The first determination is often whether the incident is domestic or international and whether a US or multinational response is necessary. Because there are no international boundaries in cyberspace, other nations can be affected by incidents detected on US information systems. For this reason, CERTs are connected globally in order to facilitate communication and cooperation.

The nature of the response to a cyber-attack may further involve an interagency approach, which could include elements of national power (diplomatic, economic, or military) rather than informational power. For example, in 2001, when a US reconnaissance aircraft collided with a Chinese Air Force fighter jet off Hainan Island, Chinese hackers launched an information assault on the United States, involving both overt and covert actions. The US government response was diplomatic, trying to secure the release of the US aircrew and assuage Chinese concern that the incident was intentional. Meanwhile, US citizens, in this case "good" hackers, responded to the Chinese information assaults with "hack-backs" of their own without US government complicity, targeting Chinese government websites (Wallace 2001). While most of these attacks were simply a nuisance, aimed at defacing websites and making a political statement, they did demonstrate that when it came to cyberspace, anything goes, and the government has little ability to control the private sector. Also, the uncoordinated response to the incident further demonstrated the need for increased cooperation through influence rather than coercion. The potential for a private citizen's actions to provoke a governmental response could increase tensions and lead to physical and not just cyber confrontation. Such was the concern when **hacktivist** groups like Anonymous took it upon themselves to attack IS websites, declaring their own war on the terrorist organization in cyberspace (Muhammad 2017).

FOR EXAMPLE

WachulaGhost

Omar Mateen, a lone-wolf terrorist who claimed allegiance to IS, attacked the Pulse nightclub in Orlando, Florida in June 2016, killing 49 and wounding 58. His attack was considered a hate crime, as well as a terrorist attack, since it targeted the LGBTQ community. In response, a gay hacktivist who called himself WachulaGhost responded with a cyber-attack on IS websites, defacing them with gay porn. He claimed to have taken down over 200 IS Twitter accounts as well. He is quoted saying, "I did it for the lives lost in Orlando...Daesh [IS] have been spreading and praising the attack, so I thought I would defend those that were lost. The taking of innocent lives will not be tolerated." (Cuthbertson 2016)

8.4.1.5 Restore

Depending on the complexity of the cyber-attack, the ability to Restore operational capacity could range from something as simple as shutting down and rebooting a computer to something as complex as implementing a contingency plan for restoring power, such as by rerouting the power grid. If the attack involves the use of computer viruses, the affected CERTs may issue patches or **information assurance vulnerability assessments (IAVAs)**, directing system administrators of the necessary remedial actions required to restore the affected information systems. Because incidents of cyber-warfare or cyber-terrorism could lie beneath the radar scope, meaning they may not be visible to most end users, many remedial actions also fall within the Restore function, involving fixes that are made without public awareness. Cyber-warriors in both the public and private sector are charged with defending our nation's critical infrastructure from the effects of these attacks, and they pride themselves on their ability to find solutions and fix problems quickly without disruptions of basic services that put Americans at risk.

Finally, the end result of any coordinated response to a cyber incident must also focus on deterrence in order to prevent future attacks. The approach taken by many countries lately is not to passively wait for the next attack to occur. Rather, hacktivists, corporations, and government agencies are taking more offensive, proactive roles in responding to the threat of cyber-attacks from criminals, terrorists, and nation-states.

8.4.2 The US Military Response to Cyber-Warfare

In the mid-1990s, the US military recognized the growing threat of cyber-warfare to both its informational architecture and the nation's critical infrastructure. Because DoD installations in the United States were dependent on civilian infrastructure for communications, transportation, energy, water, and the full range of logistical support, the DoD recognized that a threat to any of these critical systems would directly impact the military's ability to deploy forces against foreign threats and actors. To make matters worse for military planners, the operational environment for these infrastructures was not a series of buildings or hard sites that could be secured with concertina wire and a guard force. Rather, these infrastructures were composed of complex information systems, which presented a whole new set of challenges for security planners. These planners were now faced with the difficult question of how to defend critical infrastructures "over here" in order to even begin to get military forces deployed "over there" for the next conflict.

Recognizing these new challenges, the DoD began a series of training exercises aimed at testing the vulnerabilities of our nation's critical infrastructures and the information systems on which they depended. The first operational-level exercise, which was conducted in June 1997, was called Eligible Receiver. This exercise involved using National Security Agency (NSA) "hackers" operating as an adversary to attack defense and other government information systems, while also conducting simulated attacks on civilian infrastructure (Robinson 2002). The lessons learned from the exercise showed serious problems with defending the critical information systems and infrastructures on which the DoD (and the nation) depended against cyber-attacks by adversaries who use asymmetrical means to defeat (or simply neutralize) our nation's military strength indirectly.

Later, in December 1998, the Department of Defense took the initiative to create an operational unit to specifically deal with the threat toward DoD information systems posed by cyber-warfare. The Joint Task Force–Computer Network Defense (JTF-CND) was formed as a field operating agency, based in Arlington, Virginia, at the Defense Information Systems Agency (DISA). The JTF-CND would later move to operational control of US Space Command (SPACECOM) in Colorado Springs, Colorado, as a result of changes to the DoD's Unified Command Plan (UCP) that took effect on October 1, 2000 (Information Warfare Site 2003). The JTF-CND originally focused only on the defensive aspects of Information Operations (IO) in the military's evolving information warfare doctrine. The JTF-CND would eventually evolve into the aforementioned JTF-Global Network Operations (JTF-GNO) in May 2005, responsible for both offensive and defensive aspects of Information Operations, as part of the organization's realignment under operational control of the **US Strategic Command (USSTRATCOM)** in Omaha, Nebraska. The JTF-GNO also integrated DISA's former GNOSC and served as the focal point for the DoD's CERT operations.

In 2009, the Department of Defense stood up **US Cyber Command (USCYBERCOM)** as a sub-unified command under USSTRATCOM. USCYBERCOM

plans, coordinates, integrates, synchronizes and conducts activities to: direct the operations and defense of specified Department of Defense information networks and; prepare to, and when directed, conduct full spectrum military cyberspace operations in order to enable actions in all domains, ensure US/Allied freedom of action in cyberspace and deny the same to our adversaries. (USSTRATCOM 2016)

It comprised service elements from all branches of the military: Army Cyber Command (ARCYBER), Fleet Cyber Command (FLTCYBER), Air Force Cyber Command (AFCYBER), and Marine Forces Cyber Command (MARFORCYBER). Although not part of the Department of Defense, Coast Guard Cyber Command (CGCYBER) does have a direct support relationship to USCYBERCOM, as a part of the Department of Homeland Security.

As a supporting command to the five regional combatant commands, USCYBERCOM has created the **Cyber Mission Force** (CMF) to augment the assigned forces to those regional commands, providing technical expertise on cyber operations. The Cyber Mission Force also includes **cyber protection teams** (CPT), whose primary mission is to provide computer network defense support (Figure 8-3).

Before these operational changes took place, the DoD was moving forward with the development of military doctrine to deal with information-age cyber-warfare threats. Although individual service components began considering information warfare as a viable mission area in the mid-1990s, it was several years before the DoD recognized the need to issue joint doctrine with regard to Information Operations (IO). DoD had previously issued IO policy guidance in the form of a classified DoD directive in 1996. Yet, it was not until the release of Joint Publication 3-13, *Joint Doctrine for Information Operations*, on October 9, 1998, that joint commands began to organize their staffs around the need for IO planning and execution, as well as education and training (Armistead 2004).

Information Operations emerged from previous joint doctrine involving command and control warfare, based on lessons learned after the first Gulf War and the

Figure 8-3

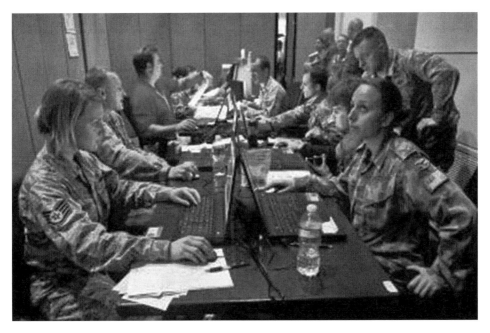

Department of Defense Cyber Protection Team. Source: Photo Courtesy of Senior Airman Brett Clashman, DoD (2015).

effectiveness of new information-based technologies for intelligence collection and targeting. IO expanded on the traditional "pillars" of command and control warfare (psychological operations, military deception, electronic warfare, physical destruction, and operations security) by adding computer network defense and the two related activities of public affairs and civil affairs (Department of Defense 1998). IO became the means by which DoD elements would conduct cyber-warfare, initially focused on defensive aspects of the cyber threat. It later expanded to include offensive cyber-warfare planning and execution under the broader category of Computer Network Operations (CNO).

The terrorist attacks against the Pentagon and the World Trade Center in September 2001 provided the impetus for broader DoD organizational changes that impacted the military's ability to carry out and defend against cyber-warfare. The threat posed by al-Qaeda and other international terrorist groups to the US homeland caused the DoD to create a new joint command, US Northern Command, dedicated to the homeland defense mission of the DoD, in support of the nation's overall homeland security effort. This change to the Unified Command Plan (UCP), signed by President Bush in May 2002, further eliminated the US Space Command in Colorado Springs, Colorado, moving most of the space and Information Operations roles of the military to US Strategic Command (USSTRATCOM) in Omaha, Nebraska. Under USSTRATCOM, operational control for all aspects of Information Operations, including computer network attack and computer network defense, were consolidated into new organizational structures and responsibilities. The JTF-CND came under USSTRATCOM's control, for example. Each of the services transformed existing IO organizations into IO "commands" in order to provide the service components in support of the joint command structure.

The military's information-age transformation signals recognition that threats to the nation's (and military's) information systems will remain. Whether the threat of cyber-warfare comes from a terrorist organization or a nation-state, the DoD's reorganization at the joint combatant command level, as well as the service component level, will better position the military to face these information-age threats. However, one significant problem remains: The DoD does not control access to, nor does it defend, the nation's critical infrastructures on which military power rides. Whether it's the nation's rail and transport system, global telecommunications architecture, or power grid, the DoD is dependent on having access to these systems. Even the DoD's logistics system cannot function in getting troops and supplies to Iraq or other future conflict areas without the help of commercial transportation and private companies like FedEx or UPS. A cyber-attack on any of the information systems that manage these critical infrastructures would have devastating effects on our military's ability to provide for our nation's defense both here and abroad.

Because cyber-terrorism and cyber-warfare are relatively new concepts, the nature of the threat posed by terrorists or even nation-states using technology in this manner remains controversial. Some critics argue that our nation's infrastructure is not that vulnerable to these types of attacks, because the infrastructure is so complex and has multiple redundancies built into it, such as with the power grid and telecommunication networks. They also contend that our economy is resilient to potential cyber-attacks and such efforts would only prove a temporary setback, as evidenced by the events of 9/11 (Ranum 2004). On the other hand, members of the Congress, the military, and others charged with providing for our nation's defenses against all enemies do not take the threat lightly and continue to reassess and reevaluate both the capability and intent of our adversaries to harm us in cyberspace.

8.4.3 The New Battlefields of Cyber-Warfare

This chapter has focused on the threats in cyberspace posed by criminals, terrorists, and nation-states. However, as the tools available for conducting cyber-warfare have become more widely available and even more anonymous, it becomes harder to distinguish who or what is behind a cyber-attack. Also, the sources of the attacks have become more disperse, not just targeting critical infrastructure or defense websites. We have seen nation-states, such as North Korea, involved in a sophisticated cyber-attack on Sony Pictures, over the release of the movie, "The Interview," which negatively portrayed its leader, Kim Jong-un. The attack was successful in causing Sony to pull the movie from its release in theaters due to threats (Peterson 2014). As a business, Sony was still reeling financially from a hack on its PlayStation Network in 2011, which compromised personal data of millions of users. More recently, the involvement of Russian hackers in the 2016 US presidential elections, poses a new type of threat to democratic countries, as it appears the Russian government was behind the attacks on the nation's political system, attempting to influence the outcome of the vote (Lipton et al. 2016). There has also been evidence Russia tried to influence elections in other European countries in 2017 (Frenkel 2017).

In 2010, the United States also changed the nature of cyber-warfare by conducting a cyber-attack against Iran's nuclear program, in an attempt to disable, or at least delay, Iran's ability to develop nuclear weapons. The operation, codenamed **Olympic Games**, was evidently an offensive computer network attack, coordinated with Israel, using the **Stuxnet** virus to infect the SCADA control systems at the Natanz nuclear site in Iran (Sanger 2013; Zetter 2014). Although not publicly admitted by the Obama administration, the attack was a major step forward in the conduct of cyber-warfare by nation-states targeting the critical infrastructure of another nation-state. What made the Stuxnet virus particularly virulent was the use of a zero-day code that would infect every Windows operating system developed since 2000, making it impossible to stop (Zetter 2014). Also, it was impossible to contain, spreading beyond the nuclear facilities in Iran to Europe and even the United States. As General Michael Hayden, former head of the CIA and NSA, was quoted saying, "we have let the genie out of the bottle" (Zero Days 2016).

The US Stuxnet virus, Russian hacking, Chinese cyber-warfare, Iranian and North Korean cyber operations, and even some hacktivists and cyber criminals operating in cyberspace all point to what are being called **advanced persistent threats (APTs)**. These are a new kind of cyber threat due to the fact that they employ advanced technology and sophisticated research and intelligence collection operations to be able to target the adversary. They are persistent since they employ a number of tools and techniques to attack the target and defeat its defenses. And they are threats due to the capability and the intent of the actors employing them (Kessler 2014, 234–235). Google was the target of the first APT in 2009, named Operation Aurora, which was believed to have been conducted by Chinese military hackers, part of a secret "hacking army" called Chinese Cyber Unit 61398. In 2014, The US government actually charged five Chinese People's Liberation Army (PLA) officers who were part of the unit with conducting cyber espionage against US companies (Kumar 2014). It seems like today, regarding cyber-warfare, everyone is a combatant, as well as a potential target (Mims 2017).

SELF-CHECK

- Define CERT.
- The five functions of the Computer Security Framework are disable, degrade, detect, deny, and destroy. True or false?
- To which military command is US Cyber Command a sub-unified command?
  - a. US Space Command
  - b. US Northern Command
  - c. US Central Command
  - d. US Strategic Command
- Olympic Games was the code word for the operation to place the Stuxnet virus into Iranian nuclear facilities. True or false?

SUMMARY

Former Secretary of Defense Donald Rumsfeld categorized the threats our nation faces in the future as "known knowns, known unknowns, and unknown unknowns" (Rumsfeld 2006). With regard to threats in cyberspace, much remains within the "unknown unknowns" category, because the most significant attacks we have experienced to date may still be unknown. The consequences may only come to light after the fact or after a policy or operational decision is made based on insufficient knowledge. Such situations have happened before. However, in cyberspace, the consequences may not become "known knowns" until it is too late, and the repercussions of those actions could have far-reaching implications.

In this chapter, you learned how to assess information-based threats to our nation's critical infrastructure. You evaluated the difference between capability and intent with regard to threats in cyberspace. In addition, you appraised the consequences of cyber-crime, cyber-terrorism, and cyber-warfare and their impact on our nation's information systems, and you learned how to judge our nation's defensive and offensive capabilities concerning cyber-warfare. While many uncertainties about the nature of the threats we face in cyberspace still remain, our nation and others continue to develop cyber-defenses and offensive cyber operations against the threats we currently face, as well as those we anticipate.

KEY TERMS

Advanced persistent threat (APT)	A sustained attack on a specific target that employs many types of tools from a hacker's tool kit and adapts to the defenses put up to thwart it.
C4I	The organizational architecture used by the US military; stands for command, control, communications, computers, and intelligence.
COMPUINT	Abbreviation for computer intelligence, or what we can learn from analyzing computer traffic, e-mail, websites, hard drives, etc.
Computer emergency response team (CERT)	One of several organizations that provide the supporting mechanisms necessary for researching and responding to computer security threats.
Computer network attack (CNA)	The offensive component of computer network operations, in which the intelligence and espionage function is changed into a hostile action.
Critical Infrastructure Assurance Office (CIAO)	Federal center for coordinating the ISAC process and encouraging the private sector to cooperate with the government in protecting itself against cyber-terrorism and threats from man-made and natural disasters.
Cyberspace	The notional environment in which digitized information is communicated over computer networks.
Cyber-crime	A crime committed or facilitated via the Internet or any criminal activity involving computers and networks.
Cyber Mission Forces (CMF)	Military units provided by USCYBERCOM to support computer network operations by the regional combatant commands.
Cyber Storm	A Department of Homeland Security exercise to simulate a coordinated cyber incident response, including information sharing mechanisms, procedures for establishing situational awareness, public and private organizational decision making, and public communications during a cyber-related incident of national significance.

Cyber protection team (CPT)

Military forces deployed by USCYBERCOM to provide computer network defense support to the Department of Defense regional combatant commands.

Cyber-terrorism

The use of computer-based operations by terrorist organizations conducting cyber-attacks that compromise, damage, degrade, disrupt, deny, and destroy information stored on computer networks or that target network infrastructures.

Cyber-warfare

Involves the actions by a nation-state or non-state actor to attack and attempt to damage another nation's or non-state actor's computers or information networks through, for example, computer viruses or denial-of-service attacks.

Defense Advanced Research Projects Agency (DARPA)

Agency within the Department of Defense that created the foundations of the modern Internet in the 1960s. It was originally known as ARPA—Advanced Research Projects Agency.

Defense Information Systems Agency (DISA)

Home of the original NOSC established by the Department of Defense; also called the Global NOSC or GNOSC because it looked at the global information infrastructure.

Denial-of-service (DOS) attack

Most common type of CNA, in which an individual computer or entire network is rendered useless, such as by the actions of a virus.

Hacktivist

A computer hacker whose activity is aimed at promoting a social or political cause.

Information assurance vulnerability assessment (IAVA)

An assessment issued by a CERT that directs system administrators regarding the necessary actions required to restore information systems affected by a cyber-attack.

Information Sharing and Advisory Council (ISAC)

One in a number of groups established by the federal government in 1998 to foster public–private partnerships in all sectors of the nation's critical infrastructures.

Joint Task Force–Global Network Operations (JTF-GNO)	The organization created from the Global NOSC after 9/11 to generate new military command and control capabilities for dealing with cyber threats. It is no longer in existence, since the formation of US Cyber Command.
National Cybersecurity and Communications Integration Center (NCCIC)	A coordination center for monitoring cyber-attacks against the country's critical infrastructure, run by the Department of Homeland Security.
National Infrastructure Protection Center (NIPC)	Federal operations center created in 1998 for tracking cyber-attacks on the nation's critical infrastructure, run by the Department Justice. It is no longer in existence since the formation of the Department of Homeland Security.
Network Operations Security Center (NOSC)	One of a number of centers established by government and the private sector to provide indications and warning capability in cyberspace.
Olympic Games	Codename for a joint US–Israeli operation to implant the Stuxnet virus into Iranian nuclear facilities.
Steganography	The practice of embedding messages or files in computer websites.
Stuxnet	Name of the computer virus that was implanted into Iran's nuclear facilities to degrade the country's ability to produce nuclear weapons.
Top Officials (TOPOFF)	A national-level domestic exercise with an international component, designed to strengthen the nation's capacity to prevent, protect against, respond to, and recover from large-scale terrorist attacks involving weapons of mass destruction (WMD).

US Cyber Command (USCYBERCOM)   Located in Ft. Meade, Maryland, it is a subordinate command of USSTRATCOM, providing cyber support capabilities to the regional combatant commands.

US Strategic Command (USSTRATCOM)   Located in Omaha, Nebraska, one of nine regional and functional combatant commands, with responsibility for information operations and for USCYBERCOM.

ASSESS YOUR UNDERSTANDING

Go to www.wiley.com/go/Kilroy/Threats_to_Homeland_Security to assess your knowledge of the basics of cyber-crime, cyber-terrorism, and cyber-warfare.

Summary Questions

1. Cyber-warfare is conflict only between nations using information-based weapons. True or false?

2. Threats are defined as possessing both capability and intent. True or false?

3. The Internet was invented by Al Gore. True or false?

4. CERTs are located only in the United States in order to detect and respond to cyber-attacks. True or false?

5. Saddam Hussein was the source behind the Solar Sunrise computer hacking incidents in 1998. True or false?

6. Information Operations (IO) emerged from previous joint doctrine involving command and control warfare. True or false?

7. Which of the following is not a part of our nation's critical infrastructure?
   (a) Banking and finance centers
   (b) Water supplies
   (c) Power facilities
   (d) Manufacturing centers

8. The greatest threat, at all security levels, is posed by which of the following?
   (a) Institutional hackers
   (b) Insiders
   (c) Organized crime
   (d) Recreational hackers

9. An example of a terrorist organization using steganography would involve which of the following?
   (a) Embedding a coded message on a computer website
   (b) Hacking into a government website to deface the site
   (c) Leaving a coded message at the scene of a terrorist attack
   (d) Providing false information on captured computer files

10. The US-CERT falls under which federal agency?
    (a) Department of Justice
    (b) Department of Defense
    (c) Department of Homeland Security
    (d) US Cyber Command

Applying This Chapter Questions

1. If you were a system administrator and asked to construct a cyber-defense model for your government agency or private company, what critical processes would you include?

2. You have detected some unusual activity on your computer, such as strange characters and e-mails. This concerns you because your company is responsible for the computerized switches (SCADA) that control the rail tracks up and down the East Coast. To whom should your report this activity and why?

3. As a county or city manager of a small rural community in the Midwest, you may feel safe from terrorist incidents, particularly cyber-terrorism. Yet, your community depends on a number of critical infrastructures that could be impacted by cyber-attacks. Compile a list of all the critical infrastructures in your community that could be susceptible to cyber-terrorism, and select the four most essential to your community's safety and security.

4. You are a military officer assigned to US Cyber Command, helping to coordinate our nation's cyber-defenses. You have been asked to speak to a local Rotary Club about threats in cyberspace. Explain the Department of Defense contribution to fight cyber-terrorism.

YOU TRY IT

Defending Cyberspace

You work at a Network Operations Security Center (NOSC) for a Department of Defense agency. You've been advised that one of your subordinate commands has been attacked by a computer virus, which is causing all the connected information systems on that base to crash and individual operators to lose critical information on their operating systems. Evaluate what you would do and how.

Cost Versus Risk at the Office

Your private company needs to update its computers and servers. You've researched a number of options and recommended a secure replacement system. Your boss tells you the computer operating system you've selected costs too much and to look for cheaper options. What do you do? Generate a policy memo to your boss explaining the cost versus risk involved in going with a less expensive operating system.

9

WEAPONS OF MASS DESTRUCTION AND DISRUPTION
Understanding Weapons That Can Create a Catastrophic Event

Christopher J. Ferrero

Department of Politics, Coastal Carolina University, Conway, SC, USA

Starting Point

Go to www.wiley.com/go/Kilroy/Threats_to_Homeland_Security to assess your knowledge of the basics of weapons of mass destruction.
Determine where you need to concentrate your effort.

What You'll Learn in This Chapter

▲ The difference between conventional and radiological terrorist incidents

▲ The types and sources of radiation and radiological/nuclear contamination

▲ The types and sources of chemical and biological weapons

▲ The consequences and management of weapons of mass destruction events

After Studying This Chapter, You'll Be Able To

▲ Evaluate the types of chemical, biological, nuclear, and radiological weapons and the nature of their employment

▲ Assess the availability and applicability of weapons of mass destruction by terrorist groups

▲ Estimate the consequences of the use of a weapon of mass destruction in creating a catastrophic event

▲ Assess the threat of terrorists using weapons of mass destruction and the potential impact on the United States

Threats to Homeland Security: Reassessing the All-Hazards Perspective, Second Edition.
Edited by Richard J. Kilroy, Jr.
© 2018 John Wiley & Sons, Inc. Published 2018 by John Wiley & Sons, Inc.
Companion website: www.wiley.com/go/Kilroy/Threats_to_Homeland_Security

INTRODUCTION

Since the catastrophic events of September 11, 2001, national and homeland security officials have been concerned about the potential nexus of terrorism and **weapons of mass destruction (WMD)**. President George W. Bush's 2002 National Security Strategy stated that "[t]he gravest danger our [n]ation faces lies at the crossroads of radicalism and technology" (White House 2002). The technology to which the 2002 Strategy referred is that related to the production and dissemination of chemical, biological, radiological, and nuclear weapons. Thirteen years later, President Barack Obama's 2015 National Security Strategy noted that

> [n]o threat poses as grave a danger to our security and well-being as the potential use of nuclear weapons and materials by irresponsible states or terrorists…Vigilance is required to stop countries and non-state actors from developing or acquiring nuclear, chemical, or biological weapons, or the materials to build them. (White House 2015)

While perspectives on the scope of homeland security have evolved in the nearly two decades since 9/11, the need to focus attention and resources on WMD remains constant. The WMD threat is a prominent homeland security issue whether one prefers the inclusive all-hazards perspective or the more exclusive, terrorism-centric approach. A major reason it retains prominence is embedded in the very phrase used to describe this category of weapon: *mass destruction*. No matter how low the probability that a terrorist group or state actor might successfully execute a WMD attack against the US homeland, the impact (should it occur) is likely to be immense. Effects could range from the destruction of cities and towns and the deaths of millions to less apocalyptic but very serious scenarios such as infectious disease outbreaks, widespread chronic illness, displacement of hundreds of thousands, and paralysis of the economy through contamination or other long-term disablement of critical economic centers or transportation nodes. This latter scenario prompts some to occasionally modify the WMD acronym to mean **weapons of mass disruption**.

Whether we speak of these weapons in terms of mass *destruction* or mass *disruption*, we remain concerned about the same technologies and materials, namely, chemical agents, biological agents, radiological material and contaminants, nuclear bombs and warheads, and any explosive devices used in conjunction with them. As such, this suite of threats is often referred to in literature and government documents as **CBRNE** (chemical, biological, radiological, nuclear, and explosive) instead of WMD. Whichever acronym you encounter, the meaning is fundamentally the same.

In this chapter, you will learn about and evaluate the different types of WMD and the nature of their employment. You will assess the availability of these deadly materials to terrorist groups and potentially threatening state actors. Finally, you will assess the potential impact of an attack on the United States using chemical, biological, radiological, and nuclear weapons.

9.1 Chemical Weapons and Their Consequences

The Federation of American Scientists distinguishes **chemical weapons (CWs)** as weapons that "use the toxic properties of chemical substances rather than their explosive properties to produce physical or physiological effects on an enemy"

(FAS n.d.). The dissemination of chemical weapons may or may not involve the use of explosives; their defining trait is their toxicity and the attendant effects on the human body. Moreover, chemical weapons are distinct from biological weapons (BWs) insofar as they are not specifically of biological origin. Many of the world's most dangerous chemical weapons and agents were invented in government laboratories during the mid-twentieth century.

Of the weapons of mass destruction addressed in this chapter, chemical weapons have historically been the most readily available and the most commonly used. Their ease of acquisition and handling relative to other WMD agents and their use in conventional warfare during the twentieth century and in the Syrian Civil War (2011–?) generates concern that terrorist groups will continue to view them as a low-cost, effective means to accomplish their objectives. Chemical weapons attacks are far from notional; they are phenomena that humanity has witnessed very recently. Fortunately, the 1993 Chemical Weapons Convention (CWC) and its enforcement body, the Organization for the Prohibition of Chemical Weapons (OPCW), have significantly reduced the availability of chemical weapons and their precursors. The CWC is an international treaty that bans the development, stockpiling, and use of chemical weapons and mandates the destruction of the world's existing chemical weapons stockpiles and precursor agents. As of January 2016, the OPCW had overseen the destruction of 91% of the world's declared chemical weapons agents and 58% of declared munitions, as well as the dismantlement of 100% of declared chemical weapons production facilities (CWPFs). The OPCW won the Nobel Peace Prize for this work in 2013. Work remains, however, and the threat of chemical weapons has not gone away (Organization for the Prohibition of Chemical Weapons 2016a).

FOR EXAMPLE

The Organization for the Prohibition of Chemical Weapons

The Organization for the Prohibition of Chemical Weapons, or OPCW, is based in The Hague, Netherlands. All states party to the CWC submit declarations of their chemical weapons and any chemical weapons production facilities (CWPFs) to the OPCW. The OPCW provides monitoring, oversight, and technical assistance to the dismantling of chemical weapons stockpiles and any associated facilities. Member states have the primary responsibility of dismantling their own chemical weapons and infrastructure, but other states party to the CWC are obligated to provide assistance to those states that may lack the resources or expertise to safely fulfill their treaty obligations. For example, the United States destroyed many of the chemical weapons surrendered by Syria after its 2013 accession to the CWC. The OPCW and CWC provide regulations to ensure that CW disposal is safe for people and the environment. Chemical weapons may not be dumped at sea, be buried, or be burned in open pits. Chemical agents can either be chemically neutralized or undergo controlled incineration. CW munitions, such as shells and warheads, may be cut apart. For comprehensive information on the status of global chemical weapons, their disposal, and the regulation of their precursors, visit the OPCW website: www.opcw.org.

9.1.1 History of Chemical Weapons Use

The modern history of chemical weapons begins with World War I. Both sides used toxic chemical vapors on the battlefield on multiple occasions. The Germans used the blistering agent mustard gas and the choking agent chlorine gas, while the French employed the blistering agent phosgene. Dissemination methods included the use of projectiles, shells, and simple dissemination from open containers via the wind. After World War I, many nations signed the Geneva Protocol (1925) banning the use of chemical weapons in warfare. However, this did not stop Japan from using such weapons against China nor Italy against Ethiopia in the 1930s. Even the United States refused to ratify the Protocol until 1975. In fact, many countries acquired chemical weapons capabilities. Fortunately, the spirit of the Geneva Protocol largely held during World War II, in which no battlefield chemical weapons were used. Nazi Germany did, however, use chemical agents to commit mass murder in its concentration camps and was later revealed to have been developing battlefield chemical agents much deadlier than those used in World War I. One such agent was the nerve agent sarin. During the Cold War, both the United States and the Soviet Union built large stockpiles of chemical weapons. Today, the United States and Russian Federation are both adherents to the Chemical Weapons Convention, but due to the vastness of their arsenals, complete disarmament in either country is unlikely before 2020.

Saddam Hussein, who ruled Iraq from 1979 to 2003, used mustard and nerve agents against Iran during the Iran–Iraq War of 1980–1988. More than one million Iranians suffered CW-related casualties during the war. Saddam also used CW against his own people, notably in a 1988 attack on Iraqi Kurds that killed over 5000 people in just one day (ABC News 2006). The last major incidence of chemical weapons use in the twentieth century occurred in 1995, when the Japanese terrorist organization Aum Shinrikyo used sarin gas in a Tokyo subway, killing 13 and injuring over 5000 (Fackler 2012).

In late 2012, the first allegations were made of chemical weapons use in the Syrian Civil War. In June 2013, the US Intelligence Community assessed with high confidence that the Syrian government, controlled by the regime of Bashar al-Assad, had used chemical weapons against opposition forces multiple times during the previous year. On August 21, 2013, a large-scale sarin attack victimized thousands of people in suburban Damascus. The United States estimated 1500 deaths from the attack, and the NGO Doctors Without Borders, which networked with hospitals in the area, estimated 3600 cases of symptoms consistent with a nerve agent attack. Symptoms included paralysis, difficulty breathing, convulsions, and foaming of the mouth. A United Nations (UN) report in September 2013 corroborated claims by medics and Western intelligence agencies that sarin had been used in the attack (Arms Control Association 2014).

The August 2013 sarin attack, widely ascribed to the Assad regime, nearly prompted American military action against the Syrian government. Instead, Russia brokered an agreement whereby Syria acceded to the Chemical Weapons Convention and subjected itself to disarmament under OPCW supervision. By June 2014, all of Syria's declared chemical weapons had been removed from the country for safe decommissioning elsewhere, and all of its declared CW production facilities had been rendered inoperable.

Despite this successful disarmament operation, rudimentary chemical weapons continued to be used in the Syrian Civil War, and some sophisticated chemical weapons appear to have remained. Disarmament relies on thorough accounting by, and the good faith of, the disarming entity. Only that which is declared is disarmed. Verification by international monitors can be hindered by noncooperation, deception, or difficulty in safely accessing war zones where weapons may be present. Negligence and human error may also occur.

Evidence suggests that Syria withheld some of its advanced chemical agents. The OPCW confirmed in 2015 that it found traces of sarin and VX nerve gas at a military facility that had not been declared by Syria as part of its chemical weapons program (Arms Control Association 2016b). Then, on April 4, 2017, the Syrian government launched another major sarin attack on civilians—this time in Khan Sheikhoun. More than 80 people died, including several children (Osborne 2017). The attack, which was similar to the 2013 sarin attack, prompted the United States to launch a cruise missile strike against the Syrian air base from which the sarin attack had been launched.

While the use of the outlawed and highly lethal sarin agent captured the world's attention in 2013 and again in 2017, many more Syrians suffered from the use of a more mundane agent. The Assad regime resorted to the use of chlorine barrel bombs only months after completing the handover of its declared weapons stocks in 2014. Chlorine has common industrial and consumer applications, and thus its possession is not prohibited under the CWC. Its weaponization is, however, a violation of the treaty. This iteration of chemical warfare exemplifies the problem of dual-use technology. Many of the ingredients of chemical, biological, and nuclear/radiological weapons have peaceful and legitimate uses—as well as deadly ones. Therefore, the availability of deadly substances cannot be eliminated, and by extension, the possibility of unsophisticated but deadly attacks remains.

Chlorine is a choking (pulmonary) agent and can be deadly for children and those with poor lung function. The OPCW confirmed the use of chlorine in attacks in Syria in September 2014. The Syrian American Medical Society documented 161 chemical weapons attacks in Syria through 2015, most involving chlorine (Syrian American Medical Society 2016).

The vast majority of chemical attacks in Syria were attributed to the Assad regime, but increased reporting through 2015 and 2016 suggested their use by terrorists engaged in Middle Eastern conflicts—specifically the Islamic State (IS).

9.1.2 Chemical Agents and Their Effects

Chemical agents are generally categorized as nerve agents, blister agents, and choking agents.

9.1.2.1 Nerve Agents

Nerve agents are the most lethal of chemical weapons agents. They cause multiple types of injury by attacking the central nervous system. In gaseous form, they can be inhaled or absorbed through the skin. In liquid form, they can be ingested.

> ### FOR EXAMPLE
>
> **Terrorist Use of Chemical Weapons**
>
> In late 2016, a joint United Nations–OPCW investigation unit known as the Joint Investigation Mechanism (JIM) determined that, despite the Assad regime's continued use of chemical weapons, only IS could have carried out a specific mustard gas attack in Marea, near the northern Syrian city of Aleppo, on August 21, 2015 (Fox News 2016). Press reports indicate that the al-Qaeda-affiliated jihadist group then known as al-Nusra had stolen a large cache of chemical weapons from an unguarded depot in Syria (Doornbos and Moussa 2016). Despite Assad's partial cooperation with the OPCW in 2014 and 2015, Western intelligence agencies never believed that Assad had surrendered "every single bit" of his chemical arsenal (Fox News 2016). Assad's use of sarin gas against Khan Sheikhoun on April 4, 2017, bears this out. The likely continued presence of chemical weapons in Syria also suggests that the world may witness future instances of acquisition and use by terrorists operating in the war-ravaged country.

Nerve agents typically work by blocking an enzyme (acetylcholinesterase) necessary for the proper functioning of the central nervous system. The eyes and lungs absorb nerve agents particularly quickly, and widespread systemic effects may occur within 1 min of exposure. Some common signs of exposure are pin-pointed pupils, muscular twitching or convulsions, bodily secretions, slurring of speech, salivation, and foaming of the mouth. An appropriate first response to such symptoms is the injection of 2 mg of atropine.

Common nerve agents include the following:

▲ Tabun (GA)
▲ Sarin (GB)
▲ Soman (GD)
▲ Cyclosarin (GF)
▲ Methylphosphonothioic acid (VX)

VX is specially designed to be persistent. "G" agents are nonpersistent but may be mixed with other substances to increase their persistence. Enhanced persistence prolongs exposure, resulting in worse injury and more difficult cleanup. In other words, increased persistence increases an agent's power as a weapon of mass destruction (death and injury) and as a weapon of mass disruption (contamination).

9.1.2.2 Blister Agents

Blister agents, or vesicants, burn and blister those parts of the body with which they come into contact. Typically this would be the skin but may also include the eyes and even the lungs (via inhalation). Exposure to these agents is typically not lethal but may be extremely painful and may cause secondary infections that could be lethal. Blister agents may be particularly attractive to terrorists for a few reasons. First, blister agents tend to be persistent. This is especially true of mustard agents. Mustards are very persistent in cold and temperate climates. These conditions characterize most of the United States. As such, mustard would be a good choice for a chemical weapon of mass disruption. Moreover, symptoms of mustard exposure are usually delayed, allowing for widespread, unnoticed dissemination of the agent and subsequent escape by a perpetrator before authorities recognize that an attack has occurred.

Common blister agents include the following:

▲ Sulfur mustard/yperite (HD)
▲ Nitrogen mustard (HN)
▲ Lewisite (L)
▲ Phosgene (CX)

9.1.2.3 Choking Agents

Choking agents, also known as pulmonary agents, attack lung tissue and the respiratory system. Phosgene is the deadliest of these agents; it accounted for 80% of all chemical weapons-related fatalities in World War I. Symptoms typically appear immediately and include coughing, choking, and tightness in the chest. Chlorine, another choking agent, has been used extensively in the Syrian Civil War, as noted earlier. Its dual-use nature makes it very difficult to regulate, and dissemination can be achieved by rudimentary methods.

Common choking agents include the following:

▲ Phosgene (CG)
▲ Diphosgene (DP)
▲ Chlorine (Cl)
▲ Chloropicrin (PS)

9.1.2.4 The Dual-Use Problem

As already noted with regard to chlorine, some chemicals that can be used as CW also have legitimate applications. Any such agent, compound, or technology that can serve both military and civilian purposes is known as dual-use. The choking agents phosgene and chlorine are both common industrial chemicals and are thus good candidates for future weaponization by terrorists due to their availability. Another example of a deadly dual-use chemical agent is hydrogen cyanide, which is used worldwide in the manufacture of acrylic polymers. This is an example of what is known as a blood agent. It harms the target by preventing the transfer of oxygen to tissues via the bloodstream. While the CWC and the OPCW have prohibited the weaponization of dual-use chemicals and disarmed the world of most extremely lethal nerve agents, many opportunities remain for those seeking to perpetrate a chemical weapons attack.

> **FOR EXAMPLE**
>
> ### Chemical Weapons Training
>
> The US military prepares its forces for dealing with the effects of chemical weapons on the battlefield by various means, including the use of chemical protective equipment, such as gas masks and special uniforms with charcoal liners, as well as specialized training. Most veterans will recall their experiences in the "gas chamber" during basic training, when they are required to remove their gas masks and be exposed to CS (riot control) gas. They are also instructed on the use of atropine injectors as a means to counteract the effects of nerve agents. Military personnel are also trained to recognize the use of chemical weapons on the battlefield and to mark areas as being contaminated and by what type of agent—persistent or nonpersistent. They also learn how to decontaminate themselves and their equipment. A full description of the types of measures employed can be found in the *U.S. Armed Forces Nuclear, Biological, and Chemical Survival Manual*, Appendix C, which also provides detailed information regarding specific chemical agents and effects. (Couch 2003)

9.1.3 The Threat of Chemical Weapons and Terrorism

The Chemical Weapons Convention (CWC) and the Organization for the Prohibition of Chemical Weapons (OPCW) have greatly reduced the chemical weapons threat since the end of the Cold War. Only three notable countries—Israel, Egypt, and North Korea—are not OPCW member states. The only member state in poor standing at the time of this writing is Syria, which is accused of using sarin and rudimentary chlorine chemical weapons after acceding to the CWC.

Verification of complete compliance with chemical weapons prohibitions and laws is difficult, particularly given the dual-use nature of some weaponizable chemicals. The OPCW is widely respected for its work, but small quantities of chemical weapons may remain in countries that have officially disarmed—either by deceptive design or by error. Some optimism is in order when looking at broad trends in CW capabilities since the 1990s. Three countries in the Middle East—a region rifed with anti-American terrorist sentiment and activity—have been disarmed of large quantities of the world's most dangerous chemical weapons. The United Nations successfully dismantled the bulk of Iraq's chemical weapons in the 1990s. The Iraq Survey Group (ISG), which was charged with looking into Iraq's WMD capabilities after the 2003 Iraq War, reported that Iraq's CW capability had not been reconstituted, as many had feared. In 2014, Syria surrendered a very large quantity of its most dangerous chemical weapons, and in 2016, Libya surrendered over 800 tons of dual-use precursor chemicals in order to ensure their denial to terrorist groups operating in that unstable and war-ravaged country. Libya's former dictator Muamar Qaddafi began disarming Libyan chemical weapons in 2003.

However, this optimism must be tempered with caution. Hazards remain in the realm of CW. Sophisticated agents may remain in countries like Syria and Iraq—countries that have been contested and partially ruled by Islamist terrorists. A *New York Times* investigation suggested that nearly 5,000 chemical munitions dating to the early 1990s were found in Iraq after the 2003 Iraq War and that a CIA program had to be launched to buy loose chemical munitions on the Iraqi black market (Nuclear Threat Initiative 2015a). A former Syrian jihadist also reported in 2016 that he had participated in a jihadist raid of a Syrian base near Darat Izza in northern Syria, from which the terrorists took barrels full of chlorine, sarin, and mustard gas (Doornbos and Moussa 2016).

In addition to the threat posed by loose chemical weapons falling into the wrong hands, the availability of dual-use chemicals remains a problem. The CWC regime partially addresses this problem by promoting multilateral monitoring and regulation of the trade in industrial chemicals in order to reduce the likelihood that dangerous precursors will fall into the hands of non-signatory states or terrorist groups. Yet regulation and monitoring of the dual-use chemicals trade does not guarantee that a determined actor will not acquire the agents necessary for at least a disruptive attack. Toxic chemicals may be acquired overtly or undercover, and their relative ease of handling, when compared with biological agents, makes them an attractive option.

The relative ease of dissemination also makes chemical weapons an attractive option to terrorists. The most common method of dissemination is through the use of explosives. Terrorist organizations are adept at facilitating explosions, though some of the chemical agent may be incinerated through this method, reducing the toxicity of the attack. Syria, as noted earlier, resorted to dropping "barrel bombs" packed with metal cylinders of chlorine gas from helicopters. Another relatively simple method of dissemination is the exploitation of wind patterns. A terrorist could simply take the lid off a barrel or canister on a windy day. A more sophisticated approach would be to use spray tanks, particularly attached to an airplane or UAV, for more tailored dissemination over a larger area. In addition to obtaining chemical weapons or agents, there is the potential for terrorist organizations to attack commercial chemical storage or production facilities. By using conventional explosives against these facilities, terrorists can create a WMD effect through the release of toxic chemical fumes into the atmosphere, which, depending on atmospheric conditions, can affect large population centers in the United States and elsewhere. Communities located near such facilities are vulnerable to these types of attacks, as evidenced by accidental explosions that have occurred in the past. For instance, the worst industrial accident in the United States occurred on April 17, 1947, in the port of Texas City, Texas (35 miles from Houston), when a fire in the hold of a cargo ship, the *Grandcamp*, led to a series of explosions. The explosions were a result of the cargo the ship was carrying: ammonium nitrate, sulfur, and other toxic chemical products. The explosion was of such magnitude that it also destroyed nearby petroleum refining facilities and other cargo ships. The resulting physical damage, as well as fires and toxic clouds that lasted for 4 days, eventually killed over 500 people and wounded 3500 others (Texas City Disaster n.d.).

SELF-CHECK

- Because chemical weapons have been banned by the Chemical Weapons Convention, they no longer exist in the world today. True or false?
- Chemical agents include which of the following?
  a. Blister agents
  b. Choking agents
  c. Nerve agents
  d. All of the above
- Define WMD.
- Sarin is an example of a chemical agent that affects the body by attacking the central nervous system. True or false?

9.2 Biological Weapons and Their Consequences

Humans have attempted to employ **biological weapons** (weapons consisting of biological or living organisms or toxins) since long before there was any scientific knowledge of the causes of disease. The bodies of disease victims were used to poison water or to spread disease by contact, and bodies were even catapulted into besieged cities. In one example, the Venetian historian Gabriel de Mussis described the siege of Kaffa on the Crimean coast by the Tartars in 1345. After a three-year siege, plague broke out among the Tartars, probably carried in from Asia by rats in their own ships. In 1348, Kaffa finally fell after the Tartars catapulted their plague dead over the walls and into the city. In another case, in 1422, infected cadavers and manure were catapulted into the city during the siege of Carolstein (Derbis 1996). These methods were inglorious and barbaric means of spreading death and thus are not often reported in the documented history, poems, and songs relating battles in our past. Modern international legal conventions and norms ban the use of these methods of death and destruction. Of course, determined groups, such as terrorists, may readily ignore international agreements and norms if doing so seems to support their objectives.

9.2.1 History of Biological Weapons Use

Some epidemiologists attribute the 1352 epidemic of bubonic plague in Europe, known as the "Black Death," to the early crude attempt at biological warfare described earlier in the siege of Kaffa. After Kaffa fell, refugees fleeing by ship may have initiated this European pandemic by traveling from seaport to seaport (Derbis 1996). During the siege of Kaffa (the present-day city of Feodosia in Ukraine), the Tartars flung dead plague victims over the city's wall, spreading the disease throughout the city. The plague took a large toll on everyone involved, including the Tartars, so they lifted the siege. Among the first places that refugees from Kaffa landed was Genoa, Italy, from which the plague spread throughout the Italian peninsula and across the entire continent of Europe.

Deliberate transmission of disease through contamination of water, as well as through fomites (objects) such as blankets or clothing, has also occurred in history. For instance, the retreating US Confederate forces in 1864 contaminated the water supply of their pursuers by driving sick farm animals into ponds and shooting them.

FOR EXAMPLE

Biological Warfare in the Americas

A famous story of biological weapon use is that of the Spanish conquistador Francisco Pizarro, who in 1533, during his conquest of what is now Peru, is said to have spread smallpox (an unknown disease in South America at that time) by dispensing infected clothing to the natives. This tactic was also used again in the French and Indian War in North America during the 1750s. As the Native Americans gained strength in this war, a commander-in-chief of the British forces devised a plan to offer blankets from Fort Pitt's smallpox hospital to the Native American fighters besieging the fort as a peace offering. Within months, it was reported that smallpox was raging in the Ohio River Valley and that the direct threat of the local Indian tribes had dissipated (Jones 2007).

During World War I, in addition to the chemical warfare mentioned previously, soldiers on both sides tried to spread diseases of horses (glanders) to devastate enemy cavalry. Fifty thousand horses in the French Army alone were infected with this condition. Because the mortality and morbidity of the disease rendered horses incapable of performing service, this was a serious and costly problem.

Biological weapon research was extensively carried out during World War II, but such weapons were not used in major battles. For instance, England developed anthrax as a weapon against beef and dairy cattle in an operation called "Operation Vegetarian." The anthrax was packed in five million "cakes" to be dropped over grazing livestock in Germany, thus further demoralizing the already starving population. The island of Gruinard, which was used for testing the anthrax, was so contaminated that it was off-limits until the late 1980s. The conventional military campaign known as "Operation Overlord" was so successful at hastening the end of the war that Operation Vegetarian was never deployed. It is also suspected that the use of air power and the potential of seeing chemical or biological weapons rained down upon populations of soldiers or civilians kept leaders from using these weapons on each other.

More recent cases of biological weapons use since World War II have included the use of ricin as an assassination weapon in London in 1978 and the accidental release of anthrax spores in Sverdlovsk in 1979. In the London incident, the ricin was delivered via a capsule in an umbrella. The victim was injected with the tiny pellet while waiting for a bus. The assassination technology was supplied by the Soviet Union.

In late September of 2001, just weeks after the terrorist attacks of September 11, a series of anthrax-tainted letters mailed in the United States caused the evacuation of government offices and disruption of the US Postal Service. Members of the Congress were targeted, but none were harmed. However, 5 people died and 22 became sick. The first victim of handling the anthrax-tainted mail was a clerk at a small newspaper in Boca Raton, Florida. The tainted mail was traced to post offices in Florida; New York; Washington, DC; New Jersey; and Connecticut. Some post office facilities in Washington, DC, were closed for over a year (NPR 2011). People were quarantined, mail was microwaved, and radiation was used at some postal centers. The antibiotic Cipro was given to a large number of potentially exposed people in Florida; New York; Washington, DC; New Jersey; and Connecticut as a prophylactic against possible exposure. The perpetrator was never brought to justice. The attack remains the most recent real-life illustration of how biological weapons can be used as weapons of mass disruption, killing a few while generating profound fear, draining resources, and compromising the function of daily life and American institutions.

9.2.2 Biological Agents and Their Effects

Biological agents can harm all forms of life, including people, animals, and plant life/agriculture. There are many biological agents that exist today, both in natural form and in research laboratories throughout the world. They range from bacteria to viruses to toxins and may be formulated into powders, solids, liquids, or aerosols for purposes of weaponization. A list of major biological agents of traditional concern is found in Table 9-1.

The conduct of a biological weapon attack may not be immediately detected due to incubation periods and the inability of medical personnel to properly diagnose symptoms once they appear. For example, cutaneous anthrax, which infects by penetrating the skin, has an incubation period of up to 7 days. Inhalation of anthrax is rarely diagnosed in time for effective treatment, causing a high mortality rate. According to the Federation of American Scientists, "an epidemic of inhalation anthrax in its early stage with nonspecific symptoms could be confused with a wide variety of viral, bacterial, and fungal infections" (FAS n.d.).

Only when enough people fall sick to a disease, with common symptoms, does the medical alert system kick in, allowing for the proper diagnosis, treatment, and containment of the disease. Since 9/11, the medical profession has taken notice of the threat of biological agents being used by terrorists, and many hospitals across the country are conducting exercises for their personnel to better detect a possible biological outbreak and respond in a timely and appropriate manner. New and extensive challenges remain, however, as discussed in the next section.

Table 9-1: Biological Agents

Common name	Scientific name
Bacterial agents	
Anthrax	Bacillus anthracis
Brucellosis	Brucella spp
Glanders and melioidosis	Burkholderia mallei, Burkholderia pseudomallei
Plague	Yersinia pestis
Q-fever	Coxiella burnetii
Tularemia	Francisella tularensis
Viral agents	
Smallpox	Variola virus
Venezuelan equine encephalitis	Alphavirus
Viral hemorrhagic fevers	Hemorrhagic fever virus
Biological toxins	
Botulinum	N/A
Ricin	N/A
Staphylococcal enterotoxin B	N/A
Mycotoxins	N/A

Source: From Anderson (2008).

9.2.3 The Threat of Biological Weapons and Terrorism

As with chemical weapons, the international community's response to biological weapons has been to seek a ban on their production and use. Although the 1925 Geneva Convention Protocols recognized the need for a restriction on the use of biological weapons on the battlefield, it wasn't until 1972 that the United Nations drafted the Biological Weapons Convention (BWC), seeking to end the production and use of such weapons. The United States signed the BWC in 1972; however, President Nixon had already unilaterally ended the US offensive biological weapon program in 1969, vowing then to never use biological weapons. The United States subsequently destroyed its stockpiles of biological weapons. The **US Army Medical Research Institute of Infectious Diseases (USAMRIID)**, located at Ft. Detrick, Maryland, continues to research biological weapons and their use, maintaining small strains of agents for the strict purpose of developing defenses against such weapons.

Fewer countries developed biological weapons than developed chemical weapons. Two noteworthy countries that developed offensive BW capabilities are the Soviet Union/Russia and Iraq. The Soviet Union had an offensive BW program for over 15 years in contravention of the BWC. Its successor state, Russia, cooperated with the United States in the 1990s and early 2000s to dismantle its bioweapons arsenal, but the thoroughness of this disarmament remains uncertain. The BWC lacks the institutionalized support for monitoring, verification, and assistance that the OPCW provides to the CWC regime. It relies more deeply on the good faith of its signatories.

Iraq is another country that made noteworthy biological weapons development efforts after the 1975 entry into force of the BWC. According to defectors and former Iraqi regime officials, Baghdad began an offensive BW production effort in 1985. It produced and tested anthrax, botulinum toxin, aflatoxin, and ricin in the run-up to the January 1991 Gulf War (Nuclear Threat Initiative 2012). Concern over continued Iraqi bioweapons programs—partially driven by fabricated intelligence about mobile BW labs—contributed to the decision to invade Iraq in 2003. Despite the misinterpretation and exaggeration of the threat that Saddam Hussein's WMD programs posed in 2003, UN inspectors consistently voiced skepticism that Iraq had declared the totality of its BW stockpile in the 1990s. The Iraq Survey Group (ISG), an American body commissioned to evaluate the presence of WMD in Iraq after the fall of Saddam, similarly hedged in its report on the status of Iraq's BW arsenal. Though most of its bioweapons and weaponizable materials seem to have been destroyed during the 1990s, Iraq's biological weapons have not been verified as having been completely dismantled. Rudiments of the program may remain. Complications in verifying the status of BW during the occupation of Iraq included the large size of the country, the lack of security and strong governance, and the destruction of many records of the Saddam Hussein regime.

The current Russian and Iraqi governments are not expected to purposefully employ biological weapons, but the possibility cannot be discounted that terrorists could acquire BW-related agents, supplies, and blueprints that are legacies of these countries' programs. Doing so, however, would be hardly necessary for a terrorist to perpetrate a biological weapons attack on the United States. Developments in biotechnology and bioengineering have opened the door to would-be bioterrorists to develop deadly agents in their own laboratories. In 2003, the Human Genome Project completed the first full sequencing of human DNA. The project revealed how the human body was biologically engineered. It was but one watershed in the scientific progression toward the ability to genetically engineer biological organisms. Another watershed—with implications for bioweapons—occurred in 2010, when biologist J. Craig Venter engineered a virus based on the phi X174 genomic code. Phi X174 is a virus that infects bacteria. Venter's team inserted their man-made DNA into an artificial bacterial cell and watched as it came alive and replicated.

Venter's project is an example of **synthetic biology**, a technology by which biologists can use DNA sequencing data to modify and even create biological agents and organisms. As Laurie Garrett of the Council on Foreign Relations puts it, "the biologist has become an engineer, coding new life forms as desired"

(Garrett 2013). DNA sequences are data, much like the ones and zeros used in computing. If you arrange the ones and zeros differently, different outcomes are produced. A terrorist skilled in synthetic biology could acquire DNA sequencing code for harmful agents and insert that code into harmless bacteria, producing deadly organisms virtually from scratch. In 2006, the British newspaper *The Guardian* successfully purchased a small segment of the smallpox genome (DNA sequence) and had it delivered to a post office box. Open and black markets in genetic data—not just the activities of elite government labs—constitute a target for monitoring, regulation, and defense.

While the tighter control of not just biological agents but also genetic coding may seem an obvious imperative, managers of the issue must grapple with the culture of sharing that predominates in the natural sciences. An example illustrates the tension between security and sharing quite well. In 2011, scientists modified the H5N1 flu, commonly known as bird flu, into a possible human-to-human agent. Ron Fouchier, one of the scientists, deemed the resultant virus "very dangerous." The US National Institutes of Health convened an advisory board that urged the scientific journals *Nature* and *Science* to withhold publication of Fouchier's and another scientist's papers so as to deny terrorists the deadly recipe they had concocted. The papers were published by these journals anyway in 2012 (Garrett 2013).

The free flow of scientific data is presumed to be beneficial overall, as scientists learn from each other's mistakes and build upon each other's successes for the ostensible good of humanity. But the democratization and proliferation of highly empowering data poses increasing threats as well. Terrorists could now more literally play God by engineering bioweapons from strings of data and the *Escherichia coli* used in high school and college science classes everywhere.

Codes of conduct are emerging within the scientific community to manage the problem of dual-use biotechnology, including the vetting of purchasers of gene sequences. Such emergent norms remain a thin layer of defense, however. Future regulations may require stricter tagging and accounting. Says Garrett, "[t]he trade in genomic sequences should be transparent and traceable" (Garrett 2013).

Challenges for terrorists remain, of course. These include recruiting scientifically adept partners, engineering, handling, and dissemination. Delivery methods could include the fomites of the past, human carriers, insect carriers, and weapons systems such as rockets, aerial bombs, and spray tanks. If successful, terrorists could mount a devastating attack. Millions could die, and communities and infrastructure could be paralyzed. The US Congress' Office of Technology Assessment offers one such horrific scenario. It estimates that 100 kg of aerosolized anthrax released from a low-flying aircraft over a large city on a clear, calm night could kill one to three million people.

Terrorists know the destructive and disruptive potential of biological weapons and have looked into acquiring or developing them. For example, British security arrested a Pakistani microbiologist in 2000 for seeking biological samples and equipment for use in an al-Qaeda bioweapons plot. As scientific advances empower more people, a terrorist BW attack will become a more plausible threat to the US homeland. It is an issue that requires the attention of policymakers, regulators, and intelligence and homeland security operators.

FOR EXAMPLE

Terrorist Ideas and Their Potential Impact

From 2013 to 2016, West Africa experienced the worst Ebola outbreak in its history. More than 10 000 people died, according to the Centers for Disease Control and Prevention (CDC). Ebola delivers a miserable death by internal bleeding. It is contracted by coming into contact with the bodily fluids of a host or by being bitten by a bat carrying the virus. Its mortality rate exceeds 90%, and there is no cure. During this outbreak period, a laptop was retrieved from an IS hideout in Tunisia. The laptop contained documents advocating for and instructing jihadists in the execution of a biological attack. Among the trove was a set of instructions for weaponizing bubonic plague. In October 2014, jihadist websites began openly discussing the possibility of using Ebola in an attack against the West. Meanwhile, members of blue ribbon commissions in the United States, including former Senator Jim Talent and former Secretary of Homeland Security Tom Ridge, warned that the federal government is under-prepared to respond to a biological weapons attack. Problems include a lack of clarity over jurisdiction and a lack of diagnostic tests and vaccines for likely bioweapons agents (Vicinanzo 2015).

SELF-CHECK

- **Which of the following is not classified as a biological agent?**
  a. Sarin
  b. Ricin
  c. Viruses
  d. Bacteria
- **What is the USAMRIID?**
- **Russia has verifiably dismantled all of the biological weapons built by the Soviet Union. True or false?**
- **Define synthetic biology.**

9.3 Nuclear and Radiological Weapons and Their Consequences

Nuclear terrorism and the use of **radiological weapons** (weapons consisting of radiological material) arguably produce more fear than scenarios involving the other WMD discussed previously. There are a few reasons:

▲ A nuclear weapon explosion is much more powerful than any conventional explosive, conjuring images of Hiroshima and Nagasaki.

▲ Even a crude radiological attack could result in contamination that would last longer than biological or chemical contamination and thus cause greater disruption through the disabling of critical nodes.

▲ Health effects can be long lasting, delayed, and incurable.

Before 9/11, we tended to think of nuclear incidents in terms of accidents at nuclear facilities. The effects of the 1986 Chernobyl accident are still very visible in the environment surrounding the Chernobyl nuclear power plant in Ukraine (see Figure 9-1). Three Mile Island, near Harrisburg, Pennsylvania, is another nuclear accident that plays a large part in our perception of nuclear power gone awry, though there were no lasting environmental effects from that incident in 1979. Incidents like these are still of concern in the post-9/11 era, though more for the potential of terrorist sabotage than for the potential of additional accidents. Another area of major concern is the use of nuclear material in a bomb—whether an actual nuclear weapon that generates massive devastation by triggering a nuclear reaction or a more rudimentary radiological weapon (**dirty bomb**) that uses conventional force to disperse radiological materials that could kill, contaminate, and terrorize.

Figure 9-1

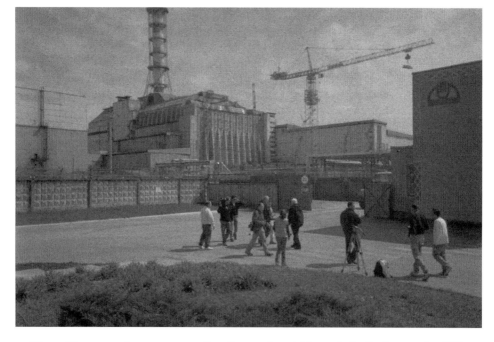

View of the sarcophagus surrounding the reactor at Chernobyl, Ukraine, on the 20th anniversary of the disaster in 2006. Source: Photo courtesy of Richard Kilroy (2006), Photograph [Chernobyl Nuclear Site, Ukraine], personal collection.

> ## FOR EXAMPLE
>
> ### The Chernobyl Nuclear Accident
>
> The worst nuclear power accident in history occurred on April 26, 1986, in Chernobyl, Ukraine, which was at that time part of the USSR. The accident was caused by human error, as engineers at the plant ignored safety procedures while going through a series of tests on reactor number 4, leading to a chain reaction in the reactor core, a massive explosion, and a partial meltdown. At least 30 people died in the initial explosion and exposure, and over 135 000 were exposed to excessive radiation as the first responders (called liquidators) tried to contain the damage. The nearby city of Pripyat (50 000 residents) had to be evacuated. Today, Pripyat remains a ghost town, and the entire area within 30 km of the accident site remains mostly uninhabited.
>
> The exact health effects of the Chernobyl disaster remain in dispute. Official International Atomic Energy Agency (IAEA) reports state that only 56 deaths can be directly attributed to the accident, while groups like Greenpeace put the figure in the tens of thousands. Regardless of this disagreement, the accident directly impacted the growth of nuclear power sources both in the United States and abroad, as many nations considered the benefits of cheap energy to not be worth the risk of a nuclear accident.

9.3.1 Radiological Materials and Their Effects

Fissile material is capable of sustaining a nuclear fission chain reaction—the mechanism used in nuclear detonations. The fissile materials used in nuclear weapons are **highly enriched uranium (HEU)** and **plutonium**. The control of these radioactive fissile materials is thus central to global and homeland security. HEU and plutonium stockpiles exist throughout the world, although bomb construction requires technical skill that cannot be taken for granted. Besides HEU and plutonium, nearly 40 radioactive elements have been discovered, some of which could be accessed and used in a radiological "dirty bomb" attack.

Before proceeding any further, let us answer a few questions about nuclear material and radioactivity. First, *what do we mean by radioactive?* Let's use uranium to illustrate. Radioactive isotopes (types of atoms) are created by nuclear fission (breakdown) of the natural element uranium-235 (U-235). Radiation is produced as particles are lost. Thus, the term **radioactive** refers to materials that give off atomic particles and produce radiation energy at a certain rate (Anderson 2008).

Second, what are the health effects of exposure to radiation? All exposure for humans carries at least a small risk of damage to health. Exposure to routine, natural background radiation encountered in daily life is too insignificant to harm most people. However, radiological emergencies such as nuclear plant failures or terror attacks may expose people to a dangerous, widely varying amount of radiation, depending upon the nature of the incident, the type of radiation involved, and even the weather. When assessing the amount of exposure in any situation, a number of factors must be considered, including the following:

▲ The nature of the radiation
▲ The strength of the source
▲ The biological sensitivity of the exposed area
▲ Exposure factors such as time, distance, and shielding from the source

Calculating these factors is called a dose assessment (Anderson 2008). Doses of human-absorbed radiation are measured in a unit called a gray (Gy). According to the Mayo Clinic,

> [s]igns and symptoms of radiation sickness usually appear when the entire body receives an absorbed dose of at least 1 Gy. Doses greater than 10 Gy to the whole body are generally not treatable and usually lead to death within two days to two weeks. (Mayo Clinic n.d.)

Table 9-2 shows signs and symptoms of radiation sickness. Early symptoms may subside, creating the illusion that the person is no longer sick, but additional symptoms may manifest later. More information on handling the health implications of a radiological attack can be found in Section 9.3.4.

Third, the basic question is how do nuclear weapons work? When a nuclear bomb is exploded, the **fissile material** experiences a chain reaction of rapid nuclear changes (either fission or fusion of atomic nuclei), resulting in the release of several types of radiation. After the blast energy is released, a shock wave and fierce wind are produced, and radioactive particles are spread throughout the blast area and into the air. The particles can travel worldwide from any nuclear explo-

Table 9-2: Signs and Symptoms of Radiation Sickness

	Mild exposure (1–2 Gy)	Moderate exposure (2–6 Gy)	Severe exposure (6–9 Gy)	Very severe exposure (10 Gy or higher)
Nausea and vomiting	Within 6 h	Within 2 h	Within 1 h	Within 10 min
Diarrhea	—	Within 8 h	Within 3 h	Within 1 h
Headache	—	Within 24 h	Within 4 h	Within 2 h
Fever	—	Within 3 h	Within 1 h	Within 1 h
Dizziness and disorientation	—	—	Within 1 week	Immediate
Weakness, fatigue	Within 4 weeks	Within 1–4 weeks	Within 1 week	Immediate
Hair loss, bloody vomit and stools, infections, poor wound healing, low blood pressure	—	Within 1–4 weeks	Within 1 week	Immediate

Source: From Mayo Clinic (n.d.).

sion depending on winds and weather. The size of the bomb can range from the size of those used in Nagasaki (21 kt, known as "Fat Man") and Hiroshima (15 kt, known as "Little Boy") to thermonuclear bombs that pack a punch of over 50 Mt (Anderson 2008). A radiological "dirty bomb" does not use the energy of an atomic chain reaction to produce an explosion. Instead, conventional explosives are used to produce a blast that disseminates radioactive material. The impact of such a bomb would be less than the impact of a true nuclear weapon but could expose large numbers of people to harmful radiation and cause subsequent sickness.

9.3.2 History of Nuclear Material Discoveries and Weapons Development

Sources place the beginning of the "Atomic Age" in 1895, with the discovery of X-rays by Wilhelm Roentgen of Germany (Atomic Archive n.d.). One year later, in 1896, French physicist Antoine Henri Becquerel discovered radioactivity. In his experiments, he found that uranium could produce "rays" that would pass through paper and glass to darken a photographic plate and that these rays possessed an electric charge. Then, in 1897, J. J. Thomson of Britain discovered the electron, and in 1899 Ernest Rutherford discovered two kinds of rays emitting from radium: alpha and beta rays. Thus, at the end of the 1890s, the "Nuclear Age" was well under way.

In the 1900s, further parts of the nuclear picture were discovered. Radioactive decay theory was published by Ernest Rutherford and Frederick Soddy, who also coined the word "isotope." The discovery of natural radioactivity won Becquerel and Pierre and Marie Curie a Nobel Prize in 1904. In 1905, Albert Einstein published the special theory of relativity ($E=mc^2$). By 1919, Rutherford was credited with inducing the first artificial nuclear reaction by bombarding nitrogen gas with alpha particles, thus obtaining atoms of an oxygen isotope along with protons.

By the end of the 1920s, Heisenberg, Max Born, and Schrodinger had formulated quantum mechanics and the uncertainty principle. The cyclotron was developed, and atomic transmutations (nuclear reactions) became much easier to create. In the 1930s, this equipment, along with a high-voltage accelerator, was used to discover deuterium, and in 1934 Enrico Fermi unknowingly achieved the world's first nuclear fission using these past discoveries. By 1939, President Franklin D. Roosevelt learned that Einstein had suggested the possibility of a weapon using uranium fission. Fusion was also recognized as a source of the sun's energy in the same year.

In the 1940s, German scientists also began conducting tests of nuclear fission, with the goal to produce a fission weapon. In 1941, American physicists confirmed that a newly discovered element, plutonium, was fissionable and usable for a bomb. In December of the same year, President Roosevelt authorized the secret Manhattan Engineering Project, later to be called the Manhattan Project, to build a nuclear bomb.

By 1945, a successful test of the first atomic bomb, the Trinity test, was carried out in Alamogordo, New Mexico. In August of the same year, "Little Boy," a uranium bomb, was dropped on Hiroshima, Japan. Between 80 000 and 140 000 residents were killed. Three days later, "Fat Man," a plutonium bomb, was dropped on Nagasaki. About 74 000 people were killed. The world gasped at the news. By the end of 1946, the Atomic Energy Commission (AEC) took over the nuclear weapons program from the US Army. Before the end of the decade, the Soviet Union successfully tested its first nuclear weapon.

In the 1950s, hydrogen fusion bombs (thermonuclear bombs), intercontinental ballistic missiles, and atomic-powered submarines were developed. In 1957, the United Nations **International Atomic Energy Agency (IAEA)** was created. This was motivated by the fact that there were now enough nuclear facilities in the world to warrant inspection by a multinational group to ensure that civilian reactors and plants were being used for peaceful purposes. The IAEA is today charged with monitoring compliance with the **Nuclear Nonproliferation Treaty (NPT)** and is often referred to as the United Nations' "nuclear watchdog."

By the end of the 1960s, five countries had nuclear weapons: the United States, USSR, United Kingdom, France, and China. In 1968, in recognition of the danger posed by nuclear weapons proliferation, all but a few of the world's states signed the Nuclear Non-proliferation Treaty, or NPT. The treaty created two classes of states. The five established nuclear powers signed on as nuclear weapon states (NWS). They committed to make good faith efforts toward nuclear disarmament, though no time frame was mandated. All other states signed on as non-nuclear weapon states (NNWS). They committed to not acquire nuclear weapons and to allow international monitoring of all civilian nuclear energy programs on their soil. The IAEA, mentioned earlier, serves this monitoring function. The NPT remains the bedrock of the global nuclear nonproliferation regime. It faces challenges, however. Three states that never signed the NPT have nuclear weapons: Israel, India, and Pakistan. North Korea withdrew in 2003 and is now assessed to have nuclear weapons. Iran remains a member of the NPT as of 2018; it has been suspected since the 1990s of covertly attempting to acquire a nuclear weapon. Other countries that once had clandestine nuclear weapon programs include Iraq, Libya, South Africa, and Syria.

The two largest nuclear powers, the United States and the Soviet Union, conducted a series of arms control negotiations and agreements from the 1970s to the 2000s. Talks initially aimed at slowing the growth of the superpowers' arsenals. Eventually they turned toward reduction. The number of nuclear weapons peaked over 60 000 in the 1980s. The global stockpile of nuclear warheads stood at approximately 15 500 in 2015 (International Panel on Fissile Materials 2015).

9.3.3 The Threat of Nuclear Weapons and Terrorism

The most straightforward way to perpetrate a nuclear attack, including for a terrorist organization, would be to acquire and use an existing nuclear weapon. The approximately 15 500 nuclear warheads that exist today are allocated among nine countries. Russia has the most; North Korea the least. Table 9-3 shows the number of warheads in each country as of 2016.

The US government has long been concerned about terrorists acquiring a nuclear warhead. Post-Cold War instability in Russia prompted worry about "loose nukes" from the former Soviet Union. Uncertainty about the loyalties of military and intelligence personnel in Pakistan raises the specter of Pakistani warheads falling into the hands of Islamist terrorists. Concern that "rogue states" would pursue nuclear covert action through terrorist allies helped prompt a war against Iraq in 2003 and talk of war against Iran. Even where no sympathies lie with criminals and terrorists, the physical security of warhead and fissile material stockpiles can vary and may be a cause for concern across the globe.

Table 9-3: 2016 Estimated Global Nuclear Warhead Inventories

Country	Warheads
Russia	7300
United States	7100
France	300
China	260
United Kingdom	215
Pakistan	140
India	110
Israel	80
North Korea	8

Source: Data from Arms Control Association (2016a).

Besides acquiring an existing weapon, a terrorist organization may attempt to build its own. This would be difficult, but it is not implausible. Countries such as Libya and Iran have encountered many technical difficulties in their efforts to acquire nuclear weapons. Still, nuclear experts express concern about the potential for non-state actors to achieve what even some states have not. The International Panel on Fissile Materials (IPFM), an independent group of experts on nuclear proliferation with members from 17 countries, assesses that a bomb design of the type used by the United States on Hiroshima may be within the capability of terrorist groups.

As previously noted, fissile material is the radioactive fuel needed for a nuclear weapon. The fissile materials used in nuclear weapons are highly enriched uranium-235, or HEU, and plutonium-239. HEU is created by spinning low-enriched uranium (LEU) in machines called centrifuges, which separate the U-235 isotope useful for weapons from the more common U-238 isotope. A concentration of about 90% U-235 is considered bomb grade, although a smaller and cruder weapon could be made with uranium enriched to 20%—the level to which Iran enriched prior to the Joint Comprehensive Plan of Action (JCPOA), an agreement that limited its nuclear program in 2015. HEU may be used for civilian applications, but most peaceful uses of uranium only require a low level of enrichment (about 5%). Such LEU could be used in a dirty bomb radiological attack. In short, the more highly enriched the uranium, the more potent a nuclear detonation it could cause. Plutonium, meanwhile, is a by-product of the irradiation of uranium in nuclear reactors. The American nuclear bomb dropped on Nagasaki was a plutonium weapon. India, Pakistan, and North Korea are assessed to use plutonium for at least some of their nuclear weapons.

Acquiring fissile material—either HEU or plutonium—is crucial to any attempt to craft one's own nuclear weapon. These fissile materials would also be strong candidates for use in a dirty bomb radiological attack should insufficient quantities of fissile material, low uranium enrichment grade, or inadequate know-how prevent the manufacture of a chain-reaction weapon. The global disposition of fissile materials is thus an important place to look for indications of the potential threat of a nuclear or radiological attack. How much fissile material is there, and where is it?

The IPFM estimates that "the global fissile material stockpile today is sufficient for more than 200 000 simple implosion-type fission nuclear weapons, each with an explosive yield exceeding those of the Hiroshima and Nagasaki weapons" (IPFM 2015). Uranium is more plentiful than plutonium. The global stockpile of HEU at the end of 2014 was about 1370 tons. The overwhelming majority of this is in the nuclear weapon states. However, a total of 27 non-nuclear weapon states possess about 15 total tons of HEU, and highly enriched uranium is used in civilian reactors in over 100 locations worldwide. The vast majority of uranium used in the civilian nuclear programs of the NPT's non-nuclear weapon states, or NNWS, is provided by the nuclear weapon states, or NWS. Only 11 countries worldwide have civilian uranium enrichment programs, one of which is Iran. The fact that most countries purchase and use uranium enriched in the NWS creates doubts about Iran's claim that it needs an independent enrichment capability to fulfill its civilian nuclear needs. The 2015 Joint Comprehensive Plan of Action (JCPOA), an agreement between Iran and world powers led by the United States, significantly reduced Iran's stockpile of uranium. Under the agreement, Iran kept only about 600 lbs. (300 kg) of LEU and shipped 25 000 lbs.—much of it enriched to 20%—to Russia for down-blending and safekeeping. Meanwhile, the deal allowed Iran to continue enriching small quantities of uranium, but only to 3.7% U-235 for 15 years. Most assessments of Iran suggest that it seeks the latent ability to rapidly build and deploy a nuclear weapon. This is known as a "breakout capability." Some politicians, activists, and analysts suggest that Iran would supply a nuclear weapon to a terrorist organization. Such behavior would be consistent with its routine use of terrorist proxies during the life of the Islamic Republic. However, most Iran experts assess the theocratic regime as too pragmatic and cautious to employ nuclear weapons either directly or through terrorists.

Pakistan, another country that raises terrorism concerns, is estimated to have a stockpile of 3 tons of HEU as of 2015. It also likely possesses about 200 kg of plutonium. The global stockpile of plutonium in 2015 was about 500 tons according to the IPFM. About half of this has been produced for weapons, and about 98% resides in the NWS. Increased production of both HEU and plutonium is likely in the coming years in Pakistan, India, and North Korea. Precisely measuring their fissile material stockpiles is and will likely remain difficult due to their not being members of the NPT. Israel's stockpile is likewise hard to precisely measure. Despite proliferation to these countries, the overall amount of global fissile material has declined since the United States and Russia began reducing their nuclear stockpiles in the 1990s. The United States retains approximately 40 tons of HEU to be down-blended under existing agreements.

Clearly, global fissile material stocks are extensive. While many are under reliable safeguards, a clear possibility exists that terrorists could illicitly acquire fissile material through theft, collaboration with government or military insiders, or covert state sponsorship. The target quantities for generating a nuclear detonation are 35 lbs. of uranium-235 or 9 lbs. of plutonium-239. Deadly and disruptive effects could be achieved with less, however.

A theft or black market sale of these ready-made materials to terrorists is probably the most serious nuclear terrorism threat to the world today. Nuclear proliferation expert Matthew Bunn calls the security measures in place at dozens of HEU and plutonium storage sites around the world "dangerously inadequate, amounting in some cases to no more than a night watchman and a chain-link fence" (Bunn 2009). The illicit acquisition of HEU or plutonium would be the biggest step required for terrorists to build a nuclear bomb. A study by Congress's Office of Technology Assessment determined that

> a small group of people, none of whom [has] ever had access to the classified literature, could possibly design and build a crude nuclear explosive device…Only modest machine-shop facilities that could be contracted for without arousing suspicion would be required. (Bunn 2009)

Any radioactive material, including low-level waste from medical facilities, could also be used in a dirty bomb. Examples are technesium-99m, iodine-131, and tritium H_3. Cleanup and reentry into the affected area after a dirty bomb explosion would be a long process. Because terrorists are interested in disrupting (if not destroying) societies, this would appear to be an attractive option. It would be relatively limited, yet extremely disruptive.

Should terrorists succeed in acquiring or assembling a nuclear weapon abroad, they would face the challenge of transporting it into the United States. One option they may pursue is to place such a bomb on a container or cargo ship and detonate it upon arrival in a major port. Given terrorists' historical propensity to use aircraft, placing a nuclear or radiological bomb on an inbound flight cannot be discounted either. Fissile material may be easier to smuggle into the United States than an assembled bomb but still faces the challenge of detection by special monitoring equipment. Port and border security are essential to homeland defense. Its value and importance includes attentiveness to the threat of infiltrated fissile materials so as to dissuade terrorists from even attempting such an operation.

Finally, instead of detonating a bomb, terrorists may attempt to sabotage nuclear facilities inside the United States. There are 100 commercial nuclear power reactors licensed to operate within the United States as of 2018; most are located in densely populated parts of the Midwest and East Coast. One method of attack would be aerial, such as flying a small plane into a nuclear facility. Emergent UAV technology might also present a threat. And as cyber threats emerge, terrorists or other enemies may try to perpetrate remote kinetic attacks on American nuclear facilities. Using the Stuxnet virus in the early 2010s, the United States and Israel physically damaged Iran's uranium centrifuges (see Chapter 8). Terrorists may similarly try to damage nuclear facilities—but on a far greater level and for the purpose of taking human life.

9.3.4 Managing Radiological Incidents and Their Aftermath

A tremendous explosion, high winds, heat, and a "mushroom cloud" would indicate a true fission or fusion weapon attack. However, the first thing those who experienced a nuclear attack in Japan remember is the bright, blinding light (Takakura 2010). This is the least likely method of terrorist radiological attack according to most experts. The second and more likely attack would be the use of a conventional explosive with a "dirty" radioactive package included. Radioactive material would thus be scattered across the debris field. Victims would be killed or injured by the explosion, and people and the environment would be contaminated by the radioactive material to a distance that would depend on the size of the explosion and the weather patterns at the site. Detection of the radiation in an attack by a dirty bomb might be delayed until emergency personnel with detection devices arrived.

To prepare for either type of attack, the first defense, if there is warning, would be to seek shelter from the blast. The penetration ability of blast fire and radiation can be deflected by terrain features such as hills, mountains, fallen trees, caves, or a good foxhole. Quickly seeking the best shelter available in the case of a brief warning is the best a person can do in the case of a nuclear blast. Reinforced concrete structures offer the most protection, followed by reinforced masonry brick houses, and finally other structures. Once inside a structure, getting below ground can reduce radiation by a factor of 10 (Couch 2003). The "duck and cover" drill of the 1950s remains a simple rule of action that is still pertinent today following warning of a nuclear attack.

Immediately following a nuclear attack or a radiological dirty bomb explosion (if it is detected), emergency personnel and victims must assume radioactive contamination. Covering your mouth with a wet cloth reduces the contaminants entering the body. Unfortunately, radiation sickness symptoms other than nausea and vomiting may not appear until days after exposure. However, medical, military, and hazardous material (HAZMAT) personnel may have personal dosimeters that indicate exposure levels and can be used to predict gamma radiation.

HAZMAT personnel must be relied upon in case of a nuclear blast or a dirty bomb to ensure isolation and decontamination of victims and to evacuate the affected area. Decontamination will involve the following processes:

1. Decontamination of the individual
2. Decontamination of casualties and victims
3. Decontamination of the uninjured public
4. Decontamination of the environment (i.e., filtering drinking water)

Rapid washing of the hair and skin and discarding of clothing can remove 95% of radiological contamination. It is seldom possible for a living patient to contaminate or threaten medical personnel. Therefore, contaminated victims' wounds should be rinsed and cleaned so that particulate material is removed. Any radioactive debris material emitting alpha, gamma, or beta rays can cause extensive local damage in a wound site and could be redistributed in the bloodstream to damage internal organs as well. Usually burns will accompany wounds, and because radioactive materials can be embedded in a charred area, excision of the wound is appropriate. Burn protocols should be observed by medical personnel, except that radioactive debris and tissue should be safely handled and disposed of by radiation technical personnel.

Treatment following a radiological attack would have to include more than just physical medical care and decontamination as described earlier. Treatment of the aftereffects of undetected exposure would require a well-organized network of medical, emergency, public, and military communication. Mental health concerns have also recently been shown to be very important. Communication to the public to combat fear and hysteria would be of paramount importance. As in any emergency situation, whether a natural disaster, an all-out war, or a terrorist attack, a smoothly operating command and control protocol system in civilian and military organizations is critical. Communication to the public should be an integral part of this protocol.

Education of all members of society on risks, actual dangers, current personal protection actions, and family action plans is crucial in preparing against a radiological threat. Locations of local shelters, local emergency communication, medical treatment protocol in radiological emergency situations, and long-term effects are also important preparations that need to be made. Breaking through the apathy of the public regarding the likelihood of a nuclear or radiological attack will be a difficult task but also a critical one. Because of this apathy, the public is not very aware of the special catastrophic effects of a nuclear or radiological attack. In addition, very little information is provided to the public by any level of government. Local health departments, local emergency management offices, and other agencies are consumed with preparations for natural disasters and managing the effects of other environmental hazards. Scenarios for nuclear attack do not have a high priority in preparedness drills because the risk for nuclear attack is lower than for other forms of attack. The proven unpredictability of terrorists, however, should warn us that what seems the most unlikely form of attack is potentially the one that will be next on the terrorist agenda.

SELF-CHECK

- People exposed to very severe levels of radiation show symptoms immediately. True or false?
- Define fissile material.
- Which of the following is the combination of a conventional explosive with radioactive material?
  a. Gray
  b. Fusion bomb
  c. HAZMAT
  d. Dirty bomb
- According to the Arms Control Association, which countries are known to have stockpiles of nuclear weapons?

SUMMARY

But even as Third Wave armies hurry to develop damage-limiting precision weapons and casualty-limiting non-lethal weapons, poorer countries are racing to build, buy, borrow, or burgle the most indiscriminate agents of mass lethality ever created; chemical and biological as well as atomic. Once more we are reminded that the rise of a new war form in no way precludes the use of earlier war forms—including the most virulent weapons.

—Alvin and Heidi Toffler, *War and Anti-War: Survival at the Dawn of the Twenty-first Century* (1993)

Even though the previous passage was written in 1993, these futurist authors predicted the dawn of the terrorist age with an eerie accuracy. According to FEMA, the effect of biological, chemical, and nuclear weapons of mass destruction relies on their punch per pound. To produce the same number of deaths within a square mile, they estimate that it would take 705 000 lbs. of fragmentation cluster bomb material; 7000 lbs. of mustard gas; 1700 lbs. of nerve gas; 11 lbs. of nuclear material in a crude nuclear fission weapon; 3 oz of botulism toxin type A; or half an ounce of anthrax spores. These numbers starkly demonstrate the power of chemical, biological, and nuclear materials as weapons of mass destruction when compared with simple conventional explosives. Explosive devices of all kinds can be used in conjunction with these weapons in innumerable combinations.

In this chapter, you evaluated the types of chemical, biological, and nuclear/radiological weapons and the prospects for their employment. You assessed the availability and applicability of weapons of mass destruction by terrorist groups and estimated the consequences of the use of WMD in creating a catastrophic event. In addition, you assessed the threat of terrorists using WMD and the potential impact on the United States.

Technological developments in the twentieth and now the twenty-first century have generated tremendous hope and possibility for humanity. The nuclear, chemical, and biological fields are essential to human development and the human future. These fields are already playing roles in producing sustainable alternative fuels, reducing food insecurity, and prolonging human life while enhancing its quality. Yet as with the ancient discovery of fire, these fields can also produce great peril and must be handled with extreme care.

The ever-present dark side of human nature, as well as the global security climate in the second decade of the twenty-first century, suggest a real risk that these technologies may be used against rather than for the benefit of humanity. The democratization of knowledge in the Internet age, coupled with the emergence of DIY bioengineering, suggests that a high priority must be placed on vigilance. Responsible governments, including the United States, must manage the intelligence challenge of monitoring the spread and use of WMD-related technologies and detecting their illicit diversion. New generations of professionals in the national and homeland security fields must work to not only understand the evolving WMD threat but also coordinate with each other to ensure that responses to any such future threats or incidents prevent the mass destruction that gives these frightening weapons their name.

KEY TERMS

Biological weapons	Weapons consisting of biological or living organisms or toxins.
CBRNE	An acronym standing for chemical, biological, radiological, or nuclear explosives. Some government agencies use this term instead of WMD.
Chemical weapons	Weapons consisting of toxic or otherwise harmful chemicals not specifically of biological origin.

Dirty bomb	A conventional explosive used to spread radioactive material.
Fissile material	Uranium-235 or plutonium-239, the primary material used to trigger the chain reaction involved in a nuclear explosion.
Highly enriched uranium (HEU)	One of the primary ingredients for building a nuclear bomb.
International Atomic Energy Agency (IAEA)	The United Nations agency charged with inspecting nuclear reactors and power plants throughout the world.
Radiological weapons	Weapons consisting of radiological materials.
Synthetic Biology	The manipulation of DNA to alter or create living organisms.
US Army Medical Research Institute of Infectious Diseases (USAMRIID)	Institute located at Ft. Detrick, Maryland, that researches biological weapons and their use and maintains small strains of agents for the purpose of developing defenses against them.
Weapons of Mass Destruction (WMD)	A phrase commonly used to describe a class of unconventional weapons that can cause massive destruction to populations and infrastructure, including nuclear weapons, chemical weapons, biological weapons, and sometimes ballistic missile delivery vehicles. It is frequently written as the acronym WMD.
Weapons of Mass Disruption	A phrase that suggests WMD can cause great harm without causing great destruction. Mass disruption to life and economic activity can be unleashed by the amateurish use of rudimentary nuclear, radiological, chemical, or biological weapons. Direct casualties may be low, but the political and economic impact may be massive.

ASSESS YOUR UNDERSTANDING

Go to www.wiley.com/go/Kilroy/Threats_to_Homeland_Security to assess your knowledge of the basics of weapons of mass destruction.

Summary Questions

1. The term weapons of mass disruption (WMD) implies that very large numbers of people would die in any attack. True or false?

2. The United States still reserves the right to use biological weapons if attacked with such weapons. True or false?

3. The radiological materials required to construct a dirty bomb are impossible to obtain; thus, the possible use of such a weapon by terrorist organizations is slim. True or false?

4. Which of the following has been used most frequently?
   (a) Chemical weapons
   (b) Nuclear weapons
   (c) Radiological dirty bombs
   (d) Biological weapons

5. Which of the following are fissile materials?
   (a) Plutonium-239
   (b) Uranium-235
   (c) Neither (a) nor (b)
   (d) Both (a) and (b)

6. Which kind of chemical weapon did Syria use against its own people in its civil war?
   (a) Sarin
   (b) Chlorine
   (c) VX
   (d) (a) and (b) only

7. Which of the following are not biological weapons materials?
   (a) Tabun
   (b) Anthrax
   (c) Plague
   (d) West Nile virus

8. What is the first thing you would notice in a nuclear explosion?
   (a) A terrible odor in the air
   (b) A blinding light
   (c) A loud explosion noise
   (d) A mushroom-shaped cloud

9. Which of the following ways can a chemical weapon enter the body?
   (a) Through the lungs
   (b) Through the skin
   (c) Through the blood
   (d) All of the above

10. How can you partly protect yourself from the blast wave from a nuclear explosion?
    (a) Climb a tree
    (b) Get inside a building
    (c) Get in a ravine
    (d) Put on protective clothing

Applying This Chapter

1. You are serving in the State Department on a counter-proliferation task force. What countries would you be most concerned about with regard to developing nuclear weapons in the future? What would be the "indicators" you would be looking for to determine such a capability? What policy options exist for helping deter nations from seeking to develop nuclear weapons capability?

2. In a classroom discussion, another student makes the point that nuclear terrorism is not a serious concern in the United States because it would be virtually impossible to smuggle a nuclear weapon into the country. How would you respond? What other scenarios would you offer of methods—other than the use of a nuclear bomb—that terrorists could use to create a WMD effect within the United States?

3. Your local community is planning a training exercise to prepare for a possible biological terrorism incident. What considerations would you recommend including for such an exercise? What local agencies and individuals would your include in this exercise? Why?

4. There is no international organization like the IAEA or the OPCW to monitor compliance with the Biological Weapons Convention. If one were established, what sorts of activities would it have to monitor and regulate?

5. CBRNE agents require a delivery mechanism. What are some delivery vehicles that might pose a threat? Are there any widely available consumer products, such as quadcopter drones, that might pose a risk? Should any consumer products be regulated in order to help reduce the threat of a terrorist or lone-wolf WMD attack?

How to Build a Bioweapon

Research the latest developments in Do-It-Yourself (DIY) synthetic biology. Figure out what you would need to create a biological weapons agent in your garage. What kind of biological weapons agent might be the easiest to create and use in a terrorist attack?

Radiological Sources

Analyze the availability of sources of radiological material that could be used in the construction of a dirty bomb. Identify countries where such sources exist and evaluate the nature of the safeguards employed to protect these sources. What policy recommendations would you make for the United States to help countries do a better job of protecting these sources of radiation?

10

DOMESTIC TERRORISM
Understanding the Role of Law Enforcement and the Nexus between Crime and Terrorism

Daniel Masters
International Studies, University of North Carolina, Wilmington, NC, USA

Starting Point

Go to www.wiley.com/go/Kilroy/Threats_to_Homeland_Security to assess your knowledge of the basics of domestic terrorism.
Determine where you need to concentrate your effort.

What You'll Learn in This Chapter

▲ The nature of the domestic terrorist threat facing the United States, including the unique challenge of leaderless resistance
▲ The problem of convergence between terrorist organizations and criminal organizations and the challenges this presents to law enforcement
▲ The nature of counterterrorism in the United States including countering violent extremism

After Studying This Chapter, You Will Be Able To

▲ Assess the different types of terrorist threats, including that of lone wolves
▲ Evaluate the domestic terrorist threat facing the United States
▲ Judge countering violent extremism (CVE) for its value and detriments
▲ Critically evaluate the rule of law foundations for US counterterrorism policies

Threats to Homeland Security: Reassessing the All-Hazards Perspective, Second Edition.
Edited by Richard J. Kilroy, Jr.
© 2018 John Wiley & Sons, Inc. Published 2018 by John Wiley & Sons, Inc.
Companion website: www.wiley.com/go/Kilroy/Threats_to_Homeland_Security

INTRODUCTION

On December 2, 2015, Syed Rizwan Farook and Tashfeen Malik went on a shooting spree (and planned bombing) at the Inland Regional Center in San Bernardino, California. The perpetrators were a married couple. Farook was an American-born citizen of Pakistani descent, and Malik was a Pakistani-born lawful permanent resident (Turkewitz and Mueller 2015). The San Bernardino attack is notable for elevating concerns over "homegrown violent extremists." The couple was not radicalized in an overseas training camp and sent to the United States. There is no indication that the couple was directed by a foreign terrorist organization (FTO). They lived and worked in the United States. They radicalized through their own interactions and through access to online content supporting "martyrdom" and "jihadism." The only conclusion left is that radicalization of Americans is possible, and this represents a different layer of threat than we have previously faced in the area of domestic terrorism. The nature of this threat can be termed **leaderless resistance**, known more commonly as "lone-wolf terrorism." As leaderless resistance captures more of our attention, we must be mindful that it is only one part of the profile of terrorism in the United States. The larger profile includes **homegrown terrorist groups (HTGs)** whose members originate within the US borders and conduct operations against targets in the United States. HTGs have existed for a long time and exist in many different forms. Historically HGT has not been considered a dominant threat. However, events like San Bernardino, the Bataclan attack in Paris, *Charlie Hebdo*, Brussels attacks, Nice truck attack, etc. have moved perception of this threat to the forefront. The increased attention to HGTs, though, has not displaced concern over **foreign terrorist organizations (FTOs)** where operatives originate in countries outside the United States and penetrate the network of homeland security to plan and conduct operations against internal targets. Alternatively, we have the **foreign organizers** that include foreign recruiters that penetrate the US security network to raise funds and recruit operatives for operations against the US and other national interests overseas. Taken together, these three areas form the general snapshot of terrorism in the United States.

As terrorist groups flatten their organizations (i.e., move toward networks and leaderless resistance), they make gains in organizational security. The trade-off is increasing interplay between two types of organizations. Specifically we observe increasing interaction between terrorist groups and criminal syndicates. The depths of integration between such organizations are difficult to determine. We are certain of higher rates of interaction and appropriation as terrorist organizations increasingly flatten their structures and encourage cells to become more operationally and financially independent. The convergence of criminal and terrorist organizations does present an enhanced problem for security forces and law enforcement.

The rise in, and attention to, leaderless resistance requires new thinking about how best to counter terrorism. It is no longer feasible to only harden likely targets or tighten border security as a measure against terrorism. Today we need to consider a different type of **counterterrorism policy** (set of laws, agencies, and programs targeted at controlling and reducing terrorist threats) that can effectively address the homegrown terrorists, foreign terrorists, and foreign terrorist organizers. An emerging policy known as **countering violent extremism (CVE)** seeks to pick off radicalized individuals in the planning stages and on a deeper level to counterprogram extremist messages in the "radical milieu." CVE is a version of counterinsurgency premised largely on the strategic goal to isolate terrorists from their supporters and defuse their political message (Kiras 2013). CVE has demonstrated successes, but it has detractors as well. The biggest critique is that CVE employed in the preplanning and planning stages of terrorist events amounts to entrapment. We need to explore CVE completely in order to see where its merits lay.

In this chapter you will learn the context of domestic terrorism beginning with a snapshot of terrorism across space and time from the eighteenth to twenty-first centuries. Next you will analyze leaderless resistance and other dimensions of homegrown terrorism. You will then learn of foreign terrorists and foreign terrorist organizers and the threat they represent, as well as the nexus between organized crime and terrorism and the challenge this poses for law enforcement and counterterrorism policy. Finally, you will review US counterterrorism policy following this discussion with a particular focus on CVE as a mode of reacting to extremist violence in the United States.

10.1 Terrorism in the United States: Across Time and Space

Domestic terrorism in the United States has a long and varied history. It shows geographic variation, and we observe distinct periodicity. There was a peak in activity in the 1970s, followed by a decline in the 1980s. There is a slight rebound in terrorism in the 1990s, and since 2000 we seem to have hit a period of stability, or no dynamic change. Forty-four percent of terrorist activity in the United States takes place in major urban centers, with New York City; Washington, D.C.; and Los Angeles leading the way (Webb and Cutter 2009). What is important to remember is that as much as terrorism has changed in space and time, it has also shifted in content as well. In the 1970s there was a Western focus of terrorism driven by the Weather Underground, Symbionese Liberation Army (SLA), and the Black Panthers. The terrorist groups rose up on the remnants of the civil rights protests and anti-Vietnam social movements. Today terrorism in the United States is most likely to reflect right-wing extremism (usually in the form of white nationalism) and Islamist-inspired lone-wolf terrorism.

10.1.1 Eighteenth- to Twentieth-Century Terrorism

To begin this discussion it is useful to revisit our working definition of terrorism from Chapter 6: "The use of violence directed at civilians to instill fear and coerce other groups that are not the immediate target of the attack." Based on this definition a major terrorist event took place on December 16, 1773, by a group known as the Sons of Liberty. Led by Samuel Adams, a group of men masqueraded as Mohawk Indians and boarded ships owned by the East India Company in Boston Harbor, broke open the tea chests, and threw them into the harbor. The act was conducted in protest of the Tea Act of 1773 that granted the East India Company preferential business rights in the American colonies. This event is heralded as the *Boston Tea Party* that provoked the Coercive Acts, restricting American trade and moving the American colonies closer to its revolution against Britain. Historically this event is treated as a defining moment, an act of patriotism, and a refusal to submit to British domination. However, as discussed in Chapter 6, the definition of terrorism is often subject to the context yielding the adage "one person's terrorist is another's freedom fighter." The Sons of Liberty are treated as freedom fighters in the American context, but by our definition of terrorism, their actions during the Revolutionary War can be seen as examples of terrorism in the United States.

Following the American Revolution popular discontent grew around the weak national government under the Articles of Confederation and in particular the inability of this government to pay its war debts, especially salaries to those who fought in the war. Poor economic conditions in Massachusetts combined with this general discontent led to Shays' Rebellion (1786–1787). A group called the Regulators led by the Revolutionary War veteran and farmer Daniel Shays began by freeing people from the statewide Debtors Prisons and escalated to closing down the Debtors Courts to prevent the state government from seizing land from poor farmers. In the early stages, the rebellion was low key and took the form of protests and demonstrations rather than violence. When the Massachusetts government was able to field a militia to put down the Regulators' revolt, it devolved into guerrilla warfare and terrorism. The rebellion demonstrated the weakness of the American government at the time and led to the Constitutional Convention in 1787 that brought about a new and more stable form of government.

With the renewed stability of the US government established in the 1790s, rebellious and terrorist activity fell off. During the early nineteenth century, the new government settled into its business and defined its new powers. Meanwhile, state governments continued with the detailed duties of regulating social life in the United States. However, the seeds of future conflict were sewn over the issue of slavery and the relative power of state governments versus the national government to regulate, even outlaw, slavery. Political division and accommodation were the order of the day until John Brown's raid on Harpers Ferry, Virginia, in 1859. Brown's army of 18 people took prominent citizens hostage and raided the federal arsenal in Harper's Ferry with the intent to liberate slaves in Virginia and then lead them as an army to liberate all the slaves in the American South. The raid failed, and John Brown's army was decimated. But the event polarized popular opinion over slavery and contributed to the onset of the Civil War (1861–1865) (Griset and Mahan 2003).

Following the Civil War political violence in the United States did not come to an end. Throughout the later nineteenth century, hostilities remained high and were directed toward the Native American population by the US government during the Westward movement (Griset and Mahan 2003). Additionally, there was significant conflict between local and federal government forces against the labor movement in the late nineteenth and early twentieth centuries. The most significant terrorist movement of this period was the Molly Maguires, an organization of Irish immigrants working in the mining industries in Pennsylvania. The organization was formed in Ireland to fight against landlords for tenants' rights. In the United States, they used intimidation and violence against the coal mining industry to ensure equality and employment opportunities for Irish Catholics. The organization finally disbanded in 1877.

At the turn of the twentieth century, a prominent terrorist threat emanated from Europe in the form of the Anarchist Syndicate (a.k.a. the Anarchists). The Anarchists were in many ways the precursors of today's al-Qaeda, as they operated as a loosely allied network of cells throughout Europe and the United States from 1878 to 1914. Their campaign was not centrally planned or coordinated, yet they accomplished much mayhem during their time. The Anarchists routinely bombed cafes, theaters, and parades. Their most notable action was the assassination of President William McKinley in 1901. This assassination is one among a number of heads of state that fell to the Anarchists. From the Anarchist threat the first international conventions against terrorism were conceived. In an agreement known as the Petersburg Protocols (1904), signatories were required to gather information on known Anarchists in their countries and share the information with other signatories. The United States declined to participate in this cooperative arrangement for a number of reasons, primarily the lack of the necessary administrative structures to gather and disperse information to the Protocol's members. In short, the lack of a centralized police or investigative service prohibited US involvement. The Bureau of Investigations (later the Federal Bureau of Investigation (FBI)) would not exist for another five years (Jensen 2010).

At the same time as the Anarchists campaign, terrorism in the rural South rose quickly. In particular the Ku Klux Klan (KKK) ratcheted up a campaign of fear and intimidation against the black population. The KKK had existed since 1865, and its campaign of racist terrorism lasted for much of the time from 1865 to the mid-twentieth century. In conjunction with KKK activities, there were racially motivated events including the Wilmington, North Carolina, Race Riot (1898); the Atlanta Race Riot (1906); the Rosewood, Florida, massacres (1920–1923); and the Tulsa Race Riot (1921). All involved terrorism by white supremacists against the local black populations.

10.1.2 Late Twentieth-Century Terrorism

Following World War II, there was a noticeable lull in terrorist violence in the United States. Racial tensions and lower key racial intimidation continued in the American South, albeit not at the levels seen in the early 1900s. The next evolution of terrorism began in the 1960s through the early 1990s. The confluence of the Civil Rights Movement and the anti-war movement brought about the next wave of terrorism. On the left, groups such as the Weather Underground and the Symbionese Liberation Army (SLA) formed out of the anti-war movement and specifically on the fringes of the Students for a Democratic Society (SDS), a group of students affiliated with the **New Left**, a political movement that takes form following the presentation of *Port Huron Statement* calling for the creation of a participatory democracy in the United States (Roberts 2012). Such groups agitated for an end to the Vietnam War and "democratization" of the United States in a more socialist form. On the fringe of the Civil Rights Movement, we observe groups like the Black Panthers dedicated to racial equality and socialism in the United States. Many of these groups were very short lived, and most of the time their activities were more criminal than political (especially for the SLA). Also, ethno-national terrorism emerged for the first time in the United States in the form of the *Fuerzas Armadas de Liberación Nacional* (Armed Forces of National Liberation or FALN) and *Movimiento Independentista Revolucionario Armado* (Independent Armed Revolutionary Movement or MIRA) of Puerto Rican nationalists dedicated to establishing an independent and socialist Puerto Rico (Griset and Mahan 2003).

In the midst of this terrorist activity, the most active threat came from the anti-Castro Cuban refugee population in Florida and around the United States. Groups like *El Poder Cubano*, Secret Cuban Government, Secret Organization Zero, Omega-7, Cuban Action Commandos, and the Luis Biotel Commandos (among others) conducted numerous terrorist operations in Miami, New York, Washington, Chicago, and Los Angles from the late 1960s to the early 1980s. Cuban terrorist organizations account for 32% of all terrorist activity in the United States from 1968 to 2006 (MIPT 2006). During the late 1970s the anti-Castro Cuban movement devolved into **émigré terrorism** (where a foreign victim is killed by a foreign terrorist group) as various groups engaged in gang-like wars to establish dominance in the United States.

One of the most active groups during the late twentieth century was the Jewish Defense League (JDL). The JDL was founded by Rabbi Meir Kahane in 1968 in New York City and served primarily to protect the Orthodox Jewish population. In the 1970s the group evolved and initiated a campaign of terrorism against targets associated with the Palestinian Liberation Organization (PLO) and Soviet targets in the United States to protest the treatment of Soviet Jews. Kahane left the United States for Israel after the group was founded, but remained the official leader of the JDL until 1985, when the JDL assassinated the leader of the Arab-American Anti-Discrimination Committee. Kahane decided to step down after this event. In 1987, the JDL was infiltrated and many group members were arrested and convicted of various crimes. Since then the JDL has officially abandoned terrorism, but incidents continued, and plots had been uncovered as late as 2002 (MIPT 2006).

Foreign terrorist operations in the United States had been predominantly émigré terrorism similar to that observed in the anti-Castro Cuban movement during the 1970s. From 1978 to the early 1980s, there was a wave of terrorism from the Croatian Freedom Fighters against Croat nationalists in the United States. Also, we observe émigré terrorism among Serbian Nationalists, Taiwanese, Vietnamese, Iranian, and Armenian–Turkish communities. The majority of foreign terrorist attacks in the United States from 1955 to 1998 were émigré terrorist incidents of some form (Hewitt 2000).

In addition to émigré terrorism, foreign terrorist groups penetrated the United States during the early 1970s to conduct operations against US targets. The major foreign terrorist activities during this time involved Palestinian groups like Black September (responsible for the 1972 Munich Olympic kidnappings in Germany) and other Palestinian Liberation Organization (PLO)-based groups. Most activities from the Palestinian groups occurred in 1972–1973 in the wake of the Munich attack. The Japanese Red Army conducted one operation inside the United States in 1988, and the Armenian Secret Army for the Liberation of Armenia (ASALA) conducted two operations, mostly émigré in nature. Random Arab groups have conducted operations as well, including Syrian Socialists and the Liberation Army 5th Battalion responsible for the 1993 World Trade Center bombing (linked to al-Qaeda).

10.1.3 Early Twenty-First-Century Terrorism

As the twentieth century came to a close, there were notable changes taking place in domestic terrorist activity. One is that the numbers of terrorist incidents began a steep decline. This followed the global trend during the late 1980s and 1990s, with a net decline in terrorist incidents. The phenomenon is driven largely by two coalescing events: the collapse of the Soviet Union (causing a drop in ideological terrorism worldwide) and new efforts to negotiate peace settlements in long-standing ethno-national conflicts (e.g., Northern Ireland, Israel–Palestine, and Sri Lanka). These trends were bolstered by law enforcement efforts that infiltrated the anti-Castro Cuban groups and the JDL. Another change we observe is parallel trends in the increasing scale of terrorist attacks (globally and domestically), the rise of ecoterrorism (domestically), a shift in terrorist activity from major urban areas to smaller cities, towns, and suburbs (domestically), and the rise in lone-wolf terrorism and public mass shootings. All these trends coming together suggested a major shift in terrorist activity similar to what we observed beginning in the 1960s with the rise of the New Left.

The new scale of terrorist attacks was first noted in 1993 with the first bombing of the World Trade Center in New York City. The Liberation Army 5th Battalion conducted this operation on February 5, 1993, by planting a high powered car bomb in the parking garage of the World Trade Center in New York detonating it at 12:17 p.m. during lunch when the potential casualty rate could be maximized. Fortunately, the explosive device was not significant enough to cause the damage intended by the terrorists; only six people were killed. The attack had the potential to cause much more damage though. Prior to this attack most terrorist attacks in the United States and abroad tended toward shock value rather than carnage. This particular incident indicated a shift in intended lethality, one that would become the signature feature of terrorism in the late 1990s and early twenty-first century.

At the end of the twentieth and beginning of the twenty-first century, there was a significant debate over the direction of terrorism in the post-Cold War era. Most analysis suggested then, and now, that religious and right-wing terrorism was on the rise (Enders and Sandler 2000; Hoffman 1998). Many believed that white supremacy groups and antiabortion terrorism would dominate the United States in the late 1990s (Carlson 1995). This perception was bolstered by the events of April 19, 1995, when Timothy McVeigh and Terry Nichols detonated a car bomb outside the Alfred P. Murrah Federal Building in Oklahoma City, killing 168 people. This single terrorist attack broke the long-standing record for the deadliest terrorist attack, domestic or international, surpassing the bombing of the King David Hotel in Jerusalem (1946) by the Jewish group Irgun. The Oklahoma City bombing shocked the United States particularly because it was committed by homegrown terrorists, not an foreign terrorist organization. Combining this attack with a slight surge in attacks by white supremacists like the Aryan Nations against immigrants, and the surge in bombings of abortion clinics and assassinations of medical professionals providing abortions, led to the conclusion that right-wing and homegrown terrorism was on the rise. Adding fuel to the fire was the 1996 bombing of the Atlanta Olympics by Eric Rudolph, a person wanted for a series of attacks against abortion clinics in Alabama.

By 1998, the uptick in right-wing extremism was surpassed by the rise of **ecoterrorism**, which involves groups conducting terrorist operations in order to influence domestic policy regarding land development, environmental policy, and animal testing. The Earth Liberation Front (ELF) and the Animal Liberation Front (ALF) were the most active ecoterrorist groups during this time. The ELF alone conducted dozens of arsons and bombings throughout the American West, Midwest, and Virginia. With the rise of the ELF, we note a dramatic shift in terrorist operations away from major urban centers, the traditional battle grounds for terrorism, and into the interior: suburbs and rural areas. This shift reflected the nature of targets for the ELF as it worked to prevent unchecked land development on the fringes of many cities. At the same time, this shift away from the major urban center also meant the ELF and ALF activities often went unnoticed by the larger population. The absence of national media coverage meant most often these events were treated as normal criminal activity rather than a dominant terrorist threat.

The September 11, 2001, attacks by al-Qaeda on the World Trade Center in New York and the Pentagon in Washington, D.C., add to the dimensions of terrorism in the United States during this period. Al-Qaeda is an anti-globalization religious terrorist group dedicated to preserving the sanctity of the Muslim holy sites in Saudi Arabia and the Middle East, and, as part of its campaign, attacked US interests in Saudi Arabia, the Middle East, and the Muslim World. The 9/11 attacks were the first and, to this point, the only successful foray into the US homeland. This single attack surpassed all other terrorist attacks in history as the most destructive in terms of loss of life, injuries, and economic damage. This attack also pushed forth a major shift in US counterterrorism policy that had previously viewed terrorism as an emerging threat, best handled through good policing and prosecution of suspected terrorists, to a major threat to national security best handled through a **war model** (militarization of a terrorist conflict) rather than a **criminal justice model** (police, courts, laws, and prisons). The attack also led the United States to engage in war with Afghanistan (2001) and Iraq (2003). The perception of the dominant terrorist threat to the United States was that of another large-scale al-Qaeda operation.

Meanwhile, since 9/11 we have observed an uptick in violence committed by homegrown extremists, not formally affiliated with any terrorist organization. These "lone wolves" seemed to represent a new terrorist threat to the US landscape; however, the lone-wolf threat had been present. The Oklahoma City bombing (1995) by Timothy McVeigh represented the most noteworthy terrorist attack in US history with the highest casualty rate and highest amount of economic damage caused by a lone-wolf attack. More recently, our attention has moved toward lone wolves due to the increasing number of violent events. We have observed an increase in such lone-wolf attacks by American Muslims since 9/11. Events like the Ft Hood shooting (2009), San Bernardino shooting (2015), the foiled events by Jose Padilla (May 2002) and John Walker Lindh (November 2001), and the Boston Bombing (2013) have captured the attention of many Americans. The idea that a citizen, or US resident, can be so easily radicalized, plan, and commit attacks against other American citizens raises alarms. Lone-wolf terrorism is perceived to be increasing (Alakoc 2015). The actual level of threat is difficult to gauge as attacks and fatalities tend to express aspects of the threat. With regard to fatalities we know lone-wolf terrorism accounts for about 26% of terrorist fatalities in the United States (1978–1999) and 14% of fatalities in Western Europe (1995–2012) (Phillips 2015). However, compared with fatalities of organization-based terrorism, we know that terrorist groups are about 113% more fatal than the lone wolf (Phillips 2015). It is the nature of the attacks, and the difficulty in identifying individuals with only loose affiliations with terrorist organizations abroad, which represent a potentially horrifying prospect for the continuation of such terrorist events in the United States.

A different branch of extremist violence also seems to peak during the same time period as **lone-wolf terrorism**, that of mass public shooters, for example, the Sandy Hook Elementary shooting in Connecticut (2012), the Pulse nightclub shooting in Orlando (2016), the EAME church shooting in Charleston, SC (2015), the Umpqua Community College Shooting (2015), or the Aurora Colorado shooting (2012). The mass public shooter tends to randomly attack strangers and bystanders at specifically symbolic target venues (Lankford 2016). Symbolic meaning of the target (person, or persons, or place) holds meaning to the individual shooter as source of conflict, personal grudge, or trauma (Lankford 2016). In this regard the mass public shooter is difficult to differentiate from lone-wolf terrorists. We often see public officials struggle with how best to define such events when the line between a lone-wolf terrorist and a public mass shooter is difficult to discern. The main demarcation between the lone-wolf terrorist and the mass public shooter is the nature of the target audience. The lone-wolf terrorist is attempting to speak to a larger audience (to instill fear, panic, and terror). The mass public shooter is expressing their violence toward a personal target that holds meaning mostly to themselves (Lankford 2016). Where confusion sets in is when a mass public shooter evokes symbolic statements the leave the impression they are part of a larger conspiracy. For instance, the Pulse nightclub shooter, Omar Mateen, swore allegiance to the Islamic State in Iraq and Syria (IS) before the shooting, yet there is no firm evidence to link Mateen to IS (Doornbos 2016). These are all forms of extremist violence but are differently motivated.

FOR EXAMPLE

Nidal Hassan, Terrorist or Not?

On November 5, 2009, Army Major Nidal Hasan engaged in a mass shooting on the Army base at Ft. Hood, Texas, killing 13 and wounding 32 others. The event today remains one of the murkier events of terrorism in US history. Major Hasan was prosecuted for murder and attempted murder charges, not terrorism-related charges. Yet the event is often cited as an example of lone-wolf terrorism in the United States. Prosecutors seek to have the event categorized as a terrorist event, and events databases, like the Global Terrorism Database (START), list the event as a terrorist event. Hasan professed the killing spree as justified in order to protect the Islamic World from US attacks. Moreover, Hasan attempted to communicate with Anwar al-Awlaki, an interlocutor for al-Qaeda. The Obama administration went to lengths to not have the event classified as terrorism and to instead have it officially labeled as a workplace shooting. US Representative John Carter stated, "I was embarrassed by the initial ruling it was a work place violence issue" (Fernandez and Blinder 2014).

This brief historical overview of terrorism in the United States gives us an idea on the nature and evolution of the domestic terrorist threat. This picture, though, is only partially complete. There are many terrorist events that take place in the United States from the late 1960s through the present. Many attacks are single events, or small clusters of events, that did not evolve into a persistent terrorist threat. Much of the terrorism in the United States comes from groups that we would not expect. And much of the terrorism in the United States is actually conducted against non-US targets. In order to flesh out this picture of domestic terrorism, we need to analyze the trends beyond the dominant terrorist groups and events in history.

SELF-CHECK

- Terrorism in the United States during the 1970s formed on the edges of the civil rights and anti-war movements. True or false?
- Émigré Terrorism is defined as
    a. A foreign terrorist attacking domestic targets
    b. Domestic terrorist attacking foreign targets
    c. Gang-related terrorism
    d. Foreign terrorist organization assassinating a foreign victim
- Define ecoterrorism.

10.2 Homegrown "Leaderless Resistance" and Foreign Terrorists

The history of terrorism in the United States shows the threat is varied. We know that the primary terrorist threat to the United States has been homegrown terrorism, primarily from right-wing groups, environmental groups, and single-issue terrorist groups (e.g., abortion clinic bombers). However, one form of terrorism has emerged as a prominent concern: the lone wolf. In the mid-2000s a debate arose between Marc Sageman and Bruce Hoffman, two notable scholars on international terrorism, about the nature of the threat facing the United States in the post-9/11 world. Hoffman argued that centralized organizations like al-Qaeda and al-Qaeda in the Arabian Peninsula (AQAP) would be the dominant terrorist threat. The capability, in particular of groups like AQAP, seemed to be increasing and showed daring inventiveness with attempts such as placing explosives into printers headed in an airplane cargo hold (Hoffman 2008). Sageman, meanwhile, argued that terrorist organizations were decentralizing, leading to radicalization of spontaneously self-organizing groups and individuals who opt to pursue terrorism (Sageman 2008). While the debate over which threat is most prominent is still not entirely settled, it certainly appears that decentralized groups have surged to become the most salient threat. Lone-wolf terrorism accounts for about 26% of terrorism-related fatalities in the United States from the late 1970s to the 1990s (Phillips 2015). Nonetheless, there has been an increase in these attacks across the country and Europe. The nature of the attacks by the lone wolf differs significantly from what we might call standard terrorism conducted by networked or hierarchical organizations. For instance, targets are less symbolic and more personal. The lone-wolf event seems fixated on increased casualties and martyrdom. In short, lone wolves represent a bigger threat today than in the past. They represent a level of radicalization and organization that is difficult to detect, and efforts to counter such threats risk infringing on basic civil liberties central to a country's polity like the United States. In addition to the lone-wolf threat is the foreign terrorist and foreign terrorist organization. These threats may not capture as much attention as lone wolves right now, but they remain a source of threats to homeland security we need to understand.

10.2.1 Understanding Leaderless Resistance

Lone-wolf terrorism is an expression of **leaderless resistance** or a form of violent engagement by individuals or small groups outside the formal structure of any organization. More precisely, lone-wolf terrorism is an attack carried out by persons that operate individually and do not belong to an organization or network and whose actions are conceived and directed without any outside command (Weimann 2012). Leaderless resistance is an adaptation promoted largely by the radical right and white supremacy groups in the United States. Leaders and followers in these groups believed they were penetrated by law enforcement. Given the problems with organizational security people like Joseph Tommasi and William Pierce called for people to attack the state and to do so without mass action. These revolutionaries must be prepared to act alone (Kaplan 1997). The radical right was very bounded in their attempt to employ leaderless resistance. It was understood that (i) public support would not come, (ii) movement leaders will not openly approve of leaderless resistors, and (iii) many of the targets chosen make it difficult to disentangle ordinary crime from leaderless resistance (Kaplan 1997).

Recent history instructs us that leaderless resistance is not the behavior of only radical right and white supremacy groups. Over the past decade or more, we have observed a number of lone-wolf attacks coming from within the American Muslim community. From 2001 to 2011, 61 individuals were involved in terrorist plots with domestic targets (Lutz and Lutz 2013). During the 1980s, the American-based al-Furqa group conducted a number of operations against religious institutions across the United States and Canada (Vidino 2009). In the 1990s we observed the al-Khifa organization (founded by al-Qaeda) started channeling American Muslims to train and fight with various jihadist organizations overseas to places like Afghanistan and Pakistan. The flow of American Muslims to overseas training and fighting increased in the post-9/11 world. It is this flow of recruits, channeled by the foreign terrorist organizers, which absorbed much of our attention in the 2000s. However, this uptick in foreign organizing activity should not displace the very real fact that most attacks planned and conducted in the United States during this time came from purely homegrown, operationally independent individuals and clusters (Vidino 2009). Examples include John Walker Lindh and Jose Padilla, which were not true lone wolves as they possessed significant organizational contacts. However, people like Ronald Allen Grecula, Michael Curtis Reynolds, Amir Abdul Rashid, and Nidal Hassan represent clear cases of individuals who were radicalized into violent jihadism without any outside assistance (Vidino, 2009). The radicalized lone wolves come from both the immigrant and American Muslim communities. The United States has been slow to recognize the rise in homegrown violent extremism in its many forms. This slow start is attributable, namely, to problems in identifying the potential source of threat.

10.2.2 Origins of Lone Wolves

Profiles of terrorists have rarely been accurate. People are often recruited counter to a profile type. Profiles are even less accurate when it comes to leaderless resistors or lone wolves. The difficulty sorting out violent radicals begins with efforts to sort the violent from the nonviolent radical and understanding who is most prone to violent radicalization. In short, where are the lone wolves coming from? Our discussion on this centers on the challenge to understand the process of radicalization itself in order to counter it.

Radicals of all types tend to share very similar outlooks toward the world. They display a cynical distrust of government, believe conspiracy theories about the government, and express a deep outrage over the foreign policy of the United States (Bartlett and Miller 2012). Additionally, radicals of all types share a keen perception of social discrimination, which leads to periods of uncertainty about their own identity. Where we do observe difference in the nonviolent radical versus the violent radical is in the context of which these beliefs are developed and nurtured. Nonviolent radicals watch many of the same videos and read many of the same radical textbooks as violent radicals. Nonviolent radicals though are exposed to these messages as part of a critical thinking education that involves group discussion and challenges to the ideas (Bartlett and Miller 2012). Violent radicals are exposed to such messages in a way that supports the ideology and actions called for, which suggests there is something else taking place.

There is pull toward violent radicalization beyond ideas; it is an emotional pull. Violent radicalization seems to derive from subcultures where in-group peer pressure is strong rendering violent action an obvious route (Bartlett and Miller 2012). The role of the subculture is best explained by Max Taylor and John Horgan (2012) in their description of the **community of practice** informal social learning environments "within which members exchange experience and views, developing each other's tacit knowledge into conversations and knowledge that allow for its transmission" (134). The community of practice provides a framework for the emergence of ideology and social control. Ideology interacts with behavior wherein ritual and practices become expressions of one's faithfulness to an ideology.

The community of practice is best understood in the context of the **radical milieu**, a social environment that shares perspectives, approves of violence (to some extent), and provides support to violent groups morally and in some cases logistically (Malthaner and Waldmann 2014). It is useful to think of the radical milieu as an environment where one, or many, social movements are interacting. Militants emerge as part of a process of political outbidding between violent and nonviolent groups over attention and followers.

The community of practice is nested within the radical milieu. On the edges of social movements, individuals participating in the movement meet, pulled together by the movement. As they meet, these individuals discuss the movement, its objectives, and even its tactics. As discussion unfolds, people share stories with each other relating to experiences that reflect expressions of social discrimination of some form. The shared messages develop into an image of a common set of experiences. The perception of shared experience is then explained as part of a larger conflict that reflects ideological content. Thus, radical ideas emerge and spread.

The direction of our discussion so far has focused on radicalization more broadly. We must now turn our attention to how this helps us to understand lone wolves. Getting from the radical milieu and communities of practice to lone wolves is a series of organizational and individual adaptations. Even as groups like al-Qaeda, AQAP, and the Islamic State of Iraq and Syria (IS) have assumed a larger role in this universe, we see that violent radicalization, from the organizational side, remains at its core a strategic adaptation. Flattening the organization pushes operational activities away from the core, while still maintaining the ability to threaten the target state. The core terrorist organization sends out messages through the Internet or through individuals placed in organizations within communities to facilitate individual contact (e.g., placing radical clerics in community mosques in the United States). The flattened organization though does not facilitate any direct control or facilitation between the organizational core and operational units. In other words the two entities (terrorist organization and individual terrorist) seem completely unrelated, except a sense of shared ideas and motivation.

However, information on lone wolves captured in a variety of datasets suggests that lone wolves are rarely completely autonomous, particularly in their radicalization. Most lone-wolf terrorists display a detectable pattern of activities with social movements, pressure groups, or violent organizations. The evidence also suggests a large number of loner attackers have prior military experience but have since left the service or have criminal convictions (Gill et al. 2014). What seems apparent is that at some point the individual breaks with the organization. This may be due to an inability to integrate into the group. In the group setting lone wolves are often described as "loners" or socially isolated. This social isolation seems to be correlated with detectable patterns of mental illness, which runs higher among lone-wolf terrorists than among terrorists associated with an organization (Gruenewald et al. 2013). Data tell us that at some point the loner either separates from the group or is expunged for some reason (Gill et al. 2014). In either instance, the separation may serve as a precipitating event for a loner attack (McCauley and Moskalenko, 2014). Most evident of the lack of complete autonomy for lone wolves is the evidence that in most cases other individuals where aware of the beliefs of the lone wolf and had knowledge of their intent, and in some cases assisted in planning of an attack (Gill et al. 2014).

10.2.3 Assessing the Lone-Wolf Threat in the United States

Returning to our foundation that lone wolves are a strategic and operational adaptation, we note that the lone wolf is an ideal tactical asset. The lone wolf is difficult to detect and free from processes that would discourage creativity and

---

FOR EXAMPLE

Databases on Lone-Wolf Terrorism

Learning about terrorism can be a challenge as events are spread across the globe, and information from media outlets in different countries is not very reliable. The problem of lone-wolf terrorism has raised another set of problems. What we refer to is the small-n problem, or few cases available to generate a comparative study in order to learn about lone-wolf terrorism. Over the past five years, this problem has slowly seen a change. Two major databases have been released on lone-wolf terrorists and non-terrorist extremist violence in the United States. The first is the US **Extremist Crime Database (ECDB)** developed by Jeff Gruenewald and William Parkin, both affiliated with START (National Consortium for the Study of Terrorism and Responses to Terrorism). The database tracks ideologically and non-ideologically motivated crimes committed by extremists (Freilich et al. 2014). A second database is the **Terrorist and Extremist Violence in the United States (TEVUS)** produced through a grant from the Department of Homeland Security to START. TEVUS includes within it the American Terrorism Study (ATS). The TEVUS dataset contains information on incidents, residences, and pre-incident activities including geocoded addresses for actual events (Fitzpatrick et al. 2017). You are encouraged to access these open-source datasets and begin work researching extremism in the United States on your own.

---

other organizational constraints (Phillips 2015). In many ways, so long as radicalization can be managed at a distance, it would seem the lone wolf is the next obvious wave of terrorism in the United States. Before we jump to that conclusion, let us keep in mind that lone-wolf terrorism has surged, but not completely supplanted violent activity from more centralized terrorist organizations. In fact data on organized terrorism versus lone-wolf terrorism suggests key advantages to organized terrorism remain strong. However, there is space where the lone-wolf terrorist has the clear tactical advantage.

Studies on terrorist activities and suicide terrorism find that terrorist organizations increase lethal effectiveness of suicide missions, and lethality of non-suicide terrorism as well (Alakoc 2015; Phillips 2015). The terrorist organization is better able to plan, supply, and carry out an attack than lone wolves. The rate of attack is equally higher for the organized terrorist group over the lone wolf. These conclusions make sense. In spite of organizational connections and other relationships to assist in planning, lone wolves are more burdened to supply and conduct an operation. Terrorist organizations achieve a level of specialized labor for operations increasing their rate of attack and overall lethality. However, this finding does have its limitations.

In cases where the counterterrorist capacity of a country is very high, lone-wolf terrorism gains a distinct advantage. States with high counterterrorism capacity can intercept communications, monitor, and interrupt activities, making organized terrorism difficult to carry out (Phillips 2015). In this environment, the lone wolf gains a tactical advantage. Lone wolves do not have organizational communications to intercept; their likelihood of being caught in a sting operation is low. Moreover, the standard police tools like routine policing of neighborhoods, informant networks, and surveillance are more effective against organizations than individuals (Phillips 2015). What this suggests is a country like the United States is a better environment for lone-wolf terrorism, which bears out the historical data well. The United States has a long history of leaderless resistance from the radical right and white supremacy, which is now being replaced by Islamist-oriented lone wolves like Nidal Hassan, the San Bernardino attackers, and others. The wave of lone-wolf terrorism, threatening as it is, should not distract our entire attention. Foreign terrorist organizations and foreign organizers remain a vibrant threat on the American stage.

10.2.4 Foreign Terrorist Organizations

The foreign terrorist threat inside the United States, historically, consists of two types of groups: first, émigré terrorism, where terrorist operatives infiltrate the US borders to conduct targeted assassinations against foreigners of the same nationality, and second, the foreign terrorist organization that infiltrates the US borders to conduct operations against US-based targets. The former is historically the more common of the two. However, the latter captures the majority of our attention in the present climate.

Émigré terrorism involves attacks by foreigners on foreign targets inside the United States (Hewitt 2003). In this context, terrorist activity is not motivated by contextual political factors inside the United States. Rather the United States provides a convenient venue for foreign groups to carry out operations against political targets. The event, in most instances, has more direct political meaning to foreign audiences than it does to a domestic audience. The question that drives most interest in this type of terrorist activity is "why a particular venue is chosen for operations?" Is there something special about the United States that made it a venue for Cuban terrorism, for example? The United States or any country may be chosen as a specific environment for émigré terrorism. This may be because access to weapons is easier, criminal networks needed to handle logistical issues are more present, or a certain political group is present and may hold a preferential status in the country. Take the example of Cuban émigré terrorism. Anti-Castro Cubans hold a preferred political status in the United States as a reflection of interests in the Cold War. However, pro-Castro Cubans also exist in the US setting the stage for competition between the two groups to protect interests. A large portion of émigré terrorism in the United States is driven by competition between pro- and anti-Castro Cuban factions from the 1960s to the 1980s (Hewitt 2005). Until 9/11 émigré terrorism posed the dominant foreign terrorist threat in the United States. That is to say, from the 1950s to the late 1990s, there were 38 émigré terrorist deaths in the United States, accounting for 7.6% of all terrorism-related deaths and 48% of deaths related to *foreign* terrorist activity (Hewitt 2000).

Since the 1990s, foreign terrorism in the United States has been most often linked to Islamic groups from the Middle East. Activity by Islamic groups is very low and, until 9/11, accounts for only 11 deaths, 2.2% of all terrorism-related deaths, and 14% of all deaths related to foreign terrorism (Hewitt 2000, 5). In the

1970s, such terrorist activity was related to the PLO and Black September, but these attacks were émigré terrorism rather than foreign terrorism. During the 1990s and 2000s, Islamic terrorist activity is linked to al-Qaeda and al-Qaeda-associated movements (AQAM) (Fitzpatrick et al. 2017). Al-Qaeda has been connected to two successful operations in the United States, the 1993 bombing of the World Trade Center and the 9/11 attacks. Beyond this activity, foreign terrorism inside the United States truly is very rare.

Saying that foreign terrorist activity against the United States is rare is not entirely accurate. A more complete picture of terrorist activity globally demonstrates that the United States or US interests are common terrorist targets throughout the world. However, few groups attack US interests on the US homeland. Rather, most terrorist activity against the United States is conducted overseas. Since the United States has a dominant government, military and business presence in Europe, the Middle East, Asia, and Latin America, terrorist groups can easily attack the United States without the encumbrance of trying to infiltrate US homeland security. Even al-Qaeda restricted much of its terrorist campaign against the United States initially to American targets overseas. Examples include the Kobar Towers bombing (1996), the US Embassies in Kenya and Tanzania (1998), and the USS Cole in Yemen (2000).

Relatively speaking, foreign terrorism, as it relates to direct threats to the US homeland, is not a dominant threat. The number of foreign terrorist attacks in the United States attacks is very low compared with other countries around the world. Attacks like 9/11 are certainly exceptions to this rule. Since 9/11, there has been a concerted effort on the part of the US government to ensure that similar terrorist operations have little chance of success. The fortunate side benefit of the increased homeland security effort is likely to be a reduction in all forms of foreign terrorist activity in the United States. As terrorist watch lists are improved and border security strengthens, the ability of émigré terrorists to operate inside the United States will decline as well. It is too early to tell the full impact the post-9/11 reforms will have, but the potential benefits are great.

10.2.5 Foreign Organizers

As we turn to foreign organizers, our attention shifts from groups and their operations to individuals and organizations that set up shop to raise funds and recruit people for terrorist operations overseas. Organizing involves two primary functions: resource mobilization and finding individuals willing to support the cause of a terrorist group. **Resource mobilization** involves raising cash to fund operations and purchase weapons and munitions for operations. **Recruitment** is often related to finding couriers that can transfer resources into the foreign environment.

The American environment is good for terrorist organizers. This is not to say that Americans are lining up to join terrorist groups all over the world. But, if an American can be recruited, the US passport offers the most flexibility for free travel in and out of foreign countries. Virtually unlimited travel allows individuals from the United States to carry money all over the world to fund operations. For terrorist organizations, it is best to have people already within the organization carry out their courier functions. However, terrorist watch lists are constantly updated, making it difficult for foreign terrorists to be certain they can infiltrate the US border security. Furthermore, passport technology is getting more complex, making it difficult to forge passports. It is then better to recruit Americans with US passports in order to circumvent the border security (Emerson 2003). Foreign organizers recruit within immigrant communities inside the United States to find people that may have sympathy for the group's causes and convince them to serve in a minor capacity, like transferring money. For example, Mohammed Salah, a naturalized American from Chicago was recruited by Hamas to carry money into Israel and the occupied territories to support Hamas operations (Emerson 2003). Given the large and varied immigrant communities within the United States, many terrorist groups from many countries will have the potential to find recruits inside the United States. This is not to say that all immigrants are potential terrorist threats. Rather, terrorists have found a way of turning America's immigrant culture into a potential resource. This perception of threat likely serves as the motivation for the Executive Orders (2017) issued by President Trump to ban people traveling to the United States from six (previously seven) majority Muslim countries.

In addition to providing recruits, the United States provides fertile ground for raising funds. Much of the way terrorists raise money involves illegal economic activity such as selling forged goods like DVDs, handbags, and t-shirts (CNN 2005) and identity theft. In one example, Hezbollah set up a scheme where they purchased cigarettes in outlets in North Carolina and resold them for profit in Michigan (Emerson 2003). In addition to this, terrorist groups have established legitimate businesses and invest money in stock markets. Terrorist organizations have also established charitable organizations that pretend to serve the interests of women and children in war-torn regions of the world, only to collect the money and send it along to the terrorist operatives. For example, companies like Microsoft, UPS, and Compaq have donated to the charity Benevolence International Foundation that fronts al-Qaeda (Raphaeli 2003).

To move the money around the world, terrorists have developed a number of schemes beyond the individual courier. One option used by terrorists is the traditional banking system. A group will establish an account, and operatives throughout the world have money transferred from the central account into individual accounts in the bank's subsidiaries. There are also alternative funds transfer systems. Diplomatic channels have been used by transferring funds and equipment through diplomatic pouches that are free from customs inspections (Raphaeli 2003). The **informal funds transfer system (IFTS)** (commonly known as the Hawala or remittance system) operates like an informal Western Union. A remitter gives money to an intermediary who then instructs a contact in the receiving country to distribute the money to a predetermined recipient in the local currency. The transfers are all informal and do not generate paper tails or bookkeeping records of transfers (Raphaeli 2003). In this system a terrorist organization can append its transfer to that of a remitter to move money to operational cells in the field.

In short, within the United States foreign organizers have a plethora of opportunities available to gather resources, organize, and recruit for operations overseas. Much of the activities of foreign organizers play upon the generous civil liberties environment in the United States. Freedoms of speech, press, and assembly, all make it possible to find and recruit people as needed and to gather resources from individuals and corporations inside the United States. In addition, the liberal business environment that encourages foreign investment and free flow of capital makes it easier for groups to move resources in and out of the United States. A cautionary note is required here though. The liberal business and political environment may be abused by foreign terrorist organizers; however, it is also one of the primary barriers we have to ensure that terrorist groups rarely establish themselves as long-term threats to domestic security. Investigative processes have improved, and laws have been adjusted to meet the emerging terrorist threat. The activities of foreign organizers simply alert us to the existing gaps in the security network. This provides us with the opportunity to fill the gap, while balancing the interests of security against the US historic traditions of a generous civil liberties environment.

This analysis of the domestic terrorist threat is instructive in a number of ways. The broad trends suggest that America's primary terrorist threat is the homegrown terrorist. Right-wing and religious terrorists groups have been the dominant threat for much of the past 50 years. Terrorism is moving away from urban centers to rural areas of the United States. The US security establishment, though, is increasingly worried about the rise in lone-wolf terrorism as terrorist organizations decentralize. Lone wolves are harder to detect and counter. The threat presently remains more in its potential. Many lone-wolf attacks are thwarted. Those that do occur capture the public's attention and increase the sense of insecurity among the broader population. Foreign terrorist organizations, which typically dominate the public discourse on terrorism in the United States, is actually not as dominant of a threat. Events like 9/11 do contradict this conclusion. But if to set aside al-Qaeda's activities, most foreign terrorism is émigré terrorism, not foreign groups infiltrating and attacking US-based targets. Finally, the United States does have a problem with foreign organizers. Terrorist organizations like Hamas, Palestinian Islamic Jihad, al-Qaeda, and the Provisional Irish Republican Army (to name a few) have long used the US environment to recruit, gather resources, and send those resources into operational fields overseas. Organizing activities range from illegal to legal activities. As our knowledge of the activities of foreign terrorist organizers increases, we will be better positioned to address the threat within the boundaries of our legal and political traditions. This analysis of the domestic threat does raise an important question on how groups are able to form and operate in a country like the United States.

SELF-CHECK

- Define community of practice.
- Which of the following best defines lone-wolf terrorism?
  a. Leftist radicals
  b. White supremacy
  c. No centralized organizational connections for planning and operations
  d. Deep organizational connections for planning and operations
- US-based targets are the most common targets for foreign terrorists. True or false?

10.3 Crime and Terrorism

The tail end of our discussion from the previous section on foreign terrorist organizers and the activities they engage in brings us to a related topic of increasing concern to counterterrorism professionals in the United States and across the world, namely, the nexus of organized crime and terrorist organizations (Dishman 2005; Makarenko 2004; Mullins and Wither 2016; Picarelli 2006). Terrorist organizations have long been thought of as organizations that live hand to mouth on donations from supporters or taxes extracted from communities they occupy. Over time terrorist organizations have learned other means for capturing resources. These activities include illegal sales of counterfeit goods, kickback schemes, "security" rackets, and even using charitable fronts as a way in which to capture donations to enable terrorist actions. In short, we are observing terrorist organizations beginning to intrude on space traditionally reserved for criminal organizations. At the same time we also see an increase in violence by criminal organizations. Violence is part of the trade. But what is different is (i) the use of terrorists as operatives to conduct operations and (ii) the deployment of violence to promote politically relevant causes that further the interests of the criminal organization (Dishman 2005). The boundary between terrorist groups and criminal organizations has always been thin. Today it seems that it is highly permeable and may not actually exist as a boundary in some cases. The question then is why is this convergence taking place? What does it look like and what does it mean?

10.3.1 Why Would Terrorism and Crime Converge?

Convergence between terrorist organizations and criminal organizations is often attributed to the move to "flatten" organizations. Flattening is another term for decentralization of an organization's operations and support away from the command node to the operational nodes. Flattening has certainly expedited convergence, but we must recognize that convergence was well underway before flattening occurred.

The main drive for convergence was the winding down of the Cold War. As the intense competition between the United States and the Soviet Union came to an end, the resource environment for terrorist organizations shrank dramatically. The United States and the Soviet Union often supported terrorist groups in different parts of the world as part of a larger "proxy war" with each other. Terrorist groups could inflict enough damage to force a country to react, but not enough to escalate toward war. Moreover, sponsorship of terrorist organizations was clandestine, making it virtually impossible to trace support from either superpower to a terrorist organization. After the Cold War ended, the United States and Russia pulled back from support of these groups, creating a major resource shortfall for many organizations. The 1990s bear this history out as we observe a major collapse in terrorist activity beginning in 1992–1993 (Picarelli 2006). It is during this time that terrorist organizations began to live hand to mouth and to tax their local populations more. However, these methods did little to make up for the gap caused by the collapse in state sponsorship (see Chapter 6).

Two things happened at once. First, a large number of terrorists became slack labor in a market where their skills were not very transferable into other trades.

Criminal organizations, however, found these skills very useful, and began to bring in former terrorists as contracted employees (for limited operations) or as part of the permanent military infrastructure for the organization. Second, terrorist organizations were forced to adapt or die. While many did die in the early stages, a number of organizations adapted by integrating criminal activities into their organizations. Terrorist organizations began contracting as security companies in their local cities to assist private establishments. Often these activities devolved into racketeering schemes. Terrorist groups began to take over drug smuggling operations in war-torn areas like Afghanistan (Dishman 2005). Meanwhile, criminal organizations began to see value in violent challenges to the government and its authority as a way to better ensure survival and expand operations.

The environment in the 1990s was ripe for transformation of the old models of organization. Terrorist organizations had to find a way to survive. Also criminal organizations gained in the benefit of available security personnel. However, the convergence of these two organizations sped up as terrorist organizations began flattening in the 2000s. Decentralization was understood primarily as a security measure for the terrorist organization, even criminal organizations.

The hierarchical core of the organization would no longer serve as command and control for the entire organization. Planning and logistics would flow to operational cells distributed around the world. Leaderless resistance would become the norm where individuals, or small cells, would conduct an operation and a parent terrorist organization would claim responsibility. To facilitate decentralization, terrorist cells had to quickly develop resources. Many cells learned fast on how to participate in credit card fraud, counterfeiting, and smuggling of various items ranging from drugs and cigarettes, to people. In short, each operational cell had to develop a business plan to facilitate operations. Hence convergence became the new norm for terrorist group organization.

10.3.2 Where Terrorism and Crime Converge and Why It Matters

The departure for this discussion is first knowing the difference between these two organizations and then how that difference matters, or matters less. The main difference between terrorist organizations and criminal organizations is that terrorist groups use violence as a way to advance interests in the public sphere. Thus, we would define the interests of the terrorist organization as a class of public good. Criminal organizations, on the other hand, seek profit from activities that are outlawed in a country. As the organizations come together, violence is deployed to protect markets and organizational interests. In this sense, violence has a purely private good character.

The public versus private good element for each organization is often treated as the frim boundary between these two organizations. In the past any crossover between the two organizations was done on the basis of a business-based alliance (Makarenko 2004). Criminal organizations provide logistic support for terrorist organizations. For instance, the criminal unit can locate forgers for passports or arms dealers for weapons and explosives. Moving in the other direction terrorists can be hired by criminal organizations to plant bombs or conduct assassinations.

> ### FOR EXAMPLE
>
> ### Deadly Alliances: ELN, FARC, and the KLA and Criminal Organizations
>
> The nexus of terrorist organizations and organized crime comes in many forms. One particular manifestation is in the form of an alliance where the terrorist group, or its personnel, is hired by the criminal organization to carry out acts of violence consistent with the criminal organization's interests. In Colombia, the National Liberation Army (ELN) was hired by the Medellin Cartel to plant car bombs through Bogota in 1993 because the cartel lacked the capabilities to do it themselves. The Revolutionary Armed Forces of Colombia (FARC) has served the interests outside criminal groups, including Mexican drug traffickers to move cocaine through Mexico into the United States (Makarenko 2004). Meanwhile, the Kosovo Liberation Army (KLA) and its political wing the Kosovo National Front (KLF) linked up with the Pristina cartel, who funneled tens of millions of dollars into the KLA, where it would then be used to buy arms for KLA operations (Makarenko 2004). In all three cases we see the terrorist organization and the criminal group interacting to advance each other's interests.

Alliances, though, have grown more complicated. Terrorist organizations appear to be forging long-term alliances with criminal organizations in order to assist in money laundering, counterfeiting, and access to smuggling routes. Criminal organizations seem to seek out terrorists to destabilize the political environment and undermine law enforcement. A terrorist group can provoke harsh arrest and detention policies to thwart terrorism, which often undermines public trust in law enforcement. This level of alliance is considered interaction, and though more complex today than in the past, it really is similar to how these organizations have always worked together. Where we see concern developing is through **appropriation** where one organization incorporates the methods of the other and takes those activities "in-house" (Mullins and Wither 2016). With regard to terrorism, we have observed appropriation for a period of time, at least as early as the 1980s when terrorist organizations in Latin America moved in to the illegal drug trade to raise revenue, giving rise to the name **narco-terrorism**. Sendero Luminoso (SL) in Peru is known for virtually taking over the transfer of coca plants from farmers to drug cartels. SL would protect the farmers from the cartels, and in exchange the farmers would pay SL for their protection and to serve as a price negotiator. Appropriation in the opposite direction is best exemplified by the Medellin and Cali Cartels in Columbia that used beheadings and car bombings as part of a war between each other and to push the government away from extradition agreements with the United States (Mullins and Wither 2016).

Appropriation is a major concern as it complicates the security issue on multiple fronts. Efforts to counter criminal appropriation of terrorism, or terrorist appropriation of criminal activity, now require counterterrorism strategies and anti-organized crime policies. In one way the more complex nature of the organizations provides a wider set of laws to use in prosecuting members of the organizations. However, the methods used to police organized crime differ substantially from those used in counterterrorism, which, for instance, is heavily based on intelligence gathering in order to identify targets of interest and then to infiltrate and take down targets. Intelligence information is useful for connecting the dots between people and activities. It relies on information from informants, some of which are paid. The quality of the information is largely hearsay, and hearsay intelligence information is not very useful in courtrooms where evidentiary rules are very high. Conversely, police may capture information on pending terrorist operations, but in order to act, they need evidence to get warrants for search and seizure. The investigation may take time, a luxury that is not always available when attempting to counter terrorism.

The convergence of criminal and terrorist organizations is a product of changes in the international system as a result of the end of the Cold War and efforts to better secure the core of a terrorist organization (decentralization). The result is that previous patterns of alliance and interaction between terrorist groups and criminal outfits has deepened to the point of convergence, or appropriation, where activities previously reserved for one group are being taken over by the other group. As a result, counterterrorism faces new challenges. These challenges are added to the complication caused already by the rise of leaderless resistance (lone-wolf terrorism). In the next section we will discuss the US response to terrorism, in all its forms. We will focus attention on countering violent extremism, the lead agency approach, and how the United States places its criminal justice system on the forefront of counterterrorism domestically.

SELF-CHECK

- Define appropriation.
- Which of the following are not ways in which terrorist and criminal organizations cooperate?
  a. Terrorists serve as military capacity for criminal organizations.
  b. Criminal organizations provide logistical support for terrorists.
  c. Terrorists destabilize the political environment for criminal groups.
  d. Criminal groups provide loans to terrorists.
- Terrorist activity relates to public goods, while criminal activity relates to private goods. True or false?

10.4 The US Domestic Response to Terrorism

As mentioned in the introduction, the variety of terrorist threats the United States faces (homegrown terrorists, foreign terrorists, and foreign organizers) means the United States must operate a flexible counterterrorist policy. In this section we will explore elements of this flexible response. Since this chapter is primarily about domestic terrorism, the majority of our discussion is centered on domestic responses to terrorism. This involves the criminal justice system as the centerpiece of our system. The Posse Comitatus Act of 1878 prohibits the use of federal troops (the military) to conduct police and security operations inside the boundaries of the United States. Posse Comitatus has been loosened somewhat over the years to allow for the military to participate in limited terrorist response situations, employing what is called Military Aid of Civilian Powers (MACP) (Wilkinson 2000). In such cases the military may serve temporarily as airport security (as they did following 9/11) or help with disaster recovery after the 9/11 attacks. For the most part, the United States has forsaken the use of the military as the primary counter-terrorist tool, thus eliminating the war model. Rather the United States has opted for the criminal justice model to address its domestic terrorist threats. Still, employing the criminal justice model is difficult as numerous government agencies come into play, and many state governments may be involved. The rise in concern over lone-wolf terrorism has prompted community-based counter-radicalization efforts termed countering violent extremism. It is a combined effort by local, state, and federal law enforcement and community outreach to interrupt lone-wolf operations, or counterprogram extremist messages. To manage the complex of local, state, and federal agencies with a portfolio related to counterterrorism, the United States opted for the **lead agency approach** combined with the Department of Homeland Security (DHS) and the National Counterterrorism Center to ensure some level of order and accountability. In this section we will learn about countering violent extremism (CVE), police and counterterrorism, and the lead agency approach model.

10.4.1 Countering Violent Extremism (CVE)

The law enforcement capabilities in the United States, relative to terrorism, focus primarily on detecting threats and thwarting attacks being planned (Connor and Flynn 2015; Dishman 2005). Such activities are best for countering organized terrorism by a group. This is not to say lone wolves cannot be caught through such methods. It is just that there are fewer opportunities with lone wolves to intercept communications and intersect with those planning operations. Adaptations are being made though in order to enhance law enforcement tactics for lone wolves. This strategy, referred to as **countering violent extremism (CVE)**, intended to create strategic messaging that encourages identification of radicalized individuals and counter-messaging of extremist content and literature. The CVE program is located in the Federal Bureau of Investigations (FBI) countering violent extremism Office. CVE is premised largely on counterprogramming extremist messages. However, CVE efforts can and, to some degree, do include the use of agent provocateurs to trigger radicalized individuals toward action in order to capture violent radicals. It is this part of the CVE program that remains most controversial. We will return to this discussion later.

Counterprogramming is the centerpiece of CVE. As we understand it, radicalization contains two pieces: cognitive (ideas) and behavioral (actions) (Neumann 2013). Violent extremists are not always as ideologically rigid as nonviolent extremists. Yet we know that violent extremists are exposed to radical ideas, and one that accepts radical ideas has a higher likelihood of becoming a behavioral extremist.

Moreover, those exposed to extremist messaging are not simply exposed to ideas. Often extremist messages contain information and instructions on how to procure weapons and build explosive devices (Connor and Flynn 2015). Hence, the extremist message is about ideas and means. Thus, the goal is to contest the extremist message circulating in likely target populations. The core message is to promote values of the country related to freedom and democracy and to illustrate how the extremist goals seek to take advantage of, and undo, civil liberties gains (Neumann 2013).

There are barriers to counterprogramming. Foremost, the message cannot come from the US government; otherwise it is dismissed as propaganda. The messages need to come from respected community leaders (Connor and Flynn 2015). In this way, direct intervention by respected community leaders can take place to provide an alternative, less violent view of the world and the role of the people in the United States. In the event that counterprogramming fails for individuals, the community leaders are better able to direct law enforcement resources toward an emergent violent extremist.

We are more certain that counterprogramming efforts do work. Case studies in the Sahel region of Africa show that in communities exposed to counterprogramming, videos and messages display an observable difference in radicalized behavior (Aldrich 2014). At the same time radicalized beliefs remain relatively unchanged between groups exposed to the message and those not exposed. These methods though take time. And while time is not always on the side of the counterterrorist professional, we need to recognize that radicalization is not an overnight process, so counter-radicalization should not be held to a higher standard.

In spite of the observable benefits to CVE, there are some areas of danger to be mindful of. The core of CVE is to counterprogram messages from violent radical organizations. At the same time, the process of countering the message does bring forth information on potential assailants. CVE has taken on prevention in the form of event disruption. **Event disruption** is when resources are devoted to behavioral radicals focusing on individual intentions to break the law (Neumann 2013). To dig into those individuals that are adopting violent extremist behavior, there is a tendency to resort to agent provocateurs that will intercept radicals and offer enabling assistance to conduct a terrorist operation (Vidino 2009). All the while, law enforcement agencies gather evidence on the individual about to commit the crime in order to build a case and arrest them before an event takes place. This form of operation is a "sting" and is often times characterized as entrapment by law enforcement luring people to commit acts of violence they likely would not have pursued without the encouragement (Connor and Flynn 2015). This critique is important as sting operations risk relationships with community leaders and can serve as a vehicle for further radicalization of people in the community.

In short, countering violent extremism has an important role for taking on the lone wolf. Lone wolves are difficult to identify. Sting operations can be used to isolate individuals willing to conduct violent operations. Yet, the deeper value of CVE is in the counterprogramming of extremist messages. Evidence suggests counterprogramming works to alter behavior in a radicalized environment. But just as any counterterrorism policy, CVE is only one of many that the United States deploys. We now turn our attention to the broader counterterrorism effort underway.

10.4.2 The Lead Agency Approach and Counterterrorism

Inside the United States there are over 20 federal agencies and any number of 50 states that potentially hold jurisdiction over any single terrorist event. Managing all the involved parties is difficult. Given that all federal agencies are under the direction of the president of the United States, this would seem to be one way to control the situation. However, President Eisenhower is famous for saying "motivation is the art of getting people to do what you want them to do because they want to do it" (Eisenhower n.d.). Federal agencies have various interests in either participating in or avoiding terrorist situations. Budgetary concerns, jurisdiction, and mission all influence the decisions of agencies to get involved with terrorism. If bureaucratic leaders believe there is a positive budgetary payoff, they will likely join in the effort. However, if taking on counterterrorist duties means doing more, with the same budget, leaders may balk to defend their own agencies interests. Budgets are but one excuse. The gist of this situation is that there may often be too many agencies trying to get involved, or avoiding responsibility, making it difficult to manage counterterrorism operations.

To provide some order to the mess, a vice presidential commission led by George H.W. Bush established the lead agency approach (1985) to handle terrorist threats. Under the lead agency system, the federal agency with jurisdiction over the terrorist situation is determined by the loci of the event. Domestic terrorism falls to the Department of Homeland Security and Federal Bureau of Investigations (FBI); Bureau of Alcohol, Tobacco, and Firearms (ATF); and the Drug Enforcement Agency (DEA). Foreign terrorist threats are assigned to the US Department of State and the Department of Defense. Aviation terrorism (e.g., hijackings) is assigned to the Federal Aviation Administration.

In the post-9/11 world, the United States has reworked much of its organization to combat terrorism, both domestically and internationally. One feature missing before 9/11 was any single agency or bureaucratic leader with clear responsibility and accountability over terrorism and counterterrorism. The lead agency approach provided a modicum of coordination for activities related to terrorism and counterterrorism. However, for most the 1980s and 1990s, there was no clear authority. Under the Reagan and George H.W. Bush administrations, counterterrorism was a collective responsibility of the National Security Council (NSC). Under the Clinton administration, a specific individual was identified within the NSC to oversee counterterrorism. However, this National Coordinator for Security, Infrastructure Protection, and Counterterrorism did not have an independent secretarial portfolio, meaning no budget, no personnel, and no real authority to order agencies to cooperate for counterterrorism. Moreover, the areas of responsibility under the National Coordinator position are wide ranging and make the charge too broad to effectively deal with. Such "czar"-like positions work better when the charge is narrow and focused.

As noted in Chapter 3, following 9/11 the George W. Bush administration established two new bureaucratic entities to provide accountability and clear authority for counterterrorism. The first, and most prominent, is the Department of Homeland Security (DHS). The role of DHS is to manage border security against foreign terrorists attempting to gain entry into the United States to conduct terrorist operations or to organize for terrorist operations overseas. In addition to this function, DHS is assigned with the duty of managing rescue and recovery efforts in the wake of a terrorist attack. In addition to DHS, the National Counterterrorism Center (NCTC) was created in 2004 to provide the larger picture on existing and emerging terrorist threats domestically and globally. The NCTC took over the functions of the Office for the Coordinator for Counterterrorism inside the US Department of State. It falls under the Office of the Director of National Intelligence (ODNI). The NCTC's primary duties are to collect all available intelligence on terrorist activities and to coordinate and direct strategic operational planning in response to terrorist threats. Combined, DHS and the NCTC provide a more unified command and clearer accountability in relation to counterterrorism and response and recovery efforts inside the United States. These federal entities though are not the very front line of counterterrorism in the United States. These agencies simply provide leadership and accountability. The front line for domestic counterterrorism is the criminal justice system at both the federal and state levels.

10.4.3 Police and Counterterrorism

The United States prides itself in being a nation based on the rule of law. As such, a conscious decision was made long ago to address terrorism as a criminal activity and to apply the rule of law to terrorist behavior in order to allow the rule of law to govern counterterrorist efforts. By turning to the criminal justice system (the system of laws, police, courts, and prisons) as the primary tool for counterterrorism, the United States is making a clear statement about terrorism: terrorists are criminals, not political actors pursuing legitimate grievances. Defining terrorism this way tentatively diminishes social or political grievances, thereby defining our motivation. Such an approach is valid as terrorist behavior presents a direct threat to society, and this threat can extend to the viability of the country (Chalk 1995). The United States has been slow to develop new laws that deal with terrorism specifically. The approach from the 1960s to the 1990s was to apply existing laws on murder, kidnapping, public endangerment, property damage, and so on, to acts of terrorism. Generally, the federal government held the position that crafting special legislation on terrorism redundantly outlaws these same behaviors (Donohue and Kayyem 2002). Special legislation against terrorism raises the treatment of the crime as political motivation becomes an aggravating factor yielding special sentencing rules (Walker 2000). Such legislative measures will run up against First Amendment protections on free speech and assembly (Donohue and Kayyem 2002). Moreover, by making a special case for terrorism as a distinct crime, the courtroom is transformed into a public forum for a terrorist or terrorist group to espouse their ideology.

The United States amended its legal approach to terrorism at the beginning of 1990s. This reflects the growing concern over foreign terrorists conducting operations against domestic US-based targets, in particular, the World Trade Center bombing in 1993. In 1996, the Anti-Terrorism and Effective Death Penalty Act (AEDPA) paved the way for the United States to designate a list of foreign terrorist organizations (FTOs), and criminalizes any contributions to an organization associated with FTOs. The government is allowed to deny entry to any person affiliated with a designated FTO, and the government may freeze the assets of any person or group affiliated with an FTO (Donohue and Kayyem 2002).

In addition to the AEDPA, the United States altered its laws regarding investigations and prosecution of suspected terrorists. Such measures amend rules on search and seizure, detention of suspects, admissibility of evidence, and confessional statements (Chalk 1995, 18; Wilkinson 2000, 116). The FBI Access to Telephone Subscriber Information Act (1993) gives the FBI access to telephone subscriber information without the need of a court order. New laws were crafted to aid investigations by tagging materials that could be used in terrorist operations. For instance, the Chemical and Biological Weapons Control and Warfare Elimination Act (1991) allows the Secretary of Commerce to maintain a list of goods and technology that can be used by terrorist organizations and requires such materials to include taggants and strict tacking systems in order for police and federal investigators to quickly follow the trail of a terrorist and identify suspects (Donohue 2001).

In the wake of 9/11, the US Congress passed the Uniting and Strengthening America by Providing Appropriate Tools Required to Intercept and Obstruct Terrorism Act (2001) (a.k.a. the USA PATRIOT Act) as a supplement to existing anti-terrorism legislation. The USA PATRIOT Act provides wide discretion to the executive branch to institute measures necessary to combat terrorism and eliminate the threat posed by al-Qaeda in particular. Through the USA PATRIOT Act, the G.W. Bush administration implemented several investigative strategies and prosecutorial rules to supplement the criminal justice approach to terrorism. Most are directed toward foreign terrorist threats and include warrantless wiretaps on international phone calls, regulation of foreign bank accounts that maintain correspondent accounts inside the United States (i.e., money laundering), and creation of the "enemy combatant" status for foreign terrorists as a special class of criminal not subject to traditional civil liberties protections (P.L. 107-56, 2001). Many of the programs have come under scrutiny for their potential violation of civil liberties, and negotiations are underway to define court proceeding rules for enemy combatants. Additionally, the USA PATRIOT Act includes a sunset provision that allows Congress to revisit and reauthorize or amend the legislation every five years. This ensures that there is accountability and oversight between the executive and legislative branches to prevent an excess of power by the executive (see Chapter 2).

In addition to the federal statutory record, many states have adopted corresponding legislation applied at the state level. Much of the legislation is redundant to the federal counterpart causing potential jurisdictional battles in the future. However, state governments correctly argue that a majority of terrorism takes place within states, and many groups, like the ecoterrorists (ELF), are not a major concern of the federal government leaving states with the primary responsibility to deal with the local terrorist threats. The states have been on the front line of passing laws to deal with "school terrorism," ecoterrorism, gang activity, and narcotics regulation, all of which are increasingly defined as "terroristic offenses" (Donohue and Kayyem 2002).

Overall, the legal approach to terrorism has proven useful. Between 1980 and 1996 about 327 cases were brought against individuals suspected of terrorist activities. Of these 255 were domestic terrorists and 72 were international (Donohue 2001). These numbers reflect the success of the legal system absent special terrorism legislation initiated in the 1990s. As new anti-terrorism legislation was passed and used in terrorism cases, we observe a surge in defendants using their political motivation as a defense. Immediately there were a number of acquittals of mistrials for cases involving domestic terrorism (Donohue 2001). However, allowing political motivation to arise in court cases has also proven useful for the prosecution as was the case for the World Trade Center (1993) bombings (Donohue 2001).

Supplementing anti-terrorism legislation, the United States has developed a variety of security measures that effectively harden likely terrorist targets or enhance the rights of victims of terrorist offenses. The Transportation Security Act (1974) requires air carriers to develop new security measures aboard aircraft. Supplementing this act, the FAA introduced the "Sky Marshal" program to place armed guards aboard aircraft to prevent hijackings. Compensation programs have been established for the families of terrorist victims. The Foreign Sovereign Immunities Act (1976) allows US citizens to bring civil suits against foreign countries involved with or sponsoring terrorist acts. To build domestic preparedness, the Clinton administration issued Presidential Decision Directive 39 requiring the Marine Corps to develop the Chemical and Biological Incident Response Force. Similar measures have branched out into the Department of Health and Human Services, the Federal Emergency Management Agency (FEMA), the Defense Department, and the Department of Justice (Donohue 2001).

The biggest areas of coverage missing in the United States is a specially designated security service that collects intelligence on suspected terrorists and dispenses it to local and federal instigative authorities to pursue (see Chapter 12). The United States has opted more for traditional local law enforcement in this area. Police units typically have advantages in community intelligence. Over time police personnel develop networks of informants that provide information that directs investigation and surveillance. This community intelligence is needed to focus the counterterrorism effort at the terrorists and away from the community. However, localized and compartmentalized information does little overall as the goal is to neutralize a terrorist organization, not just individuals. The challenge is how to centralize all the information into databases, accessible by many, to maintain focus on the broader terrorist threat. To facilitate centralization for counterterrorism, many countries have developed specialized security services that are specifically designed to collect and disseminate information to meet terrorist challenges (Chalk and Rosenau 2004). Examples include *Direction de la Surveillance du Territoire* (DST) in France; MI5 in Britain; *Bunderkriminalant* (BKA) and *Persone, Institutionen, Objekte, Sachen* (PIOS) in Germany; *Cesid Gaurdia Civil* and *Policia Nacional* in Spain; and Australian Security Intelligence Organisation (ASIO) in Australia (Chalk 1995). The security service collates intelligence data and disseminates it to international intelligence services and local police (Wilkinson 2000). Moreover, the agency does not have a complementary law enforcement or military role. Rather the security service provides information to direct police action (Chalk and Rosenau 2004). The role of the security services is very narrow in definition: preemptive information gathering designed to prevent new groups from emerging or entrenching in society. In addition to this narrow role, the security services will also provide information directed as specific homeland threats, which will help with target hardening by directing resources to the most vulnerable targets.

Given the US experience with the Counterintelligence Program (COINTELPRO: 1956–1971), the tendency inside the government is to avoid repeating past mistakes. However, the need is still present. To fill this gap the United States created the National Counterterrorism Center (NCTC) and combined with the Office of the Director of National Intelligence (ODNI), which ideally will provide a nexus point where all intelligence, foreign, and domestic. Once the intelligence is consolidated, it can then be distributed to the appropriate local or federal agencies to guide counterterrorism efforts. The system is still very new, and time is needed to coordinate the activities of agencies that were previously independent.

FOR EXAMPLE

COINTELPRO and the Church Commission

The FBI's Counterintelligence Program (COINTELPRO), established in 1956, was the implementation of the Smith Act of 1940, which prohibited groups and individuals from advocating an overthrow of the US government. COINTELPRO initially targeted the American Communist Party. Since Communist ideology advocates violent revolution to overthrow capitalist regimes, this seemed a perfect target for monitoring. However, COINTELPRO went beyond investigations of political groups deemed potential threats to the security of the United States. COINTELPRO investigated several social and political movements including the New Left student movement during Vietnam and the Reverend Martin Luther King during the Civil Rights movement. In addition to the investigations, COINTELPRO engaged in misinformation campaigns to discredit these social groups. These aggressive disruptive campaigns included purposely circulating disruptive rumors and dirty tricks to prevent meetings from taking place. The effort destroyed the American Communist Party and was seen as a success. The program was kept intact well into the 1970s when it was finally revealed to the public through a Freedom of Information Act request. Upon this revelation, the US Congress quickly organized a commission to investigate COINTELPRO. The Church Committee investigation revealed the nature of COINTELPRO and the abuses of power associated with it. By the end of the Church Committee hearings, COINTELPRO was a shadow of what had been. Various Supreme Court decisions required that the FBI must have evidence of subversive activity before initiating an investigation. FBI agents came to believe proactive investigations were the quickest way to kill a career. By 9/11 the FBI had all but given up surveillance of political groups because its history demonstrated abuse of power rather than good intent.

The overall effort to invest in law enforcement-based counterterrorism is good investment. Expanding capabilities of law enforcement yields benefits beyond counterterrorism. At the same time evidence shows us that fatalities and casualties associated with terrorism decline when countries provide sufficient financial support for law enforcement (Danzell and Zidek 2013).

Summarizing US counterterrorism efforts, we can say that the policies continue to be in a state of flux. The United States has made drastic changes to its laws and policies regarding counterterrorism over the past 50 years. From the 1960s to the 1990s, terrorism was treated exclusively as a local crime issue, especially for homegrown terrorists. This tactic has been very effective. As the homegrown and foreign terrorist threats mounted, the laws and policies changed to reflect the rising saliency of the issue in the political system. The uncoordinated efforts of the federal government were first reorganized in the 1980s with the rise of international terrorism. New laws were implemented in the 1990s to define terrorist offenses and apply new sentencing requirements for individuals convicted of committing acts of terrorism. In the post-9/11 world, the federal government mounted a major reorganization to meet the terrorist threat, placing counterterrorism policy as a major national policy. The Department of Homeland Security was created along with the National Counterterrorism Center. The Office of the Director of National Intelligence was a new addition to the intelligence community to better serve national interests by combining all available intelligence to direct counterterrorism efforts (see Chapter 12). The rights of terrorist victims are now secured. In all countries, counterterrorism responses tend to reflect the most recent attack. In the United States a decision was made to think proactively about terrorism, not just react. At the state level, governments are passing new laws to define terrorist offenses in order to supplement their battles against homegrown terrorists. Gaps still exist, and there remain many gaps we may not even be aware of. The test is always the ability of the government to diffuse terrorist threats before they manifest. To date, the United States, in cooperation with its allies, has diffused terrorist plots to bomb airplanes en route from London, a plot to bomb the New York City subway and tunnel system, and Faisal Shahzad's attempted bombing of Times Square (NYC) in 2010, among many other examples of foiled plots. The counterterrorism system today is better, more comprehensive than in the past. Yet, emerging threats like radicalized lone wolves requires new thinking. This is being met with the development of countering extremist violence programs designed to disrupt events and counterprogram extremist messages. Today's counterterrorism system is more comprehensive, but it is an evolving system.

SELF-CHECK

- Which of the following government bureaucracies is not involved in domestic counterterrorism?

  a. Department of Homeland Security

  b. Department of Defense

  c. Federal Bureau of Investigations

  d. Bureau of Alcohol, Tobacco, and Firearms

- CVE involves counterprogramming extremist messages to target audiences. True or false?

- The Posse Comitatus Act of 1878 prohibits which of the following?

  a. Terrorism

  b. The FBI from harassing political groups

  c. Federal troops from police and security operations inside the United States

  d. The federal court system from being used in terrorism cases

SUMMARY

Much of the national discourse on terrorism revolves around AQ, IS, and other Islamic fundamentalist terrorists operating in the Middle East, Central Asia, and the Sahel in Africa and the threat they present to US interests. When we turn our eye to the domestic terrorist situation in the United States, a very different picture emerges. Domestic terrorism has a long history in the United States. Terrorist activity began as early as the colonial period and continues to this day. Many terrorist groups attack foreign targets inside the United States, not US-based targets. Additionally, many foreign terrorists operating inside the United States are engaged in émigré terrorism against foreign targets, not US targets. During the 1990s and early 2000s, the terrorist threat in the United States comes from the ecoterrorist groups like Earth Liberation Front. The United States has faced separatist terrorist challenges from Puerto Rican terrorist groups during the 1960s and 1970s. And on occasion foreign terrorist organizations have infiltrated the US security network and conducted major operations including the 9/11 attacks. The terrorist threat is varied including homegrown terrorists, foreign terrorist organizations, and foreign organizers. Since 9/11, the terrorist threat and extremist violence in the United States has evolved. Lone-wolf terrorism, and autonomous cell terrorism, presents a potentially large threat inside the United States, as certain individuals seem prone to cognitive and behavioral radicalization. We explored leaderless resistors (lone wolves) that represent a unique challenge related to processes of radicalization and planning operations. Lone wolves are difficult to detect and intercept. The lone-wolf threat though accounts for 26% of domestic terrorist fatalities in the United States (Phillips 2015). An added layer to extremist violence in the United States is the rise of mass public shooters who are not terrorists in the strict sense of the definition. Instead, the mass public shooter represents a threat similar to the lone wolf. They can more easily evade detection during their planning stages, making it more difficult to disrupt these events.

In this chapter we also explored the convergence of criminal organizations and terrorist organizations. The end of the Cold War and tactical decisions to decentralize terrorist operations has pressured terrorist cells into developing a revenue flow, often from illicit sources. Appropriation of criminal behavior by terrorists has been met with an equal appropriation of terrorist behavior by criminals. Criminal groups will now use violence in order to influence social policy related to outlawed activities. The nexus of terrorist and criminal organizations creates new challenges in counterterrorism. The approaches to countering criminal organizations and terrorist organizations are different. The tools and methods used to counter a terrorist organization are built around infiltration and intelligence gathering. Law enforcement attempts to collect evidence on criminal activities for prosecution of offenders. The two approaches are not entirely at odds, but they are far from perfect complements. Moreover, the multiple intersecting jurisdictions involved with any counterterrorism case add actors to the picture, making coordination of effort more problematic.

Finally, in this chapter we reviewed counterterrorism policy in the United States that shows a strong tendency toward the criminal justice model for confronting the threat of domestic terrorism. The United States prides itself as a nation of laws and relies on this approach to deal with terrorist threats inside the homeland. The response to terrorism over the years has been very fragmented as many home-grown terrorists were treated a regular criminals prosecuted at the local level. This policy suited the United States very well until the 1980s and 1990s. The proliferation of international terrorism, and the growing threat that international terrorism may penetrate the homeland, prompted various reorganizations of government, new laws, and finally new federal departments and agencies inside the United States in order to meet the threat of domestic terrorism. Gaps may still exist in the counterterrorism shield, but, to date, the system has proved to work very well. In time we may see if new vulnerabilities exist. No state can completely eliminate its exposure to terrorism; however, the United States appears to have done a good job at minimizing the risk.

KEY TERMS

Appropriation	When one organization (criminal or terrorist) incorporates the methods of the other and takes those activities in-house.
Community of practice	Informal social learning environment where members exchange views and experiences, developing tactic knowledge that allow for its transmission.
Countering violent extremism (CVE)	Strategic messaging campaign that encourages the identification of radicalized individuals and counter-messaging extremist content and literature.
Counterterrorism policy	Set of laws, agencies, and programs targeted at controlling and reducing terrorist threats.
Criminal justice model	Using the system of police, courts, laws, and prisons to address a terrorist situation.
Ecoterrorism	A form of terrorism where the group attempts to influence domestic policy regarding land development, environmental policy, and animal testing.
Émigré terrorism	A form of foreign terrorism where a foreign victim is killed by a foreign terrorist group inside the boundaries of a different country.
Event disruption	When resources are devoted toward behavioral radicals focusing on individual intentions to break the law.

Extremist Crime Database (ECDB)	A database on illegal violent incidents involving at least one suspected perpetrator that subscribes to an extremist belief system.
Foreign organizers	Foreign terrorist recruiters and agents that raise funds and recruit operatives from inside the United States for operations against US and other national interests overseas.
Foreign Terrorist Organization (FTO)	A type of terrorist group whose operatives originate outside the United States, penetrate homeland security to plan and conduct operations against internal targets. Officially listed as FTOs by the US State Department.
Homegrown Terrorist Group (HTG)	A type of terrorist group whose members originate within United States and conduct terrorist operations against targets in the United States.
Informal funds transfer system (IFTS)	A foreign remittance system where a person gives money to an intermediary who then instructs a contact in the receiving country to distribute the money to a predetermined recipient in the local currency.
Lead agency approach	A counterterrorism policy where the federal agency with jurisdiction and accountability is determined by the loci of the threat (domestic, international, or aviation).
Leaderless resistance	A form of violent engagement by individuals or small groups outside the formal structure of any organization.
Lone-wolf terrorism	An attack carried out by persons that operate individually whose actions are conceived and directed without any outside command.
New Left	A political movement that takes form following the presentation of *Port Huron Statement* calling for the creation of a participatory democracy in the United States.
Radical milieu	Social environment that shares perspectives, approves of violence, and provides support to violent groups.

Recruitment	Finding couriers that can transfer resources into foreign environments.
Resource mobilization	Raising cash to fund operations and purchase weapons and munitions.
Terrorist and Extremist Violence in the United States (TEVUS)	A database portal that compiles information on behavioral, geographic, and temporal characteristics of extremist violence in the United States (1970–present).
War model	Militarization of a terrorist conflict.

ASSESS YOUR UNDERSTANDING

Go to www.wiley.com/go/Kilroy/Threats_to_Homeland_Security to assess your knowledge of the basics of domestic terrorism.

Summary Questions

1. The domestic terrorism problem is primarily a result of foreign terrorists operating on American soil. True or false?

2. After 9/11 the United States reorganized its counterterrorism policies by creating the Department of Homeland Security and National Counterterrorism Center. True or false?

3. US counterterrorism policy is based on the criminal justice model using laws, courts, police, and prisons to handle terrorists rather than the military. True or false?

4. Who of the following is NOT an example of a lone-wolf terrorist?
   (a) Nidal Hassan
   (b) Amir Abdul Rashid
   (c) Omar Mateen
   (d) John Walker Lindh

5. Leaderless resistance is based on a philosophy that clearly states that public support will not come, and movement leaders will not openly approve of attacks. True or false?

6. What differentiates lone-wolf terrorists from mass public shooters?
   (a) Violence is targeted at property or individuals that are personally meaningful, not politically meaningful.
   (b) They radicalize outside a formal organizational structure.
   (c) They attack random strangers that have symbolic meaning.
   (d) Conduct all preparation and planning for an event by themselves.

7. Countering violent extremism seeks to counterprogram extremist messaging and disrupt planning. True or false?

8. What must be avoided in counterprogramming extremist messages?
   (a) The message must provide an alternative, less violent view of the world and its people.
   (b) The message cannot come from the target government, like the US government.
   (c) The message must be carried forward by respected community leaders.
   (d) Trust in community leaders to direct police resources to emergent violent extremists.

9. The two things that drove convergence of criminal organizations and terrorist organizations is the sudden increase of terrorist "labor" as terrorism declined in the 1990s and terrorist organizations adopted a more hierarchical organizational structure. True or false?

10. Appropriation means
   (a) Terrorist groups and criminal organizations formally merge into a single organization.
   (b) Criminal organizations and terrorist organizations compete with each other for influence.
   (c) One organization incorporates the methods of the other and takes those activities "in-house."
   (d) Criminal organizations and terrorist groups negotiate separate spaces for their operations.

Applying This Chapter

1. You are asked to explain when and where to employ a countering extremist violence (CVE) policy for a police department in a major urban center. In doing this, what specific things should be a part of the program to make CVE work?

2. In the course of an investigation on a small group of radicals, you discover, through a paid informant, that the people hope to conduct a terrorist attack on a major venue in the city. You also discover these same people are running drugs in that city in order to fund their operations. Begin planning an event disruption. Think about the best way to engage the radicals (sting operation or counter-messaging). What are the benefits to either approach, and what are the limitations? Also you wish to direct police resources at the drug trafficking to cut off resources to the group. What is the major challenge you face in passing the information along to the police?

3. A mass shooting has taken place in an industrial park in your city. A location the represents your city's main connection to the world through e-commerce. The new media are quickly gathering as you begin to set up a command center. What message(s) need to be communicated and controlled? Keep in mind you do not know yet if this is a terrorist event or a mass public shooting.

YOU TRY IT

Lone-Wolf Terrorism in America

Write a paper that compares several lone-wolf terrorist events. You can draw upon either the ECDB or TEVUS databases to gather information. You can construct the project to compare individuals involved with lone-wolf terrorism or communities where lone-wolf terrorism takes place (or is planned).

Counterterrorism

Analyze CVE counterterrorism policy. Is CVE useful for any and all terrorist situations? What are the primary challenges to counterprograming extremist messages? Take an example of CVE in operation (in the United States or abroad) and evaluate the way in which CVE is employed.

11

ENABLERS OF MASS EFFECTS
The Impact of the Information Age on Threats to Homeland Security and the All-Hazards Perspective

Carmine Scavo

Department of Political Science, East Carolina University, Greenville, NC, USA

Starting Point

Go to www.wiley.com/go/Kilroy/Threats_to_Homeland_Security to assess your knowledge of the basics of enablers of mass effects.
Determine where you need to concentrate your effort.

What You'll Learn in This Chapter

▲ The ways information and ideas are transmitted in the information age

▲ The role the media plays in shaping perceptions

▲ The ways terrorists can use the Internet to further their aims

▲ The role of educational institutions in shaping generational views toward terrorism

After Studying This Chapter, You'll Be Able To

▲ Evaluate why the information age benefits terrorist organizations in communicating their messages to domestic and international audiences

▲ Propose different media sources for an informational requirement

▲ Evaluate the role of ideas in the international battle against terrorism

▲ Assess the impact of the Internet on terrorist capabilities and threats

Threats to Homeland Security: Reassessing the All-Hazards Perspective, Second Edition.
Edited by Richard J. Kilroy, Jr.
© 2018 John Wiley & Sons, Inc. Published 2018 by John Wiley & Sons, Inc.
Companion website: www.wiley.com/go/Kilroy/Threats_to_Homeland_Security

INTRODUCTION

The word **enabler**, as it appears in the title of this chapter, can have several different meanings. First, it can mean anything that assists in the creation of mass effects—an institution or process that makes it possible for mass effects to occur when they would not have occurred otherwise. Or, the word can mean an institution or process that allows the mass effect to have a greater effect than it would have had otherwise. "Enabler" could also mean an institution or process that is utilized by those who might cause mass effects.

The institutions and processes we will discuss in this chapter include the media (including social media), the Internet, and educational institutions. All of these can make it easier for mass effects to happen; they can help mass effects become larger than they might have been otherwise, and they all have also been used by terrorists and others to further their aims. Before looking at these institutions and processes, however, we'll look at the roles that information and ideas play in mass effects. In this discussion, it is important to remember that any approach to emergency and disaster management is heavily dependent on information to assist first responders in determining actually what is happening, who (if anyone) might be responsible for the act, and what can be done to address the situation.

Thus, in this chapter, you will assess the role of the information age in facilitating the spread of messages—both those messages that legitimately should be spread in times of emergency or disaster and those messages that terrorists would like to spread to further their aims—both domestically and internationally. You'll also become familiar with the role of ideas and values in modern world culture and evaluate the role of decision-making rules of thumb in assessing the likelihood of potential disastrous events in the United States. Finally, you'll evaluate the assets and limitations of the Internet as a tool for terrorists.

11.1 The Power of Information and Ideas

We live in a global society—the world is linked together through a variety of mass media that make it possible for virtually everybody on the planet to be able to witness an event within a few minutes or hours of its occurrence. More than one billion people—some 40% of the people on Earth—watched live on television, on the Internet, or on mobile devices, as Germany beat Argentina in overtime in the 2014 FIFA World Cup Soccer final match in July. Another one billion watched India beat Pakistan in a semifinal Cricket World Cup match in Adelaide, Australia. Other sporting events—the Olympics, the Super Bowl, and so forth—draw somewhat smaller but still impressive audiences. While broadcast or cable television coverage of live events remains strong, more and more people are reporting that they rely on social media as sources of information. A recent Pew Research Center survey of the American public reports, for example, that 62% of American adults report viewing news on social media with 18% reporting they view such news often (Gottfried and Shearer 2016).

The number of people who are watching breaking news also seems to be increasing, although finding accurate numbers globally is difficult since it involves aggregating television, the Internet, and mobile source information from over 200 countries around the world.

Although ours is a global society, there is also a tremendous amount of local variation in how people view problems, solutions, and so on. For example, religion plays a much more important role in determining how people in some parts of the world (Middle East, Latin America) view social and political reality than it does in other parts of the world (Northern Europe). The political scientist Ronald Inglehart has developed a series of questions in which he attempts to measure individuals' value orientations. He classifies these on a materialist–post-materialist dimension. **Materialists** are people who are concerned with personal survival—providing for themselves or their families, making a good salary, and all the "perks" that come along with that salary. **Post-materialists** are those who are more concerned with what some call "higher goals"—preserving and protecting freedom of speech and more self-expression type values. In addition, Inglehart and others (Inglehart and Baker 2000) have described more traditional values and values associated with change and "modernism." The cultural values map in the following text (Inglehart and Welzel 2015) shows more than 65 nations around the world arrayed on these 2 dimensions. Countries in the lower left-hand corner of the map are those where the populations (as measured by answers to questions in the World Values Survey) are more traditional and materialistic, while countries in the upper right-hand corner are those where the populations are more post-materialistic and less traditional. One can see the United States' position as high on self-expression values but also somewhat more traditional than other English-speaking countries like Canada, New Zealand, or Great Britain (Figure 11-1).

There also seems to be a growing and powerful anti-globalism movement across the world. The 2016 British vote to leave the European Union, the election of nationalist candidates in Poland, Macedonia, and the Philippines, and the election of Donald Trump as President of the United States demonstrate a powerful backlash against global society with candidates making the appeal to voters that conditions in their individual countries have suffered as a result of too much attention to the conditions of people in other parts of the world and not enough attention to people in their own countries. Often the focus of this backlash has been immigration with calls to limit the number of refugees entering a country and also limiting the number of people entering the country in less-than-legal ways (Bonikowski 2016; Podobnik et al. 2016).

This focus on values and the way that values influence one's view of the world should not surprise anybody—information and ideas are extremely powerful in determining what happens in our world. According to the nineteenth century French writer Victor Hugo, nothing is as powerful as an idea whose time has come. But how do we know that the idea's time has actually come? The contest over the control of information, the interpretation of information, and the role of ideas is one that is never ending. When two people who do not have a shared worldview discuss controversial issues, it often seems they are talking past each other—they do not share a common frame of reference through which the issues can be debated.

For many years, the dominant model of American politics has been the pluralist model—this model assumes that various groups compete in the political arena using money, numbers of members, access to leadership, and so on as resources in the group competition. This model is as old as the foundation of the American republic—in Federalist 10, James Madison defended the US Constitution as an

Figure 11-1

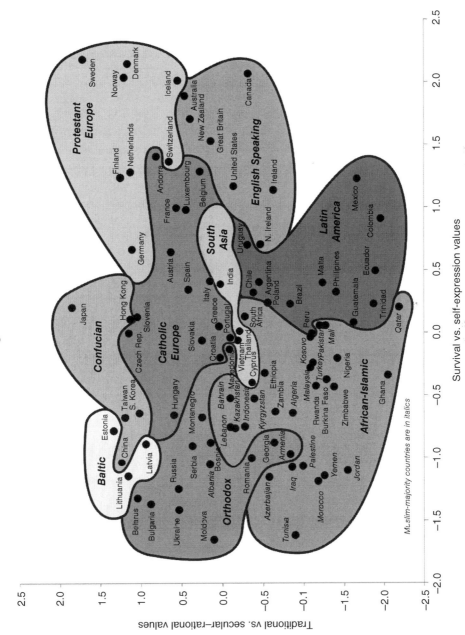

Inglehart–Welzel cultural map. Source: From Inglehart and Welzel (2015), www.worldvaluessurvey.org.

attempt to cure the mischief of faction. The pluralist model is so deeply engrained in the US society that it is difficult at times to think that it may not be entirely accurate. But we do know that one thing that the model neglects is the power of ideas (Kingdon 1984). There are many times where it can be shown that a new and different idea that may not be popular (but that may be right) is accepted by more and more people, eventually becoming a dominant worldview.

In this different type of competition, politics plays a much more complicated role than it does in the simpler pluralistic universe. If money or access or other resources are the most important things in determining success in any political competition, the "haves" in the world have a tremendous advantage over the "have-nots." And yet we know that often the "have-nots" can win based on the power of their ideas, not on their own innate political power. For example, while the Apartheid government in South Africa had almost a monopoly on political force, the anti-Apartheid forces had a much more positive idea—that people should not be separated simply because of the color of their skin. This idea eventually won when the Apartheid government was replaced in 1994 by a government composed of all races.

The classic reference in discussing the battle of ideas in modern world culture is Samuel Huntington's book *The Clash of Civilizations and the Remaking of World Order* (1996). Huntington wrote that with the end of the Cold War, the dominant form of conflict had changed from ideology to culture and religion. And Huntington also wrote that Western civilization was at an intellectual disadvantage in this clash since it assumed that liberal democracy was the only remaining ideology after the end of the Cold War and so simply assumed there was no alternative. Huntington thought that Chinese culture represented one major intellectual threat to Western culture, but Islam represented another. The major point, however, is that the threat is not so much military or economic as it is intellectual and idea based as the generalized themes of these cultures contest for large-scale popular adoption.

How does this happen? How does one set of ideas supplant another? Malcolm Gladwell (2000) describes one such process in his book *The Tipping Point*. Gladwell and others (Grodzins 1958; Schelling 1978) have developed a model where ideas influence a few people who influence a few more until at some point, one additional person adopts the new idea and then, suddenly, everybody does. The environment turns over from one state to another. Think of an avalanche: A small amount of snow and ice breaks loose in the mountains and nothing happens. In a different place, a small amount of snow and ice breaks loose and begins to slide, picking up additional snow and ice. At some point, the amount of snow and ice is enough to let the whole side of the mountain come down, taking trees, houses, and unfortunate people with it.

11.1.1 Ideas and Terrorism

In a 2015 speech, President Obama said "we have to confront squarely and honestly the twisted ideologies that these terrorist groups use to incite people to violence. We need to find ways to amplify the voices of peace and tolerance and inclusion, and we especially need to do it online…We are not at war with Islam. We are at war with people who have perverted Islam" (Davis 2015, A1). This battle of ideas involves creating a positive alternative to the image of world society that terrorists would like people to believe. Examine the map of political values described earlier. Look for countries that we might think are places where terrorism could arise. In which section of the map do these countries tend to be clustered? Many are in the lower left-hand section—where traditional and survival values dominate. In other words, these are countries in which there are a large number of poor people who at the present time seem to have little hope they can better themselves. This may partially be the result of poor education, poor economic development opportunities, or a worldview that ignores physical accomplishments in the current world but instead focuses on rewards that may be granted in the afterlife. When people lack education, they have a hard time succeeding in a world where education is valued. Where economic development opportunities are lacking, even educated people may not succeed since there are few venues to exercise one's education. And where a people's worldview replaces physical, material rewards in the current world with promises of rewards in the afterlife, those same people may focus on all kinds of actions that make them worthier for those promised rewards rather than taking actions to improve their or their children's material conditions.

What is the positive alternative that the United States and the Western world can offer to the have-nots of the Middle East and other areas that may be hotbeds of potential terrorism? Certainly one thing is material comfort—it is absolutely true that the nations of North American and Europe have the highest standards of living of all nations in the world. And yet, if one does not think that such material comfort is important or if one thinks that it is beyond one's possible reach, what does this promise mean? Indeed, one might ask why a person might want to continue his or her life if there is no promise for improvement in the current life but only a possibility of reward in the afterlife.

If this battle of ideas is framed as a battle between true believers and a decadent Western culture, true believers have an upper hand. By describing to a conservative, traditional people the ways that Western societies glorify the semi-nude public display of the human body—at beaches, nightclubs, on television, and in films—the "true believer" side in the battle of ideas seizes the moral high ground. By portraying this same thing as an exercise in freedom of expression, Western societies can attempt to blunt the attack by demonstrating that simply because people can act in such ways doesn't mean that everybody does act in those ways and that the freedom that such activity exemplifies is worth more than any excess that might be its result. "I may disagree with everything you say, but will defend unto death your right to say it," a quotation commonly attributed to the French philosopher Voltaire best sums up this Western attitude of freedom of expression and tolerance for differing opinions. But this is a difficult point to make to people who have not been raised with norms of tolerance or freedom of expression.

Many times, this battle of ideas takes the form of choosing the proper term to describe a thing or event that carries with it certain connotations that the speaker wants to summon. President George W. Bush's unfortunate choice of words immediately after the 9/11 attacks—"'this crusade, this war on terrorism'—brought up images of European knights invading Moslem strongholds over several hundred years in the Middle Ages" (Ford 2001). Likewise there has been tremendous difficulty in describing who the terrorists actually are. The group we call Islamic State (IS) in this volume has also been called Islamic State in Iraq and Syria (ISIS), Islamic State in the Levant (ISIL) (the Levant being an old term describing much the lands of the Middle East), and Daesh (an acronym for the Arabic phrase *al-Dawla al-Islamiya wa al-Sham*, which translates as Islamic State of Iraq and the

Levant). Each of these has similar but somewhat different meanings. First, they all signify that the group is legitimate—it is called a state rather than an organization or a religion. Second, IS signifies the group battling against the Assad regime in Syria, while ISIL expands that meaning to include the group fighting against the legitimate government in Iraq. IS can mean both, but, again, grants statehood to the organization. Daesh became popular as a descriptor in international circles in 2015, but IS dislikes this term because it claims the word shows disrespect and has threatened "to cut the tongue of anyone who publicly used the acronym Daesh, instead of referring to the group by its full name" (Associated Press 2014). Many news sources have settled on calling the group "the Islamic State group," indicating they are not legitimatizing the organization with statehood. "The word 'state' implies a system of administration and governance. It's not a term that would be used to characterize a terrorist group or militia that is merely rolling up territory," said David Phillips of Columbia University (Associated Press 2014).

A similar battle over terminology arose during the 2016 US presidential campaign when Republican candidate Donald Trump attacked Democratic candidate Hillary Clinton and sitting President Barack Obama for their seeming refusal to use the term "radical Islamic terrorists" to describe groups like IS or al-Qaeda. Trump said

> Nor can we let the hateful ideology of Radical Islam—its oppression of women, gays, children and nonbelievers—be allowed to reside or spread within our own countries. We will defeat Radical Islamic Terrorism, just as we have defeated every threat we faced in every age before. But we will not defeat it with closed eyes, or silenced voices. Anyone who cannot name our enemy is not fit to lead this country. Anyone who cannot condemn the hatred, oppression and violence of Radical Islam lacks the moral clarity to serve as our President. (Politico 2016)

Both Clinton and Obama responded that they do not use such terms since they see the war against terrorism not to be a war against Islam and that by using the term that Trump does, they are actually hurting the US image in the Islamic world. This contest over what words to use to describe these organizations and events is an example of the larger battle of ideas—choose the wrong term and you risk being on the wrong side of history in opposition to an idea whose time has come.

11.1.2 Ideas and Disasters

Risk assessment models and matrices help evaluate hazards on the basis of the probability of their occurring and the extent of the potential damage the event might cause (see Chapter 4). Large-scale terrorist attacks, which could cause huge amounts of damage, are generally considered to be low probability events, while hurricanes, floods, tornadoes, and earthquakes are much higher probability events in areas where they have occurred before (hurricanes in East and Gulf Coast areas, tornadoes in the Midwest, etc.). Events that require the highest degree of planning are those that have high probabilities of occurring and also can cause a great deal of damage—such as a major hurricane along the Gulf of Mexico coast or a major earthquake along the San Andreas fault in Los Angeles or the Hayward fault in San Francisco. Much of risk assessment estimates the probability of an event occurring partially on the basis of how frequently that event has occurred in the past. Five-hundred-year floods cause much more damage than 100-year floods, but the former is much less probable than the latter so the preparation for each is different. The Saffir–Simpson hurricane wind scale categorizes hurricanes into five categories:

Category 1 storms show winds of 74–95 mph with possible damage to roof shingles, vinyl siding, and gutters. Trees may lose large branches and may be uprooted. Power lines can be damaged.

Category 2 storms show winds of 96–110 mph with major roof damage to homes. Uprooted trees can block many roads and power loss should be expected.

Category 3 storms show winds of 111–129 mph with major structural damage to homes. Major trees may be uprooted or snapped and will block numerous roads. Power may be unavailable for several days.

Category 4 storms show winds of 130–156 mph with severe structural damage to homes. Most trees and power poles will come down. Much of the affected area will be uninhabitable for weeks or possibly months.

Category 5 storms show winds of 157 or greater mph with a high percentage of homes totally destroyed. Power will be out for weeks or possibly months (National Hurricane Center 2017b).

Each of the category storms has greater potential wind damage than the one preceding it, but it also carries a lower probability of occurring. While almost 300 hurricanes have hit the Atlantic or Gulf Coasts of the United States, only three have been Category 5 hurricanes—the 1935 Florida Keys Labor Day hurricane (before the US Hurricane Center began naming major storms), 1969s Hurricane Camille in Mississippi, and 1992s Hurricane Andrew, which cut across southern Florida (Williams et al. 2015). The Saffir–Simpson scale estimates only wind damage; hurricanes also cause much more damage through the severe flooding damage from both storm surge (the rise in sea level as a result of both the high winds and the low barometric pressure in the storm) and torrential rain (National Hurricane Center 2017a). Hurricane Katrina was a Category 3 storm, with sustained winds of approximately 120 mph, when it came ashore on the Gulf Coast in 2005, but had attained Category 5 status while out in the Gulf of Mexico. The storm surge that caused levees to collapse in New Orleans was thus a Category 5 storm surge (nearly 28 ft—a record storm surge hitting the United States), while the winds from the hurricane had decreased to Category 3 levels. Accompanying that storm surge was 8–12 inches of rain, enough alone to cause major flooding in low-lying areas. Additionally, Katrina spawned some 43 tornadoes throughout Alabama, Florida, Georgia, Louisiana, and Mississippi (Knabb et al. 2011).

One way that ideas become involved in the risk assessment process is in the evaluation of various events' probability. There are many ways that these probabilities can be estimated—the most common is through experience as stated earlier. But assessing the probability of an event through how commonly it has occurred in the past means that the probability of events that are new or extremely unusual cannot be assessed. This can be the situation with nuclear, biological, chemical, or radiological terrorist events. Since these have never occurred in the United States and have only occurred extremely rarely elsewhere, figuring out their likelihood is problematic, to say the least. With these types of events, even sophisticated decision makers often resort to using heuristics (rules of thumb): the **representativeness heuristic** (assessing the probability of an unknown event on the basis of how it represents an event we know), the **availability heuristic** (assessing the probability of an event by how clearly we can imagine events like it), and the **vividness heuristic** (events that contain vivid descriptions or images are often viewed as more probable than those that are more abstract) (Kahneman and Tversky 1973; Nisbett and Ross 1980). These heuristics often work well for us but sometimes their use can result in wrong conclusions. Here are examples of each leading to a potential wrong conclusion:

▲ **Representativeness heuristic:** Which of these two series of events is more probable (likely)? XXXXXXOOO or XXOXXOOXX. Many people will say the second one is more probable because it looks "more random" than does the first, but the correct answer is that they are both equally probable since they contain six X's and three O's.

▲ **Availability heuristic:** People asked what the probability of dying in a plane crash is after there has actually been a plane crash will generally say it is higher than those asked when there hasn't been a plane crash recently.

▲ **Vividness heuristic:** On the basis of National Highway Traffic Safety Administration (NHTSA) ratings of automobiles, you decide to buy the safest rated car. Your best friend then calls you and says, "Don't buy that car—a friend of mine almost died in a crash when she was driving that make of car!" How does this new piece of information change your decision? If you are like many people, this vivid piece of information will dramatically affect your decision but it really shouldn't since this is one case compared to the many involved in developing the NHTSA ratings.

You can see how each of these would work in estimating the probability of natural disasters or terrorist events. Even sophisticated disaster managers might not correctly estimate these probabilities if they are working in areas where there are few preexisting cases.

FOR EXAMPLE

Hurricane Katrina

The Federal Emergency Management Agency (FEMA) developed a report in 2001 (McGray 2005) that concluded that a major hurricane hitting New Orleans was one of the three most likely disasters that might occur in the United States (the other two were an earthquake in San Francisco and a major terrorist event in New York City). So it should have come as no surprise when Hurricane Katrina hit New Orleans in 2005. But emergency management officials at the federal, state, and local levels were slow in responding to Katrina partially because they could not imagine the consequences of such a powerful Category 3 storm (availability). People along the Gulf Coast thought that if they moved their cars inland of the CSX railroad tracks that run near the coast through Mississippi and Louisiana, their cars would not be flooded. This natural berm had protected cars when Hurricane Camille had hit in

1969 (representativeness). After Katrina, aerial photos of the Gulf Coast showed some 10 000 flooded cars that had been parked just north of the CSX tracks (Allen 2006). The vivid depiction of the destruction from Hurricane Katrina and the disorganized governmental response to this storm led to the appointment of US Coast Guard Admiral Thad Allen as the principal federal officer (PFO) on the scene. Allen's success in organizing the relief effort in New Orleans led to the appointment of Coast Guard Admiral Brian Peterman to spearhead possible relief efforts before the Hurricane Ophelia hit the North Carolina coast later in 2005, even though the Category 1 Ophelia caused relatively little damage to coastal North Carolina (vividness).

SELF-CHECK

- Define enabler.
- Post-materialists are people who are concerned with personal survival. True or false?
- Prior to 9/11, which of the following did FEMA believe was not one of the three most likely disasters to occur in the United States?

  a. Hurricane in New Orleans

  b. Earthquake in San Francisco

  c. Terrorist attack in New York City

  d. Chemical spill in Houston
- Most damage in hurricanes is caused by the strong winds they generate. True or false?

11.2 Media and Terrorism

Modern mass media have evolved from a time 200 years ago when newspapers dominated news delivery mechanisms, to 100 years ago when radio became dominant, to 50 years ago when three major television networks—ABC, CBS, and NBC—dominated the airwaves, to the current time of television and the Internet cooperating and competing with each other for followers. Each change in news delivery mechanisms has meant quicker dissemination of information and more decentralization in how information is delivered. In the 1990s, cable and satellite television allowed for a much broader array of actors on the broadcast spectrum and gave rise originally to venues like CNN, Fox News, MSNBC, and other news outlets that crafted their messages to a narrower audience than the earlier mass broadcasters did. More recently, niche marketing or narrowcasting (Parsons 2003) evolved to become a much more popular source of information for the public.

More recently all types of television news have been challenged by social media-based news sources, and both television news and newspapers have had to adapt to a world in which many people get their daily news from their computers, tablets, or smartphones. Viewership of television news in the United States and the United Kingdom has declined by three to four percentage points a year since 2012, which is directly comparable with the losses in readership that newspapers suffered a decade earlier. Most of those who have abandoned television news are younger people, resulting in the audiences for television news shows being much older than the average age of the population (Nielsen and Sambrook 2016). Younger people are increasingly relying on social media for their news, and social media delivers news differently than traditional media does. Fully 90% of 18–29-year-old Americans make use of social media, while only 35% of those 65 and older do, although this latter group has gone from 2% usage in 2005 to 35% usage in 2015 (Perrin 2015).

11.2.1 The Internet and Terrorism

The Internet is an anarchic, decentralized environment—there is little external regulation of the content and procedures that take place in this virtual environment and almost anybody can contribute. The Internet is also easy to use and it allows for almost complete anonymity in communications—individuals can make themselves known by screen names or aliases or they may simply be known only by their Internet Protocol (IP) addresses. While external monitors (government, university web administrators, corporate supervisors, etc.) can trace where individual users have gone on the Internet and where they currently are, this monitoring is very resource intensive, and for the majority of cases, it makes little sense. And even when it may make sense, a user can work through proxy servers to disguise his or her IP addresses or can "spoof" another user's profile and send out materials as if they were coming from the second user's computer. Only in a totalitarian society or when there is a known threat does it make sense to monitor one's Internet usage. And even though it is possible to monitor where users go in the Internet, it is much less possible to control what they post. Researchers and students both have fallen victim to inaccurate or false information posted on Internet websites—often with humorous results. But the use of the Internet by terrorist groups is not humorous; it is instead powerful, dangerous, and widespread. Gabriel Weimann, a researcher at the United States Institute of Peace, conducted a six-year research project on how terrorists use the Internet. In Weimann's view, the "internet is in many ways an ideal arena for activity by terrorist organizations" (Weimann 2004, 3).

While a great deal of attention has been paid to the possibility of cyber-terrorism, Weimann writes that terrorist groups use the Internet in more mundane ways that can be just as dangerous. These are psychological warfare, publicity and propaganda, data mining, fundraising, recruitment and mobilization, networking, sharing information, and planning and coordination (Weimann 2006).

Psychological warfare: Terrorism is a form of psychological warfare, which the US Department of Defense defines as "the use of propaganda and other psychological actions having the primary purpose of influencing the opinions, emotions, attitudes, and behavior of hostile foreign groups in such a way as to support the achievement of national objectives" (Joint Publication 3-53 2003). The Internet, because of its attributes previously described, is almost the perfect venue to carry out this type of warfare. Weimann discusses the threat of cyber-terrorism—or more accurately "cyberfear." This occurs when "concern about what a computer attack *could* do (e.g., bringing down airliners by disabling air traffic control systems, or disrupting national economies by wrecking the computerized systems that regulate stock markets) is amplified until the public believes than an attack *will* happen" (Weimann, 2006, 5).

Publicity and propaganda: Television, radio, and print media have some form of editorial control—at some point in the publication process, editors make decisions about what the media will carry. The Internet does not have this—terrorist websites carry anything the terrorist groups want to post there. Part of this is an act of self-creation as the underdog. Terrorist groups use websites partially because, they claim, they are being excluded from traditional media. They use words like "martyr" and "genocide" on their websites to frame issues in the way they want. They claim that they are the victims of state violence and only resort to violence in self-defense. They portray themselves as weak and their cause as inherently "right."

Data mining: This term can be defined as the use of the Internet for open-source information, which, when pieced together, provides information of intelligence value for an organization. As a result of laws and policies developed in the 1980s and 1990s, a great deal of information about government agencies in the United States has been posted on the Internet. For example, laws collectively known as "community right to know" laws required companies that stockpiled hazardous chemicals to notify residents of surrounding neighborhoods what chemicals the companies were using. Local fire departments also needed to have this information in case a fire broke out in the company facilities. When the World Wide Web became popular in the mid-1990s, many companies and government agencies concluded that it would be more efficient for them to comply with these laws and regulations by listing the hazardous chemicals they were working with on their websites. After the 9/11 attacks in the United States, different US government agencies—the Environmental Protection Agency, the Department of Energy, and so on—began advocating the removal of this kind of information from these websites because they thought potential terrorists were collecting sensitive data from them. Gellman (2002) reported that the FBI had tracked multiple casings of websites for nuclear power plants, dams, and gas facilities to computers outside the United States. Later in 2002, laptop computers seized from al-Qaeda contained some of the information that had been collected from those websites. In 2014, the FBI and the Department of Homeland Security (DHS) issued a joint warning to US military veterans that they needed to be careful in their use of social media since IS was monitoring those sites and had issued threats against US military veterans. The report called for veterans to review information they might post that could attract the attention of IS and its supporters (Feeney 2014).

Fundraising: Related to publicity and propaganda, fundraising is also an aim of terrorist websites. Weimann (2004) writes that the Irish Republican Army (IRA) website allows visitors to make donations by credit card. Often terrorist groups gather information from website users to develop a demographic profile of people they can approach for donations. Then a sympathetic front group approaches the user and asks for money for seemingly legitimate uses. This money is then forwarded to the terrorist organization. After 9/11, the US government seized the assets of several charities operating in the United States, claiming they were front groups for IS, Hamas, and al-Qaeda.

Recruitment and mobilization: Many terrorist websites have pages that are headed "what you can do" or "help in the struggle." These web pages often are recruitment devices by which the terrorist group is seeking individuals who are more devoted to their cause than the casual web browser. The user who goes to one of these pages may get an anonymous email asking if he or she would like more information or directions on how to use an anonymous chat room where details of upcoming events may be discussed. Often, training manuals are distributed to the user who can prove that he or she is genuinely interested in the terrorist group's cause or mission. These manuals might teach users how to build bombs, purchase satellite phones, and so on. Interested users are also provided with propaganda and information on the group's ideology or religious beliefs. Using information gathered from the pattern of how the individual user accesses the group's website, the group can customize the information provided to the user—different information for men and women, older people or younger, people from different countries, and so on.

Networking: Modern terrorist organizations do not often resemble the hierarchical type of structure described by Max Weber (the nineteenth century German sociologist who coined the word "bureaucracy") in his classic works on organizations. Instead these new type organizations look something like amoebae—the organization can change its shape when it is confronted by a threat or presented with an opportunity. After Afghanistan was invaded by US and other troops in late 2001, al-Qaeda morphed into what Peter Bergen (2002) has called "al-Qaeda version 2.0," a virtual organization that maintains contacts via the Internet rather than in person. Rather than being an organization with Osama bin-Laden at its head, the new al-Qaeda is composed of highly trained operatives around the world who keep in touch with each other via the Internet and who know that they can take action on their own to maximize their opportunities. This has been entitled the "leaderless resistance" by some analysts (Wallace-Williams 2006).

Information sharing: A great deal of information on the fundamentals of terrorist activity can be found on the Internet. Guides to bomb making, chemical weapons, poisons, assassinations, and so on are readily available from a variety of websites. These guides are good not only for potential terrorist organizations but also for the lone, disaffected individual who may be looking for revenge to compensate for perceived insults. Many of the more common guides—*The Terrorist's Handbook*, *The Anarchist Cookbook*, and so on—are available from a number of websites, and so when one website is shut down or convinced to stop carrying the information, users can find it elsewhere. Weimann (2004) reports that a Google search for the words "terrorist" and "handbook" found nearly 4000 hits. Al-Qaeda publishes the e-magazine *Inspire*, while IS has its own e-magazine *Rumiyah* [Rome]. Both publications are cold-bloodedly matter-of-fact in their descriptions of what potential terrorists can and should be doing. "One's attack may be to harvest a large kill count. It may be aimed at disrupting the financial stability of a specific nation. It may simply be aimed at terrorizing the enemies of Allah and depriving them of a peaceful sleep. Accordingly, as the objective of the attack varies, the *mujahid* must choose a method that best suits the operation at hand" (Rumiyah 2016, 10). *Inspire* runs articles such as "The Successful Pressure Cooker Bomb" (*Inspire* 2016), which provides in-depth illustrated instructions not only on how to build a pressure cooker bomb (like the one used in the Boston Marathon bombing in 2013) but also where such bombs can be placed for maximum effectiveness.

Planning and coordination: After 9/11, the US government seized a laptop computer from Abu Zubaydah—the al-Qaeda operative who is commonly thought to have planned the attacks. This computer contained a large number of encrypted messages, many dated just before the September attacks. At times, the codes used in messages were very elaborate—for example, using steganography (embedding messages in graphic files)—but at other times, the codes were fairly simple. Mohammed Atta—one of the 9/11 terrorists—described the buildings targeted by the terrorists as the faculties of fine arts, law, urban planning, and engineering. And the scenario described by Gellman (2002) in the "Data Mining" section shows that al-Qaeda and other terrorist groups were gathering information in order to plan to combine conventional and cyber-terrorism attacks. A facility's website containing evacuation information could be jammed at the same time the physical facility was attacked, thus presumably maximizing casualties.

The Internet is composed of what many call the Surface Web—what most of us call the Internet—which can be searched using Google or other search engines and where many people conduct business, do their banking, and interact with educational institutions in online courses. However, the Surface Web is only about 10% of all of the Internet. The **Deep Web** is that part of the Internet that is not accessible to the general user since the information contained there does not contain hyperlinks and so can only be accessed by performing an internal search query—a search using the site's own search functions. The third part of the Internet—the **Dark Web**—is an encrypted network that allows users to interact with other users with anonymity. For example, the typical Internet user uses the Surface Web to access his or her banking information, but once logged on to the bank's website, the user is accessing the Deep Web since the information in one's bank account is not generally available to other users through search engines. While information on the Deep Web is not accessible to users who don't have legitimate access to it, information on the Dark Web is purposefully hidden since much of it is illegal or dangerous or, at the very least, socially unacceptable. One can access the Dark Web by using a browser such as The Onion Router (**TOR**)—an anonymous browser available free of charge—which promises to protect a user's anonymity by "bouncing your communications around a distributed network of relays run by volunteers around the world. It prevents somebody watching your Internet connection from learning what sites you visit, and it prevents the sites your visit from learning your physical location" (TOR 2016). While it is difficult but not impossible for authorities to trace general Internet usage across URLs around the planet, it becomes virtually impossible when the user is using TOR or a similar Internet browser. The Dark Web has thus become the home of much criminal and terrorist activity—not only planning attacks but also purchasing weapons or raising funds through online drug sales or prostitution. As one writer puts it, the Dark Web is "the place where the dregs of society dwell. You can say that it's the black market for everything, you will get stuff like drug dealing, prostitution, child trafficking, organized crime, or anything which the law will not permit" (NS 2016). The Dark Web is regularly used by Islamic terrorists, but it is also used by domestic terrorist groups in the United States and by more "common" criminals for purposes such as tax avoidance, money laundering, racketeering, and so on (Moore and Rid 2016; Zhou et al. 2005).

11.2.2 Social Media, Terrorism, and Disaster Response

It is now becoming difficult to distinguish between the traditional media of radio, television, and newspapers and online media such as the Internet or social media. Many of us have foregone paper newspapers and read electronic versions of *The New York Times* or *The Washington Post* or listen to podcasts of radio shows or stream those shows live on our smartphones or tablets. And many of us go one step further, paying little attention to traditional media but instead getting our news from online news sources that are admittedly not unbiased. If one reads a Facebook reposting of an article that ran on *The New York Times* website, would the source be considered traditional media, electronic media, or social media? While this melding of media is an occurrence in our daily lives, it is nevertheless useful to make the distinction between the Internet and social media, especially according to how individuals access the medium. The Internet was optimized to work on desktop or laptop computers; we all know the frustrations of attempting to open some Internet sites on a tablet or a smartphone. In fact, many Internet sites have parallel mobile sites or apps that work much better on tablets and smartphones. Social media generally can be directly accessed on mobile devices—in particular some social media such as Twitter are designed to work on mobile devices making accessing those media much simpler for the user who does not have access to a computer network.

Social media creates a media environment in which news delivery has evolved from a one-to-many model (where single "talking heads" deliver the evening news on television or through newspaper articles) to a many-to-many model in which each individual can become his or her own reporter. The recent innovation of Facebook Live—in which any Facebook user can hit an icon on his or her main page and begin broadcasting live through a smartphone—has created numerous opportunities for individuals to publicize/advertise/share what might be going on in their lives with the nearly 1.8 billion Facebook users in the world (Statista 2016a). Likewise a Twitter user can send a tweet instantaneously to some 317 million users in the world (Statista 2016b). And the number of users of all kinds of social media continues to grow over time.

This move from a more centralized media environment to a much more decentralized one has had a number of effects on society and the problem of terrorism. The first of these is that, as previously noted, each person has become a reporter. In 2011, a series of uprisings against governments in North Africa set off what was known as Arab Spring. Throughout those uprisings in Bahrain, Egypt, Libya, Syria, Tunisia, and Yemen, protestors made use of social media to plan events, keep each other abreast of what was going on, warn others of potential police or military retaliation, and appeal to the outside world for support (Gerbaudo 2012). Paolo Gerbaudo, an Italian freelance journalist happened to be in Tahrir Square in Cairo during a protest in July, 2011, when armed soldiers entered the square to clear it of protestors:

> A few metres to my left, I notice a young Egyptian woman standing by the fence. She was in her early twenties, with long curly black hair and a pair of designer glasses. I guessed she was from an upper-class area of Cairo like Maadi, Mohandessin or Nasr City. She seemed as distressed as I was at witnessing the attack (or daring enough) to raise a finger to stop it. Reaching into her bag, she extracted what I immediately recognized as an HTC phone, the kind with a sliding keyboard, sort of a weird marriage of an IPhone and a Blackberry. She aimed the phone's camera at the square and snapped a picture of yet another violent arrest. Then she started tapping her fingers on the keyboard. She stared for a second at the screen before clicking the 'enter' button and then furtively put the phone away as though worried she might be noticed and targeted….What might she have written in her message? Was she simply reporting what was going in the square? Or was she inciting…comrades to join in the counter-attack against the police? Or suggesting the best way to elude security when approaching the square? Or was she just recording a protest souvenir to show off to friends? Who would be reading her tweet, and how would they be reacting? Would they be inspired to join the protests, or would they be scared away? Who was she anyway? And did all this tweeting and re-tweeting really matter when it came to influencing collective action, mobilizing and coordinating people on the ground? Or was all this just an activist delusion: a way of feeling part of the action while in fact standing on the sidelines? (Gerbaudo 2012, 2)

Social media has become an important surrogate for in-person interactions and the self-selecting aspects of social media such as Facebook and Twitter, which allow individuals to consume information solely from like-minded individuals. One recent analysis of VKontakte, a very popular social networking site in central Europe that has some 350 million users, identified 196 pro-IS "aggregates" (*ad hoc* virtual communities created on social media sites) involving 108 086 individual followers between January 1 and August 31, 2015 (Johnson 2016). While the number of aggregates did not change very much over the course of the study, individual aggregates would appear and disappear. Over one set of undefined months, the rate of creation of new aggregates rose sharply—the peak coinciding with the June, 2015, attacks on Kobane in Syria by IS fighters. The researchers found a similar pattern of a spike in creation of new aggregates around the time of the onset of civil unrest in Brazil in 2013, indicating that the rapid increase in the creation of new aggregates may be a leading indicator of attacks in the real world.

Social media reaction to the Bay Area Rapid Transit (BART) officer's shooting of Oscar Grant in 2009 (made famous in the award-winning 2013 film *Fruitvale*

Station) demonstrates the reach of social media after a major event. Cellphone videos taken at the scene were viewed more than 500 000 times on YouTube over a two-day period in January. Viewers posted almost 3000 comments. Bay Area Rapid Transit (BART) officers were so concerned about the potential effects of the release of the videos that they attempted—without success—to confiscate all cellphone recordings at the scene (Anthony and Thomas 2010). The idea that any person can become a reporter on his or her own has given rise to the descriptor "citizen journalism" to mean the documenting and posting online of events by bystanders as the events are occurring (Matheson 2014).

An in-depth review of research on the uses of social media in emergency and disaster events (Houston et al. 2015) concluded that social media are used in 15 different manners. The following list provides these along with the stage of the event in which the use is most prevalent:

1. Providing and receiving disaster preparedness information: pre-event
2. Providing and receiving disaster warnings: pre-event
3. Signaling and detecting disasters: pre-event and event
4. Sending and receiving requests for help or assistance: event
5. Informing others about one's own condition and location and learning about a disaster-affected individual's condition and location: event
6. Documenting and learning what is happening in the disaster: event and post-event
7. Delivering and consuming news coverage of the disaster: even and post-event
8. Providing and receiving disaster response information and identifying and listing ways to assist in the disaster response: event, post-event
9. Raising and developing awareness of an event, donating and receiving donations, and identifying and listing ways to help or volunteer: event, post-event
10. Providing and receiving disaster mental/behavioral health support: event, post-event
11. Expressing emotions, concerns, and well-wishes and memorializing victims: event, post-event
12. Providing and receiving information about (and discussing) disaster response, recovery, and rebuilding and telling and hearing stories about the disaster: event, post-event
13. Discussing sociopolitical and scientific causes and implications of and responsibility for events: post-event
14. (Re)connecting community members: post-event
15. Implementing traditional crisis communication activities: pre-event, event, post-event

One can see that this exhaustive list mirrors much of what traditional media would do with either disasters or terrorist events; the major exception being that the mediator (television or newspaper reporter) is missing. Social media provides direct individual-to-individual interaction, allowing or requiring communities to deal with disasters on their own.

Political scientists often speak about the twin functions of mediating institutions—interest aggregation and interest articulation (Almond and Coleman 1960). Interest articulation is the actual expression of interests from the masses to the government. So, political parties, interest groups, and the media identify what is happening in the mass public and press the public's demands on government. They routinely do this by aggregating those interests—so it is unfortunate that Mrs. Smith did not receive her Social Security check, but it is a politically powerful event when a large number of Americans do not receive promised government benefits over a long period of time. Social media allows for interest articulation—both between individuals and government and between one individual and another. But social media does not routinely allow for interest aggregation—the messages are individualized and not collected into common themes. Somebody later at some time must comb through all the postings to determine what their meaning actually is. Again, a government official receiving a tweet that an individual is stuck on his or her rooftop as floodwaters surge below is valuable in providing assistance to that individual, but 1000 tweets of people stuck on rooftops during a flood requires somebody to determine who is in the greatest need and how to organize the response to that need given limited rescue resources.

Two additional effects of growing social media reliance need to be noted: first, the growing tendency for individuals to rely on information from sources that confirm their underlying beliefs than those that challenge their beliefs; and second, the tendency for individuals to contribute to the reinforcement of like-minded opinions in individuals through the interactive nature of social media. The term **homophily** describes the tendency for users online to seek out information that confirms their underlying beliefs and avoid information that confronts those beliefs. Homophily—love of the same—is a term used as early as the 1950s by sociologists to mean the tendency for people to affiliate with people who are similar to them in terms of beliefs and core values. Made popular in physical terms by Bill Bishop (2008) in his book *The Big Sort* that describes how Americans are moving into neighborhoods where residents share common values, homophily becomes even more important online since it is easier to associate with those we agree with and disassociate from those we disagree with online than physically.

The multiplicity of sources of information makes it easier for each individual to confirm their core beliefs by finding a supporting source online. In 2005, the comedian Steven Colbert coined the word "truthiness" to mean things that seem or feel true even if they may not necessarily be true. With so many news sources available online, it is now possible to "confirm" the truthiness of virtually any opinion one might hold. This has allowed nefarious content providers to develop "fake news"—online postings that resemble news articles but that are entirely fictitious in nature. In December 2016, the website AWDNews.com published a fake news article that quoted former Israeli Defense Minister Moshe Yaalon threatening that Israel would destroy Pakistan with nuclear weapons if Pakistani troops entered Syria to fight against IS (AWDNews 2016). In response the Pakistani Defense Minister Khawaja Muhammad Asif went on Twitter to write, "Israel def min threatens nuclear retaliation presuming pak role in Syria against Daesh [IS]. Israel forgets Pakistan is a nuclear state too" (Goldman 2016).

> ## FOR EXAMPLE
>
> ### Pizzagate
>
> Just before the November 2016 presidential election in the United States, articles began to appear on Facebook and other social media claiming that Hillary Clinton and her chief campaign aide John Podesta were involved in a child abuse run out of a suburban Washington DC pizzeria called Comet Ping Pong. The fake news storm even took on its own title—Pizzagate—and at one point generated some five posts per minute on Twitter. None of the information in the fake news piece was accurate, but it did not stop the report from circulating endlessly through hyperspace (Kang 2016). A real-world consequence of this social media storm was that Edgar Maddison Welch, a North Carolina resident, decided to visit Comet Ping Pong and investigate the matter himself. He arrived at the pizzeria armed with an assault rifle and confronted several of the staff who fled. He then fired a shot into the floor before being arrested by the police (Independent 2016).

A social media meme can go viral through the passage from one user to another or the posting of an article or image on Facebook or Twitter or some other social media. The meme is relayed in a fashion that resembles an illness growing in a population—one person infects two others, who infect four others, who infect eight others, and so on. In a very short period of time, the illness has reached epidemic proportions, affecting a large proportion of the population. Most often these memes are innocent—cats dancing on piano keys or being scared by zucchini placed near their food dishes—but at times the memes are nefarious, for example, videos of IS militants threatening to behead hostages. This type of posting can go viral through YouTube, Twitter, or many other social media venues.

IS in particular has become especially adept at using social media to further its cause. In general IS and other terrorist organizations use the Internet and social media as methods to post propaganda. Al-Qaeda became good at releasing tapes through **al-Jazeera**, the Arabic-language news network headquartered in Qatar. However, IS took this one step further by recognizing that mediating institutions like al-Jazeera were no longer necessary for them to communicate with the world.

> The jihadist insurgents in Syria and Iraq use all manner of social media apps and file-sharing platforms, most prominently Ask.fm, Facebook, Instagram, WhatsApp, PalTalk, kik, viper, JustPaste.it, and Tumblr. Encryption software like TOR is used in communications with journalists to obscure locational information. But circumstances conspire to make Twitter the most popular application. Specifically engineered for cellphones, it is easy and inexpensive to use. Posts (tweets) may contain images or text, links to other platforms can be embedded, and an incoming tweet can effortlessly be forwarded to everyone in an address list. Some types of social media require either 3G or Wi-Fi access but Twitter can be used in the absence of either. (Klausen 2015, 1)

Former FBI Director James Comey testified before the US Senate and described evolution from "your grandfather's al-Qaeda" to the much more modern approach of IS:

[I]f you wanted to get propaganda, you had to go find it. Find where Inspire magazine was and read it. If you want to talk to a terrorist, you had to send an email into Inspire and hope that Anwar al-Awlaki would email you back. Now all that's in your pocket….You can have direct communication with a terrorist in Syria all day and night, and so the effect of that—especially on the troubled minds and kids—it works! It's…the constant feed, the constant touching, so it's very, very different and much more effective at radicalizing than your grandfather's al-Qaeda model.

They [IS] have a highly sophisticated media effort that utilizes all the tools and techniques of modern-day, social media internet-based advertising….They're actually quite good at what they do. (Reilly 2015)

IS used social media to publicize its early military victories in Syria. In 2014, the BBC, for example, reported on how Twitter accounts reportedly linked to IS provided a running description of the group's invasion of Iraq (Irshaid 2014). Writing in *The Atlantic*, Brooking and Singer (2016) described the IS Twitter announcement of their invasion of northern Iraq in 2014, "Like most of everything today, the campaign was launched with a Hashtag [#AllEyesOnIS]." Brooking and Singer went on:

So intertwined are the Islamic State's online propaganda and real-life operations that one can hardly be separated from the other. As IS invaders swept across northern Iraq…, they spammed Twitter with triumphal announcements of freshly conquered towns and horrific images of what had happened to those who fought back. A smartphone app that the group had created allowed fans to follow along easily at home and link their social media accounts in solidarity, permitting IS to post automatically on their behalf….Media reports from the region were saturated with news of the latest IS victory or atrocity, helping to fuel a sense of the Islamic State's momentum. There was no time to distinguish false stories from real ones. Instead, each new post contributed to the sense that northern Iraq had simply collapsed in the face of the IS onslaught. (Brooking and Singer 2016, 72)

IS videos are designed to appeal to a modern generation who appreciate high quality video. "IS videos are of far higher quality than are those of other groups—we would say they are, technically, a generation ahead of most others… We would argue that, visually IS videos mimic what could be called a 'Hollywood visual style'" (Dauber and Robinson 2015). The videos excel in terms of the story they tell; the quality of editing, lighting, and composition; and the use of special effects to drive home their major points.

IS' use of social media for recruiting is legendary. In 2014, the Soufan Group, which provides security and intelligence services to governments and multinational organizations, estimated that IS had successfully recruited more than 12 000 foreign fighters from some 81 countries. A year later, the number had grown to between 27 000 and 31 000 from at least 86 countries (Soufan Group 2015), and this occurred despite Western intelligence agencies efforts to shut down IS efforts to recruit westerners.

There are many different paths that researchers have suggested individuals undertake to become radicalized Islamists. Some (Moghaddam 2005) describe the process as a staircase; others (McCauley and Moskalenko, 2008) as a pyramid; still others see a conveyor belt (Baran 2005); and often many see a distinction between radicalization of beliefs and radicalization of action (Neumann 2013). The New York Police Department (Silber and Bhatt 2007), which has one of the most successful and well-noted counterterrorism units in all of local policing, describes the process, from an al-Qaeda perspective, as having four steps:

1. **Pre-radicalization** or the situation in which individuals originally find themselves. "The majority of the individuals involved in these plots began as 'unremarkable'—they had 'ordinary' jobs, had lived 'ordinary' lives and had little, if any, criminal history."

2. **Self-identification** where individuals explore Islam, moving away from their old identity and adopt Salafi Islam as their new identity. Salafi Islam is a strict form of Sunni Islam that seeks to return to a purer form of Islam. Salafi jihadism is the belief in war against nonbelievers with the promise that victory would mean the restoration of the caliphate and correcting other Muslim's moral behavior through violence, the threat of violence, and expulsion (*takfir*) from Islam. "The catalyst for this 'religious seeking' is a cognitive opening, or crisis, which shakes one's certitude in previously held beliefs and opens an individual to be receptive to new worldviews." These triggers can include such things as job loss, perceived racism, international conflicts, or death of a close relative.

3. **Indoctrination** in which a "spiritual sanctioner" leads the individual progressively into adopting Salafi-jihadi beliefs with a conclusion that action (jihad) is required to further the cause. "While the initial self-identification process may be an individual act, ... association with like-minded individuals is an important factor important as the process deepens….[T]his self-selecting group becomes increasingly important as radical views are encouraged and reinforced."

4. **Jihadization** where individuals accept their individual duty to take action and become holy warriors. Plans begin for taking action to implement the decisions made (Silber and Bhatt 2007, 6–7).

The swift penetration of social media into most the world's consciousness has resulted in a combination of the third and fourth of these steps. It is no longer necessary for individuals to band together as groups to reinforce beliefs or to take action. IS and al-Qaeda have shifted their strategies from collective action to a campaign of encouraging "lone-wolf" attacks on Western targets. Such attacks—simple, almost random, and very difficult to detect or defend against—have some major advantages for terrorist groups like IS: they are cheap and easy; they require no planning or knowledge of the lone wolves on IS's part; they damage the psyche of a nation by demonstrating that attacks can happen anywhere at any time; and they boost IS's image since many of the perpetrators cite the group as the inspiration for their operations (Mendelsohn 2016). IS has been quick to claim responsibility for lone-wolf attacks such as trucks being driven into crowds in Nice and Berlin or a car driven into a crowd of students at Ohio State University, even though the group most likely had little to do with the planning or execution—except in the broadest way—of those attacks. An IS commentator in their magazine *Rumiyah* used the Bastille Day truck attack in Nice as an example of what IS lone-wolf attackers could do, "Observing previous vehicle attacks, it has been shown that smaller vehicles are incapable of granting the level of carnage that is sought. Similarly, off-roaders, SUVs, and four-wheel drive vehicles lack the necessary attributes required for causing a blood bath….Rather, the type of vehicle most appropriate for such an operation is a large load-bearing truck" (Rumiyah 2016, 11). One observer also notes the strategic value of IS lone-wolf attacks:

> With its defeats in Iraq, Syria, and Libya, the group is desperate for payback, and attacks by inspired supporters not only serve that purpose but are also an important force multiplier that works as a swarming tactic. A large number of uncoordinated attacks in a short period of time could upset the delicate balance of freedom and security in Western societies and bolster its [IS'] political objectives, such as using anti-Islamic sentiment in the West to feed its propaganda machine. (Mendelsohn 2016)

There is controversy, however, about the concept of lone-wolf attacks and its related concept of self-radicalization. Many commentators, observing the recent truck, knife, and shooting attacks perpetrated by lone terrorists, conclude that these people self-radicalized by reading IS or al-Qaeda or other material online with little or no contact with the organizations themselves. Likewise, some terrorists such as Mohammed Merah—the al-Qaeda-inspired gunman who killed seven people in Toulouse and Montauban, France, in 2012—may have become radicalized while serving time in French prison. Merah did, however, have at least some contact with al-Qaeda in Afghanistan and Pakistan and also possibly with Islamic terrorists in prison. As one commentator noted, "One does not become 'self-radicalized' in prison….There is always a facilitator, an influence, or a catalyst. Be that literature, another cellmate, or clergy" (Dunleavy 2012). How much is the individual responsible for his or her radicalization and how much is he or she recruiting by terrorists organizations? Is the model a "top-down" one—where recruiters seek out individuals—or a "bottom-up" one—where individuals seek out information (Veldhuis and Staun 2009)? The answer to this question seems to be that the process moves in both directions; it is a two-way street. Recruiters identify approachable people on the basis of beliefs they post online or actions they take or plan to take suggesting they are open to recruitment.

A recent study of the writings of 11 lone-wolf terrorists—only 2 of whom were Islamic radicals—concluded that their writings were dominated by negative emotions, particularly anger, but they are not less cognitively sophisticated or flexible in their thinking than writings by a baseline group or by 3 peaceful activists (Martin Luther King, Jr., Mahatma Gandhi, and Nelson Mandela) (Baele 2016). Radical Islamic groups like IS or al-Qaeda allow personally disaffected individuals the opportunity to externalize their personal grievances through a process of radicalization. Lone-wolf terrorists share several attributes—they suffered a degree of psychopathology and social ineptitude, their actions were facilitated by Internet access, and they were motivated by personal grievances combined with broader goals (Teich 2013). An online IS recruiter thus could be searching social media sites for postings that exhibit high degrees of anger, resentment, and sadness and then begin an online interaction with the individual assessing his or her interest in learning more about how to address their feelings toward the world. The process would seem to mirror the process by which psychological counselors seek to build trust with clients while leading them to address their problems—with the exception that the IS recruiter's goal is to lead the individual into identification with its radical ideology and possibly to take violent action to address their personal grievances.

FOR EXAMPLE

Seduced by IS

Laura Passoni's book *In the Heart of Daesh (IS) with My Son* (Passoni and Lorsignol 2016) recounts her story of being recruited by IS. Ms. Passoni is Belgian, raised as a Catholic but converted to Islam as a teenager. She became pregnant by her long-time boyfriend who then abandoned her and her son. She became depressed and in her depression, created a Facebook alias where she posted pictures of hijab-dressed women carrying automatic weapons. An IS recruiter saw these and took interest in her, eventually convincing her to join IS. The recruiter reportedly "showed her romantic videos about life in Syria, and never the violent ones. She imagined jihadists as brave, loyal men who would take care of her and her son" (Cigainero 2016). A Tunisian man then contacted her and offered to marry her and take her to Syria; she accepted.

Once in Syria, however, she was put in communal women's quarters while her husband underwent IS training. She learned that she was there to bear children for IS. Passoni, her son, and husband eventually escaped to the Turkish border where she was repatriated to Belgium. Both she and her husband were tried and convicted of associating with a terrorist organization. He is currently serving a four-year sentence in prison, while her sentence was suspended after the court determined she truly did not understand the nature of IS. She is currently lecturing to young Belgian women about the dangers of IS recruiting.

Passoni's vivid story is not unusual. There are a fairly large number of similar stories of Americans who have been recruited by or who self-selected IS. Vidino and Hughes (2015) cite several of these: two Somali-born and one Sudanese-descent teenage girls from Denver who were in online contact with the IS recruiter Umm Waqqas. The girls attempted to fly to Syria but were intercepted by German police in Frankfurt and sent home; Hoda Muthana, an American citizen born in Yemen, who lived in Alabama left the United States for Turkey and eventually Syria where she married an IS fighter (who was later killed in an airstrike). Muthana has herself become an IS propagandist on Twitter calling for violence in the United States during national holidays; the New Yorker "Samy" who became involved online with a Muslim Brotherhood supporter in Arizona who encouraged Samy to go to Syria and join IS. Samy underwent 3 weeks of religious training and a month of military training to become "a regular employee of IS" (Vidino and Hughes 2015, 10).

SELF-CHECK

- It is easy to differentiate between traditional media, electronic media, and social media. True or false?

- There is general agreement on the process by which people become self-radicalized. True or false?

- Which of the following statements best describes the differences between IS and al-Qaeda videos?

    a. They are basically the same because they espouse similar worldviews.

    b. IS videos are much more sophisticated than those of al-Qaeda.

    c. Al-Qaeda videos are like classic rock, while IS videos are like hip-hop.

    d. IS videos are much less interesting and exciting than al-Qaeda videos.

11.3 The Role of Educational Institutions

In the worldwide contest of ideas, what role do educational institutions play? For the most part, Western educational institutions have been the home of liberal democracy. It is in Western universities that students are introduced to the history of Western intellectual thought from Plato to postmodernist theorists. The term liberal arts is used to describe this set of humanistic values that students study in Western universities. Much of this study is designed to open minds, to increase tolerance for new and different ideas, to evaluate ideas based on their merit rather than their origin, and to weigh the relative merits of contesting ideas.

In opposition to this, liberal arts approach to education is the training school approach exemplified by military basic or advanced training or much of the curriculum in medical schools or engineering schools where students need to master specific "correct" approaches in order to be certified to become practitioners. A liberal arts approach to surgery might weigh the relative merits of surgery versus nonsurgical methods for addressing the underlying problem— including alternative therapies such as acupuncture or holistic approaches. A surgeon needs to be able, on the other hand, to conduct a surgical procedure with care such that the problem is solved, while the patient does not unduly suffer. While military officers may read Clausewitz or Machiavelli or Lao-tse on theories of war and how and when wars should be fought, enlisted soldiers in basic training do not. These latter soldiers are too busy learning how to master different weapons, how to act effectively as a unit, and how to obey the orders of their superiors.

11.3.1 Alternative Educational Institutions

Training schools are not the only competition to liberal arts-based universities. Religious schools—**madrassas**—have become popular venues for the teaching of traditional Islamic ideas in many countries where Islam is a popular religion. A recent analysis by *The Financial Times* estimated that there are some six million students studying in madrassas in the three countries of India, Pakistan, and Bangladesh alone (Mallet 2015). There are both economic and religious reasons why madrassas are attractive to Moslems. First, most madrassas are free of cost to those who attend; the schools are supported by alms given by Moslem faithful and, at least in the past, by wealthy Saudi international charities like *al-Haramayn*. Second, and most likely as important as financial considerations, many Moslems prefer that their children be educated in a religious institution since some "view its traditional pedagogical approach as a way to preserve an authentic Islamic heritage" (Armanios 2003, 3). Only a small number of madrassas have been linked to terrorist groups—the United States Agency for International Development (USAID) reported that such links are "rare but worrisome" (Benoliel 2003, 12), but the larger question of the effect of the type of education being offered at madrassas is murkier. Where the schools are financed by Saudi charities, the focus of the curriculum is often on Wahhabism, a strict form of Sunni Islam. In this type of curriculum, "students are often instructed to reject the 'immoral' and 'materialistic' Western culture" (Armanios 2003, 3). Graduates of madrassas are not particularly prepared to compete for Western or international corporate jobs, and so many find employment in the religious sector in their home countries or become educators in madrassas themselves.

11.3.2 International Students in the United States

Since the early part of the twentieth century, US universities have accepted large numbers of foreign students. Today, US universities house the largest number of international students (in excess of 1 000 000) of any country in the world, although as a percentage of all university students, the percentage of international students in the United States remains low (on the order of 1%). The Institute of International Education (IIE) reports that the largest numbers of such students come from China (328 547), India (165 918), Saudi Arabia (61 287), and South Korea (61 007) with substantial numbers also coming from Canada, Brazil, Taiwan, Japan, Vietnam, and Mexico. The dominant areas of study for these students are engineering (20.8%), business administration (19.2%), mathematics, and computers sciences (13.6%) with social sciences, health professions, education, and agriculture also being popular (Project Atlas 2016). US universities like to accept international students for a variety of reasons—at times they are even better prepared to pursue university courses than US-educated students are. Students who do not speak English as a first language but who have had formal training in English often know more about the English language than native-born English speakers who have picked up the language naturally. Training in math and science in many parts of the world is more rigorous than it is in the United States, and so students coming to this country to pursue university education in those fields often are better prepared than US-educated students.

In the past, the US government made substantial investments in the education of international students through such programs as the Muskie/Freedom Support Act program that provided tuition and stipends to students from former Soviet and Eastern European states studying in fields like law, public administration, public policy, business administration, and education. When the students have completed their studies in the United States, they were required to return to their home countries to work and were forbidden from applying for immigration to the United States for at least two years. The idea behind this program and others like it was multifaceted: to contribute to the economic and political development of other countries, to expose US students to excellent foreign students with the hope that such exposure will stimulate the US students to better performance, and so on. But one goal of the program should be clear—it is in the interests of the US government to attempt to spread US values to other countries, especially those where values are currently changing. Investing resources in university students seems to be a particularly good way of doing this since, upon returning home, many of the US-educated students take positions of political, economic, and educational leadership. Most international students studying in the United States are paying their own way from personal or family funds (67%). Some (17%) received funding from the university in which they are studying, while some 7% are funded by their own country and another 7% are funded through their employment (Open Doors 2016).

FOR EXAMPLE

International Students

Why do so many international students want to study in the United States? Some 19% of the 4.1 million students studying outside their own country came to the United States—almost twice the number studying in the second most attractive country, the United Kingdom (Zong and Batalova 2016). The quality of higher education in the United States, American culture that tends to be accepting of foreigners, and the possibility of staying in the United States after graduation have all been given as reasons why the United States is so attractive to international students. But another reason may be the national exams that many countries in the world use for admission into their public universities. Alan Goodman, president of the Institute of International Education (IIE), says in the United States, "you still have an opportunity to take courses in college and pursue the career of your choice rather than the career that is chosen for you based on your exam results" (Turner 2015). For some of these students, this choice is not an easy one. Turner cites the case of a young Indian man—Shreyas Manohar—who came to the United States to study at Columbia University in New York. Originally he was going to study economics in order to go into a business or management career, but he found he had an interest in creative writing. "Whether [an international student] studies what he actually likes, or whether he does something that is practical and which he can tell his parents that is redeemable for a job later," is a choice for international students studying in the United States in the same way that it is for domestic students (Turner 2015).

The general openness of the US system to international students does come at some cost. Several of the 9/11 terrorists entered the United States with legitimate student visas. This led the US government to a major reexamination of visa requirements for students studying in the United States. One problem with pre-9/11 regulations was the lack of monitoring of what foreign students studying in US universities were actually doing—some enrolled in classes, dropped them, and then disappeared for the remainder of the semester or academic year. Others graduated from the programs to which they applied and then disappeared into the US shadow economy, working as undocumented aliens. The problem of "visa overstaying" is probably larger (in terms of numbers of people) than the problem of people sneaking across the border from Mexico or Canada. The General Accounting Office (GAO) estimated that in 2003 there were some 2 000 000 people in the United States who had overstayed legitimate business, tourist, or student visas or Border Control Crossing cards (GAO 2004). More recently the Department of Homeland Security estimated a much smaller number—nearly 500 000—who had overstayed visas after arriving by air or by sea (DHS 2016). When asked in congressional testimony about the number of people overstaying US visas, Assistant Secretary for International Affairs at DHS, Alan Bersin, responded simply "we don't know" (Nixon 2016).

After 9/11, the US government began to address the question of tracking international students in the United States for study more seriously. Since 2002, international students who enter the United States have been required to register with Student and Exchange Visitor Information System (**SEVIS**), a computerized registry of international students studying in the United States. The fee for complying with SEVIS is paid by the individual student and is typically $100. Partially as a result of increased fees and regulations on international students (as well as increased tuition and fees in the United States), the number of such students requesting visas to study in the United States declined dramatically immediately after 9/11 and has continued to decline for the years following that, although at a much lower rate. At the same time, however, international students attending universities in Europe, Australia, and China have increased dramatically.

While the US government hopes that international students who study in the United States will return to their countries to spread US values, this may not always be the case. International students studying in the United States at times face discrimination in local rentals, education of children, and even in their interactions with other students. While the goal of most international study programs is to expose foreign students to their US colleagues, international students may wind up living and socializing with people from their home countries or with other international students. For students who do not speak English as a first language, living and socializing with somebody "from home" may mean speaking a language that is much more comfortable than English. This, of course, means that their exposure to and immersion in US culture is diminished. An evaluation of the first 10 years of the Muskie/Freedom Support Act graduate program found that alumni of the program had a more democratic outlook toward the work environment and greater communication skills and were more likely to think they could influence the direction that their own society was taking in comparison with a similar group of students who had not enrolled in US graduate programs (Bureau of Educational and Cultural Affairs 2002). All of these outcomes argue that exposure to US graduate programs has very positive outcomes on these international students who returned to their home countries.

SELF-CHECK

- The quality of higher education in the United States, American culture that tends to be accepting of foreigners, and the possibility of staying in the United States after graduation have all been given as reasons why the United States is so attractive to international students. True or false?
- What is SEVIS?
- The Institute of International Education (IIE) reports that the largest numbers of international students in the United States come from which country?
  - a. China
  - b. India
  - c. Saudi Arabia
  - d. South Korea

SUMMARY

In this chapter, you examined the broad topic of enablers of mass effects and the many variations on how this term can be applied in the context of homeland security today. Clearly, in the information age, the diverse forms of media and communication available to terrorist organizations can have multiplier effects in helping them win the war of ideas. The Internet and print and broadcast media have all contributed to the spread of information about terrorism and, at the same time, serve as a means of propagating terrorist messages throughout the world as well as recruiting individuals to serve as terrorists or terrorist supporters. At the same time, you learned the ease by which information can be transmitted through modern media makes communication in times of emergency or disaster much less cumbersome than it was in the past.

You also learned that within the United States, colleges and universities serve multiple educational purposes by providing the means by which international students can learn US democratic values and pluralism, or they can serve as recruiting grounds for disenfranchised groups who face discrimination or profiling, particularly Middle Eastern students. The same schools may also serve to educate students about Homeland Security and provide academic programs that will better enable future generations of security managers, planners, and leaders the tools to effectively combat terrorism through knowledge of the threat (see Chapter 13). At the same time, these programs of study can lead to new research methods and policy choices that will aid in confronting the threat of terrorism, without alienating nations and peoples who share the same desires for peace, security, and more democratic ways of life.

KEY TERMS

Al-Jazeera	An Arabic-language news network headquartered in Qatar.
Availability heuristic	A rule of thumb in decision making that assesses the probability of an event by how clearly we can imagine events like it.
Data mining	The use of the Internet for open-source information, which when pieced together, provides information of intelligence value for an organization.
Dark Web	The encrypted network that is only accessible through special browsers such as TOR, allowing users to remain anonymous or untraceable.
Deep Web	Anything posted on the Internet that a commonly used search engine such as Google cannot find but that can be found through the use of an internal search query.
Enabler	Anything that assists in the creation of mass effects. Can be an institution or process that makes it possible for the mass effect to occur when it would not have occurred otherwise; an institution or process that allows the mass effect to have a greater effect than it would have had otherwise; or an institution or process that is utilized by those who would cause a mass effect.
Homophily	Literally "love of the same;" this term is now used to describe the tendency for online users to seek out information that confirms their preexisting beliefs and to avoid information that might contradict those beliefs.
Madrassas	Religious schools, primarily located in Muslim countries, that teach radical Islamic ideas and are often considered a potential breeding ground for terrorists.
Materialists	People who are concerned with personal survival: providing for themselves or their families, making a good salary, and all the "perks" that come along with that salary.
Post-materialists	People who are more concerned with what some call "higher goals," such as preserving and protecting freedom of speech and other more self-expression-type values.
Psychological warfare	The use of propaganda and other psychological actions having the primary purpose of influencing the opinions, emotions, attitudes, and behavior of hostile foreign groups in such a way as to support the achievement of national objectives.

Representativeness heuristic	A rule of thumb in decision making that assesses the probability of an unknown event on the basis of how it represents an event we know.
SEVIS	Acronym for "Student and Exchange Visitor Information System," a computerized registry of international students studying in the United States.
TOR	An anonymous web browser that allows users' online activity to avoid being tracked by surveillance or traffic analysis.
Vividness heuristic	A rule of thumb in decision making that assesses the probability of an event based on how vividly it is described or portrayed.

ASSESS YOUR UNDERSTANDING

Go to www.wiley.com/go/Kilroy/Threats_to_Homeland_Security to assess your knowledge of the basics of enablers of mass effects.

Summary Questions

1. Enablers of mass effects refer only to the Internet. True or false?
2. Terrorist organizations are very aware of the role the media plays in helping them frame their story. True or false?
3. Psychological warfare is a term used only to describe means of interrogation. True or false?
4. While the US government hopes that international students who study in the United States will return to their countries to spread US values, this may not always be the case and they could return to their home countries with even more extremist views. True or false?
5. Schools that propagate radical Islamic teachings are called
   (a) Ummas
   (b) Materialists
   (c) Heuristics
   (d) Madrassas
6. Of all regions of the world, Internet growth is occurring most rapidly in
   (a) Africa
   (b) Latin America
   (c) Europe
   (d) The Middle East
7. Which of the following heuristics are applicable in understanding the power of ideas and communication?
   (a) Representativeness
   (b) Vividness
   (c) Availability
   (d) All of the above
8. The encrypted network that is only accessible through special browsers such as TOR, allowing users to remain anonymous or untraceable is called:
   (a) Dark Web
   (b) Deep Web
   (c) Secret Web
   (d) None of the above

Applying This Chapter

1. You are serving as a counterterrorism analyst at the Department of Homeland Security. Your boss asks you to explain how terrorist groups are using the Internet today. How would you respond? Provide specific examples of how terrorists are using the Internet today.

2. During a college class on the politics of terrorism, a student makes a comment that due to the potential threat of terrorists using student visas as a means of entering the United States legally, your university should stop accepting international students. How would you respond? Explain your reasons for supporting or not supporting such a position.

3. You are a staffer for an influential member of the US Congress (pick your local representative) who holds a key vote in a tough new anti-terrorism law. Conduct a web search on the Internet for information about this member of the Congress. Using data mining, see what you can find out about that individual that would help enable a terrorist organization better understand how to influence his or her vote using the enablers identified in this chapter. Only use open-source, accessible information available over the Internet or other known media sources. Prepare a report back to that member of the Congress.

4. Conduct a survey on campus of how many students have seen al-Jazeera TV broadcasts or visited the network's website. Record their responses as favorable, unfavorable, or neutral with regard to its reporting on the war on terrorism.

Terrorism and the Media

Review a number of different media sources in the United States and overseas reporting on terrorism. Compare similar stories in the different media outlets and how each source frames the argument. Determine the heuristic the reporter may be assuming in his or her reporting on the subject. Also consider the source within the Inglehart–Welzel Cultural Map for content analysis and perspective.

Understanding Heuristics

Do a study on the different types of heuristics that impact people's perception of natural disasters and the role of different government agencies. Present examples of real-world events, such as Hurricane Katrina, and determine that heuristic (vividness, availability, or representativeness) best explains their perception of which government agency was the least responsive to the disaster and why.

12

HOMELAND SECURITY INTELLIGENCE
Understanding the Structure and Methods for Protecting the Nation

Jonathan Smith

Department of Politics, Coastal Carolina University, Conway, SC, USA

Starting Point

Go to www.wiley.com/go/Kilroy/Threats_to_Homeland_Security to assess your knowledge of the basics of Homeland Security Intelligence.
Determine where you need to concentrate your effort.

What You'll Learn in This Chapter

▲ The nature of intelligence and how it supports homeland security

▲ The organization of intelligence capabilities across the homeland security enterprise

▲ The uses and limitations of the main types of intelligence collection methods in homeland security

▲ The inherent tension between intelligence operations and civil liberties in the American system of government

After Studying This Chapter, You'll Be Able To

▲ Describe the role of intelligence in supporting the decision processes of policymakers

▲ Explain how information that is relevant to homeland security missions is shared between the governmental and nongovernmental actors in the US homeland security community

▲ Assess which method of intelligence collection is most appropriate to a given homeland security challenge

▲ Explain how government organizations involved in homeland security attempt to collect intelligence information without infringing on the constitutional rights of citizens

Threats to Homeland Security: Reassessing the All-Hazards Perspective, Second Edition.
Edited by Richard J. Kilroy, Jr.
© 2018 John Wiley & Sons, Inc. Published 2018 by John Wiley & Sons, Inc.
Companion website: www.wiley.com/go/Kilroy/Threats_to_Homeland_Security

INTRODUCTION

In spite of the recent focus on terrorism, threats to domestic security are not a new phenomenon. Similarly, the collection and use of intelligence information to combat these threats is also an enduring component in how governments have attempted to respond. That being said, the growing role of non-state actors as both foreign and domestic security threats has expanded the quantity and capabilities of intelligence organizations across all levels of government in the US system. This growth has not only enhanced the capabilities and level of cooperation among domestic intelligence organizations but also renewed debate over government infringement of civil liberties guarantees.

In this chapter, you will trace the growing role that intelligence plays in supporting policymakers in homeland security issues. You will also learn to distinguish from the myriad of governmental and nongovernmental actors that provide intelligence support for homeland security missions, as well as their primary mechanisms for intelligence cooperation. Additionally, you will assess the strengths and weaknesses of various methods of intelligence collection that are used by these actors. Lastly, you will explain how the concern over preserving the civil liberties and civil rights of citizens impacts the conduct of intelligence activities within the United States.

12.1 Intelligence and Homeland Security

The tension between security and liberty has a long history within the United States. The use of intelligence information by governments is intended to support the most fundamental mission of the government—protecting the lives of its citizens. However, the potential for misuse of a process that is frequently conducted in secret raises concerns about whether it adheres to the confines of the law. The case of the New York Police Department (NYPD)'s attempt to monitor Muslim communities in the years following the September 11 attacks is illustrative of both the promises and pitfalls of utilizing intelligence in homeland security missions.

12.1.1 NYPD Surveillance of Muslim Communities

Given the impact of the September 11 terrorist attacks on the city of New York, it is unsurprising that the New York Police Department (NYPD) became one of the country's most robust domestic intelligence organizations. With some informal assistance from the Central Intelligence Agency (CIA), the NYPD constructed a clandestine intelligence collection operation under an organization known as the "Demographics Unit" (Apuzzo and Goldstein 2014). Starting in the mid-2000s, the operation focused on Muslim-affiliated communities and conducted surveillance operations within 100 miles of the city including sending informants into mosques and monitoring Muslim student associations at nearby universities. The hope was that this program would serve as an early warning system to prevent a terrorist attack. Unfortunately, there is no evidence that the program ever generated a lead or triggered a terrorist investigation for the NYPD (Apuzzo and Goldman 2012). However, it did raise substantial controversy when its activities were made public by the media in 2011. The program was officially disbanded in 2014 (Weisner 2015).

The revelation that the NYPD operations were occurring outside of the city limits without coordinating with its neighboring jurisdictions led to recriminations with elected leaders from those areas. For instance, while the NYPD alerted the Newark Police Department to its activities in their area, it did not alert the city's mayor or get his authorization for their surveillance operations (Dharapak 2012). New Jersey Governor Chris Christie, while noting a need for such operations to protect the region, was critical of the operation since it led to the prospect of multiple agencies watching the same people unbeknownst to one another (Portnoy 2012). The Federal Bureau of Investigation (FBI) also indicated that these unilateral activities by the NYPD outside of the city limits damaged FBI "partnerships with Muslims and jeopardized national security" (Apuzzo and Goldman 2012).

Additionally, the New York Police Department was taken to court by the targets of these collection activities. In three federal lawsuits, the plaintiffs accused the NYPD of violating their civil liberties. They alleged that the NYPD engaged in unconstitutional discrimination by utilizing "religious identity was a permissible proxy for criminality" (Weisner 2015). In allowing one of the cases to proceed, a US Circuit Court Judge concluded that the NYPD activities were akin to the treatment of Jewish Americans during the Red Scare or Japanese Americans during World War II. As of 2016, the city had settled two of these cases out of court.

This episode illustrates the modern nature of intelligence support to homeland security. First, the issue of combating terrorism is the highest of policy priorities within the United States to a degree never before seen in American history. Since the September 11 terrorist attacks and the continuing incidents of terrorism encouraged by violent Islamic extremist entities, governments at all levels within the American system are focused on preventing and mitigating this threat. Second, given the decentralized nature of our federal system, there are multiple actors and levels of government engaged in intelligence activities. This leads to issues of collaboration and deconfliction that are less prominent in the realm of intelligence activities outside of the United States. Lastly, because intelligence collection inside the homeland is more likely to involve citizens, legal and constitutional constraints on these activities are a more prominent than in comparable operations outside of the United States.

12.1.2 What Is Intelligence?

Intelligence is fundamentally about providing an information advantage to policymakers. If you can obtain information that your adversary does not have (or information that your adversary does not expect you to have), it strengthens your ability to prevail in a conflict or competition with that adversary. As the cliché goes, "information is power." For instance, in the NYPD surveillance of Muslim communities noted at the beginning of this chapter, the intent of the program was to gather information about a terrorist attack before it occurred—and, thus, prevent it from occurring. In a non-homeland security example, the role of intelligence in the Cuban Missile Crisis (1962) is widely viewed as a strong example of what the intelligence function can provide policymakers. In that case, US reconnaissance aircraft were able to detect the presence of Soviet nuclear-capable missiles that were hidden in the forests of Cuba. By supplying this knowledge to President Kennedy before the Soviets had intended for this to be made public, the president was able to direct US policy efforts that led to a successful withdrawal of the Soviet missiles from Cuba without armed conflict.

The use of intelligence to support policymakers is not a new phenomenon. Sometimes, intelligence is jokingly referred to as "the second oldest profession" (with prostitution being the first). Examples from ancient history abound. For instance, Moses was seeking intelligence for the Israelites when they arrived at Canaan after escaping bondage in Egypt. In the Book of Numbers, he dispatched twelve spies to the area to gather information and report back. Among other things, Moses requested that these men, "See what the land is like and whether the people living there are strong or weak, few or many" (The Holy Bible NIV 1984, 355). When they returned, the information they provided was key to the Israelites choosing to not attempt an attack at that time.

As with many concepts, there can be a variety of competing definitions for the term intelligence. Common attributes that are found in these definitions are the use of secrecy in the process and the role in supporting policy (Warner 2007). One commonly used definition comes from Mark Lowenthal, a retired intelligence official. He defines intelligence as "the process by which specific types of information important to national security are requested, collected, analyzed and provided to policymakers…" (Lowenthal 2015, 10). This definition is essentially an abbreviated encapsulation of the intelligence cycle (Figure 12-1).

The **intelligence cycle** is a widely used model for understanding the process by which intelligence assessments are produced and delivered. While some scholars, such as Arthur Hulnick, have criticized the intelligence cycle as inconsistent with real-world practice, it does identify the five basic elements that are necessary for the process to work (Hulnick 2015, 90). Ideally, this cycle would start with some planning and direction, where a policymaker would pose a question or identify an information gap (this is sometimes referred to as an intelligence requirement). For instance, in the NYPD surveillance of Muslim communities, the process should have started with a policymaker asking about the likelihood of terrorist threats to the city. From there, the intelligence bureaucracy would develop and execute a plan to collect information that could assist in answering this intelligence requirement. However, **intelligence collection** often generates a large volume of information regardless of its potential value to answering the initial question. Processing and exploitation is the third step in the cycle and is tasked with sifting through the collected information to find data that is relevant and useful to addressing the intelligence requirement. This information is then passed along to the analysis and production phase of the intelligence cycle. Here the new information is combined with previous knowledge on the subject to construct a paper or oral presentation that addresses the initial question. Finally, this paper or presentation is delivered to the policymakers in the last step of the intelligence cycle, dissemination.

This process is identified as a "cycle" in order to highlight that the intelligence process is ongoing. That is, if the process does not yield sufficient information to support the policymaker, then the process starts again. Alternatively, even if the information is sufficient to answer the initial question, it may yield new questions that policymakers want the intelligence organization to address. So, the

Figure 12-1

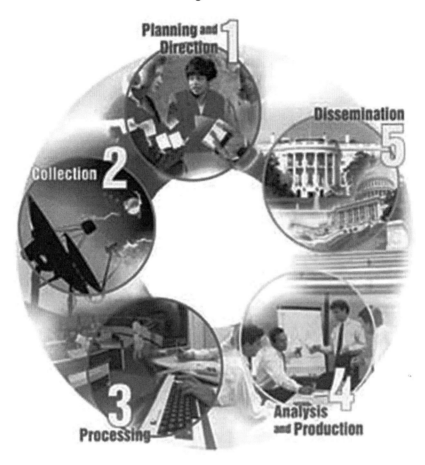

Intelligence cycle (CIA 2012, 39).

intelligence bureaucracy should be continually operating to address the needs of policymakers.

With regard to how intelligence information is collected, it can be acquired either actively or passively. Traditional conceptions of the intelligence process envision an active approach to collection. In this case, a decision maker asks a question and then the collection process allocates resources to answer that question. For instance, in the Cuban Missile Crisis example, the Air Force and Central Intelligence Agency began photo-reconnaissance flights over Cuba in response to an intelligence requirement that wanted to know the presence and extent of Soviet military activity on the island. However, in the realm of homeland security, much of the information is gathered in a passive manner known as **surveillance**. This is the continuous observation of a place, person, group, or ongoing activity in order to gather information. For instance, an immigration officer at the border may not be attempting to address an intelligence question, but their ongoing collection of information on people entering the country is recorded and may be of use to intelligence at some later point (Figure 12-2).

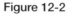

Figure 12-2

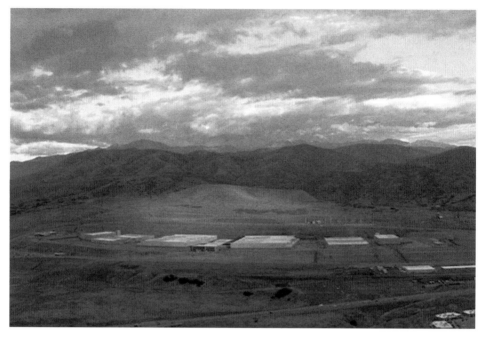

NSA Bumblehive Utah Data Center. Source: Photo Courtesy of Parker Higgins EFF (2014).

FOR EXAMPLE

The Bumblehive

Historically, surveillance has been limited by the ability to store this data. However, advances in computer technology have substantially improved the ability to store and access large volumes of information. For instance, the National Security Agency created a new data storage facility for the organization in Utah in 2012. Known as the "**Bumblehive**", it is a massive data repository to collect digital information and is projected to have a capacity of five billion gigabytes. According to one report, this facility could collect and maintain records on every phone call made in the United States for a year with only 2% of its storage capacity. (Goodwin 2016)

This process of supporting policymakers with intelligence can be done in a variety of areas. While many tend to envision national security issues when considering intelligence, it can also be used to support decision making in other areas like business and public health. So, when we are discussing the idea of homeland security intelligence, what is meant by that? This question has not been resolved to date. As Mark Lowenthal noted, "over a decade after 2001, U.S. policymakers and intelligence officers are still working out what homeland security intelligence means" (Lowenthal 2015, 371). For this chapter, we will use the idea that this term signifies an intelligence support function to homeland security. But that begs the question what is "homeland security"? The Department of Homeland Security (DHS) defines its vision as "ensuring a homeland that is safe, secure, and resilient against terrorism and other hazards" (DHS 2016). With these missions in mind, we will focus our discussion of intelligence in the counterterrorism and law enforcement intelligence domains.

12.1.3 The Limited Historical Role of Intelligence in Domestic Affairs

The application of intelligence support in the domestic arena has always been politically circumspect. The idea that government could utilize secret monitoring of US citizens has raised concerns about violating central constitutional principles of the citizenry. As one study noted, "American society with its strong sense of civil liberties has long held in disdain the conduct of intelligence operations within the United States against its own citizens" (Gerringer and Bart 2014, 75).

However, aside from an abstract concern about the potential for abuse, part of this reluctance was borne of episodes where the federal government actually engaged in inappropriate intelligence practices against its citizens. For instance, as public opinion was driven by anti-communist sentiment in the years after World War I, the Department of Justice utilized questionable legal methods to locate individuals with communist or anarchist affiliations during the **Palmer Raids**. In response to a series of terrorist bombings, Attorney General A. Mitchell Palmer tasked the recently created Bureau of Investigation (the forerunner to the current Federal Bureau of Investigation) to track and expel people who were deemed a security threat. However, the use of illegal entrapment and incommunicado detentions raised objections from Congress and other executive departments (Rosen 2013). In another example, President Hoover utilized a member of the Office of Naval Intelligence to conduct an espionage operation to steal information and monitor political opponents in 1930 (Gregory 2016, 38). As can be seen, questions about the appropriate use of intelligence operations inside the United States are not a new concern.

The idea that a domestic intelligence function was a possible threat to the American system of government was a prominent factor in how the current national intelligence community (IC) was formed in the years after World War II. Stories about the activities of the German secret police—the Gestapo—in their country provided a cautionary example about the possible impact of a domestic intelligence organization in the United States. The revelations of how this organization was utilized to identify and exterminate government opposition within the country highlighted the potential abuse that such an intelligence capability could bring to a political system. In spite of the rising threat of communism in the aftermath of World War II, policymakers wanted to avoid creating this type of organization. As Rhodri Jeffreys-Jones (1989) noted, "Truman's concern about the possible development of an American police state was the single most important factor in causing him to block early central intelligence agency proposals" (Jeffreys-Jones 1989, 30).

As a result, when a permanent national security intelligence function was established with the Central Intelligence Agency (CIA) in 1947, a bright line was drawn between the foreign and domestic arenas. The CIA was prohibited from utilizing domestic police powers. Similarly, the Federal Bureau of Investigation (FBI), which had developed extensive intelligence networks in Latin America during the war, was required to relinquish its foreign operations and focus solely on domestic work. This basic division would remain in force as new organizations joined the national intelligence community. However, while the CIA–FBI division of responsibility brought peace of mind to the governmental leadership, it also brought "alarming stories of rivalry and lack of cooperation between the external and internal guardians of security" (Jeffreys-Jones 1989, 30). This competition would be a significant problem with the rise of non-state actors in the late twentieth century.

The events of September 11, 2001, substantially altered the concerns regarding domestic intelligence organizations. However, before the rise of terrorism challenged this barrier between foreign and domestic intelligence capabilities, other trends outside of terrorism were challenging this foreign–domestic divide. For instance, the US counternarcotics effort in the War on Drugs has straddled this world of external national security threats and domestic law enforcement. Since its inception in 1973, the Drug Enforcement Agency has had an intelligence function that was tasked not only with looking at consumption of illegal drugs inside the United States but also with the cultivation and transportation that occurs outside the country. This also blurs the distinction between security and law enforcement functions. As one author noted when discussing the relationship between law enforcement and national security intelligence, "these two categories of intelligence overlap and often are indistinguishable from one another" (Smith 2014, 59).

SELF-CHECK

- Define intelligence.
- Intelligence collection is a widely used model for understanding the process by which intelligence assessments are produced and delivered. True or false?
- Which US intelligence organization was created in 1947?
  a. Army Intelligence
  b. CIA
  c. DIA
  d. FBI

12.2 The Structure of Intelligence Organizations

The availability of intelligence information in homeland security is driven by two factors: intelligence collection and collaboration with other intelligence organizations. That is, according to most concepts of the intelligence cycle—the process by which intelligence reports are created and disseminated to decision makers—intelligence collection is a central component. After all, without the raw information that is generated by the collection process, what is there to analyze or disseminate? However, intelligence information (both raw data and finished intelligence products) can also be provided by collaborative arrangements with other agencies and levels of government. As a result, this chapter discusses not only the collection methods that are usually identified in a discussion on the intelligence process but also the nature of the collaboration between intelligence-related structures in the US homeland security system.

As with any other discussion of homeland security in the United States, what is found in this area is that there is a greater need for collaboration than what is discussed in US national security. In national security intelligence, the need for collaboration is only between competing organizations within a single level of government. For example, one of the key recommendations of the 9/11 Commission was for increased collaboration between two organizations in the US Intelligence Community: the FBI and the CIA (Kean and Hamilton 2004). In contrast, understanding the homeland security intelligence environment requires an awareness of the federal–state relationship. That is, the intelligence section of the New York Police Department is ultimately controlled by the state of New York, not the US government. There is also a more significant need for understanding the role that private actors play in providing intelligence support to homeland security missions in the United States.

Another factor that complicates information exchange between organizations in homeland security is the distinction between the terms "intelligence" and "investigation." To be sure, the methods of investigation are very similar to the steps of the intelligence cycle (Smith 2014, 60). However, the different terms highlight the different contexts in how the information is utilized. While this is not an absolute distinction, intelligence tends to be more prospective in focus and investigations tend to be more retrospective. *The National Incident Management System Field Guide* highlights this difference. It defines intelligence as "information that has been evaluated and from which conclusions have been drawn *to make* informed decisions" (emphasis mine). In contrast, it defines investigation as "the systematic collection and analysis of information pertaining to factors suspected of contributing to, or *having caused*, an incident" (emphasis mine) (FEMA 2013, 34).

Historically, this distinction has complicated information sharing between domestic security organizations, particularly between law enforcement and intelligence entities. In particular, it can lead to different standards regarding how and when to gather information, as well as how to utilize that information once it is collected. As William Spracher (2014) notes, "While law enforcement aims to arrest perpetrators of a crime… and obtain a conviction, intelligence… often prefers to gain information about trends and patterns without rolling up the sources of the information too soon" (7). Hence, law enforcement is typically interested in information that can lead to successful criminal prosecutions. They must ensure that not only is the level of information sufficient to support the prosecution, but that it was also obtained properly lest it be inadmissible in court (this is legal principle known as the exclusionary rule). In contrast, intelligence organizations are typically interested in information that can warn of an upcoming event so that decision makers can take steps to avert the problem. They are typically less constrained about how the information is acquired. So, aside from any other barriers that are common for organizational collaboration (e.g., jurisdictional conflict, intergovernmental competition, etc.), the intelligence function in homeland security can also be complicated by who is collecting the information and how that information is being utilized.

FOR EXAMPLE

The Boston Marathon Bombing

The April 2013 bombing of the Boston Marathon ended with the death of one suspect and the apprehension of another. Wounded in the final shootout with police, Dzhokhar Tsarnaev was taken to the hospital for treatment. However, Tsarnaev was questioned by the FBI *before* he was read his Miranda rights. Under a Justice Department rule, a suspect can be interrogated without receiving a warning of his rights under a "public safety" exception. Indeed, the rule allows for continued interrogation for collecting valuable and timely intelligence even if that is not connected to the immediate threat to public safety (Bazelon 2013). This episode highlights a dilemma for the FBI—is their main goal prevention or prosecution?

This distinction between law enforcement and intelligence in the United States has been referred to as "the wall." Driven by revelations in the 1970s, the concept was that national security intelligence and law enforcement activities inside the United States would be distinctly separate activities to prevent the possibility of misusing intelligence resources inside the United States. However, like the blurring of the foreign–domestic divide in intelligence, the events of September 11 terrorist attacks have also complicated this distinction. The emphasis of detecting and tracking possible terrorist threats inside the United States has prompted a more robust connection between intelligence organizations and local law enforcement. Also, the recognition that terrorist entities collaborate with (or engage in their own) criminal enterprises further complicates the distinction. For instance, the Afghan Taliban utilize the opium trade to support their terror activities in that country. This crime-terror nexus means that it is an increasing difficult challenge to separate the worlds of intelligence and law enforcement. As a result, in the years since the September 11 terrorist attacks, institutional arrangements in homeland security intelligence have been in flux.

12.2.1 National-Level Intelligence Organizations

Aside from the changes in the nature of the relationship between law enforcement and intelligence, the opening years of the twenty-first century brought strong pressures to reform the US' intelligence structure. On September 11, 2001, the terrorist strikes on the World Trade Center and the Pentagon were only the beginning incidents that led to calls to improve the national-level intelligence system. Later that fall, a series of anthrax attacks carried out via the US postal system further exacerbated concerns about the ability of the intelligence community structure to identify and warn of impending dangers. These concerns about the national intelligence community grew even more as a result of the national intelligence estimate on Iraq's weapons of mass destruction (WMD) capabilities in 2003. These incidents, in conjunction with the subsequent postmortem reports of several high-profile commissions that were convened to study these issues (e.g., the 9/11 Commission, the Robb–Silberman Commission) prompted calls to reform the intelligence community. As a result, the **Intelligence Reform and Terrorist Prevention Act (IRTPA)** was signed into law in December 2004.

This legislation changed the national intelligence leadership in two significant ways. First, the head of the intelligence community was renamed from the Director of Central Intelligence (DCI) to the **Director of National Intelligence** (DNI). This was not merely a change in name, but also of mandate. Under the old system, the Director of Central Intelligence was the President's chief intelligence advisor on foreign intelligence issues. Under the new system, the DNI was responsible not only for foreign intelligence but also for the domestic and homeland security intelligence domains. The second substantial change was that the Director of National Intelligence did not have managerial control over the Central Intelligence Agency like their DCI predecessors. Under the pre-IRTPA system, the head of the IC was also dual-hatted as the director of the CIA. Some have suggested that this separation has weakened DNI's position as head of the intelligence community. For instance, Richard Posner argues that DNI's inability to hire or fire across the community or to move resources except in a circumscribed way is a sign that the IRTPA reorganization has not be successful (Posner 2006, 25).

Through the Office of the Director of National Intelligence (ODNI), this legislation mandated changes that were important to the challenge of homeland security. For example, the Federal Bureau of Investigation was charged with establishing an intelligence branch to support its national security mission. This led to a substantial growth of the intelligence function within the FBI. One book notes that two-thirds of the FBI's intelligence positions did not exist prior to this legislation (Priest and Arkin 2012). Also, the Department of Homeland Security was tasked with conducting preflight comparisons between airline passenger manifests and federal government watch lists.

The primary function for the DNI is to coordinate the activities of the intelligence community (IC). This function can be seen by the major operational centers located within the ODNI organization. For instance, one such center is the **National Counterterrorism Center** (NCTC). The vision statement of the NCTC notes that it is an operational center that leads the community by setting the standard for expertise, collaboration, and information sharing on counterterrorism issues. It is also staffed by personnel from multiple departments and agencies across the US government (NCTC 2016). This same model is utilized in the other operational centers in ODNI—the National Counterintelligence and Security Center, the National Counterproliferation Center, and the Cyber Threat Intelligence Integration Center (CTIIC). The CTIIC is the newest center, being created in February 2015, and is symptomatic of the growing importance of cyber issues in intelligence.

It is important to note that DNI's role is to coordinate, vice control the constituent organizations of the IC. Aside from being mandated as the principal intelligence advisor to the president, DNI's focus is to oversee and direct the implementation of the National Intelligence Program by leading efforts at intelligence integration (ODNI 2017). This means that the DNI does not have direct managerial control over the members of the US intelligence community outside of ODNI. This distinction severely limits DNI's ability to control the activities of the larger IC.

Figure 12-3

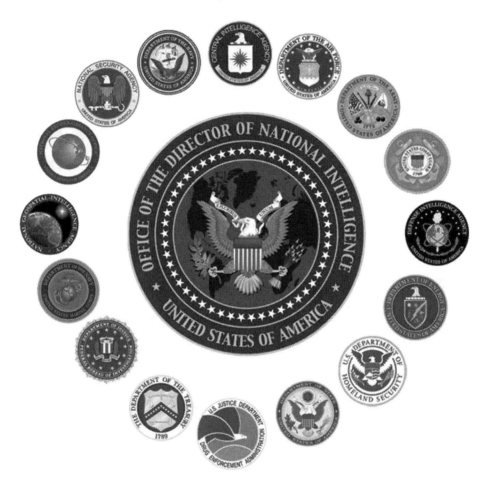

US Intelligence Community (DNI 2011).

Aside from the ODNI, there are 16 constituent organizations within the US intelligence community. The Central Intelligence Agency is the most well-known member of the IC. However, the Department of Defense (DoD) manages the largest portion of the intelligence community with eight separate organizations. Several cabinet departments—State, Energy, Treasury, and Homeland Security—have intelligence departments that serve as members of the IC as well as the Federal Bureau of Investigation and the Drug Enforcement Agency (both elements of the Department of Justice) and, lastly, the Coast Guard (while part of the Department of Homeland Security) (Figure 12-3).

Among these IC members, the Central Intelligence Agency (CIA) is the only independent agency dedicated to intelligence operations. It is important to note that CIA's mandate is focused on foreign, not domestic, intelligence. For instance, it is the lead organization for counterintelligence missions of the US government only when they are outside of the United States. The CIA is a multipurpose organization performing many different intelligence functions. The Directorate of Intelligence focuses on the production and dissemination of intelligence analysis, and the National Clandestine Service on clandestine human intelligence (HUMINT) collection and covert action operations.

While specific information is unavailable, the eight intelligence organizations within the DoD are believed to represent as much as 80% of the IC budget (Jensen et al. 2013, 66). Four of these are the intelligence components of the uniformed services and are tasked with the development of intelligence capabilities for their respective branches. For instance, the Office of Naval Intelligence supports the Department of the Navy. The 25th Air Force (known as the Air Force Intelligence Agency until 2014) provides the same function for the Air Force. The Intelligence and Security Command of the US Army and the Marine Corps Intelligence Activity have comparable missions. They are managed by their respective service secretaries and are typically focused on operational-level intelligence issues.

The Defense Intelligence Agency (DIA) reports directly to the Secretary of Defense. This organization primarily provides strategic-level intelligence analysis on military and defense issues. However, while the DIA serves as an all-source intelligence analysis organization, it also engages in intelligence collection in a number of ways. The Defense Attaché System, which provides overt human intelligence collection at US embassies abroad, is managed by this organization. More recently, the DIA established a Defense Clandestine Service that is designed to conduct espionage operations akin to the CIA's National Clandestine Service. The DIA is also the lead organization in the IC for the Measurement and Signature Intelligence (MASINT) collection program.

The Defense Intelligence Agency is separate from the military services and serves as a mechanism for coordinating and integrating the services. For instance, the DIA manages the placement of military and civilian intelligence personnel to the intelligence organizations of the combatant commands (COCOMs), such as US Central Command (CENTCOM). While the intelligence organizations of the COCOMs do not count as members of the IC, they provide substantial intelligence collection and analysis from their assigned region. One of these COCOMs—US Northern Command (NORTHCOM)—is tasked with providing military support to civil authorities within the United States, as well as protecting US interests on the continent of North America.

Beyond DIA and the services, there are three intelligence organizations within the Department of Defense that are critical to national-level intelligence collection activities. First, the National Security Agency (NSA) is the lead intelligence organization with regard to signals intelligence (SIGINT) collection and communication security. The NSA is the largest employer of mathematicians in the country and is the primary US organization for the encryption and decryption of national security information. Widely believed to be the largest (by both manpower and budget) organization within the IC, this organization also has a substantial connection to cyber intelligence issues. Indeed, US Cyber Command, a component of US Strategic Command, was created at the NSA in 2009. Additionally, the director of the NSA is dual-hatted as the commander of this military organization (see Chapter 8).

The National Geospatial-Intelligence Agency (NGA) and the National Reconnaissance Office (NRO) are the two other civilian organizations within the Department of Defense. NGA is the lead organization in the IC for geospatial intelligence (GEOINT) collection and analysis. While the mission of NGA is external to the United States, they have provided support to humanitarian operations within the country. Much of NGA's work would be impossible without the National Reconnaissance Office (NRO). A joint DoD–CIA-staffed organization whose existence was not publicly acknowledged until 1992, the NRO is a primary enabler of technical intelligence collection missions. Its mission centers on the design, construction, and operation of the nation's reconnaissance satellites.

Like the military service intelligence components of the DoD, many nonmilitary intelligence organizations are elements of an established cabinet department and are primarily charged with supporting that policy area. Hence, their specializations are connected to the organization that they serve. The Bureau of Intelligence and Research (INR) at the State Department provides all-source intelligence analysis and reporting in support of US diplomacy. The Office of Intelligence and Counterintelligence of the Department of Energy is focused on counterproliferation intelligence. The Department of the Treasury maintains an intelligence function that was created in 2004 and focuses on intelligence and counterintelligence issues that relate to the department's missions and responsibilities. This means it specializes on financial intelligence (FININT).

There are two agencies within the Department of Justice that are members of the intelligence community. The Drug Enforcement Agency joined the IC in 2006. Its Office of National Security Intelligence is charged with facilitating coordination and information sharing with other elements of the national government in counter-drug activities. The other IC agency within the Department of Justice is the Federal Bureau of Investigation. Unlike the CIA and the intelligence organizations within the Department of Defense, these organizations have missions that are more likely to involve them in domestic security operations that would relate to homeland security.

While it serves in both a law enforcement and an intelligence capacity, the FBI is mandated by federal law as the lead agency in domestic intelligence collection (Carter 2004, 16). As a result, in addition to pursuing traditional law enforcement missions like major thefts, white collar crime, and corruption, the FBI also pursues foreign espionage assets, subversives, and terrorists. In the balance between law enforcement and intelligence, the recent emphasis on counterintelligence and combating terrorism has shifted the focus of the FBI toward intelligence-related operations.

Beyond the headquarters element, there are 56 FBI field offices located throughout the United States. These offices conduct operations and investigations within their jurisdiction, and each has an associated Field Intelligence Group (FIG). These sections use linguists, analysts, and special agents to gather and assess intelligence information from their area to support the national headquarters. Additionally, each of these FBI field intelligence offices manages at least one **Joint Terrorism Task Force** (JTTF) to promote collaboration with other government organizations at the federal, state, and local levels.

12.2.2 The Department of Homeland Security and Intelligence

Within the Department of Homeland Security (DHS), there are two IC members. The Coast Guard was moved from the Department of Transportation to the Department of Homeland Security when it was formed in 2002. Its intelligence office provides support to the operational elements of the service in their maritime security missions. Within the DHS headquarters, the **Office of Intelligence and Analysis** (I&A) is the newest member to join the intelligence community and is tasked with ensuring that the homeland remains safe, secure, and resilient (Larence 2014, 9). This office does not possess any unique intelligence collection capabilities, but it does represent the primary avenue for IC collaboration with the network of fusion centers that are operated by state and local governments throughout the United States. It is also tasked with managing intelligence information in support of the Homeland Security Enterprise.

12.2.2.1 The Homeland Security Intelligence Enterprise

When the Department of Homeland Security was created in 2002, it represented the largest federal government reorganization since 1947. However, it represented more of a consolidation of functions than the creation of new ones. Twenty-two previously separate organizations were now unified under one cabinet department. A natural management question was how these offices would integrate their (sometimes overlapping) capabilities. Intelligence collection and analysis is one of those areas of concern. The headquarters element of the DHS is expected to establish mechanisms to coordinate intelligence analysis and collection within the organization. To that end, the head of the Office of Intelligence and Analysis (I&A) is mandated to serve both as the head of that particular office and as chief intelligence officer for the entire cabinet department.

Aside from the headquarters element of DHS, there are six agencies that have an internal intelligence component—Customs and Border Protection, Immigration and Customs Enforcement, US Citizenship and Immigration Services (USCIS), Transportation Security Administration, the Secret Service, and the Coast Guard. Of these, only Coast Guard Intelligence is a formal member of the IC. This collection of offices—the I&A Office in Homeland Security and its six constituent partners—represents a distinct intelligence sub-community at the federal level. The primary purpose of these resident intelligence functions is to provide tactical and operational support to their respective agencies. While these intelligence entities collaborate and share information, they do not represent a unified structure. Much like DNI's relationship to the other IC organizations, I&A is charged with fostering collaboration, vice directly managing its constituent partners. They can also provide training and access to other intelligence community resources for these agencies (Larence 2014, 21–22). So, while these constituent agencies are mandated to advise and coordinate closely with I&A, the intelligence offices of these operational components report to the heads of their respective agencies (Randol 2010, 7) (Figure 12-4).

Most of these agencies collect surveillance information in the normal course of their operational activities. For instance, Customs and Border Protection (CBP) gathers large amounts of data regarding personnel and cargo inbound to the United States. They also gain information from their disruption of illegal activities along the border (e.g., illegal immigration and drug seizures). In another example, the Citizenship and Immigration Services (USCIS) collects background information and biometric data on individuals applying for immigration benefits (Randol 2010, 34). The information that is gathered by these agencies can be stored and utilized to provide support to decision makers, as needed.

Figure 12-4

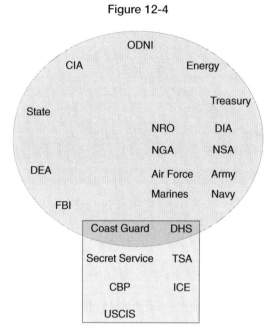

Relationship between IC and homeland security intelligence.

FOR EXAMPLE

UK Terror Plots 2007

In 2007, there were two attempted terrorist attacks in the United Kingdom. In the course of their investigations, the British authorities determined that the bombing suspects had immigrated to the United Kingdom and had been working as medical professionals. In response to this revelation, USCIS reviewed its records for individuals who had immigrated to the United States with comparable backgrounds to the UK suspects. This information was correlated with other data to produce several reports that were used to support the counterterror efforts of the intelligence community (Randol 2010, 36).

12.2.3 State, Local, and Tribal Government

In addition to the national government, there are more than 89 000 state, local, and tribal government organizations in the United States. With the growing threat of non-state actors in the post-9/11 environment, many of these organizations are developing intelligence capabilities to support their unique security requirements. Since these organizations will often be the first responders in any homeland security crisis, they also serve as a useful intelligence warning tool for national-level decision makers.

12.2.3.1 Law Enforcement

In the United States, there are more than 17 985 state, local, and tribal law enforcement organizations. Many of these organizations are quite small. Approximately half of these organizations have less than 10 full-time officers on staff and little, if any, intelligence capability. However, an increasing number of midsize forces have added collection and analysis capabilities in the years since the September 11 terrorist attacks (Steiner 2015, 51). While very few local law enforcement agencies could hope to match the capabilities of the New York Police Department, the incorporation of intelligence practices continues to reach deeper into the world of local law enforcement.

This growth is driven by a desire to reduce threats to the communities they serve. The underlying approach is influenced by a relatively new law enforcement paradigm known as **intelligence-led policing** (ILP). This is a model of law enforcement that emphasizes intelligence support in assessing and managing risk to guide operations. Its focus is on preventing crimes, as opposed to reacting to crimes that have already occurred. And since it involves forecasting criminal or illicit courses of action, the tools of intelligence analysis are essential. The ILP model gained currency in the United Kingdom in the 1990s, where two local police organizations successfully utilized analysis of previous crimes to reduce motor theft and property crime in their jurisdictions (Jensen et al. 2013, 279). This approach to policing has gained currency in US law enforcement since the turn of the century.

Beyond utilizing intelligence methods to reduce crimes in their local area, it is also important to note the "first responder" role that local law enforcement can play in homeland security. For instance, in the San Bernardino terrorist attack in December 2015, local law enforcement forces secured the scene of the initial attack. They also debriefed victims, which provided critical information for local police to locate and kill the terrorists. As James Steiner noted, local law enforcement is important to the FBI because not only does it represent a large intelligence collection network, but it is also an operational partner during emergency contingencies (Steiner 2016, 354).

12.2.3.2 National Guard

Each state—and several US territories—has a National Guard that is a military reserve force under the dual control of their local state or territorial government, as well as the federal government. Since the passage of the Dick Act of 1903, organized state militias have been required to mirror federal military forces in organization, equipment, and discipline (Stentiford 2002, 13). Under normal conditions, they are controlled by their state or territorial government under Title 32 of the US Code. However, they can be federalized under Title 10 of the US Code. Under these conditions, National Guard forces are subject to national government control and must abide by the same rules and regulations that govern the Department of Defense.

The National Guard represents a unique organization in homeland security intelligence due to their reduced restrictions in supporting state and local operations when they are not federalized. Under those circumstances, they are not subject to the restrictions of the Posse Comitatus Act, which limits the use of the US military in the domestic security domain. They often are represented in state fusion centers where their counter-drug and civil support team elements are authorized by regulation to support civil authorities. However, they are also required to provide the National Guard Bureau at the federal level with information to support situational awareness and a common operating picture (Coble 2009, 35).

12.2.4 The Private Sector

Private companies are increasingly involved in intelligence functions. Some are incorporating intelligence practices to support internal decision-making processes much like our conventional conception of the use of intelligence. However, intelligence is also potentially a service or product that can be marketed to government or other private actors.

Many large corporations in finance, energy, healthcare, and telecommunications have intelligence functions that are designed to provide security analysis and decision support to their leadership. Threat mitigation and risk assessment are common concerns, as these facilities can be the target of both criminal and terrorist attacks. For instance, the American International Group (AIG) insurance company maintains a global security operations center, which conducts security briefings and threat analysis to advance the safety and security of AIG employees and assets worldwide. The growing vulnerability of large organizations to computer network intrusion makes security and risk analysis a growing priority within the private sector.

Corporations can also incorporate intelligence analysis in order to understand their competition and the market forces that impact their profitability. In this regard, they function much like their governmental counterparts. For instance, in the mid-twentieth century, Japanese car manufacturers were attempting to expand their sales in the US automobile market. The early days were not successful. However, these firms studied production innovations in the US, as well as consumer habits and long-term resource trends. So, when instability in the Middle East led to dramatic rises in the price of gasoline—prompting customers to seek out smaller and more fuel-efficient vehicles—Japanese car manufacturers were well positioned (Walton 2010, 282). In this instance, a collection of private firms studied their current operating environment and future trends in order to guide their strategic choices for future growth.

Aside from conducting intelligence support to facilitate their own operations, some businesses also provide this to government offices on a contract basis. While the use of private contractors to augment government personnel in key functions is not new, its growth in the security sector in the wake of September 11 terrorist attacks has been profound. There are 1931 private companies that work on programs related to counterterrorism, homeland security, and intelligence in the United States (Priest and Arkin 2012, 10). According to a report in the *New York Times*, 70% of the national intelligence budget in 2013 was allocated for services provided by the private sector (Shorrock 2013).

The Department of Homeland Security was particularly reliant upon contractor support in its early years of operations due to the need to meet security requirements as rapidly as possible. In the initial DHS grant guidance for developing **fusion centers**, it encouraged the "hiring of contractors/consultants…for participation in information/intelligence sharing groups of intelligence fusion centers" (DHS 2004, 27). This involvement of private contractors in state fusion centers has raised concerns by some observers about unfair market advantage and possible violations of civil liberties (German and Stanley 2007, 2).

Some private companies also produce intelligence analysis for anyone who is willing to pay for a subscription. These organizations utilize publicly available, open-source analysis to provide insight on a variety of security issues around the globe, including homeland security issues. For instance, STRATFOR, a well-known firm in Texas, provides geopolitical analysis and consulting services to website subscribers and corporate clients. Other companies, such as Jane's Intelligence Review, KGS Nightwatch, and the Economist Intelligence Unit, provide comparable services.

12.2.5 Intelligence Collaboration

With such a broad collection of federal, state, and nongovernmental actors that could be relevant to homeland security intelligence issues, the question of how well these organizations share information is important. Given that secrecy is oftentimes viewed as a defining trait of intelligence, the idea of sharing with others can be counterintuitive. For instance, in discussing the evolution of law enforcement intelligence, some have noted that the sharing of intelligence between organizations has been limited historically (Gerringer and Bart 2014, 75). A recent study from the American Enterprise Institute echoed that sentiment when it noted, "federal, state, and local law enforcement entities outside of Washington are doing the work to gather, share and analyze information and intelligence *within several, often siloed structures*" (emphasis mine) (Mayer 2016, 1) (Figure 12-5).

The need to share information across this diverse collection of actors is widely recognized. For instance, the **National Criminal Intelligence Sharing Plan** (NCISP) was established in 2003 to promote the sharing of critical information among law enforcement personnel across all levels of government. Organizations that invite participation from other entities to share information and coordinate activities are increasingly common across the government. Several frameworks

Figure 12-5

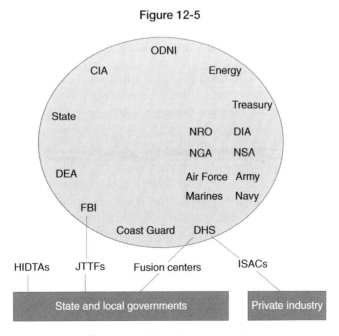

Intelligence collaboration mechanisms.

have been developed in the homeland security domain to promote collaboration among relevant federal, state, local, tribal, and private sector actors. Four will be discussed in this section: Joint Terrorism Task Forces, fusion centers, High Intensity Drug Trafficking Areas (HIDTA), and Information Sharing and Analysis Centers (ISAC).

12.2.5.1 Joint Terrorism Task Forces

The oldest of these collaborative frameworks related to homeland security is the Federal Bureau of Investigation's Joint Terrorism Task Force (JTTF) model. The first JTTF started in 1980 as a collaborative initiative between the FBI and the New York Police Department to track down the perpetrators of violent attacks within the city. With a primary focus on combating terrorism, JTTFs are investigative units that are composed of law enforcement and intelligence specialists from all levels of government in the US system.

FOR EXAMPLE

Investigating a Terror Plot 1984

The Los Angeles Joint Terrorism Task Force worked with the local sheriff's department to identify a cache of explosives that belonged to a group connected with domestic terrorist organizations such as the Weather Underground. The group had been plotting to use the explosives to conduct violent attacks to free a Puerto Rican nationalist, Oscar Lopez, from federal prison, as well as to disrupt the 1984 Summer Olympics in Los Angeles. Both plots were disrupted and an initial cache of explosives were discovered in 1985. When the second cache of explosives was found in 1986, the JTTF was able to utilize its investigative resources to connect the second cache to the group as well (Jones 1986).

Given the emphasis on protecting the homeland from terrorist attacks in the last two decades, there has been a substantial increase in the number of these task forces. There were 35 JTTFs in 2001; there are more than 100 today. In 2015, there were more than 4000 personnel from 55 federal agencies and over 500 state and local organizations working in these task forces (FBI 2015).

JTTFs have both analytical and operational components. A typical JTTF will have a collection of investigators, linguists, and analysts, as well as operational elements like Special Weapon Action Team (SWAT) personnel. As a result, JTTFs are tasked with not only investigating terrorist activities but also serving as the primary responders for these investigations. JTTFs have been utilized in seizing money in terrorist financial schemes, responding to local threats, and arresting suspicious subjects with all kinds of deadly weapons and explosives. For instance, the disruption of the plot by Christopher Cornell to attack the US Capitol in 2015 is an example of both the analytical and operational roles played by Joint Terrorism Task Forces (Savasta 2015).

Critics of these task forces are primarily concerned about the outsized role of the FBI. Some have expressed concern that the FBI's organizational culture tends to inhibit information sharing with state and local partners. There is also a concern that JTTFs are used as a method to "federalize" investigations of local law enforcement (Mayer 2016, 6).

12.2.5.2 Fusion Centers

For most states and territories in the United States, their primary intelligence organization is a fusion center. Developed in the wake of the September 11 terrorist attacks, these organizations were designed to promote better information sharing between all levels of government. These organizations are created and managed by the state or territorial entity where they reside. However, their development was promoted by the federal government by providing material support via the Department of Homeland Security. This support includes deploying federal personnel to fusion centers, training, security clearances, and connectivity to federal systems (DOJ 2016). Currently, there are 78 fusion centers located in states and major population centers across the United States. With the exception of Wyoming (where there is a criminal intelligence center in the Attorney General's Office), there is at least one fusion center within each state (Figure 12-6).

The scope of operations for fusion centers vary depending on the jurisdiction that they operate in. Some are narrowly focused on the mission of combating terrorism, but others also cover all types of criminal activity (Gerringer and Bart 2014, 76). As a result, there is a wide variety of organizational and manning structures for fusion centers across the country. For instance, one fusion center is staffed by a contingent of three personnel; another is composed of more than 250 personnel (Peteritas 2013). As one fusion center director noted, "There's an old axiom… if you've seen one fusion center, *you've seen one* fusion center" (emphasis mine) (Collier 2016).

What these fusion centers share is a focus on improving the flow of intelligence information and analysis between all levels of government. For instance,

Figure 12-6

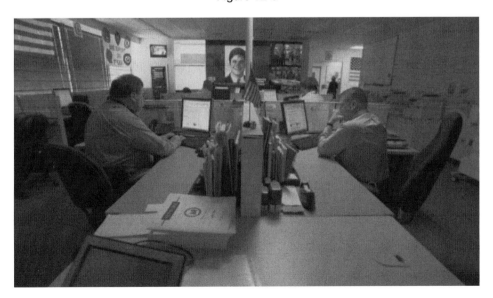

Arizona Fusion Center (FBI 2009).

fusion centers serve as a conduit for suspicious activity reports (SARs) to be passed from local government entities in their jurisdiction up to the federal government. In 2012, the National Fusion Center Association claimed that more than 22 000 SARs were generated, leading to 1000 federal inquiries or investigations (O'Harrow 2012, A1). Fusion centers also serve as an information hub for IC-generated analysis to be disseminated to state and local government actors, when appropriate.

However, there is some question regarding the effectiveness of fusion centers. One study from the American Enterprise Institute noted, "fusion centers have struggled to show meaningful utility in the information and intelligence arena" (Mayer 2016, 1). A 2012 report by the US Senate Homeland Security and Governmental Affairs Investigations Subcommittee went even further, calling them "pools of ineptitude." With regard to assisting the federal government, the investigation contended that "fusion centers often produced irrelevant, useless or inappropriate intelligence reporting to DHS, and many produced no intelligence reporting whatsoever" (O'Harrow 2012, A1).

There have been concerns that state and local partners are having difficulty in staffing fusion centers and that the personnel assigned to these organizations may not have the appropriate intelligence training (Larence 2007, 7). This has led some to question not only the quality of analysis but also the possibility that they might be a threat to the civil liberties of the citizenry. For instance, a 2009 report from the Missouri Information Analysis Center noted that bumper stickers for presidential candidate Ron Paul might be an indicator of militia activity or domestic terrorism (Greaney 2009). In another instance, the North Texas Fusion Center identified Muslim lobbyists as a potential threat. When the American Civil Liberties Union sent a note to Tennessee public schools warning them to not celebrate Christmas as a religious holiday, the Tennessee Fusion Center put the notification in its map of "terrorist events or other suspicious behavior" (Rittgers 2011).

Another concern regarding fusion centers is the degree to which they overlap with the FBI's Joint Terrorism Task Forces. Forty-two of the fusion centers are located in the same city as a JTTF; nearly two dozen fusion centers are actually collocated with local FBI organizations (Mayer 2016, 5). The two systems also overlap substantially on the mission of combating terrorism. This raises concerns about redundancy, miscommunication, and the waste of limited resources.

12.2.5.3 High Intensity Drug Trafficking Areas

Another mechanism for intergovernmental coordination in a policy area relevant to homeland security issues are the **High Intensity Drug Trafficking Areas (HIDTA)**. Established by the White House Office of National Drug Control Policy in 1990, these organizations are designed to implement intergovernmental initiatives that confront drug trafficking threats in their area. Each HIDTA is governed by an HIDTA executive board, which includes representatives of local, state, and federal law enforcement agencies in the area. By law, each HIDTA board is equally divided between federal law enforcement on the one side and state and local agencies on the other.

Within this program, there are 59 **investigative support centers (ISCs)**. A centerpiece of the HIDTA program, the ISCs facilitate information sharing, intelligence collection, analysis and dissemination, and technical and strategic support to HIDTA initiatives and participating agencies (ONDCP 2001). This capability allows their associated HIDTA to identify new targets and trends, deconflict targets and events, and more effectively manage cases (ONDCP 2016).

12.2.5.4 Information Sharing and Analysis Centers

Recognizing that more than 85% of critical infrastructure in the United States is privately owned, President Clinton issued Presidential Decision Directive 63 in 1998, which called on each critical infrastructure sector to establish a sector-specific information sharing organization. The first ISAC was created by the financial services sector in 1999. Today, there are 21 ISACs representing various critical infrastructure sectors within the United States. As with other areas of homeland security, the September 11 terrorist attacks were pivotal in the growth of ISACs. More than 75% of the ISACs in existence were established after 2001.

While specific language varies, each ISAC is intended to facilitate sharing of information between government and the private sector by gathering, analyzing, and disseminating threat information to the larger industry and government. Through the National Infrastructure Protection Plan, the Department of Homeland Security supports these organizations by providing security clearances for industry experts to assist in evaluating threat information and incidents. ISACs are also tasked with sanitizing the information that they share (Bullock et al. 2013, 164). Aside from limiting national security-protected information, they must also be cognizant of not divulging proprietary information of their members. Given that participation by private companies is voluntary, ISACs must ensure that they do not undermine the business operations of their members.

SELF-CHECK

- Define intelligence-led policing.
- High Intensity Drug Enforcement Areas are collaborative organizations that were created by the
  a. Central Intelligence Agency
  b. Department of Homeland Security
  c. Federal Bureau of Investigation
  d. White House Office of National Drug Control Policy
- All Joint Terrorism Task Forces were established after the terrorist attacks on September 11, 2001. True or false?

12.3 Methods of Collecting Intelligence Information

When discussing the area of intelligence collection, it is important to recognize the difference between **sensors** and **platforms**. Both are important to successful intelligence collection. Having the right sensor–platform combination is often the key to getting useful intelligence to support policymakers. Sensors are the means by which intelligence information is collected. For instance, one of the key ways that the United States was able to confirm that Soviet missiles had been placed in Cuba during the Cuban Missile Crisis in 1962 was from imagery intelligence. A camera captured images of Soviet missiles and associated equipment in the forests of Cuba, thereby confirming reports that had come from other sources.

However, a camera (or any other collection method) is useless if it cannot be at the right time and place to capture the information. For that, the sensor must be attached to some type of platform. Indeed, a platform might carry multiple sensors. A platform is the means by which a sensor reaches its physical location to gather intelligence information. For instance, in the Cuban Missile Crisis example noted previously, the camera was attached to a U-2 aircraft. This aircraft ensured that the camera was in the correct position at the correct time to ensure that useful intelligence information was collected. If the U-2 had placed this camera over the right location during the middle of the night or during a cloudy day, it would have not produced the intelligence information that was so valuable to policymakers in this case. Platforms can be a variety of things, primarily in the realm of transportation. Satellites, aircraft, ships, and submarines have all served as platforms for collection sensors. However, even fixed objects, like a building or a telephone pole, might serve as a platform for an emplaced sensor (e.g., a security camera).

One recent innovation in collection platforms is the use of autonomous or semi-autonomous assets. For instance, the use of unmanned aerial vehicles (UAVs) by the US government has grown in recent years. The MQ-9 Predator B UAV has been used extensively by the US military and intelligence communities in national security-related missions since the 1990s. The combination of their low-cost, long loiter time over the target, and lack of a human pilot risking capture/injury/death has driven a substantial increase in the MQ-9's usage. Advances in technology, which have expanded capabilities, as well as reducing size and cost, have also expanded the use of UAVs (Figure 12-7).

The use of unmanned aerial vehicles (UAVs) to collect intelligence over US soil has been expanding over the past decade. The US Customs and Border Protection (CBP) service has been using these platforms to monitor the border since 2006. Historically, this organization is one of the few federal agencies that are authorized to regularly operate UAVs inside the United States by Federal Aviation Administration (FAA) regulations. However, CBP frequently loaned these assets to other federal, state, and local authorities. In a period between 2010 and 2012, the UAVs were utilized for non-CBP missions 687 times. Beyond supporting border monitoring

Figure 12-7

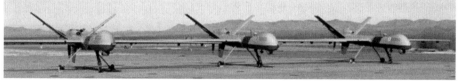

US Customs and Border Protection MQ-9 Predator B UAVs (USCBP n.d.).

activities of other agencies, CBP UAVs were employed to support disaster relief operations, search for missing persons, and identify illegal drug production areas (Whitlock and Timberg 2014, A1). However, as the value of such tools has risen and the cost to purchase declined, UAVs are increasingly being utilized by other actors inside the United States. As of 2013, more than a dozen local law enforcement organizations had applied to the FAA for authorization of operate these platforms (Horgan 2013).

Another recent platform is computer networks or "cyber." Given the increasing reliance of individuals and societies on networked computer systems to be more efficient and effective, they have also become more vulnerable to the collection of their sensitive information. Hence, the "information superhighway" is also a tool that allows individuals or machines to observe and collect information from around the world. The magnitude of this capability, as well as the potential security threat it poses, is becoming increasingly important to governments. The recent creation of US Cyber Command by the Department of Defense, the Directorate of Digital Innovation within the CIA, and the Cyber Threat Intelligence Integration Center within ODNI are but three indicators of cyber's growing relevance. As one observer noted, "cyber will become as important to the IC as overhead (satellite) systems became a half century ago" (Kojm 2016).

Beyond the platforms that are necessary for intelligence collection, this section focuses on the three most common areas of intelligence collection sensors—that which is derived from direct human contact, that which is openly available in the public domain, and that which can be observed using technology. What will be found is that, like the tools in a toolbox, each of these methods has unique strengths and weaknesses. Thus, which method of collection should be utilized is driven by the type of intelligence information being requested and the unique nature of the target.

12.3.1 Human Intelligence Collection

The collection of sensitive information by person-to-person contact is the oldest form of intelligence collection. This section will discuss the three main types of **human intelligence (HUMINT)** collection—espionage, overt collection, and interrogation. Espionage is the most notorious form of human intelligence collection and is essentially the theft of information from an adversary. This theft can take place by verbally passing along information or removing documents. Espionage is typically defined by its clandestine nature—that is, neither of the actor nor the action is detected by the adversary. The target is unaware that the information has been taken, let alone who has taken it.

While the "cloak and dagger" of espionage is what captures the popular imagination, overt collection is a far more common form of human intelligence collection. Overt HUMINT is intelligence collection where the potential adversary is well aware that their information will be passed along as intelligence information. For instance, a defense attaché in a foreign embassy is supposed to interact with members of the host country government and military. It is the key reason for their being in the country. But it is also understood that they will report to their government on any useful intelligence information that is gleaned from those conversations. In the domestic realm, **community policing** would be an example of this type of collection. Police officers interacting with members of the community are not hiding the fact that they are attempting to collect information on community concerns (indeed, quite the opposite). That information will be utilized by local law enforcement to guide decisions on future police activities in the area.

The third type of human intelligence collection is interrogation. This type of collection is defined by the fact that the information source is within the physical custody of the organization trying to collect intelligence. A criminal suspect being interviewed while in police custody and a prisoner of war being questioned by the enemy on the battlefield are both examples of this type of HUMINT. Interrogation of these types of personnel could utilize either coercive or noncoercive methods. Certainly within the United States, coercive methods of interrogation are severely limited by legal and constitutional protections for the subjects in custody.

A method of collection that is related to this type of HUMINT is document and domicile exploitation—sometimes collectively referred to as "**sensitive-site exploitation**." This is defined as the collection, identification, and evaluation of physical materials from a detained individual or location. People tend to have a lot of associated documents and items that can convey significant information about their capabilities, beliefs, and intentions. These items could be store receipts, membership cards, electronic devices, etc. For instance, in Operation NEPTUNE SPEAR, US special operations forces not only killed Osama Bin Laden but also collected a vast array of documents and computer hard drives. This information was evaluated to further the US effort to degrade al-Qaeda's network and capabilities.

Human intelligence collection has particular strengths and weaknesses. It is a particularly useful method of gaining information on adversary plans and intentions. That is, aside from simply identifying an adversary's capabilities, it can yield information about "why" the enemy is pursuing a certain course of action.

However, this method of collection is limited by two important factors. First, you must gain access to the information. The process of recruiting a source who has access to the information (or inserting an asset that does not currently have access) can be a difficult and time-consuming process. Yet, without access, HUMINT is largely impossible. Second, can the source of the information be trusted? Source credibility is a critical question that is difficult to validate. Particularly in espionage, the motivation for why someone is willing to betray their country or group by passing secrets can be critical to assessing whether the information is accurate. Indeed, it is possible that the source is providing the collector with false information because they are not betraying their country/group at all— they may be serving as a double agent. James Jesus Angleton, the head of the CIA's counterintelligence section until 1975, referred to this difficulty in assessing the motivation and credibility of human intelligence sources as a "wilderness of mirrors" (Epstein 2011, 9).

12.3.2 Open-Source Intelligence Collection

In spite of the cultural mystique of secrecy in the profession of intelligence, most of the information that is utilized in the construction of intelligence products is not secret. Newspapers, books, television programs, professional conferences, and much more can provide useful information to support intelligence analysis and decision making. The US intelligence community defines **open-source**

intelligence as "publicly available information that is collected, exploited, and disseminated in a timely manner to an appropriate audience for the purpose of addressing a specific intelligence requirement" (ODNI 2006).

Such information can be useful in a variety of ways. First, it may provide useful contextual and background information such as the leadership, rules, or basic structure of an organization. Second, the combination of multiple pieces of publicly available information may yield sensitive information. For example, in the 1970s, the United States was unable to develop stealth (radar evading) technology until researchers found an academic book written by a Soviet mathematician some 10 years earlier. The combination of this book and the previous research solved the problem. Lastly, it is possible that sensitive information may be published inadvertently in the public domain. For instance, during the Battle of Midway in June 1942, the *Chicago Tribune* published an account of the battle that made it clear that the United States had decrypted the Japanese naval code. This was a closely held secret for much of the war, and the unintentional disclosure could have been very damaging to US progress in the war (Goren 1981). However, the article appears to have escaped the notice of the Japanese.

It is also important to note that the rationale for publicly sharing information may not be the reason it is of value to intelligence personnel. For instance, propaganda videos by al-Qaeda leader Osama Bin Laden were largely intended for recruiting members, but they were also scrutinized by intelligence agencies in the United States to determine such things as the location and health of the leader. During the aerial bombing campaign in the First Gulf War (1991), Iraqi government media reports of the damage were attempting to undermine international resolve by generating sympathy for the population—intelligence personnel would use this video footage to confirm damage assessments from other intelligence sources. This means actors should exercise good operational security practices in their public communications—but, to a surprising degree, this does not happen.

The use of open-source material for intelligence collection and analysis has been widely recognized for some time. The al-Qaeda training manual (which is, itself, posted on the Internet) notes that using public sources, it is possible to gather 80% of the information about the enemy (Al Qaeda 2001). And while the 80% number is a "round number," it is not a new estimate. In 1948, the first Director of Central Intelligence, Admiral Roscoe Hillenkoetter, noted, "80 percent of intelligence is derived from such prosaic sources as foreign books, magazines, and radio broadcasts, and general information from people with a knowledge of affairs abroad" (Richelson 2015, 347).

To be sure, the Internet has substantially impacted the availability of open-source information. Since its creation as a communication network between government laboratories in 1994, it has grown as a global communication source that is accessed by more than 3.6 billion people (IWS 2016). As of 2014, there are over one billion websites on the World Wide Web (ILS 2016). This represents a quantum leap in the amount of open-source information that is available to be collected. However, this also exacerbates the "wheat vs. chaff" dilemma that is a problem in the discipline of intelligence collection. Most collection methods can gather a large volume of information, most of which is not relevant to the intelligence question that is being addressed. As a result, the processing and exploitation phase of the intelligence cycle has to sift through all of the collected data to separate the pertinent from the irrelevant material. With the growth of the Internet, the proverbial "needle" may still be in the "haystack"—unfortunately, the haystack keeps getting bigger and bigger.

Another area of open-source intelligence collection that is rising in value is **social media intelligence (SOCMINT).** Particularly when collecting information on individuals or groups, social media sites such as Facebook, Instagram, and Twitter can provide a substantial amount of information regarding patterns of behavior, known associates, locations, etc. The satirical website "The Onion" once did a farcical video that portrayed Facebook as a CIA-sponsored open-source intelligence operation (The Onion, 2011). While this has no basis in fact, the "truth in jest" from this video is that a lot of useful intelligence information can be gleaned from such social media sites.

12.3.3 Technical Intelligence Collection

Since the early twentieth century, technology has expanded our world in a number of ways. Collecting information that can be used for intelligence purposes is one of them. There are a number of collection disciplines that use technology-based sensors to derive information that can be used to support decision making. The most widely known are signals intelligence, geospatial intelligence, and measurement and signatures intelligence. Many of these sensors specialize at "**remote sensing**"—the science of collecting information about an object or area from a considerable distance. They may also require some level of science or mathematical expertise to understand and process the results of this collection.

12.3.3.1 Signals Intelligence

Signals intelligence (SIGINT) is intelligence derived from electronic signals and systems used by individuals or equipment, such as communication systems, radars, and weapon systems. This collection discipline is typically divided between the sub-fields of electronic intelligence (ELINT) and communications intelligence (COMINT).

Electronic intelligence is essentially the nonverbal side of signals intelligence. In the modern age, there is a plethora of electronic equipment that provides information to society. For instance, radar (which stands for "radio detection and ranging") systems are based at all major airports to coordinate and deconflict aircraft departing and arriving at their facility. That signal (or "ping"), and how frequently it repeats, can convey a lot of information about the capabilities of the radar without uttering a word. In the realm of homeland security, tracking cell phones via their global positioning system (GPS) signal would also be an example of this type of intelligence collection.

Communications intelligence is the more well-known branch of SIGINT. The ability to monitor conversations that are being held by telephone, radio, video teleconference, etc. can yield important information. Like HUMINT, it can potentially give important insights into what is being planned or considered by an opponent. As one former director of the National Security Agency once boasted, "imagery intelligence tells you what has happened, (communications intelligence) tells you what will happen" (Lowenthal 2015, 65).

However, for all of the potential benefits of COMINT, its value can be severely limited by at least four issues. First, the method of communication must be vulnerable to collection. The phrase "wiretapping" goes back to the days when all electronic communication was transmitted by wire or landline cable. If you could not access the wire, you could not access the communication. In contemporary times, an increasing amount of communication is transmitted via the electromagnet spectrum, thus making it vulnerable to remote-sensing COMINT methods. However, landline communication is still utilized. Second, if the intercepted communication is in a foreign language, it must be translated. This is particularly problematic if there is a large volume of collection that may contain time-sensitive information. Third, if the target is aware that their communications are being monitored, they may opt to rely on non-electronic means of communication. For instance, al-Qaeda senior leaders have largely relied on couriers in the years after the September 11 terrorist attacks in order to avoid detection. Last, if a target is concerned about monitoring but still wants to use electronic communication, they may encrypt their communications.

Encryption is the process of encoding a message so that it cannot be easily understood by an unauthorized recipient. The use of codes and ciphers to protect communications was used long before the advent of cellphones and the Internet. Records going back to ancient Greece note the use of such methods (Sheldon 1986, 40). However, advances in mathematics and computing technology have greatly increased to scope and complexity of encryption capabilities. Moreover, these technological advances have made advanced encryption systems more widely available. This means that many private companies and even individuals may have communications that are difficult to monitor even if they are intercepted. In 2016, Apple's refusal to assist the US government in decrypting the iPhone data of a terrorist killed after an attack in San Bernardino, California, further highlighted the growing availability of encryption to non-state actors (Rubin 2016, 1).

However, even with the growing complexity of encryption methods, it is still possible to gain intelligence information from intercepted communications. Sometimes it is possible to decrypt a portion of the communications, thus revealing part of the intended communication. It is also possible to make use of the trends in communications even if they are encrypted. Utilizing the idea of **traffic analysis**, it is possible to measure the volume and pattern of communication networks to gain important insights. For instance, in the years since the September 11 terrorist attacks, a surge in "chatter" among known and suspected terrorists has been used by governments as a possible indicator of an impending attack. Traffic analysis can also be used to support social network analysis of organizations (Joachim 2003). If one actor of a given organization has more connections and volume of communication with other elements, that actor is likely a critical element worthy of further investigation.

12.3.3.2 Geospatial Intelligence

Geospatial intelligence (GEOINT) is essentially the construction of maps and collection of images to support policymakers. The use of graphical representations of the physical world has been in use since ancient times. Cartography—or map making—has been used by everyone since the time of the ancient Greeks. To be sure, technological advances have made this method much more informative and widely available. For instance, software systems such as geographic information systems (GIS) create maps that not only identify the physical world but also overlay a variety of other data to facilitate intelligence analysis.

With regard to imagery collection, there are different types of imagery sensors, and each has its own benefits and problems. **Electro-optical imagery** is the most common type of imagery sensor—it produces the type of picture that you can take with a camera or cellphone. This image captures the light visible to the human eye. It can produce pictures that are very compelling—as the old saying goes, "a picture is worth a thousand words." Certainly, the electro-optical images that were captured by the U-2 aircraft in the Cuban Missile Crisis were compelling to decision makers in the US government. However, like the human eye, an electro-optical sensor is limited by environmental conditions. If there is not enough available light (e.g., during periods of darkness) or if bad weather or some other object is obstructing the target, it will not be possible to collect the imagery. This type of imagery is also most susceptible to cover, concealment, and deception activities of an adversary. If the target is hidden or its appearance manipulated to look like something else, it is possible that the analyst looking at the electro-optical image would not see the target.

Full motion video (FMV) is a relatively recent innovation for electro-optical sensors. While video recording devices have been around for some time, the use of full motion video in intelligence collection is a more recent development. The advent of drones and surveillance monitors that are able to capture and store video footage has allowed for the ability to observe behavior and monitor activities to an unprecedented degree. However, the increased volume of collection does present a challenge in processing that video footage. In 2009, one estimate of the total amount of FMV that was taken by US forces in Iraq and Afghanistan was 17 years' worth of video footage (Buxbaum 2010). As one senior military official noted about the growth of FMV, "we are swimming in sensors and drowning in data" (Magnuson 2010). The proliferation of video cameras across governments and society within the United States would suggest that this is an even larger problem in the homeland security domain.

Aside from electro-optical imagery, another type of imagery that is well known is infrared (IR) imagery, which uses a thermography device to construct an image based on variations in infrared radiation. IR imagery is useful in detecting heat sources, such as warm-blooded animals (e.g., humans) and equipment that is in (or has recently been in) operation. For instance, if a boat in port has recently operated its engine (or is currently operating its engine), that compartment will be very visible on IR imagery—even if the boat has no lights on. Since it detects variations in heat, vice visible light, IR imagery is not limited to daytime operations. Indeed, the reduction of temperature during nighttime hours makes detection more likely due to the contrast between the target and the surrounding environment (Figure 12-8).

The last type of imagery is radar-generated imagery. Radar imagery constructs an image by transmitting radio waves at a given area and measuring the return of those signals. Sometimes known by the nickname of "bloobology" since the images can appear fuzzy and out of focus, radar imagery can be taken by day or night and

Figure 12-8

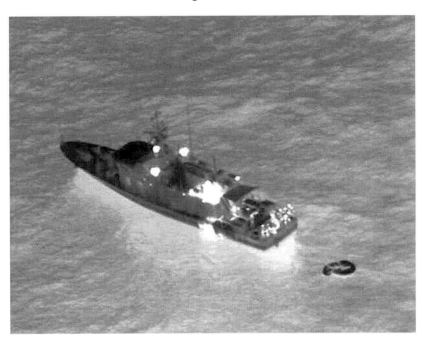

Infrared imagery of a ship at sea (US Navy 2006).

in any type of weather. Additionally, radar imagery is useful in defeating concealment measures like camouflage since the radio waves can often penetrate the
covering material.

12.3.3.3 Measurement and Signatures Intelligence

Measurement and Signatures Intelligence (MASINT) is the newest of the
technical collection disciplines. These sensors are designed to detect and differentiate specific signatures that reveal the presence of a particular material or
phenomenon. MASINT represents a diverse collection of technical collection
methods including acoustic, seismic, radiological, chemical, and more. In some
respects, it is a grouping of all technical collection methods that do not clearly fit
into the areas of SIGINT or GEOINT. As one observer noted, "whereas SIGINT is
akin to sound and IMINT to sight, MASINT is akin to touch, taste and smell"
(Seng 2007, 1).

MASINT is particularly useful in counterproliferation and bomb-detection activities. For instance, **hyperspectral imagery (HSI)** can monitor weapons of mass
destruction (WMD) activities via remote sensing. It captures emitted electromagnetic radiation that is not visible to the human eye. Using spectral analysis, an HSI
sensor can produce a product that looks like a brightly colored image. These colors
represent specific spectral signatures that are associated with particular materials.
As a result, it is possible to assess the chemical composition of materials without
directly touching them. HSI has also been used for improvised explosive device
detection during the conflicts in Iraq and Afghanistan. Aside from HSI, other
MASINT sensors can assess materials by sampling particles directly on or near the

material. A Giger counter measures radiation in this way, as well as the explosive trace detectors used by the Transportation Security Agency at most airports.

Of all the methods of technical intelligence collection, MASINT is the one that requires the most substantial technical expertise or equipment to assess the meaning of the data. For instance, the multicolored hyperspectral image is the result of a person or system converting the electromagnetic spectral readings from the sensor into a product that communicates the meaning of the data. That requires a degree of scientific expertise not common for the layman. However, if trained personnel or equipment are available to interpret the collected information, MASINT has the ability to reveal significant information that is not available via other means.

SELF-CHECK

- Define SIGINT.
- One example of technical intelligence collection is sensitive-site exploitation. True or false?
- Which of the following collection methods is not a form of human intelligence collection?
  a. Espionage
  b. Interrogation
  c. Overt HUMINT
  d. Traffic analysis

12.4 Challenges to Homeland Security Intelligence

The disclosures, and resulting controversies, from the Edward Snowden episode in 2013 are best understood as the interaction of the competing principles of security and liberty within the context of rising technology in contemporary American society. A former contractor working for the National Security Agency in Hawaii, Snowden fled to Hong Kong with a collection of sensitive documents related to government electronic-monitoring programs. In a series of interviews with *The Guardian* newspaper, he made public government programs that were substantially more robust than previously known.

Having collected hundreds of thousands of documents on electronic storage devices, the first program he revealed was known as PRISM. This program allowed for direct access to Internet accounts of individuals with a court order. However, he also revealed that a companion program, MUSCULAR, had secretly penetrated the links to data center communications for such Internet firms as Google and Yahoo. This allowed the NSA to collect from hundreds of millions of user accounts across the world, including inside the United States (Gellman and Soltani 2013, 1). Another program, known as BOUNDLESS INFORMANT, collected and mapped metadata from around the world. Snowden also revealed a secret court order that compelled Verizon to turn over the metadata of millions of US calls on a daily basis (Greenwald 2013, 1).

12.4.1 Balancing Liberty and Security in Homeland Security Intelligence

On the one hand, the enhanced need to secure the homeland in the wake of the September 11 terrorist attacks is understandable. The United States had just been attacked on US soil by a foreign adversary—and on a scale that had not happened since the Japanese attack on Pearl Harbor in 1941. Also, the nature of the threat was new. Instead of the traditional national security concern from other nation-states, the threat was from non-state actors. It was a collection of individuals that did not have to have a fixed geographic location and could easily pass through national borders undetected. And the years since 2001 have proven that this type of threat will endure for years to come.

The concern is that the tools used to monitor these potential security threats, and the lack of public awareness of their use, could run afoul of constitutional provisions that are designed to protect individuals from unnecessary government surveillance. As one study noted, "the inherent secrecy that cloaks intelligence also fosters suspicions of improper behavior by (government) and infringements upon civil liberties" (Gerringer and Bart 2014, 77). The restriction of government powers relative to the citizenry is one of the central values of the American system of government. Indeed, civil liberties protections are as old as the Constitution itself.

And yet we live in an advanced technological age that the founding fathers of the Constitution would likely find unrecognizable. From communication to finances to relationships, an increasing number of people across the world are reliant on electronic devices such as cellphones and computers. For instance, the first mobile telephone device was created in 1973; by 2011, there were more cellphones in the United States than people (Kang 2011, 1). So, the desire of government to investigate possible threats runs into long-standing legal protections for the individual—all in an age when we increasingly interact on electronic devices that are more susceptible to eavesdropping. This changing context raises the question of whether the balance between security and liberty in American society will be rebalanced in the years to come.

Civil liberties protections are primarily found in the Bill of Rights of the US Constitution. While the First and Fourth Amendments are most pertinent to surveillance, the first nine amendments largely identify the key rights that government cannot take away from the citizenry. For instance, the First Amendment to the US Constitution does not guarantee a citizen freedom of speech. Instead, it says "Congress shall make no law…abridging the freedom of speech…" (U.S. Constitution). Moreover, most of these civil liberties guarantees in the Bill of Rights are mandated as minimum requirements for state governments as well. Through the doctrine of incorporation, the due process clause of the 14th Amendment has been interpreted by the US Supreme Court to require state governments to abide by most of these constitutional protections as a minimum standard for their own conduct.

The question of the balance of security and liberty in the American system is often resolved in the US Supreme Court. As Chief Justice Charles Evans Hughes once noted, "we are under a Constitution, but the Constitution is what the judges say it is..." (Maclin 2012, xiii). None of the guarantees in the Bill of Rights are unlimited, and the Justices have frequently noted that "national security" was an exceptional circumstance. For instance, in *Katz v. United States* (1967), the court held that a person has a reasonable expectation of privacy under the Fourth Amendment in their electronic communication. However, they also noted that this limit on government surveillance did not extend to intelligence and national security issues (*Katz v. United States* 1967, 7).

The tension between liberty and security in American society is not new. For instance, given the historical concerns regarding the use of intelligence collection methods inside the United States, much of the national intelligence community is limited in their abilities to collect information inside the United States. This guidance is contained in Executive Order 12333, a document signed by President Ronald Reagan in December of 1981. In the section on the Conduct of Intelligence Activities, it is noted that

> Collection of such information is a priority objective and will be pursued (in a)... manner that is consistent with the Constitution and applicable law and respectful of the principles upon which the United States was founded. (the White House 1981)

So, for instance, the Defense Intelligence Agency is not allowed to engage in domestic intelligence collection operations unless it is approved by the Attorney General of the United States.

One of the most well-known federal mechanisms for conducting intelligence collection operations on US soil is the **Foreign Intelligence Surveillance Act (FISA)**. Initially passed in 1978 in order to facilitate more aggressive surveillance measures of espionage suspects who were working for a foreign state, the law has been amended several times since 2001 to incorporate the threat of terrorism. The law was inspired by revelations of abuses of intelligence authorities uncovered in the Church Committee hearings in the mid-1970s. Prompted by media reports from journalists such as Seymour Hersh, the committee found that government agents had acted illegally when they conducted intelligence surveillance on US citizens "without any legitimate basis or suspicion of criminal activity, much less connection with a foreign power" (Breglio 2003, 186). For instance, in COINTELPRO (a shorthand for counterintelligence program), the Federal Bureau of Investigation unlawfully monitored a wide array of domestic opposition groups, including elements of the civil rights and antiwar movements (see Chapter 10).

FISA is intended to balance the government's need to collect intelligence related to national security with a citizen's constitutional right against unlawful search and seizure contained in the Fourth Amendment. The law creates a Foreign Intelligence Surveillance Court (FISC) composed of eleven federal district court judges who are appointed by the Chief Justice of the US Supreme Court to seven-year nonrenewable terms. In secret proceedings, these judges review search warrants that are submitted by counterintelligence officials who are investigating suspects believed to be working for a foreign power against the United States. While official records are unavailable, it is reported that the FISC has approved more than 28 000 warrant requests and only denied 11 since its creation (Lowenthal 2015, 100). Some have argued that this means the forum is essentially a "rubber stamp" for the government. However, others believe that this success rate speaks to the quality of the warrants that are presented to the FISC.

FISA has been amended several times since 2001 to accommodate the changing nature of the technology and national security threats. The Uniting and Strengthening America by Providing Appropriate Tools Required to Intercept and Obstruct Terrorism (USA PATRIOT) Act of 2001 amended FISA requirements by permitting the use of roving wiretaps. Previously, warrants that authorized wiretaps were limited to a particular location. Recognizing the advent of mobile communications, these roving wiretaps allow for continuous surveillance of a given individual—even if they change location or communication methods. In response to the rising challenge of non-state terrorism, the Intelligence Reform and Terrorist Prevention Act (2004) included a "lone-wolf amendment." This adjusted FISA's definition of "agent of a foreign power" to include noncitizens acting independent of a foreign power. This was inspired by the September 11 terrorist attacks, where a suspected plotter could not be monitored under FISA because he did not meet the requirement of working for a foreign state (Turner 2005). Lastly, the FISA Amendments Act (2008) provided blanket retroactive immunity to those telecommunication companies that assisted the government in surveillance operations.

The challenge of balancing liberty and security is even more pronounced at the state and local levels. With the growth of intelligence-led policing in the United States, many local jurisdictions must reconcile restrictions on intelligence collection activities with the law enforcement function that they are attempting to advance. Using grant funding that is channeled to state and local governments through the Omnibus Crime Control and Safe Streets Act of 1968, the federal government uses the "power of the purse" to encourage local compliance with **Title 28, Part 23, of the Code of Federal Regulations**. Much like the history at the federal level, this code went into force in 1980 when it became clear that some law enforcement agencies were keeping files on political groups without any justification of probable cause.

The regulation is essentially guidance for the management of criminal intelligence records systems to ensure that they are consistent with constitutional guarantees (Carter 2004, 149). It allows for criminal intelligence to be compiled in databases that can be shared with other agencies, so long as there is reasonable suspicion that the subject is engaging in criminal behavior. As Jeremy Carter noted, the "code says you have to establish a criminal predicate, basically probable cause, to keep information on identifiable individuals" (Carter 2016).

Unless it is directly related to the charge of criminal conduct, law enforcement organizations are not allowed to retain information on a subject's religion, political views, or associations. However, this is particularly problematic with the suspicious activity reports (SAR) program that is coordinated through state fusion centers. Because of the ambiguous criteria associated with such reports, there are concerns that they can be utilized to collect information, which is beyond this scope (Schmitt 2009, A12). For instance, a report that reviewed more than three thousand SARs that were produced by the Los Angeles Police Department between

2008 and 2012 found that 80% were of no value. They included such behaviors as photographing infrastructure or asking about a building's hours of operation (Bluemel 2013).

The balance between liberty and security in the American system is likely to remain fluid. The growing use of intelligence collection methods inside the homeland will continue to erode the barrier between the law enforcement and national security communities. The continuation of non-state threats like terrorism and organized crime will continue to drive the desire of government to utilize the tools that they have at hand to address these security challenges. However, the basic civil liberties protections that are widely viewed as fundamental to our society will endure. The rise of communication technologies further complicates questions about how security and liberty should be balanced in the American system. The only sure bet is that this debate will continue to play out in the US legal system.

12.4.2 Intelligence Support to Disaster Relief

Most discussions of intelligence support to homeland security focus on law enforcement and anti-terrorism missions. However, as the use of intelligence concepts and processes has grown in new policy areas, it is important to note that they have also been applied to support disaster response and recovery efforts.

One of the first uses of intelligence collection support to disaster response operations has been the use of geospatial intelligence to monitor the extent of the damage. For instance, in 1993, FEMA requested that US Navy F-14 fighter aircraft carrying the Tactical Airborne Reconnaissance Pod System (TARPS) conduct photo-reconnaissance missions to measure the extent of flooding in the Midwest.

In the aftermath of the September 11 terrorist attacks, changes were made in US law that increased the flexibility in utilizing national intelligence assets to support major domestic emergencies and disaster response operations. Hurricane Katrina saw a significant utilization of intelligence collection assets. For instance, the National Geospatial Intelligence Agency began conducting imagery collection of critical infrastructure and port facilities before the landfall of the hurricane in order to produce more accurate damage assessments after the storm had passed (Petitjean 2013, 57). Additionally, the National Security Agency was instrumental in reuniting family members in the wake of the disaster (White House 2006, 94).

Another area for intelligence support to disaster relief operations is open-source intelligence collection. In the immediate aftermath of a disaster event, survivors and witnesses often attempt to communicate with family and friends (Metz 2016). Presuming communication networks near the disaster area are functioning, the monitoring of social media for immediate observations can improve situational awareness for decision makers and assist in maximizing the deployment of the right numbers and types of disaster assistance capabilities (Lindsay 2011, 4).

Hurricane Sandy saw this evolution grow still further with private organizations utilizing intelligence methods to plan and implement their disaster relief operations. For instance, the data management system that was used widely by the US intelligence community to support operations in Iraq and Afghanistan was utilized by private groups in support of response and recovery operations. The nonprofit organization Direct Relief International (DRI) utilized the Palantir Gotham data management system to identify at-risk counties in the United States in advance of the 2012 hurricane season. With the storm nearing landfall, DRI correlated the hurricane's projected path with flood plain maps and supply levels at partner medical clinics in the area (Palantir 2017). This allowed the organization to stage the most relevant medical supplies for the areas likely to be hardest hit by the storm (Young 2012).

Additionally, in the aftermath of the hurricane that caused more than 250 deaths and $60 billion in damage, the Palantir Gotham system was incorporated by other nongovernmental organizations to support relief operations. For instance, the disaster response organization Team Rubicon used the system to create a database for directing its operations (Streams 2012). The system not only coordinated requests with response assets but also allowed the response assets to update the organization's strategic picture by uploading reports and imagery at the scene. As one member of Palantir Technologies noted, "we are doing disaster relief in a way no one has ever done before" (Palantir 2017).

SELF-CHECK

- Define civil liberties.
- One example of a US government update to the Foreign Intelligence Surveillance Act would be Title 28, Part 23, of the Code of Federal Regulations. True or false?
- Who appoints the judges to the Foreign Intelligence Surveillance Court?
  a. The Attorney General
  b. The Chief Justice
  c. The Director of National Intelligence
  d. The President
- Which of the following technologies has been used effectively in providing intelligence support to disaster response?
  a. Palantir Gotham
  b. PRISM
  c. Facebook
  d. Bumblehive

SUMMARY

In his 1993 senate confirmation hearing, CIA Director-designate James Woolsey made the following remark:

> Yes, we have slain a large dragon. But we live now in a jungle filled with a bewildering variety of poisonous snakes. And in many ways, the dragon was easier to keep track of. (Jehl 1993, A1)

Intelligence operations in support of homeland security are reflective of this view. The growing number and capabilities of malevolent non-state actors who can transmit people, material, and ideas across national boundaries with increasing ease represents a significant security threat. The more effective and efficient use of information that is gathered in the intelligence process is one mechanism for government to meet this challenge.

Intelligence collection reflects a "toolbox" of capabilities to address policy-maker concerns. Each intelligence collection discipline represents a unique way of gathering information that contains particular benefits and problems. For instance, espionage is an important method for gathering the plans and intentions of an adversary. However, getting access to the individuals with that information and assessing the credibility of those information sources can be challenging.

The rise of new platforms such as unmanned aerial vehicles and computer networks is expanding the opportunities for gathering information. Also, the growing capabilities of electronic data storage and the proliferation of emplaced sensors (such as security cameras) are increasing the ability of intelligence to use passively collected surveillance data in new ways.

However, because homeland security takes place within a governing context that contains multiple agencies and multiple levels of government, intelligence cooperation is a critical component to the utilization of intelligence support. Even within the federal intelligence community, the structure is decentralized with relatively weak leadership. Ensuring collaborative relationships between federal, state/territorial/tribal, local, and private partners has been a major focus of homeland security efforts since 2001. However, the push for increased collaboration has created a variety of new mechanisms that lead to potential duplication of efforts. The competition between Joint Terrorism Task Forces and the state fusion centers is a prime example of this issue.

Lastly, because intelligence collection inside the United States may involve intrusive monitoring on the citizenry, it raises possible legal and constitutional conflicts that are not often an issue for intelligence activities outside of the United States. In both the areas of national security and law enforcement intelligence, governments have sought laws and regulations that strike a balance between the competing values of securing the homeland and protecting the civil liberties of individuals. However, the changing nature of the security threat since 2001 and the rise of technology have created new pressures in the efforts to achieve that balance.

In this chapter, you learned that intelligence is used to assist homeland security decision makers in making more effective policy decisions. However, given the federal structure in the US system, there are a variety of intelligence organizations outside of the intelligence community, and their ability to coordinate information and activities is a critical factor. You also learned that there are different methods for collecting information of intelligence value, each with its own unique set of strengths and weaknesses. And as the use of these methods is expanding into areas beyond combating crime and terrorism, there are ongoing debates about the legal and constitutional limits of intelligence operations in support of homeland security missions.

KEY TERMS

Bumblehive	A data storage facility built by the National Security Agency in 2012.
Civil liberties	Individual rights that are protected against governmental interference.
Community policing	A method of policing where officers are assigned to specific areas to become familiar with local inhabitants.
Director of National Intelligence	The chief intelligence advisor to the president and the coordinator of the US Intelligence Community.
Electro-optical imagery	An image constructed by measuring and transmitting variations in light levels in a given scene via electronic means.
Encryption	The process of altering a message so that it can be read only by the sender and the intended recipient.
Foreign Intelligence Surveillance Act	A 1978 federal law that stipulates procedures for the clandestine surveillance of espionage or terrorism suspects without violating the constitutional protections of the individual.
Fusion center	An intelligence coordination center controlled below the level of the national government but supported by the Department of Homeland Security.
Geospatial intelligence (GEOINT)	The construction of maps and collection of images to support intelligence missions.
High Intensity Drug Trafficking Area (HIDTA)	An organization designed to implement intergovernmental initiatives that confront drug trafficking threats in a given geographic area.
Human intelligence (HUMINT)	Intelligence information that is generated by the direct personal interaction of people.
Hyperspectral imagery	A form of spectral imaging that collects information from across the electromagnetic spectrum, including areas not visible to the human eye.
Intelligence	The process by which specific types of information important to national security are requested, collected, analyzed, and provided to policymakers.

Intelligence collection	The acquisition of specific information in support of addressing intelligence requirements of decision makers.
Intelligence cycle	A visual model designed to identify the key elements in the intelligence process.
Intelligence-led policing	A model of law enforcement that emphasizes intelligence support in assessing and managing risk to guide operations.
Intelligence Reform and Terrorist Prevention Act	A 2004 federal law that reorganized the roles and structure of the intelligence community leadership.
Investigative support center	A support organization of the High Intensity Drug Trafficking Area program that shares counter-drug intelligence across all levels of government.
Joint Terrorism Task Force	An FBI initiative that manages investigative units that are composed of law enforcement and intelligence specialists from all levels of government in the US system.
Measurement and Signatures Intelligence (MASINT)	An intelligence collection method that detects and differentiates specific signatures to reveal the presence of a particular material or phenomenon.
National Counterterrorism Center	An organization with the Office of the Director of National Intelligence that serves as the primary US government organization for integrating and analyzing intelligence pertaining to counterterrorism.
National Criminal Intelligence Sharing Plan	A federal law enforcement intelligence sharing initiative that links all levels of government in the US system.
Office of Intelligence and Analysis	The primary intelligence office within the Department of Homeland Security.
Open-source intelligence	Intelligence information that is generated from publicly available sources, such as the news media and academic conferences.
Palmer raids	A series of legally questionable operations by the Department of Justice to locate individuals with communist or anarchist affiliations from 1919 to 1920.

Platform	The means by which a sensor reaches the appropriate physical location to gather intelligence information.
Remote sensing	The detection or acquisition of information about a given object or phenomenon without physically interacting with it.
Sensitive site exploitation	The systematic review of documents and materials for intelligence purposes at a given location.
Sensor	A mechanism that detects or measures observable phenomena or records.
Signals intelligence	Intelligence information derived from electronic signals and the associated systems used by individuals or equipment.
Social media intelligence	The collection and analysis of intelligence information gathered from open-source social media networks.
Surveillance	The continuous observation of a place, person, group, or ongoing activity in order to gather information.
Title 28, Part 23, of CFR	A federal regulation designed to provide criminal intelligence sharing standards for local governments that receive federal grant funding through the Omnibus Crime Control and Safe Streets Act of 1968.
Traffic analysis	The analysis of communication attributes that does not involve the actual content of the communications.

ASSESS YOUR UNDERSTANDING

Go to www.wiley.com/go/Kilroy/Threats_to_Homeland_Security to assess your knowledge of the basics of homeland security intelligence.

Summary Questions

1. The process by which specific types of information important to national security are requested, collected, analyzed, and provided to policymakers is known as
   (a) Data
   (b) Espionage
   (c) Intelligence
   (d) Metadata

2. In 2012, the National Security Agency created a new data storage facility in the state of
   (a) Arizona
   (b) Colorado
   (c) New Mexico
   (d) Utah

3. At the national level, the intelligence community is composed of ____ separate organizations.
   (a) 5
   (b) 11
   (c) 17
   (d) 22

4. The Director of the National Security Agency (NSA) is also the commander of US Northern Command (NORTHCOM). True or false?

5. The type of organization that is designed to promote the sharing of security information among private industry in critical infrastructure sectors within the United States is known as
   (a) Fusion centers
   (b) Information sharing and analysis centers
   (c) Investigative support centers
   (d) Joint Terrorism Task Forces

6. Human Intelligence Collection would include all of the following methods except
   (a) Defense attachés
   (b) Espionage
   (c) Interrogation
   (d) Traffic analysis

7. Most forms of technical intelligence collection utilize the principle of "remote sensing." True or false?

8. Which of the following did not amend the Foreign Intelligence Surveillance Act?
   (a) Executive Order 12333
   (b) The FISA Amendments Act
   (c) The Intelligence Reform and Terrorist Prevention Act
   (d) The USA PATRIOT Act

Applying This Chapter

1. You are the governor of a small northeastern state. Your chief of staff indicates that he read on the Internet that al-Qaeda was planning to target the electrical power infrastructure in your region. Based on this scenario, identify the intelligence organizations that you would want to contact and what information you would expect them to provide. Of the organizations that you have identified, which do you expect would be most useful in assessing the likelihood of this possible threat? Explain.

2. You are an intelligence analyst attempting to assess the intentions of a radical anti-government group that maintains a secure compound in a rural area outside of Denver, Colorado. If you only had one intelligence collection method at your disposal, which type of intelligence would you select: HUMINT, OSINT, SIGINT, GEOINT, or MASINT? What sensor–platform combination would be most effective? What are the potential limitations of the method you selected? Explain and defend your choice.

3. In 2012, a report from the Senate Homeland Security and Government Affairs was very critical of fusion centers. They described them as "pools of ineptitude, waste and civil liberties intrusions." Do you agree or disagree with that assessment? Explain your response. Also, if fusion centers were eliminated, what would the impact be on the intelligence collection capabilities within the US system?

4. In Executive Order 12333, it notes that the collection of intelligence information is a priority that will be pursued in a manner "that is consistent with the Constitution and applicable law and respectful of the principles upon which the United States was founded". Based on the current amended version, does the Foreign Intelligence Surveillance Act meet that standard? Why or why not? If you were asked to make a new amendment to the existing FISA legislation, what do you think would be most important issue to address? Explain.

Intelligence Cooperation

Compare the missions and organizational arrangements of fusion centers and Joint Terrorism Task Forces. Assess which is most effective in promoting long-term cooperation between state and national intelligence organizations.

Edward Snowden Revelations

Research the disclosures made by Edward Snowden since he left US government service in 2013. Explain the intelligence collection capabilities he disclosed and evaluate the impact of these disclosures on US attempts to combat terrorism in the homeland.

13

HOMELAND SECURITY PLANNING AND RESOURCES
Understanding the Future Challenges of Homeland Security in a Federal System

Stephan Reissman

National Oceanic and Atmospheric Administration (NOAA), Silver Spring, MD, USA

Starting Point

Go to www.wiley.com/go/Kilroy/Threats_to_Homeland_Security to assess your knowledge of the basics of homeland security planning and resources.
Determine where you need to concentrate your effort.

What You'll Learn in This Chapter

▲ How the federal system of government in the United States impacts agencies that must plan homeland security activities

▲ The key documents that inform homeland security planning at the federal, state, and local levels of government

▲ The performance measures and the different models for conducting homeland security planning and resourcing

▲ How higher education has developed programs and curriculum to prepare students for careers in homeland security

After Studying This Chapter, You'll Be Able To

▲ Analyze the federal system's impact on homeland security planning

▲ Examine key documents in homeland security planning such as the Quadrennial Homeland Security Review

▲ Appraise the future of homeland security planning and resourcing

▲ Evaluate the various educational opportunities available to students interested in careers in homeland security

Threats to Homeland Security: Reassessing the All-Hazards Perspective, Second Edition.
Edited by Richard J. Kilroy, Jr.
© 2018 John Wiley & Sons, Inc. Published 2018 by John Wiley & Sons, Inc.
Companion website: www.wiley.com/go/Kilroy/Threats_to_Homeland_Security

INTRODUCTION

As a final chapter to the text, an important discussion is the future of homeland security, as both a function of government planning, resourcing, and direction and of educational programs that have emerged related to teaching about homeland security. In 2017, some might have thought that homeland security would no longer be in vogue, the Department of Homeland Security (DHS) would dissolve, and agencies, such as the US Coast Guard, would return to the Department of Transportation. Terrorism would no longer be the focus of US security policies abroad, and the focus at home would be to treat terrorism, as in much of the rest of the world, as criminal acts, rather than national security threats.

Yet, today, the world seems less secure, terrorism has not gone away, and the loss of personal freedoms and civil liberties continues to be debated. The growth in educational programs alone, related to teaching homeland security, is a testimony that reports of its death are premature. But what will homeland security look like in the future, particularly in a constrained resource environment? Will it return to an exclusive view and focus just on terrorism, or will the inclusive, all-hazards approach take on new significance, as well as structure, going forward?

In this last chapter you will learn about the challenges of doing homeland security in a federal system of government that we have in the United States. All agencies having homeland security responsibilities at the federal, state, and local levels must conduct planning using limited resources and funding to perform their mission. You will also study the processes put in place to facilitate future planning, such as the Quadrennial Homeland Security Review (QHSR). You will also comprehend the performance measures of agencies having homeland security responsibilities. You will also review what homeland security education programs are available for students considering careers in homeland security. In the end, hopefully this chapter will generate some new ideas for additional research and writing on the topic of threats to homeland security.

13.1 Basics of Homeland Security Planning

Planning is foundational to almost any enterprise, whether that be in the public or private sector. In the military, plans are developed through a process of deliberate or crisis-action planning for practically any mission area. Yet, during World War II, General Dwight D. Eisenhower is quoted as saying, "In preparing for battle I have always found that plans are useless, but planning is indispensable" (Nixon 1962, 235). In business, planning is also an important process in determining a company's missions, priorities, and resources to accomplish those missions. As one example, Liz Richards, Executive Vice President of the Material Handling Equipment Distributors Association, quoted Alan Lanier, stating that "Planning is bringing the future into the present so you can do something about it now" (Richards 2012). The danger of not planning is that "if you don't know where you are going any road will take you there" (Harrison 2002).

In this text we have seen the many faces and roles of homeland security. We see a federal agency formed from the ashes of 9/11, from pieces from many other agencies with an expressed focus on preventing terrorism in the United States. However as the

Department of Homeland Security (DHS) coalesced, it was clear that some of the organizations and functions assigned to DHS included activities that did not fit into a terrorism focus. Some practitioners and academics opt for a more "inclusive" definition of homeland security, seeing certain customs functions or citizenship functions as homeland security. Others have taken an all-hazards approach, including disaster management and even public health into the homeland security arena. And still others take a more focused approach, defining homeland security as those activities that are directly responsible for "fighting" terrorism.

It is important to note that homeland security as an endeavor is different than the roles and responsibilities of the Department of Homeland Security. DHS acts on their charge from federal statutes and authorities, budget items, and executive orders. But its requirements do not necessarily apply to state, local, and private sector homeland security organizations, freeing them to define homeland security in ways that can be more focused on terrorism or can be inclusive of other activities including disaster response and emergency management or some other combination of activities.

13.1.1 Planning for Homeland Security Activities

Identifying those activities which homeland security agencies are required to do comes from a variety of sources. Senior elected officials (the president, state governors, mayors, county executives) may set priorities. Additionally, legislatures will also weigh in (with direction and budgetary funding). Expert panels, public hearings, academic research, key stakeholder review, and other efforts will also influence how homeland security agencies develop their roadmaps. While looking at how the federal Department of Homeland Security is charged, the following identifies a number of documents that DHS uses to form its strategic direction:

▲ Program planning documents: Any items that describe the intended purpose and outcomes of the program—this could include background documents written during the development of the program (charge from senior leaders, literature reviews, initial discussions/presentations, brainstorming) (Goodykoontz et al. 2014, 27).

▲ Congressional budget justifications: Each year, DHS submits a budget justification to the Office of Management and Budget (OMB). These justifications may describe different aspects of programs that can be used for development as well (Goodykoontz et al. 2014, 27).

▲ Organizational strategic documents:
  ▲ Quadrennial Homeland Security Review (QHSR): The QHSR outlines the vision, mission areas, goals, and objectives for homeland security (DHS 2014a).
  ▲ DHS Bottom-Up Review: The Bottom-Up Review provides an overview of the alignment between DHS activities and organization and the 2010 QHSR mission priorities and goals. Identifies areas where greater alignment is needed (Goodykoontz et al. 2014, 27).
  ▲ DHS Annual Performance Report: This report identifies department-level performance measures, targets, and results for DHS missions, goals,

and objectives. Describes the performance measurement and management process in DHS (Goodykoontz et al. 2014, 27).

▲ DHS Strategic Plan for FY 2012–2016: The Strategic Plan outlines DHS goals, objectives, and performance indicators (DHS 2014b).

▲ DHS Component, Directorate, Office, or Division Strategic Plans: These documents can provide missions, goals, objectives, and (sometimes) performance measures and targets for specific organizations within DHS (Goodykoontz et al. 2014, 27).

▲ Stakeholders: Programs can be affected and influenced by outside sources. This could include perspectives and findings from partner agencies, public hearings, focus groups, and information from states, local governments, and professional associations (Goodykoontz et al. 2014, 27).

▲ Past program performance data: Examine past outcomes, including programs that are similar to this one. It is important to ensure that the outcomes still apply to the current program (Goodykoontz et al. 2014, 27).

▲ Reports from the Government Accountability Office (GAO), Inspector General (IG), and others: These entities may find problems with program activities or results. These types of reports may have recommendations based on the program review; it's important to see if the recommendations have been addressed and how these have impacted the program (Goodykoontz et al. 2014, 27).

As these inputs are examined and discussed by policymakers, strategic direction can be developed that espouses the key principles of how an organization will achieve its mission. Two of the key documents in the process are the DHS **Quadrennial Homeland Security Review (QHSR)** and the **DHS Strategic Plan 2014–2018**. Let's take a look at both of these to see how these overarching source documents disseminate their agency's strategic direction, not just for the leadership and staff at DHS but also for state and local agencies that will be working with them as well as private sector companies and the general public.

13.1.2 Quadrennial Homeland Security Review

According to the Department of Homeland Security,

> The Quadrennial Homeland Security Review (QHSR) is the Department of Homeland Security's capstone strategy document, which is updated every four years as required by law. The report offers recommendations on long-term strategy and priorities for homeland security. Each QHSR cycle entails an extensive three-year-long review process before the report is finalized and submitted to Congress. The Department strives to make the QHSR as thorough and inclusive as possible by working with a wide range of stakeholders inside and outside government, who share responsibility for safeguarding the Homeland. The QHSR will provide the strategic foundation to ensure that the Department is ready to meet future challenges. (DHS 2014a)

The first QHSR, published in 2010, was focused on developing a vision for homeland security along with introducing the key homeland security mission areas, goals, and objectives. This was one of the earlier attempts to articulate this from the DHS perspective. The second QHSR was published in 2014 and it's anticipated that the 2018 QHSR will be ready to submit to Congress in December 2017.

The 2014 DHS Quadrennial Homeland Security Review (QHSR) identified five basic homeland security missions:

1. Prevent terrorism and enhance security
2. Secure and manage our borders
3. Enforce and administer our immigration laws
4. Safeguard and secure cyberspace
5. Strengthen national preparedness and resilience (DHS 2014a)

While not all of these functions were initially envisioned as part of homeland security by its creators, as the agency has matured, we see that these missions set up the framework of how federal homeland security is defined. Let's look a little further into each of these missions and how DHS has framed them.

1. **Prevent Terrorism and Enhance Security**
   The QHSR acknowledges that "Preventing terrorist attacks on the Nation is and should remain the cornerstone of homeland security" (DHS 2014a, 6). The QHSR goes on to acknowledge that terrorism may be harder to detect and cites the Boston Marathon bombing as a changing threat from a centralized Al-Qaeda senior leadership "to centrally plan and execute sophisticated external attacks" to the rise of smaller affiliates and domestic-based attackers. It acknowledges the need for "partnering across federal, state, local, tribal, and territorial law enforcement" (DHS 2014a, 6).

2. **Secure and Manage Our Borders**
   As DHS includes border security entities, the QHSR looks for the agency to address "terrorist threats, drug traffickers, and other threats to national security, economic security, and public safety" (DHS 2014a, 6). It also discusses screening of cargo and monitoring international travel under suspicion. However it discusses the balance required to "promote and expedite lawful travel and trade that will continue to strengthen our economy" (DHS 2014a, 6–7).

3. **Enforce and Administer Our Immigration Laws**
   The QHSR reports that DHS "will continually work to better enforce our immigration laws and administer our immigration system" (DHS 2014a, 7). As one reads this section, it is hard to see how this is an homeland security activity since the agency is also working on securing and managing borders. However the tie-in appears to be made through using resources to remove "those who represent threats to public safety and national security" (DHS 2014a, 7).

4. **Safeguard and Secure Cyberspace**
   A growing threat that the QHSR explains is "illustrated by the real, pervasive, and ongoing series of attacks on our public and private infrastructure" (DHS 2014a, 7). Infrastructure protection is a significant role within DHS and includes what are called "sectors" such as energy, telecommunications, water, transportation, and financial services (see Chapter 5). All of these areas are

certainly subject to cyber-attacks in their different forms. DHS will need to work within the federal government as well as private sector agencies to support the furthering of cybersecurity capabilities.

5. **Strengthen National Preparedness and Resilience**
   This is where the all-hazards approach predominately comes in to play. While seemingly not an approach to dealing with terrorism, the QHSR discusses the improvement of "disaster planning with federal, state, local, tribal, and territorial governments, as well as nongovernmental organizations and the private sector … and how the nations; prepositioned a greater number of resources; and strengthened the Nation's ability to respond to disasters in a quick and robust fashion" (DHS 2014a, 8). In addition to the emergency management functions, DHS also uses this section to describe efforts to improve agency-wide efficiency, morale, and work processes.

13.1.3 Expanding on the QHSR: The DHS Strategic Plan

While the QHSR takes a broad view of the homeland security missions, the Fiscal Years 2014–2018 DHS Strategic Plan (DHS 2014b) looks to further define how these items should be addressed, including putting forth performance measures. Let's take a look at the strategic plan's five mission areas:

Mission 1: Prevent Terrorism and Enhance Security

The beginning of the section for mission 1 highlights the reason that DHS was founded: "Preventing terrorism is the cornerstone of homeland security" (DHS 2014b, 14). This is a daunting task with many moving parts. The challenge in developing a strategic plan that addresses this key DHS mission is to ensure that it is clearly stated and that actions proposed can be done and can be measured (which is discussed in a later part of the chapter). The plan also notes that DHS is not the only agency responsible for preventing terrorism, including federal, state, local, private sector, and even international partners. It acknowledges the need to defend against threats from actors ranging from state-sponsored terrorists to lone-wolf attackers; this calls upon a range of methods, skills, and actions to address these different threats.

Within each to these missions are goals that further elaborate on strategies that the homeland security community led by DHS will need to undertake, and within each of these goals, sub-goals highlight further actions steps. So in this plan each layer provides a little more detail as to how these missions are to be addressed. Ultimately each component within DHS, whether it is ICE or CBP or FEMA will further define their strategy for addressing these missions.

Mission 2: Secure and Manage our Borders

This mission speaks to both the movement of people to the United States (including air travel), along with international trade and the flow of goods into the country as part of the global supply chain. The mission also addresses the goal of DHS to "disrupt and dismantle transnational criminal organizations and other illicit actors" (DHS 2014b, 20). This mission further addresses protective actions such as the role of the Secret Service to protect the president and others and support the response to **National Security Special Events**, such as the Super Bowl. This is one of the areas that advocate a risk-based approach to these actions (see Chapter 4).

This mission goes on to highlight the sub-goals that involve securing the borders from all modes of transportation as well as the shipping of goods.

Mission 3: Enforce and Administer our Immigration Laws

While important for maintaining an efficient and effective system for immigration, this area of the DHS Strategic Plan does not reflect the initial mission of homeland security, preventing terrorism. However, the legislation that founded DHS brought this national function into the agency. DHS explains that "Smart and effective enforcement and administration of our immigration laws remains a core homeland security mission" (DHS 2014b, 25). This is a distinctly different function than part of the mission 1 goal of preventing terrorism but is evident in the arena of enhancing security. This mission deals more with border enforcement, immigration laws, and paths to citizenship to name some of the priorities.

Mission 4: Safeguard and Secure Cyberspace

Cybersecurity has become a major threat to both government and private sector organizations (see Chapter 8). This mission area addresses the role the DHS has in the cyberspace arena. While the agency works closely with other federal partners, they are also working with the private sector to provide support and intelligence so they can protect their systems and operations. Threats that this mission addresses includes "theft of trade secrets, payment card data, and other sensitive information through cyber intrusions to denial-of-service attacks against Internet websites and attempted intrusions of U.S. critical infrastructure" (DHS 2014b, 29).

One of the interesting challenges as the "cyber-world" evolves is the idea of how this area fits into our critical infrastructure. So much of our world is linked through cyber technology or as it is called in the Strategic Plan the "cyber-physical convergence" (DHS 2014b, 30) that cyber issues can cross over to all of our sectors in critical infrastructure and need to be addressed both on the cyber side and through critical infrastructure strategies and risk evaluation.

FOR EXAMPLE

Cybersecurity at the State and Local Government Levels

The increasing threats in cyberspace have posed a major challenge for all levels of government and the private sector. While the DHS Strategic Plan lists cybersecurity as one of the five homeland security priority mission areas at the federal level, state and local governments are realizing their own vulnerabilities in cyberspace. In the 2016 National Preparedness Report, state and local governments rated their cybersecurity preparedness with the lowest proficiency rating of 31 key functions, with only 13% reporting they were highly proficient. Although some might consider this finding to be due to the states and local communities considering cybersecurity as a federal agency responsibility. However in the same report, over 70% of the those emergency management personnel at the state and local community level believed that states were primarily responsible for cybersecurity preparedness that impacts those communities, not the federal government (24).

Mission 5: Strengthen National Preparedness and Resilience

This mission focuses on disaster response and emergency management using more of the all-hazards approach that has been discussed previously. This mission is attached to our efforts not only to address terrorism but also to address threats such as from hurricanes, earthquakes, pandemics, and oil spills. This mission also looks beyond the law enforcement realm but to the work of the myriad of agencies that are involved with these hazards such public works, public health and medical, transportation, and public utilities. This mission also expands the approach to address not only the response to an incident but encompasses the "before" actions in the form of preparedness and mitigation strategies and how we deal with the aftermath through recovery.

The approach is one that relies on the efforts of what is called the whole community approach, which DHS explains as calling "for the investment of everyone—not just the government—in preparedness efforts. Whole Community is a means by which emergency managers, organizational and community leaders, government officials, private and nonprofit sectors, faith-based and disability organizations, and the general public can collectively understand and assess the needs of their respective communities as well as determine the best ways to organize and strengthen their assets, capacities, and interests" (DHS 2014b, 35). Whole community involves multiple layers of government and takes the philosophy that the federal response is but one part of how we as a nation respond to a disaster or other emergency and that for the most part, the federal response supports the state and local agencies and is not (despite what we see in movies) in charge of what is going on.

In addition to these five missions there is also a section that addressed an area called "Mature and Strengthen Homeland Security." This section addresses information sharing and dissemination across the agency as well as human resources, personnel, and agency development and "ensuring that the Department invests and operates in a cohesive, unified fashion, and makes decisions that are transparent and collaborative to drive the Secretary's strategic guidance to results" (DHS 2014b, 40). These address those essential supporting activities that keep an agency moving forward.

13.1.4 Final Thoughts on the QHSR

Willis (2014) warns about five homeland security trends that need to be considered by DHS as they move forward through the QHSR process. These included addressing "terrorism fatigue," the idea that "law enforcement and domestic security operations had become too focused on terrorism at the cost of addressing other public safety issues such as drug violence, public health, or crime" (1). At the same time he does acknowledge that terrorism is a real threat, citing both domestic and international events. So a difficult balance of addressing public safety issues beyond terrorism must be considered while knowing that risks and threats from terrorism must be factored into policy and planning decisions. A greater emphasis on enhancing risk management will be helpful for determining policy priorities.

Additionally, analysts at the Heritage Foundation (Carafano et al. 2013) discuss how the QHSR should impact on the focus of DHS. Their commentary goes beyond the broad categories of the DHS enterprise to look at areas like modernizing the Coast Guard; strengthening intelligence, counterterrorism, and information sharing; rethinking aviation security and refocusing FEMA to address truly cata-strophic events; and centralizing management authority. They warn that while organizational changes often include major reorganizations of the agency, they would be better addressing their recommendations and the findings of the QHSR to improve the organization.

SELF-CHECK

- Define the QHSR.
- Which of the following is not one of the mission areas of the QHSR and DHS Strategic Planning document?

  a. Prevent terrorism

  b. Safeguard and secure cyberspace

  c. Defend the North American homeland

  d. Strengthen national preparedness and resilience

- Annually, DHS submits a budget justification to the Office of Management and Budget (OMB), which frequently describes the intent behind various programs, both within the components and at DHS headquarters. True or false?

- Whole community involves single layers of government and takes the philosophy that the federal response is the primary part of how we as a nation respond to a disaster or other emergency. True or false?

13.2 Coordinating Homeland Security Planning

While DHS is the agency that coordinates the actions of the federal government in the arena of homeland security, it is not the only agency involved in the delivery of homeland security. All federal agencies have some role to play in homeland security. Additionally DHS's activities are directly tied in with state and some local homeland security, law enforcement, and emergency management activities. Therefore DHS, as it plans to address its multiple functions, will require resources, inputs, and actions from many partners. In order to plan for how DHS will address homeland security in the United States, DHS needs to include these partners in its planning for how the government will address homeland security. Presidential directives have established a process for how this planning is supposed to take place that accounts for multiple **stakeholders.** Under the Obama administration, **PPD-8** was the Presidential Policy Directive that dealt with homeland security planning and national preparedness, requiring the development of a national preparedness system and a national preparedness goal (DHS 2011). Planning can be defined as "conducting a systematic process engaging the whole community as appropriate in the development of executable strategic, operational, and/or com-munity-based approaches to meet defined objectives" (DHS 2015, 8). There are three levels of planning: tactical, operational, and strategic. Your role within an agency often defines the type of planning that you do.

Strategic planning is focused more on the requirements of an agency, its long-range goals, and priorities and identifies responsibilities to carry out these goals and priorities. It looks at more of the "What do we do?" issues of an agency rather than the "How do we do them?" type issues. Operational planning identifies personnel, resources, and assets needed to execute the objectives of the strategic plan. It goes further into the "How" of what an agency does. Tactical planning is more detailed, situationally based, and more specific, focused on the day-to-day operations of a situation. The following discussion will look at strategic planning designed to execute agency (or interagency) policies.

13.2.1 The Six-Step Planning Process

One of the most important characteristics of successful planning efforts is the use of a defined planning process. A predetermined and agreed-upon process must be used by a planning group so that the methods are clear to all even as the information and material gathered is being generated. It is also important to plan in teams so that the key stakeholders are involved and that there are different specialists involved in the process with a variety of skill sets and perspectives. Including the stakeholders in the process also aids in gaining consensus and approval. Another benefit is the establishing of relationships among agencies and planners that can also be leveraged during an event or during day-to-day activities.

While there are several different versions of planning processes in use, for the most part, they have similar characteristics and steps used to meet the goal of developing a plan. The diagram that follows represents the six-step planning process as used by FEMA and other agencies in the National Incident Management System (NIMS), Comprehensive Planning Guide (CPG) 101, and the FEMA Regional Planning Guide. Let's briefly look at each aspect of the process (Figure 13-1):

Figure 13-1

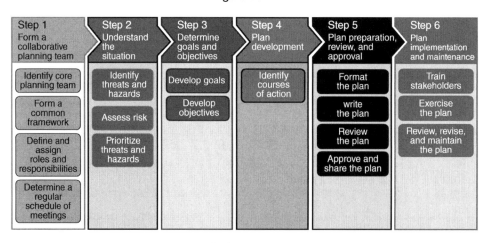

Six-step planning process. Source: Federal Emergency Management Agency (2010).

Step 1: Form a Collaborative Planning Team. It is important to obtain the right types of experts and agency representatives as the process begins. These people may vary depending upon the type of situation that is being addressed. Some planners may remain throughout the process, while others may have a short tenure in the plan development.

Step 2: Understand the Situation. This step seeks to understand the background of the problem that requires the plan to be developed and involves direction from the senior leaders as to what success is for this plan. The planners will need to research the situation so that they understand the issues at hand. They will develop the facts and assumptions about the plan's background and discuss a risk assessment/analysis so that a baseline agreed-upon situation statement is developed and understood by the participants.

FOR EXAMPLE

Facts and Assumptions: What's The Difference?

Facts and assumptions are used to help define the planning problem. Facts "are verified pieces of information, such as laws, regulations, terrain maps, population statistics, resource inventories, and prior occurrences. Initial resource availability and capabilities are key facts that should be included" (FEMA 2013). Assumptions "consist of information accepted by planners as being true in the absence of facts in order to provide a framework or establish expected conditions of an operational environment so that planning can proceed. Assumptions are used as facts only if they are considered valid (or likely to be true) and are necessary for solving the problem" (FEMA 2013). So in an actual disaster, a fact may be that FEMA has a (quantities of) prepositioned supplies in storage for a disaster (water, food, cots, etc.). An assumption that links to this fact is that critical transportation routes and infrastructure will be disrupted by the incident or by secondary effects, such as populace movement and emergency response efforts (FEMA 2016b, 10).

So while FEMA has large amounts of critical supplies ready to go, it must plan for disruptions in the access routes to get them to the affected populations. This could be through dividing up these supplies and prepositioning them (if there is warning) in different parts of the anticipated area of impact so that some supplies can get through (FEMA 2016b).

Step 3: Determine Goals and Objectives. Goals and objectives must be developed in order to clearly indicate the desired end state—what the plan is looking to achieve. Goals and objectives help to ensure that the multiple departments, agencies, and organizations involved in a planning effort and, ultimately in the plan's execution, understand the shared direction of the plan.

Goals are broad, general statements that indicate the intended solution to problems identified in **Understand the Situation.** *Objectives* are more specific and are actions carried out during the execution of the plan. Determining goals and objectives lead to developing a mission statement for your plan (FEMA 2013). The mission statement does not address how the action should occur. The "how" is used in developing the courses of action (COAs). After developing the mission statement, a best practice is to ensure that senior leadership has reviewed and endorses the statement and that the goals and objectives are aligned with the desired end state. It is important to keep senior leadership apprised of the direction of the planning process a periodic interval so that the planners can be sure that they are not planning in a vacuum and they have "interim buy-in" of the leadership (FEMA 2010).

Step 4: Develop, Compare, and Select Courses of Action. In order to achieve the goals and objectives defined previously, the planning team will develop courses of action (COAs). Often at least two COAs are developed, but it could be more depending upon senior leader guidance or even that the planners determine that there are multiple options. COAs are evaluated in order to determine their strengths and weaknesses and are ranked. The COA that will best meet the objectives is selected as the concept of operations for the plan (FEMA 2010).

Step 5: Develop the Plan. Once the COA is determined then the next step is to develop an executable plan. There is often a predetermined format that will be used by the team (there are multiple styles that can be used). As part of the development of the plan, the team should ensure that they have involved key stakeholders (as best as the situation and the sensitivity of the plan will permit). After comments and concerns are adjudicated and the plan refined, the team needs to ensure that the plan is compliant with any applicable regulatory requirements (FEMA 2010). The plan then goes for a senior leader review and will hopefully receive official approval.

Step 6: Implement, Evaluate, and Revise the Plan. After the plan is approved and disseminated, training will need to be developed so that the agencies will be able to perform the tasks identified in the plan they are required to do. Some of these training events will be done internally to the organization, but multi-organizational training events and exercises will help to familiarize how different agencies will work together in an incident and will aid in evaluating the effectiveness of the plan.

Planning is a cyclical process. After exercises and real events, an after-action review and corrective action process should take place that should lead to an update of the plan, which incorporates any lessons learned. Additionally planners should consider a review and update of the plan if there are certain triggers such as a change in operational requirements, change in hazards or threats, or even if applying lessons learned from an incident from another jurisdiction may improve the existing plan.

So now we have a plan, people are trained and ready to go, and perhaps even executing aspects of the plan; now there are questions to be addressed:

▲ Are we meeting the direction and goals of the strategic plan?
▲ Can we develop measurements to demonstrate how we are performing?
▲ How do we improve our performance?

One of the steps is through developing performance measures. This is an important next step so that the people executing the plan, the stakeholders, senior leadership, and partners can assess how well the plan is meeting the intent of the process.

13.2.2 Performance Measurement: The Challenging "Art" of Measuring Success in Homeland Security Planning

For some organizations, **performance measures** are based on counting a certain number of items and then determining methods to improve the number of products manufactured. While this might work for certain industries, for programs that have structural complexities like homeland security, these measures cannot be based on counting individual "things" but will actually become an effort to figure out how to measure for "results"—what activities, or combination of activities, best demonstrate how the work is being accomplished.

Performance measures are used to "inform key program management decisions such as setting program priorities, allocating resources, or identifying program problems and taking corrective action to solve them" (Goodykoontz et al. 2014, 16). This requires us to ask and answer difficult questions to help us understand how we are doing our jobs.

Many of the activities of government in general, and homeland security in particular, defy measurement of specific activities to determine success. For these activities we may need to examine multiple activities to summarize success or develop "proxy" measures to address performance. This section will discuss an overview of how to think about performance measurement.

As we think about performance measurement, it is important to consider the adage: "What gets measured gets done." People will typically prioritize the activities that their management is tracking. The challenge of the organization is to develop both measurements and activities that are directly linked to the agency's key missions so that what is measured is also what people are working on. It is essential for agencies to identify these activities and promote it among their staff and stakeholders. It is also possible that all key activities cannot be measured. This may be due to staffing, time, or cost issues, so it is important to measure what will demonstrate how the program is moving toward its purpose.

Let's look at some of these key concepts in performance measurement. The goal of measures is to give managers and leadership data and information about a program's performance so that they can make decisions based on evidence rather than on "a good guess." Measures can examine areas like cost, timeliness, and customer satisfaction. The goal is to determine if the intent of the program is being met and that the outcomes match the stated goal. Determining outcomes in homeland security is often not straightforward. For example, if an agency is tasked with deterrence of potential terrorists, it may be difficult to measure this directly. Proxy measures would need to be developed by extrapolating information from other agency activities. Another example would be the deployment of supplies in a disaster. While the timeliness of applying these supplies is important, it is also critical to measure which supplies were sent and how were they used.

There are many challenges in performance measurement and many questions that need to be pondered as they are developed. The following highlights many of the questions that need to be considered when looking at homeland security measures (or many other performance measures for that matter).

Questions to Consider in the Development of Performance Measures

▲ How do I determine what is actually important to measure?

▲ How do I know if my measures are outputs or outcomes?

▲ How are the two different?

▲ Is it worth measuring inputs or processes?

▲ What external factors are likely to affect my measurements?

▲ How can I properly identify the expected outcomes for my program?

▲ What if I have no control over the intended purpose or strategic direction of my program?

▲ If I'm measuring a challenging topic like resilience, how can I break the topic down to better understand it?

▲ What methods can I use to measure outcomes that are not directly observable, such as undetected border crossings?

▲ How do I know that the measures I created are actually valid for what I am trying to measure?

▲ What are some likely limitations that may constrain my measurement efforts?

▲ How can I overcome these limitations, or work within them?

▲ How many measures should I use?

▲ What data sources can I use to measure performance?

▲ Once I have data on my outcome variables, how do I determine whether it was my program that caused those effects, or some external factor(s)?

▲ If my program is just one of several programs or activities contributing to the same outcome, how do I know the effect my program had?

▲ What if I am not the program's only owner? (Goodykoontz et al. 2014, 18–19)

13.2.3 SMART Measurement

One popular way to develop measures is through the use of the "**SMART**" mnemonic/framework (Doran 1981). Additionally, "Developing specific, measurable objectives requires time, orderly thinking, and a clear picture of the results expected from program activities. The more specific your objectives are, the easier it will be to demonstrate success" (OKGOV n.d.).

While there are some differences in what the letters represent in the mnemonic depending upon the model, essentially a "SMART" measure is one that is:

▲ Specific

▲ Measurable

▲ Attainable/achievable

▲ Relevant/realistic

▲ Time bound/timed/timely

Specific: This is the who, what, where, and why of what is being accomplished. Sometimes we include "how" in the measure. Verbs such as "coordinate" or "facilitate," are not good to use as they are vague and difficult to measure. Verbs such as "train" or "increase" are better as they can clearly indicate what will be done.

Measurable: The measure should be quantifiable and something that can be measured. Because activities are not always easy to measure, sometimes we will need to look for "proxy measures" that represent what we want to measure. We also want to be concerned about the burden of the data collection effort as well as the cost to collect and interpret.

Attainable/achievable: The objective should be accomplished with available resources. Also it is important to use a measure based on an activity that is within the program's control. It makes it challenging to measure an activity and achieve success when the program is reliant on outside influences to achieve. In that case measurements must be adjusted to address those parts of the program that can be controlled.

Relevant: Addressing (and measuring) this objective's impact must move the desired goal or strategy along. It must tie into the program's responsibilities.

Time bound: A specified and reasonable time frame must be part of the measure. Target dates are important, but also periodic checks along the way help to prevent a last-minute rush.

SELF-CHECK

- Describe the six-step planning process.
- Which of the following is not one part of the SMART mnemonic for performance measurement?
    a. Strategic
    b. Measurable
    c. Achievable
    d. Relevant
- When developing a plan you only need to inform senior leadership once the plan has been completed because they are typically so busy. True or false?
- When developing a plan, you need to develop only one course of action (COA). True or false?

13.3 The Logic Model: A Process Framework to Visually Demonstrate the Performance Measurement Process

Another helpful tool in performance measurement and planning is the use of the logic model process. The **logic model** accounts for agency missions, inputs, processes, activities, outputs, and outcomes in a way that creates a visual depiction of a program from initial inputs through near-term, intermediate, and long-term outcomes.

It can be used as a tool to gather input from multiple stakeholders and lends itself to being used at group meetings to help visually depict a program. It is often used by public health programs that have similar challenges to homeland security of complexities and hard to define measures. "Program logic model is defined as a picture of how your organization does its work—the theory and assumptions underlying the program. A program logic model links outcomes (both short- and long-term) with program activities/processes and the theoretical assumptions/principles of the program" (W. K. Kellogg Foundation 2004).

13.3.1 Components of a Logic Model

Using a logic model as a tool to facilitate discussion among practitioners and key stakeholders enables them to develop a "visual roadmap" that allows the participants and the stakeholders to know "what will get measured" and "what should get done"—it is transparent and something that can be posted and shared to develop a common understanding of what is expected. A logic model consists of five components:

1. **Resources** include the human, financial, organizational, and community resources a program has available to direct toward doing the work. Sometimes this component is referred to as inputs.
2. **Program activities** are what the program does with the resources. Activities are the processes, tools, events, technology, and actions that are an intentional part of the program implementation. These interventions are used to bring about the intended program changes or results.
3. **Outputs** are the direct products of program activities and may include types, levels, and targets of services to be delivered by the program.
4. **Outcomes** are the specific changes in program participants' behavior, knowledge, skills, status, and level of functioning. Short-term outcomes should be attainable within 1–3 years, while longer-term outcomes should be achievable within a 4–6-year time frame. The logical progression from short-term to long-term outcomes should be reflected in impact occurring within about 7–10 years.
5. **Impact** is the fundamental intended or unintended change occurring in organizations, communities, or systems as a result of program activities within 7–10 years (W. K. Kellogg Foundation 2004, 2).

By developing a logic model, managers have an effective way to define the work and display the flow and key sections of a program and how to measure it. Performance measures can be drawn from any of the parts of the model's components, but with the graphic depictions of the process, you can see how the measures fit in the overall program. For example, it is possible that your work activities may not achieve the desired outcomes. This may also be true for outputs that may look important during planning but may turn out not to achieve the desired outcomes. By visually depicting the program in the logic model, these outcomes (impacts, long-term results) are the only justification for doing the work in the first place, the successful achievement of mission or program goals.

A completed logic model can also be used for program orientation and training so that new participants or stakeholders can understand the goals of the program (Zantal-Weiner and Horwood 2010).

A challenge is to ensure that outputs are linked to outcomes. The fact that program managers administer grants and that the funds are distributed may not create a safer working conditions or better skills by a first responder. The problem is that outputs are not always simply connected to the program's outcomes (Fleming and Goldstein 2012). For example, if a program manager after program administers more grants, does this result in grantees being able to deliver faster results (and is speed of the result even the issue to measure)? If program managers only measure outputs (grants given), the data will not tell them or their stakeholders what they really need to know: whether the program is accomplishing what it was intended to accomplish. Measuring program results, and measuring them well, is vital to effective performance measurement—and ultimately to effective performance management.

The following is the frame of a logic model. You can see how the different components flow and the prompts that you might use while developing the contents of each component (Figure 13-2).

The logic model is an excellent process to develop performance measures, incorporate input from disparate stakeholders, and create a visual model of a program. This visual model serves to enhance accountability as it is clear to readers and stakeholders what a program intends to do and how it will note success. Facilitating and developing a strong logic model takes time and practice and can add to the direction of an agency.

FOR EXAMPLE

Public Safety Canada's Use of Logic Models

Public Safety Canada (PSC) was stood up shortly after the United States created the Department of Homeland Security. Its functions mirror some of those of DHS, to include emergency management. The use of a logic model was part of a nationwide evaluation of a major emergency prevention/mitigation and preparedness initiative in Canada. In Canada, Public Safety Canada has a central role to provide the leadership and coordination necessary to prepare for a whole-of-government (federal) emergency response. The model sought to link what the initiative was is funded to do (activities) with what the activities are intended to produce (outputs) and what they intend to achieve (outcomes) (PSC 2012).

Ultimately, the evaluation (including development and application of the logic model) found that "Public Safety Canada's mandated activities related to a whole-of-government approach are not duplicated by other organizations; however, federal and provincial/territorial organizations suggest that there are opportunities for improved synergy with federal regional offices and provinces/territories" (PSC 2012). To see an example of how Canada's PSC applied the Logic Model view this link: https://www.publicsafety.gc.ca/cnt/rsrcs/pblctns/vltn-ffctv-crrctns-2010-11/index-en.aspx#a2.5

Figure 13-2

Program action—logic model

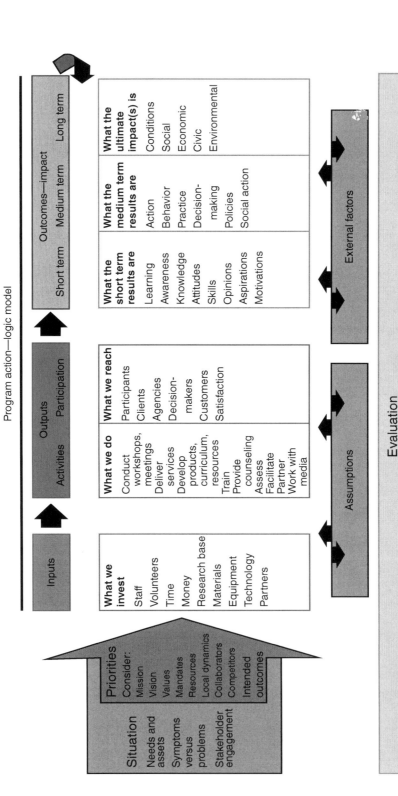

Logic model. Source: University of Wisconsin Extension (n.d.).

13.3.2 Challenges in Performance Measurement

One of the challenges in measuring emergency preparedness and response is that based on the unpredictable nature of the requirements for emergencies and disasters, there is always something more could be done. Increasing spending may not be the best way to use limited government funds. So attempts made to measure preparedness often involve inputs particularly, not outcomes, "providing relief to disaster victims when and where it is needed" (Jackson 2008, vii). For example, developing and using checklists for response efforts tells you what is available and what was used, but not how well the resources were used to help an impacted community. A look at overall systems of delivery using "Reliability Assessment" measures can be helpful as a tool for preparedness evaluation (Jackson 2008, 12).

Real-time evaluation during emergencies can be a helpful process but is complex. It is possible with this that immediate effects of interventions can be assessed and potentially corrections can be made rather than waiting for a post-event review of lessons learned (Brusset et al. 2010).

Of course in addition to the difficult challenge of measuring the "right things"—it's also important to understand your program well enough to be aware of those areas that you do not typically look at that can creep up and "bite you," sometimes called "snoozing alligators" (Frost 2000). That is one of the reasons periodic evaluations and reassessments of plans are done.

One of the key challenges in performance measurement in homeland security, especially in disaster/emergency management, is due to low numbers of major incidents that test programs and systems. While this is, overall, a good thing for society, it may mean there is less data to note trends and if the courses or actions taken are effective. This means, in part, that a robust system to adapt and refine programs and plans must be part of an homeland security system of preparedness.

SELF-CHECK

- Which of the following is not one of the five components of the logic model?
  - a. Resources
  - b. Outputs
  - c. Inputs
  - d. Outcomes
- The logic model serves as a visual depiction of a program. True or false?
- Outputs and outcomes are the synonymous. True or false?
- When you cannot directly measure an outcome, you can try to develop proxy measures that can represent the outcome you are looking to examine. True or false?

13.4 Education in Homeland Security

When the first edition of this book was published in 2008, homeland security studies were a field in its early childhood. The field has grown and matured fast since the early 2000s with new programs that span the fields of international relations, public administration, criminal justice, emergency planning, computer programming, and the sciences. More universities are now offering undergraduate and graduate education in homeland security studies, and the demand for qualified security studies professionals has grown dramatically. However, because the field is still young, it has not yet found a true home. The US Department of Education Classification of Instructional Programs (CIP) codes are used to report higher education programs. Security studies programs are coded as 45.0902 (National Security Policy Studies), 43.0301 (Homeland Security Policy), 43.0302 (Crisis/Emergency/Disaster Management), and 43.0303 (Critical Infrastructure Protection) (NCES n.d.). Security-related courses can also be offered in programs in cybersecurity (CIP code 11.1003, 29.0207, or 43.0116) or in military science (two-digit CIP code 28). Because of the multidisciplinary nature of the field, these courses are scattered through academic institutions.

The Center for Homeland Defense and Security (CHDS) reports 445 homeland security programs, which include associates, bachelors, masters, and doctoral degrees and certificate programs on its University and Agency Partnership Initiative web page (CHDS 2017). FEMA reports 310 institutions of higher education that provide graduate or undergraduate programs in emergency management (FEMA 2016a). Employment opportunities exist with the federal government, state governments, and private sector security companies and in the nonprofit sector for students whose academic work focuses on these areas.

Students entering the field of homeland security or emergency management not only need to know both the basics of homeland security and emergency management but also need to have the larger skills of a university-educated person. These are the ability to write, to think, to do basic mathematics, to be familiar with computer programs, and to communicate verbally, in writing, and in the new multimedia environment. Knowledge of American government, the international environment, and some expertise in a foreign language are particularly useful. The **National Security Education Program** (NSEP) identifies 60 critical languages as designated by the US Department of Defense, State Department, Department of Homeland Security, and the US Intelligence Community as especially valuable for students entering the field of national security. These include Arabic, Azerbaijani, Bangla, Chinese, Hindi, Indonesian, Japanese, Korean, Persian, Punjabi, Russian, Swahili, Turkish, and Urdu (NSEP n.d.).

13.4.1 Homeland Security Education Core Curricula

In looking at a variety of sources on homeland security education, a few trends appear. There is still no set definition of homeland security among these institutions. This is consistent with the field of homeland security as a whole. This means that there is not a core curriculum agreed upon for homeland security education. There is also not an educational group to accredit these programs for homeland security. While the institutions that offer homeland security degrees are accredited (for the most part), the homeland security programs are not formally accredited—there is not a process to do so. Homeland security degree programs can be found in schools of public administration, public health, criminal justice, and others.

So what are the most important things to study in an homeland security degree? Topics in law enforcement, terrorism, critical thinking, policy development, public–private partnerships, federalism, intelligence, and biological threats are found in many homeland security educational programs. Of course for a student interested in studying homeland security, it is important to select a program that best suits a student's need. However, it could be argued that certain elements of an homeland security program, say, at the bachelor's level, should have some core elements that can be agreed upon. That would go to the creation of a "culture of homeland security," which acknowledges certain consistent educational sections. There would be plenty of space for electives, but a common core would go toward creating a culture of homeland security and perhaps a common language.

Let's look at two examples of homeland security curricula to see the range in educational programs. Penn State University offers a Master of Professional Studies in Homeland Security, delivered fully online with some optional elements of residency. It is 33 credits with several specializations and includes a 9-credit common core curriculum that all students complete together regardless of their specialization. Students can then choose to take what is called the "Base Program in Homeland Security" or can specialize in one of six options:

▲ Public health preparedness
▲ Geospatial intelligence
▲ Information security and forensics
▲ Cyber threat analytics and protection
▲ Counterterrorism
▲ Agricultural biosecurity and food defense

While the students may specialize in a variety of areas, the online program has all students participating in a "Unifying Core Curriculum" that includes certain educational goals and objectives:

▲ Understand major policies and legislation that shapes homeland security in a globalized society.
▲ Become familiar with organizations that play a key role in the implementation of homeland security policies and administration and recognize the interactions among them.
▲ Understand the way in which a person or group responds to a set of conditions so as to prevent and respond to incidents and catastrophic events when needed.
▲ Recognize the impact that catastrophic events, both natural and man-made, have on society and the domestic and global economy.
▲ Identify and assess potential threats, vulnerabilities, and consequences.
▲ Apply leadership skills and principles that are necessary for producing and acting on information of value within a collaborative setting.
▲ Communicate effectively in the context of particular institutional cultures.
▲ Use, conduct, and interpret research and data effectively in decision making.
▲ Practice ethics and integrity as a foundation for analytical debate and conclusion.
▲ Develop an appreciation of the cultural, social, psychological, political, and legal aspects of terrorism and counterterrorism. (Penn State World Campus n.d.)

So while there are a variety of courses that the student can take at Penn State, the master's program is looking for the student to understand some broad areas of homeland security as a policy network and address aspects such as legislation, human behavior, emergency management, leadership, and communication, interpreting research, ethics, terrorism, and counterterrorism. Some of these are base courses that ensure comprehensive understanding of the broader context for homeland security policies and practice.

Another school, Eastern Kentucky University (EKU), offers an undergraduate Bachelor of Science in Homeland Security through the College of Justice and Safety. Through a strategic planning process, EKU instituted a multidisciplinary program that focuses on the following three disciplines or "pillars": disaster management, intelligence studies, and security operations/management. Students take courses in each of these areas as part of the core curriculum for the program and then concentrate in one or more of the pillars based on their interests by enrolling in minors and university certificates. The program also emphasizes professional skill development in critical and creative thinking, information literacy, oral and written communications, interpersonal relations, and teamwork and leadership (EKU 2017).

The following core and supporting course requirements demonstrate a range of key homeland security areas:

- ▲ Introduction to homeland security
- ▲ Physical security
- ▲ Disaster preparedness and response
- ▲ Critical infrastructure protection
- ▲ Security management
- ▲ Critical problem analysis
- ▲ Cyber security
- ▲ Risk analysis
- ▲ Policy and legal analysis
- ▲ Intelligence process
- ▲ Homeland security technology
- ▲ Disaster resilience
- ▲ Geographic information systems
- ▲ WMD/hazardous materials
- ▲ Strategic planning and leadership (capstone)
- ▲ One of multiple terrorism course offerings

Additionally the EKU Homeland Security Program encourages students to leverage approximately 30 credit hours of electives toward completing a minor or certificate in one or more of the aforementioned concentrations (Eastern Kentucky University n.d.).

There is some overlap in the objectives of the two programs even though there is not a national core curriculum. Homeland security is a very broad area and these two programs (and others) are looking to provide a wide range of offerings.

That being said, when looking at an undergraduate experience, there can be a question of whether an undergraduate degree in homeland security is too specialized, and perhaps a more general degree in public policy/administration or criminal justice might be better for a student. However, if homeland security is a person's career goal (and/or if they are already working in homeland security), then undergraduate studies in this area may be right for them. For example, approximately 20% of EKU's students enter private sector security positions (e.g., corporate, retail, contract, etc.) following graduation. The degree program balances a traditional liberal arts education with vocational/practical knowledge and experience, so students are prepared for entering the workforce.

The same can be asked about the master's level. Does a more general Masters in Public Administration (MPA) present a student with a more crosscutting view of the public sector? Is adding a core or a major in homeland security to an MPA sufficient? Or does it pay to study for a master's that is all about homeland security? While there is not one correct answer (we call it "situationally dependent"), the introduction of core topics covering a range of areas related to homeland security can help students, faculty, and the field of homeland security better define itself.

13.4.2 Research in Homeland Security: Trends and Future Thoughts

There is no dearth of research topics for the Homeland Security Enterprise. To start with there is the vantage point of the "overarching" area of homeland security. While some of these topics have been discussed in the text, further "drilling down" by researchers can help policymakers prioritize homeland security activities during these times of scarce finances and competing resources. This leads to the challenge to develop research questions and studies that branch off from topics such as the following:

▲ How is homeland security different from law enforcement or intelligence?
▲ How is it best to organize and prioritize homeland security components and functions?
▲ What is the role of the private sector in homeland security?

But homeland security research is not limited to policymaking and prioritization decisions. It can also get into specific subsections of homeland security and look to answer operational questions as well as theoretical questions. For example, in the area of transportation, a 2016 Congressional Research Services study looked at "Transit and Passenger Rail Security," highlighting the challenges of security where "stations… are designed primarily for easy access" (CRS 2016, 15) rather than today's tightly controlled airports.

While an extensive network is in place for security for air passengers and those working in airports, millions of passengers travel each weekday on both trains and busses. The Transportation Security Administration (TSA) established "goals and objectives for a secure transportation system." The three primary objectives for reducing risk in transit are as follows:

▲ Increase system resilience by protecting high-risk/high-consequence assets (i.e., critical tunnels, stations, and bridges).
▲ Expand visible deterrence activities (i.e., canine teams, passenger screening teams, and antiterrorism teams).
▲ Engage the public and transit operators in the counterterrorism mission (CRS 2016, 44).

Researchers can look at these three objectives and examine how they have been addressed or implemented and if the intentions of senior leadership are being met. Research like this can lead to a sharing of best practices, changes in funding of programs, and reprioritization of policy options.

Another area that is challenging is in the area of research in disaster and emergency management. A lot of disaster research is post hoc, in which researchers typically are not able to do real-time operational research. Often these are retrospective studies based on qualitative interviews or based on data collection after the event. It is a challenge to get researchers to the field during an event as there can be issues of safety of the researchers and prioritization of the use of resources. In a chaotic situation, logistics of providing supplies and responders to a resource-constrained environment would take precedence over supporting researchers whose contribution the event will not be seen until long after the event is over. While there is some deployment of researchers to study activities in the field, better educating the response community of the value of research to aid improvement of practice and sharing existing programs that use deployed researchers in the field is an area for improvement in homeland security research.

FOR EXAMPLE

Homeland Security Centers of Excellence

One entity coordinating research efforts in homeland security the Department of Homeland Security Science and Technology (S&T) Centers of Excellence (COE). "The COE network is an extended consortium of hundreds of universities conducting groundbreaking research to address homeland security challenges… the COEs work closely with the homeland security community to develop customer-driven, innovative tools and technologies to solve real-world challenges. COE partners include academic institutions; industry; national laboratories; DHS operational components; S&T divisions; other federal agencies; state, local, tribal and territorial homeland security agencies; and first responders. These partners work in concert to develop critical technologies and analyses to secure the nation."

Current COEs include the following:
- Arctic Domain Awareness Center of Excellence (ADAC)
- Borders, Trade, and Immigration Institute (BTI)
- Center for Visualization and Data Analytics (CVADA)
- Center of Excellence for Awareness and Localization of Explosives-Related Threats (ALERT)
- Center of Excellence for Zoonotic and Animal Disease Defense (ZADD)
- Coastal Resilience Center of Excellence (CRC)
- Critical Infrastructure Resilience Institute (CIRI)
- Food Protection and Defense Institute (FPDI)
- Maritime Security Center of Excellence (MSC)
- National Center for Risk and Economic Analysis of Terrorism Events (CREATE)
- National Consortium for the Study of Terrorism and Responses to Terrorism (START) (DHS n.d.)

There is no dearth of research needed, but there are limited funds, researchers, and data. The furthering of homeland security needs solid research to prevent operational decisions that are based on "that's how we always did it" instead of based on case studies, data, operational research, and many dedicated researchers.

SELF-CHECK

- What is the National Security Education Program?
- There is no need for research in homeland security. True or false?
- The DHS S&T Centers of Excellence coordinate multiple centers studying homeland security topics. True or false?
- Which college offers an undergraduate Bachelor's degree in homeland security?
  a. University of North Carolina Wilmington
  b. Eastern Kentucky University
  c. Coastal Carolina University
  d. East Carolina University

SUMMARY

In this chapter we learned that homeland security, as both a practical endeavor and a federal agency, remains in the public consciousness and continues to play a central role in countering terrorism. The five federal homeland security strategic missions, namely, prevent terrorism and enhance security, secure and manage our borders, enforce and administer our immigration laws, safeguard and secure cyberspace, and strengthen national preparedness and resilience, form the backbone for how DHS carries out its role. While debate may continue regarding if these should be the missions of DHS (along with debating what homeland security really entails), for now these missions continue to be executed by DHS under the Trump administration.

We also learned that the requirements for planning, measurement of activities, education, and research continue to expand in need and complexity. Scarce public dollars means that agencies need to do a better job at understanding (and explaining) their roles and being able to demonstrate success. Applying techniques to arrive at SMART measures and the application of logic models as tools to evaluate a program and to depict its efforts to stakeholders are techniques used in government, nonprofit, and private sectors and can add to homeland security activities.

Colleges and universities have added homeland security education programs offering certificates and associate, bachelor's, master's, and doctoral degrees. While currently there is not a "set" curriculum for homeland security education, we do see some coalescence of areas of concentration and in course offerings.

In the area of research of homeland security, both enterprise-wide organizational research and specialized research continue, with the federal government taking a leadership role in funding these efforts. Real-time field research, while it does have complexities, will add to the understanding of homeland security activities and aid in evaluation and service improvement.

Ultimately a public that is informed about the missions of agencies performing homeland security function, as well as a transparent means to demonstrate how these missions have been accomplished, will help further the understanding of public safety in an homeland security world.

KEY TERMS

DHS Strategic Plan	Document that provides additional details and performance measurements for implementing the mission areas of the QHSR. Usually issued for four years to correspond with the current QHSR, which is from 2014 to 2018.
Logic Model	A process/tool/display that can be used to tie all of the items in use for performance management that can help develop performance measures.
National Security Education Program	A major federal initiative designed to build a broader and more qualified pool of US citizens with foreign language and international skills.
National Security Special Event	An event of national or international significance deemed by the US Department of Homeland Security (DHS) to be a potential target for terrorism or other criminal activity. These events have included summits of world leaders, meetings of international organizations, presidential nominating conventions, and presidential inaugurations.
Performance measures	Used to inform key program management decisions such as setting program priorities, allocating resources, or identifying program problems and taking corrective action to solve them.
PPD-8	The Obama administration Presidential Policy Directive that deals with national preparedness required the development of a national preparedness system and a national preparedness goal.

Quadrennial Homeland Security Review (QHSR)   Document produced by the Department of Homeland Security every four years that identifies mission objectives to guide planning and resourcing for DHS but also other federal, state, and local agencies with homeland security responsibilities.

SMART   A mnemonic/framework for goal of objective setting that stands for specific, measurable, attainable/achievable, relevant/realistic, and time bound/timed/timely.

Stakeholders   Individuals, groups, organizations, government departments, businesses, or anyone with a stake or a vested interest in an agency, program, or project.

ASSESS YOUR UNDERSTANDING

Go to www.wiley.com/go/Kilroy/Threats_to_Homeland_Security to assess your knowledge of the basics of homeland security planning and resources.

Summary Questions

1. Universities can play an important role in educating students about the nature of threats today and the all-hazards nature of homeland security by offering courses and programs of study in this new academic discipline. True or false?

2. When you develop a response plan, it is important to keep your senior leaders informed as to the progress so that they can advise you on if the plan is meeting their strategic direction. True or false?

3. How many courses of action should you develop while writing a plan?
   (a) One
   (b) Two
   (c) At least two
   (d) Three unless the plan only involves a short operational period

4. The whole community approach empowers those affected by disasters by referring to them as "disaster victims." True or false?

5. Even though you might not measure them, it is important to keep an eye on "snoozing alligators." True or false?

6. Strategic planning is focused on "How will we get something done." True or false?

7. DHS addresses cybersecurity as a key part of their strategy. True or false?

8. Which of these is one of the steps in the six-step planning process?
   (a) Understand the situation
   (b) Plan development
   (c) Form a collaborative planning team
   (d) All of the above

Applying This Chapter

1. During a college class on homeland security, a student makes a comment that it is likely that in the future the university would not be offering a degree program in homeland security since the term will go away. How would you respond? Explain your reasons for supporting or not supporting such a position.

2. You are assisting your local homeland security director with an evaluation project to demonstrate how effective your agency is at responding to disasters. You realize that there is no data to directly answer the question. What can you do to account for that what you have been asked to measure?

3. You are part of a "collaborative planning team" developing a plan for your local public health agency's response to a pandemic flu outbreak. What are three facts that you can make for the plan, and what are three assumptions that you might have to make?

4. While chatting with your fellow students in between classes, one tells you that he is going to apply for a master's degree program in homeland security while another student says he was going to go for a master's in public administration. Help them think through the "pros and cons" of each type of degree program.

YOU TRY IT

Homeland Security Education

Do a web search on colleges offering programs of study related to homeland security. Categorize them on the basis of the predominant academic discipline under which they fall (e.g., which academic department) and their main focus (terrorism, emergency management, all-hazard, interdisciplinary, etc.). Also determine who you think their main target audience is for this type of degree (e.g., full-time student, adult learner, resident vs. distance learning, etc.).

Form a Core Planning Team

For each of the five homeland security missions, namely, prevent terrorism and enhance security, secure and manage our borders, enforce and administer our immigration laws, safeguard and secure cyberspace, strengthen national preparedness and resilience, develop a list of the disciplines you would want to have on your core planning team (first step in the planning process).

REFERENCES

Preface Works Cited

Clapper, J. R. 2014. Current and Projected National Security Threats to the United States. January 9. Testimony before the Select Committee on Intelligence. Washington, DC: US Government Publishing Office.

Chapter 1 Works Cited

Barnett, T. P. M. 2004. The Pentagon's New Map: War and Peace in the Twenty-first Century. New York: Putnam.

Barnett, T. P. M. 2005. Blueprint for Action: A Future Worth Creating. New York: Putnam.

Bowden, M. 1999. Black Hawk Down: A Story of Modern War. New York: Atlantic Monthly Press.

Brower, C. 2002. The commander-in-chief and TORCH, address given at the Franklin D. Roosevelt Presidential Library, Hyde Park, New York, November 12. http://www.fdrlibrary.marist.edu/cbtorch.html (accessed June 23, 2006).

Bush, C. G. 1905. Uncle Sam – "What particular country threatens us, Theodore?" March 12. *New York World*. Am 3056 (489), Houghton Library, Harvard University.

Civil War Trust. n.d. Antietam. September 16, 1862. http://www.civilwar.org/battlefields/antietam.html?tab=facts (accessed July 15, 2016).

Department of Defense. 1989. Soviet Military Power. Washington, DC: US Government Printing Office.

Department of Defense. 2015. Global War of terrorism service (GWOT-S) medal – approved operations. Office of the Under Secretary for Personnel and Readiness. http://prhome.defense.gov/Portals/52/Documents/RFM/MPP/OEPM/docs/GWOT-S%20Medal%20-%20Approved%20Ops%20-%202015%2003%2011.pdf (accessed August 2, 2016).

Foley, H. 1969. Woodrow Wilson's Case for the League of Nations. New York: Kraus.

Threats to Homeland Security: Reassessing the All-Hazards Perspective, Second Edition.
Edited by Richard J. Kilroy, Jr.
© 2018 John Wiley & Sons, Inc. Published 2018 by John Wiley & Sons, Inc.
Companion website: www.wiley.com/go/Kilroy/Threats_to_Homeland_Security

Gaddis, J. L. 1990. Strategies of Containment: A Critical Appraisal of Postwar American National Security Policy, New York: Oxford University Press.

Glasser, S. B. 2017. Trump National Security Team blindsided by NATO speech. *Politico*. June 5. http://www.politico.com/magazine/story/2017/06/05/trump-nato-speech-national-security-team-215227 (accessed June 8, 2017).

Griffith, J. 1997. In Pursuit of Pancho Villa 1916–1917. The Journal of the Historical Society of the National Guard of Georgia, 6 (3–4).

Hamilton, A., J. Madison, and J. Jay 1961. The Federalist Papers. New York: New American Library.

Hammes, T. X. 2004. The Sling and the Stone: On War in the Twenty-first Century. St. Paul, MN: Zenith.

Hennigan, W. J. 2016. White House releases part of secret drone 'playbook.' *The Sun News*, August 7: 7A.

History Guide. n.d. George Kennan: The sources of Soviet conduct (1947). http://www.historyguide.org/europe/kennan.html (accessed March 22, 2007).

Jentleson, B. 2004. American Foreign Policy: The Dynamics of Choice in the Twenty-first Century, 2nd ed. New York: Norton.

Jordan, A. A., Taylor, W. J. Jr., and M. J. Mazarr 1998. American National Security, 5th ed. Baltimore, MA: Johns Hopkins University Press.

Kagan, D. 2001. While America Sleeps: Self-delusion, Military Weakness, and the Threat to Peace Today. New York: St. Martins.

Kagan, R. and W. Kristol, eds. 2000. Present Dangers: Crisis and Opportunity in American Foreign and Defense Policy. New York: Encounter.

Lipowicz, A. 2010. Huge size of DHS contractor workforce leaves senators 'astonished'. *FCW*. March 1. https://fcw.com/articles/2010/03/01/dhs-has-too-many-contract-employees-senators-charge.aspx (accessed August 1, 2016).

McCaskill, N. D. 2016. Trump promises wall and massive deportation program. *Politico*. August 31. http://www.politico.com/story/2016/08/donald-trump-immigration-address-arizona-227612 (accessed September 1, 2016).

Miller, G. 2011. Under Obama, an emerging global apparatus for drone killing. *Washington Post*. December 27. https://www.washingtonpost.com/national/national-security/under-obama-an-emerging-global-apparatus-for-drone-killing/2011/12/13/gIQANPdILP_story.html (accessed August 2, 2016).

Morgenthau, H. J. 1948. Politics among Nations: The Struggle for Power and Peace, 1st ed. New York: Knopf.

National Security Strategy. 2010. White House. May. National Security Archive. http://nssarchive.us/NSSR/2010.pdf (accessed August 1, 2016).

National Security Strategy. 2015. White House. February. National Security Archive. http://nssarchive.us/wp-content/uploads/2015/02/2015.pdf (accessed August 1, 2016).

National Strategy for Combating Terrorism. 2003. White House. February. https://www.cia.gov/news-information/cia-the-war-on-terrorism/Counter_Terrorism_Strategy.pdf (accessed November 7, 2017).

National Strategy for Counterterrorism. 2011. White House. June. https://obamawhitehouse.archives.gov/sites/default/files/counterterrorism_strategy.pdf (accessed November 7, 2017).

National Strategy for Homeland Security. 2007. Homeland Security Council. Homeland Security Digital Library. https://www.hsdl.org/?view&did=479633 (accessed August 2, 2016).

PBS. n.d. Korematsu v. United States (1944). http://www.pbs.org/wnet/supremecourt/personality/landmark_korematsu.html (accessed July 27, 2016).

Rumer, E. 2016. Russia and the security of Europe. Carnegie Endowment for International Peace. June 30. http://carnegieendowment.org/2016/06/30/russia-and-security-of-europe-pub-63990 (accessed August 1, 2016).

Salam, R. 2014. We never should have left Iraq. *Slate*. June 12. http://www.slate.com/articles/news_and_politics/politics/2014/06/iraq_sunnis_and_shiites_the_u_s_should_never_have_withdrawn_its_troops_in.html (accessed August 1, 2016).

Siasoco, R. V. and S. Ross. 2006. Japanese relocation centers. http://www.infoplease.com/spot/internment1.html (accessed July 27, 2016).

Snow, D. M. 2004. National Security for a New Era: Globalization and Geopolitics. New York: Pearson Longman.

Tuchman, B. 1966. The Proud Tower: A Portrait of the World before the War 1890–1914. New York: Macmillan.

Walsh, N. P. 2016. US special forces take the fight to ISIS in Libya. *CNN*. May 26. http://www.cnn.com/2016/05/18/middleeast/libya-isis-us-special-forces/index.html (accessed August 2, 2016).

White, M. 2003. Historical atlas of the twentieth century. http://users.erols.com/mwhite28/coldwar1.htm (accessed July 18, 2006).

White, J. R. 2014. Terrorism and Homeland Security, 8th ed. Belmont, CA: Wadsworth.

Williams, W. A. 1978. Americans in a Changing World: A History of the United States in the Twentieth Century, New York: Harper and Row.

Chapter 2 Works Cited

1900 Storm. n.d. https://www.1900storm.com/facts.html (accessed November 7, 2017).

Bea, K. 2006. Federal Stafford act disaster assistance: Presidential declarations, eligible activities, and funding," Congressional Research Service Report RL 33093. April 28. https://digital.library.unt.edu/ark:/67531/ https://digital.library.unt.edu/ark:/67531/metacrs8988/m1/1/high_res_d/RL33053_2006Apr28.pdfmetacrs8988/m1/1/high_res_d/RL33053_2006Apr28.pdf (accessed November 7, 2017).

Breeden, S. 2016. Responders: Matthew a reminder of Floyd, but with better preparation. *Daily Reflector*. Greenville, NC. October 13. http://www.reflector.com/News/2016/10/13/Responders-Matthew-a-reminder-of-Floyd-but-with-better-preparation.html (accessed October 14, 2016).

Broughton, E. 2005. The Bhopal Disaster and its Aftermath: A Review. Environmental Health, 4, 6. http://www.pubmedcentral.nih.gov/articlerender.fcgi?tool=pubmed&pubmedid=15882472 (accessed January 19, 2007).

Canton, L. 2013. "All-hazards" doesn't mean "plan for everything." *Emergency Management*. August 7. http://www.emergencymgmt.com/emergency-blogs/managing-crisis/Allhazards-Doesnt-Mean-Plan-for-Everything.html (accessed September 30, 2016).

Carrns, A. and B. McKay. 2005. New Orleans Levee System has been Key to Survival. Wall Street Journal (August 31). http://old.post-gazette.com/pg/05243/563080.stm (accessed January 10, 2018).

Center for Chemical Process Safety. n.d. About CCPS. http://www.aiche.org/CCPS/About/index.aspx (accessed January 19, 2007).

City of Los Angeles. 1928. St. Francis Dam disaster. Historical photo collection. Department of Water and Power. http://dbase1.lapl.org/images/dwp/ws///1001830.jpg (accessed June 14, 2017).

CNN. 2006. Apex mayor: Fire fizzling. Evacuees can't go home yet. *CNN*. October 6. http://www.cnn.com/2006/US/10/06/plant.fire/index.html (accessed January 19, 2007).

Department of Homeland Security. 2006. DHS introduces new regulations to secure high-risk chemical facilities. Press release. December 22. http://www.dhs.gov/xnews/releases/pr_1166807052891.shtm (accessed January 19, 2007).

Department of Water and Power. n.d. City of Los Angeles photo archive. http://www.lapl.org/collections-resources/visual-collections/department-water-power-photo-archive (accessed June 14, 2017).

England-Joseph, J. 1998. "Disaster assistance: Information on federal costs and approaches for reducing them. Testimony before the Subcommittee on Water Resources and Environment, Committee on Transportation and Infrastructure, House of Representatives, March 26.

Epic Disasters. n.d. The United States' worst earthquakes. http://www.epicdisasters.com/deadlyusearthquake.php (accessed January 15, 2007).

Federal Emergency Management Agency. n.d. FEMA history, http://www.fema.gov/about/history.shtm (accessed January 15, 2007).

Gannon, M. 2005. AIR worldwide estimates total property damage from hurricane Katrina's storm surge and flood at $44 billion. http://www.iso.com/press_releases/2005/09_29_05.html (accessed January 15, 2007).

Glasser, S. B. and J. White. 2005. Storm exposed disarray at the top. *Washington Post*, September 4.

Global Security. n.d. Weapons of mass destruction civil support teams. http://www.globalsecurity.org/military/agency/army/wmd-cst.htm (accessed January 19, 2007).

Gregory, P. A. 2015. Reassessing the Effectiveness of All-Hazards Planning in Emergency Management. Inquiries Journal/Student Pulse, 7 (06). http://www.inquiriesjournal.com/a?id=1050 (accessed September 30, 2016).

Homeland Security Wire News. 2015. Fusion centers, created to fight domestic terrorism, suffering from mission creep: Critics. April 25. http://www.homelandsecuritynewswire.com/dr20150421-fusion-centers-created-to-fight-domestic-terrorism-suffering-from-mission-creep-critics?page=0,0 (accessed October 14, 2016).

Infoplease. n.d. Americas worst disasters. http://www.infoplease.com/ipa/A0005349.html (accessed January 15, 2007).

Johnstown Area Heritage Association (JAHA). n.d. An overview of the 1889 tragedy. http://www.jaha.org/attractions/johnstown-flood-museum/flood-history/ (accessed November 7, 2017).

Lowder, M. W. 2006. FEMA disaster response operations and cross border events. Trilateral Conference on Preparing for and Responding to Disasters in North America, San Antonio, TX, November 7.

Miskel, J. F. 2006. Disaster Response and Homeland Security: What Works and What Doesn't. Westport, CT: Praeger Security International.

National Fire Prevention Association, NFPA 1600: Standard on Disaster/Emergency Management and Business Continuity/Continuity of Operations Programs (February 2016).

National Oceanographic and Atmospheric Administration. 2002. Hurricane Andrew: Ten years later. http://www.noaa.gov/hurricaneandrew.html (accessed January 15, 2007).

Organization for Economic Cooperation and Development. n.d. Chemical accidents, http://www.oecd.org/about/0,2337,en_2649_34369_1_1_1_1_1,00.html (accessed January 19, 2007).

Ortmeier, P. J. 2005. Security Management: An Introduction, 2nd ed. New York: Pearson, Prentice Hall.

Pickering, K. 2017. Photograph [U.S. Army Multimedia: South Carolina National Guard 43rd Civil Support Team trains to respond to real world incidents] Washington, DC: US Army. https://www.army.mil/article/184142/south_carolina_national_guard_43rd_civil_support_team_trains_to_respond_to_real_world_incidents (accessed June 19, 2017).

Pocock, E. n.d. Disasters in the United States: 1650–2005. http://www.easternct.edu/depts/amerst/disasters.htm (accessed January 19, 2007).

Quotlr. n.d. 18 Best Frederick the great quotes. http://quotlr.com/author/frederick-the-great (accessed October 14, 2016).

Ramsay, J. D. and L. Kiltz. 2014. Critical Issues in Homeland Security. Boulder, CO: Westview Press.

Schleifstein, M. 2009. Study of Hurricane Katrina's dead show most were old, lived near levee breaches. The Times Picayune (NOLA.com). August 29.

Sensenig, D. and P. Simpson. 2008. Chemical fire in Apex, North Carolina. US Fire Administration Technical Report USFA-TR-163/April. https://www.usfa.fema.gov/downloads/pdf/publications/tr_163.pdf (accessed December 30, 2016).

South Carolina Emergency Management Division. 2013. South Carolina hazard mitigation plan. October. http://www.scemd.org/files/

Mitigation/State_Hazard_Mitigation_Plan/1_SHMP_FINAL_2013. pdf (accessed November 7, 2017).

Sylves, R. 2006. President Bush and Hurricane Katrina: A Presidential Leadership Study. Annals of the American Academy of Political and Social Science, 604 (1), 26–56.

Tiwari, J. and C. Gray. n.d. US nuclear weapons accidents. http://www.cdi. org/Issues/NukeAccidents/accidents.htm (accessed January 19, 2007).

United States Environmental Protection Agency. 2006. Kanawa drill to test emergency responders. http://yosemite.epa.gov/opa/admpress. nsf/93216b1c8fd122ca8cb2dc/3f8af06ebf12afca852571ed006d5d 94!OpenDocument (accessed January 22, 2007).

United States Geological Service. 2004. The Mississippi valley-"whole Lotta Shakin' goin' on". http://quake.wr.usgs.gov/prepare/factsheets/ NewMadrid/ (accessed January 15, 2007). Archived October 11, 2013. http://web.archive.org/web/20041106230247/http://quake. usgs.gov/prepare/factsheets/NewMadrid/SeismicZone.gif (accessed July 31, 2017).

United States Senate. 2012. Federal support for and involvement in state and local fusion centers. Permanent Subcommittee on Investigations. Committee on Homeland Security and Governmental Affairs. October 3.

Weden, M. L. 2016. Defining an 'all hazards' approach to hospital emergency management, *Intermedix*. September 9. https://www. intermedix.com/blog/defining-an-all-hazards-approach-to-hospital-emergency-management (accessed March 3, 2017).

Wilkman, J. 2016. Floodpath: The Deadliest Man-Made Disaster of 20th-Century America and the Making of Modern Los Angeles, 1st ed. New York: Bloomsbury Press (Kindle Edition).

Wilks, A 2016. SC to get $65 million in federal aid for Hurricane Matthew recovery. *The State*. December 29. http://www.thestate. com/news/politics-government/article123531014.html (accessed December 30, 2016).

Williams, R. 2009. Earthquake hazard in the New Madrid seismic zone remains a concern. US Geological Service Fact Sheet 2009–3071. August. https://pubs.usgs.gov/fs/2009/3071/pdf/FS09-3071.pdf (accessed November 7, 2017).

Chapter 3 Works Cited

Alvarez, L. and R. Perez-Pena. 2016. Orlando gunman attacks gay nightclub, leaving 50 dead. *The New York Times*. June 12. http:// www.nytimes.com/2016/06/13/us/orlando-nightclub-shooting. html (accessed January 3, 2017).

Anderson, J. E. 2000. Public Policymaking, 4th ed. Boston, MA: Haughton Mifflin Company.

Bahamonde, M. 2005. Photograph [FEMA Multimedia: Hurricane Katrina Flooding in New Orleans]. Washington, DC: Federal Emergency Management Agency. https://www.fema.gov/media-library/assets/images/45883 (accessed June 26, 2017).

Bahler, B. 2008. Photograph [FEMA multimedia: Florida Logistics Center Team]. Washington, DC: Federal Emergency Management Agency. https://www.fema.gov/media-library/assets/images/53457.

Bell, B. 2016. Political will and creative approaches needed for future disasters demands. In The Book of the States, 2016. Lexington, KY: The Council of State Governments.

Bellavita, C. 2008. Changing Homeland Security: What is Homeland Security? Homeland Security Affairs, IV (2).

Bender, D. J. 2015. Congress Passes the Cybersecurity Act of 2015. Western Springs, IL: The National Law Review. http://www.natlawreview.com/article/congress-passes-cybersecurity-act-2015 (accessed January 3, 2017).

Boccia, S. 2016. Not out of control: Analysis of the federal disaster spending trend (Master's Thesis). Monterey, CA: Naval Postgraduate School.

Booher, A. 2005. Photograph [FEMA Multimedia: National Guard Response to Hurricane Dennis]. Washington, DC: Federal Emergency Management Agency. https://www.fema.gov/media-library/assets/images/44857 (accessed June 26, 2017).

Curry, A. and R. Spaulding. 2006. Central California Area Maritime Security Committee: Putting Security to the Test. The Coast Guard Journal of Safety and Security at Sea: Proceedings of the Marine Safety and Security Council, 63 (1).

Cybersecurity Act of 2015, Consolidated Appropriations Act, 2016, Pub. L. 114-113, Div. N.

de Vogue, A. and L. Jarrett. 2017. Trump admin appeals travel ban case to Supreme Court. CNN. June 2. http://www.cnn.com/2017/06/01/politics/trump-travel-ban-supreme-court/index.html (accessed June 3, 2017).

Disaster Mitigation Act of 2000, Pub. L. 106-390.

Disco, J. 2016. Photograph [DHS Multimedia: New York City Skyline]. Washington, DC: US Department of Homeland Security. https://www.dhs.gov/photo/skyline-lower-manhattan-new-york-harbor (accessed June 26, 2017).

Dye, T. 2005. Understanding Public Policy, 11th ed. Upper Saddle River, NJ: Pearson Education.

Eastern Kentucky University. 2017. Homeland Security Program Guide, 2017–2018. Richmond, KY: Eastern Kentucky University.

Environmental Protection Agency. 2016. Deepwater Horizon – BP Gulf of Mexico Oil Spill. Washington, DC: Environmental Protection Agency. https://www.epa.gov/enforcement/deepwater-horizon-bp-gulf-mexico-oil-spill (accessed January 3, 2017).

Federal Civil Defense Act of 1950, Pub. L. 81-920.

Federal Disaster Relief Act of 1950, Pub. L. 81-875.

Federal Emergency Management Agency. 2007. Robert T. Stafford Disaster Relief and Emergency Assistance Act, as Amended, and Related Authorities (FEMA 592). Washington, DC: US Department of Homeland Security.

Federal Emergency Management Agency. 2011. A Whole Community Approach to Emergency Management: Principles, Themes, and Pathways for Action (FDOC 104-008-1). Washington, DC: US Department of Homeland Security.

Foster, C. 2006. Regional Solutions to Homeland Security. State News, 49 (2), 9–12.

Foster, C. 2017. Homeland Security Traditions. Eastern Kentucky University Homeland Security Degree Programs Briefing Materials, EKU.

Foster, C. and G. Cordner. 2005. The impact of terrorism on state law enforcement – Final report (grant no. 2003-DT-CX-0004 awarded by the National Institute of Justice, US Department of Justice). June. Lexington and Richmond, KY: The Council of State Governments and Eastern Kentucky University.

Foster, C. and C. J. Kinsella. 2004. Homeland Security Brief: Order the Quarantine! Assessing State Health Powers and Readiness. Lexington, KY: The Council of State Governments.

Friedman, T. L. 2005. The World is Flat: A Brief History of the Twenty-First Century. New York: Farrar, Straus and Giroux.

Fulfilling Rights and Ensuring Effective Discipline Over Monitoring Act (USA FREEDOM Act) of 2015, Pub. L. 114-23.

Godschalk, D. R., T. Beatley, P. Berke, D. J. Brower and E. J. Kaiser. 1999. Natural Disaster Mitigation: Recasting Disaster Policy and Planning. Washington, DC: Island Press.

Homeland Security Act of 2002, Pub. L. 107-296, 116 Stat. 2135.

Johnson, J. 2016. Fifteen years after 9/11: Threats to the homeland. Written Testimony of DHS Secretary Jeh Johnson for a Senate Committee on Homeland Security and Governmental Affairs Hearing. September 27. Washington, DC: US Department of Homeland Security. https://www.dhs.gov/news/2016/09/27/written-testimony-dhs-secretary-johnson-senate-committee-homeland-security-and (accessed January 5, 2017).

Kettl, D. F. 2014. System under stress: The challenge to 21st century governance, 3rd ed. Los Angeles, CA: Sage (CQ Press).

Kilroy Jr., R. J. ed. 2008. Threats to Homeland Security: An All-Hazards Perspective, 1st ed. Hoboken, New Jersey: J. Wiley and Sons.

LaMotte, S. 2016. CDC issues historic travel warning over Miami Zika outbreak. CNN. August 3. http://www.cnn.com/2016/08/01/health/cdc-miami-florida-zika-travel-warning/ (accessed January 3, 2017).

Lynch, P. 2011. Photograph [FEMA Multimedia: Humane Society Provides Assistance to Animals]. Washington, DC: Federal Emergency Management Agency. https://www.fema.gov/media-library/assets/images/59799 (accessed June 26, 2017).

Maritime Transportation Security Act of 2002, Pub. L. 107-295.

McDermott, T. 2004. Ronald Reagan remembered. CBS. June 6. http://www.cbsnews.com/news/ronald-reagan-remembered/ (accessed May 22, 2017).

McElreath, D. H., C. J. Jensen, M. Wigginton, D. A. Doss, R. Nations and J. V. Slyke. 2014. Introduction to Homeland Security, 2nd ed. Boca Raton, FL: Taylor & Francis Group (CRC Press).

McEntire, D. A. 2015. Disaster Response and Recovery: Strategies and Tactics for Resilience, 2nd ed. Hoboken, NJ: John Wiley & Sons, Inc.

Melillo, J. M., T. C. Richmond and G. W. Yohe, eds. 2014. Climate Change Impacts in the United States: The Third National Climate Assessment: US Global Change Research Program. Washington, DC: US Government Printing Office. http://nca2014.globalchange.gov/ (accessed January 5, 2017).

Miller, R. 2006. Hurricane Katrina: Communications and Infrastructure Impacts. In Threats at Our Homeland: Homeland Defense and Homeland Security in the New Century – A Compilation of the Proceedings of the First Annual Homeland Defense and Homeland Security Conference, ed. B. Tussing. Carlisle Barracks, PA: US Army War College.

Murphy, G. R. and C. Wexler, C. 2004. Managing A Multijurisdictional Case: Identifying the Lessons Learned from the Sniper Investigation. Washington, DC: Police Executive Research Forum.

National Academy of Sciences. 2012. Disaster Resilience: A National Imperative. Washington, DC: The National Academies Press.

National Commission on Terrorist Attacks Upon the United States. 2004. Media kit/photograph [9/11 Commission]. National Commission on Terrorist Attacks Upon the United States [Independent, Bipartisan Commission Established in Public Law 107-306, November 27, 2002]. http://govinfo.library.unt.edu/911/press/index.htm (accessed June 26, 2017).

National Emergency Management Association. 2011. State Emergency Management Director Handbook. Lexington, KY: National Emergency Management Association.

National Emergency Management Association. 2016. NEMA 2016 Biennial Report. Lexington, KY: National Emergency Management Association.

National Flood Inurance Act of 1968, Title XII of the Housing and Urban Development Act of 1968, Pub. L. 90-448.

National Homeland Security Consortium. 2016. 2016 National Issues Brief. Lextington, KY: National Emergency Management Association.

New York State Division of Homeland Security and Emergency Services. 2014. New York State Homeland Security Strategy, 2014–2016. Albany, NY: New York State Division of Homeland Security and Emergency Services.

Office of the Director of National Intelligence. n.d. Members of the IC. Washington, DC: Office of the Director of National Intelligence. https://www.dni.gov/index.php/intelligence-community/members-of-the-ic (accessed January 5, 2017).

Phillips, B. D. 2016. Disaster Recovery, 2nd ed. Boca Rotan, FL: CRC Press/Taylor and Francis Group.

Plano, J. and M. Greenberg. 1985. The American Political Dictionary, 7th ed. New York, NY: Holt, Rinehart, and Winston.

Port of Los Angeles. 2017. Photo Gallery [Security]. Los Angeles, CA: Port of Los Angeles. https://www.portoflosangeles.org/newsroom/photo_gallery.asp (accessed June 26, 2017).

Post-Katrina Emergency Management Reform Act of 2006, Title VI of the Department of Homeland Security Appropriations Act, 2007, Pub. L. 109-295.

Reaves, B. A. 2011. Census of state and local law enforcement officers, 2008 (NCJ 233982). Washington, DC: Bureau of Justice Statistics, US Department of Justice.

Reaves, B. A. 2012. Federal law enforcement Officers, 2008 (NCJ 238250). Washington, DC: Bureau of Justice Statistics, US Department of Justice.

Rice, D. 2016. Why the W.Va. floods were so deadly and destructive. *USA Today*. June 27. http://www.usatoday.com/story/weather/2016/06/27/west-virginia-floods-storm-train/86429020/ (accessed January 11, 2017).

Robert T. Stafford Disaster Relief and Emergency Assistance Act of 1988, Pub. L. 100-707.

Rural Policy Research Institute. 2009. Demographic and Economic Profile: Nonmetropolitan America. Columbia, MO: Rural Policy Research Institute. http://www.rupri.org/Forms/Nonmetro2.pdf (accessed January 5, 2017).

San Francisco Department of Emergency Management. n.d. SF72. San Francisco, CA: San Francisco Department of Emergency Management. http://www.sf72.org/home (accessed January 5, 2017).

Schenck v. United States. 1919. 249 US 47.

Schneider, R.O. 2016. Managing the Climate Crisis: Assessing Our Risks, Options, and Prospects. Santa Barbara, CA: Praeger/ABC-CLIO.

Select Bipartisan Committee to Investigate the Preparation for and Response to Hurricane Katrina. 2006. A Failure of Initiative, 109th Congress, Report No. 109-377. Washington, DC: House of Representatives.

Simpkins, B. and C. Foster. 2017. Introduction: Technology securing the homeland. In Homeland Security Technologies for the 21st Century: Practical Applications and Emerging Trends, eds. R. Baggett, C. Foster and B. Simpkins. Santa Barbara, CA: Praeger/ABC-CLIO.

Sylves, R. 2015. Disaster Policy and Politics: Emergency Management and Homeland Security, 2nd ed. Washington, DC: CQ Press.

The White House. 2017. Executive Order 13780: Protecting the Nation from Foreign Terrorist Entry Into the United States. Washington, DC: The White House. https://www.whitehouse.gov/the-press-office/2017/03/06/executive-order-protecting-nation-foreign-terrorist-entry-united-states (accessed June 3, 2017).

The White House Office of Homeland Security. 2002. National Strategy for Homeland Security. Washington, DC: The White House.

Tussing, B. 2012. Defense support of civil authorities. In Introduction to Homeland Security, eds. K. G. Logan and J. D. Ramsay. Boulder, CO: Westview Press.

Uniting and Strengthening America by Providing Appropriate Tools Required to Intercept and Obstruct Terrorism Act (USA PATRIOT Act) of 2001, Pub. L. 107-56.

US Census Bureau. 2012. Growth in Urban Population Outpaces Rest of Nation, Census Bureau Reports. Washington, DC: US Department of Commerce. https://www.census.gov/newsroom/releases/archives/2010_census/cb12-50.html (accessed January 5, 2017).

US Department of Agriculture. 2016. Population & Migration: Overview. Washington, DC: US Department of Agriculture. http://www.ers.usda.gov/topics/rural-economy-population/population-migration.aspx (accessed January 11, 2017).

US Department of Commerce. 2017. Photographs [National Ocean Watch: Economic Sectors]. Washington, DC: US Department of Commerce. https://www.commerce.gov/media/photo/enowecono micsectorsphotos-1800x1521jpg (accessed June 26, 2017).

US Department of Homeland Security. n.d. About the Campaign "If You See Something, Say Something." Washington, DC: US Department of Homeland Security. https://www.dhs.gov/see-something-say-something/about-campaign (accessed January 3, 2017).

US Department of Homeland Security. 2010. Quadrennial Homeland Security Review Report: A Strategic Framework for a Secure Homeland. Washington, DC: US Department of Homeland Security.

US Department of Homeland Security. 2012. Photograph [DHS Multimedia: US Coast Guard Response Training]. Washington, DC: US Department of Homeland Security. https://www.dhs.gov/photo/response-boat-training-chesapeake-bay-uscg (accessed June 26, 2017).

US Department of Homeland Security. 2013. National Response Framework, 2nd ed. Washington, DC: US Department of Homeland Security.

US Department of Homeland Security. 2015. National Preparedness Goal, 2nd ed. Washington, DC: US Department of Homeland Security.

US Department of Homeland Security. 2016a. Notice of Funding Opportunity (NOFO): Fiscal Year 2016 Emergency Management Performance Grant Program (EMPG). Washington, DC: US Department of Homeland Security. https://www.fema.gov/emergency-management-performance-grant-program (accessed January 11, 2017).

US Department of Homeland Security. 2016b. Notice of Funding Opportunity (NOFO): Fiscal Year 2016 Homeland Security Grant Program. Washington, DC: US Department of Homeland Security. https://www.fema.gov/fiscal-year-2016-homeland-security-grant-program (accessed January 11, 2017).

US Department of Homeland Security. 2016c. National Protection Framework, 2nd ed. Washington, DC: US Department of Homeland Security. https://www.fema.gov/media-library-data/146601730905 2-85051ed62fe595d4ad026edf4d85541e/National_Protection_ Framework2nd.pdf (accessed November 7, 2017).

US Department of Homeland Security. 2016d. Our Mission. Washington, DC: US Department of Homeland Security. https://www.dhs.gov/ our-mission (accessed January 3, 2017).

US Global Change Research Program. n.d. Glossary. Washington, DC: US Global Change Research Program. http://www.globalchange. gov/climate-change/glossary (accessed May 17, 2017).

US Government Accountability Office. 2015. High-Risk Series: An Update (GAO-15-290). Washington, DC: US Government Accountability Office.

Waugh, W. 2000. Public Administration and Emergency Management. Emmitsburg, MD: Federal Emergency Management Agency.

Weisman, S. 2016. Ransomware? Bad news, it's getting worse. *USA Today*. May 7. http://www.usatoday.com/story/money/columnist/2016/05/07/ ransomware-bad-news-s-getting-worse/83876342/ (accessed January 3, 2017).

Chapter 4 Works Cited

Ander, S. and A. Swift. 2013. "See something, say something" unfamiliar to most Americans. *GALLUP*. http://www.gallup.com/ poll/166622/something-say-something-unfamiliar-americans.aspx (accessed June 14, 2017).

Baker, G. W. and D. W. Chapman, eds. 1962. Man and Society in Disaster. New York: Basic Books.

Bates, F. L. and W. G. Peacock. 1993. Living Conditions, Disasters and Development: An Approach to Cross-Cultural Comparisons. Athens, GA: University of Georgia Press.

Bloomberg. 2015. Bloomberg Poll, November 2015. Cornell University, Ithaca, NY: Roper Center for Public Opinion Research.

Bolin, R. C. 1982. Long-Term Family Recovery from Disaster. Boulder, CO: University of Colorado Institute of Behavioural Science.

Bolin, R. C. 1993. Household and Community Recovery After Earthquakes. Boulder CO: University of Colorado Institute of Behavioural Science.

Buzan, B. 1991. People, States, and Fear: An Agenda for International Security Studies in the Post-Cold War Era. Boulder, CO: Rienner.

California Governor's Office of Emergency Services. 2014. State of California threat and hazard identification and risk assessment (THIRA). http://www.caloes.ca.gov/PlanningPreparednessSite/ Documents/01%20THIRA%20Summary%202014%20Final%20v2. pdf (accessed June 14, 2017).

Committee on Disaster Research in the Social Sciences/National Research Council of the National Academies. 2006. Facing Hazards and Disasters: Understanding Human Dimensions. Washington, DC: National Academies Press.

Congressional Research Service. 2015. USA FREEDOM act reinstates expired USA PATRIOT act provisions but limits bulk collection. *CRS Legal Sidebar*. June 4, 2015. https://www.fas.org/sgp/crs/intel/usaf-rein.pdf (accessed June 20, 2017).

Cutter, S. L., L. Barnes, M. Berry, C. Burton, E. Evans, E. Tate and J. Webb. 2008. A Place-Based Model for Understanding Community Resilience to Natural Disasters. Global Environmental Change 18(4): 598–606.

Dorman, A. and J. Kaufman, eds. 2014. Providing for National Security: A Comparative Analysis. Stanford, CA: Stanford University Press.

Drake, B. 2013. Homeland Security Is Viewed Favourably by Americans Ahead of Jeh Johnson's Hearing. Pew Research Center. http://www.pewresearch.org/fact-tank/2013/11/13/senate-committee-considers-new-leader-for-the-favorably-viewed-homeland-security-department (accessed June 14, 2017).

Dynes R. 1970. Organized Behavior in Disaster. Lexington, MA: Heath-Lexington Books.

Dynes, R., E. L. Quarantelli, and G. Kreps 1972. A Perspective on Disaster Planning. Columbus, OH: The Ohio State University Disaster Research Center.

Federal Emergency Management Agency. 1997. Multi-Hazard Identification and Risk Assessment: A Cornerstone of the National Mitigation Strategy. Washington, DC: Federal Emergency Management Agency.

Federal Emergency Management Agency. 2008. National response framework. https://www.fema.gov/pdf/emergency/nrf/nrf-core.pdf (accessed June 20, 2017).

Federal Emergency Management Agency. 2013a. Hurricane sandy: FEMA after-action report. https://www.fema.gov/media-library-data/20130726-1923-25045-7442/sandy_fema_aar.pdf (accessed June 21, 2017).

Federal Emergency Management Agency. 2013b. Including building codes in the National Flood Insurance Program. Fiscal year 2013 Report to Congress Impact Study for Biggert-Waters Flood Insurance Reform Act of 2012. Washington, DC. https://www.fema.gov/media-library-data/1385728818014-f08e55ee835906501039 95b2c66e2285/Incl_Bldg_Codes_NFIP2.pdf (accessed November 7, 2017).

Federal Emergency Management Agency. 2013c: Information sheet: Threat and hazard identification and risk assessment. https://www.fema.gov/media-library-data/1388146249060-7b2abfe6be10c67c 4070ed42deaaadf1/THIRA_Information_Sheet_20131104.pdf (accessed June 14, 2017).

Federal Emergency Management Agency. 2016. National preparedness system. https://www.fema.gov/national-preparedness-system (last updated December 20, 2016, accessed October 26, 2017).

Federal Emergency Management Agency. 2017a. Hazus. https://www.fema.gov/hazus (last updated March 27, 2017, accessed October 26, 2017).

Federal Emergency Management Agency. 2017b. Plan. https://www.fema.gov/plan (last updated March 28, 2017, accessed October 2017).

Harvey, F. P. 2008. The Homeland Security Dilemma: Fear, Failure and the Future of American Insecurity. New York: Routledge.

Kowalski, K. M. 2008. A Pro/Con Look at Homeland Security: Safety vs. Liberty After 9/11. Beverly Heights, NY: Enslow.

Lindell, M. K. and R. W. Perry. 1992. Behavioral Foundations of Community Emergency Planning. Washington, DC: Hemisphere.

Lindell, M. K. and R. W. Perry. 2000. Household Adjustment to Earthquake Hazard: A Review of Research. Environment and Behavior 32: 590–630.

Lindell, M. K. and C. Prater. 2003. Assessing Community Impacts of Natural Disasters. Natural Hazards Review 4: 176–185. 10.1061/(ASCE)1527-6988(2003)4:4(176).

Lyman, E. 2004. Chernobyl on the Hudson? The health and economic impacts of a terrorist attack at the Indian point nuclear plant. September. http://www.ucsusa.org/global_security/nuclear_terrorism/impacts-of-a-terrorist-attack-at-indian-point-nuclear-power-plant.html (last modified September 2004, accessed October 26, 2017).

McCreight, R. 2015. Examining the strategic hybrid threat: Technology, terrorism, transnational criminal organizations, and old enemies after 2015. In Cross-Disciplinary Perspectives on Homeland and Civil Security: A Research-Based Introduction, ed. A. Siedschlag. New York: Peter Lang.

Mileti, D. S. 1999. Disasters by Design: A Reassessment of Natural Hazards in the United States. Washington, DC: Joseph Henry Press.

Miskel, J. 2006. Disaster Response and Homeland Security: What Works, What Doesn't. Westport, CT: Greenwood Publishing Group.

National Oceanic and Atmospheric Administration. 2006. Vulnerability Assessment Techniques and Applications (VATA). http://hsc.usf.edu/nocms/publichealth/cdmha/toolkit_dm/GLOSSARY/NOOA--Vulnerability%20Assessment%20Techniques%20and%20Applications.htm (accessed December 25, 2017).

National Oceanic and Atmospheric Administration, Office for Coastal Management 2017. Vulnerability assessment. https://coast.noaa.gov/digitalcoast/topics/vulnerability-assessments.html (accessed July 17, 2017).

Office of the Director of National Intelligence. 2017. Statement for the record: Worldwide threat assessment of the US intelligence community. Senate Select Committee on Intelligence. Daniel R. Coats, Director of National Intelligence. May 11. https://www.dni.gov/files/documents/Newsroom/Testimonies/SSCI%20Unclassified%20SFR%20-%20Final.pdf (accessed June 14, 2017).

Pew Research Center. 2013. Most expect "occasional acts of terrorism" in the future. Six-in-ten say post-9/11 steps have made country safer. http://www.people-press.org/2013/04/23/most-expect-occasional-acts-of-terrorism-in-the-future (accessed June 14, 2017).

Pew Research Center. 2015. Beyond distrust: How Americans view their government. Broad criticism, but positive performance ratings in many areas. http://www.people-press.org/2015/11/23/beyond-distrust-how-americans-view-their-government (accessed June 14, 2017).

Philpott, D. 2015. Understanding the Department of Homeland Security. Lanham, MD: Bernan Press.

Pitchford, P. 2006. Air ban on liquids lightened. *Press-Enterprise*. September 25. Page A-1.

President's Commission on Aviation Security and Terrorism. 1990. Report of the President's Commission on Aviation Security and Terrorism. Washington, DC. http://www.peacefare.net/wp-content/uploads/2013/08/Pan-Am-103-report.pdf (accessed June 14, 2017).

Ramsay J. D. and L. Kiltz. 2014. Introduction. In Critical Issues in Homeland Security: A Casebook, eds. J. D. Ramsay and L. Kiltz. Boulder, CO: Westview.

Ryan, W. R. 2015. The role of intelligence in homeland security. In Cross-Disciplinary Perspectives on Homeland and Civil Security: A Research-Based Introduction, ed. A. Siedschlag. New York: Peter Lang.

Siedschlag, A., ed. 2015. Cross-Disciplinary Perspectives on Homeland and Civil Security: A Research-Based Introduction. New York: Peter Lang.

Smith, S. K., J., Tayman, and D. A. Swanson. 2013. A Practitioner's Guide to State and Local Population Projections. Dordrecht: Springer.

Sorokin, P. A. 1942. Man and Society in Calamity: The Effects of War, Revolution, Famine, Pestilence upon Human Mind, Behavior, Social Organization and Cultural Life. New York: Dutton.

State of New Jersey. 2012. Christie Administration Releases Total Hurricane Sandy Damage Assessment of $36.9 Billion. http://www.state.nj.us/governor/news/news/552012/approved/20121128e.html (published November 26, 2012).

Steiner, J. E. 2015. Homeland Security Intelligence. Thousand Oaks, CA: CQ Press.

The National Commission on Terrorist Attacks Upon the United States. 2004. 9/11 commission report. http://www.9-11commission.gov/report/911Report.pdf (accessed June 14, 2017).

United Nations Office for Disaster Risk Reduction (UNISDR). 2015. Sendai Framework for Disaster Risk Reduction 2015–2030. http://www.unisdr.org/files/43291_sendaiframeworkfordrren.pdf (accessed December 25, 2017).

US Customs and Border Protection. 2017. CBP facilitates record level of travelers and modernizes trade systems in FY2016. https://www.cbp.

gov/newsroom/national-media-release/cbp-facilitates-record-level-travelers-and-modernizes-trade-systems (accessed June 14, 2017).

US Department of Homeland Security. n.d. National terrorism advisory system. https://www.dhs.gov/national-terrorism-advisory-system (accessed June 14, 2017).

US Department of Homeland Security. 2006. Securing our nations rail systems. https://www.hsdl.org/?view&did=476518 (accessed July 19, 2017).

US Department of Homeland Security. 2008. National Response Framework. Washington, DC. https://www.fema.gov/pdf/emergency/nrf/nrf-core.pdf (accessed June 20, 2017).

US Department of Homeland Security. 2010. Quadrennial homeland security review report: A strategic framework for a secure homeland. https://www.dhs.gov/sites/default/files/publications/2010-qhsr-report.pdf (accessed June 14, 2017).

US Department of Homeland Security. 2011. Risk management fundamentals: Homeland security risk management doctrine. https://www.dhs.gov/sites/default/files/publications/rma-risk-management-fundamentals.pdf (accessed June 14, 2017).

US Department of Homeland Security. 2013a. NIPP 2013: Partnering for critical infrastructure security and resilience. https://www.dhs.gov/sites/default/files/publications/national-infrastructure-protection-plan-2013-508.pdf (accessed June 14, 2017).

US Department of Homeland Security. 2013b. Threat and Hazard Identification and Risk Assessment Guide. Comprehensive Preparedness Guide (CPG) 201, 2nd ed. https://www.fema.gov/media-library/assets/documents/26335 (accessed June 14, 2017).

US Department of Homeland Security. 2014a. The 2014 quadrennial homeland security review. https://www.dhs.gov/sites/default/files/publications/2014-qhsr-final-508.pdf (accessed June 14, 2017).

US Department of Homeland Security. 2014b. Overview of the national planning frameworks. https://www.fema.gov/media-library-data/1406718145199-838ef5bed6355171a1f2d934c25f8ad0/FINAL_Overview_of_National_Planning_Frameworks_20140729.pdf (accessed June 14, 2017).

US Department of Homeland Security. 2015a. National Preparedness Goal, 2nd ed. https://www.fema.gov/media-library-data/1443799615171-2aae90be55041740f97e8532fc680d40/National_Preparedness_Goal_2nd_Edition.pdf (accessed June 14, 2017).

US Department of Homeland Security. 2015b. Presidential Policy Directive/PPD-8: National Preparedness. https://www.dhs.gov/presidential-policy-directive-8-national-preparedness (last published September 23, 2015).

US Department of Homeland Security. 2016. National preparedness report. https://www.fema.gov/media-library-data/1476817353589-987d6a58e2eb124ac6b19ef1f7c9a77d/2016NPR_508c_052716_1600_alla.pdf (last accessed June 14, 2017).

US Department of Homeland Security Risk Steering Committee. 2010. DHS Risk Lexicon. 2010 edition. https://www.dhs.gov/sites/default/files/publications/dhs-risk-lexicon-2010_0.pdf (accessed June 14, 2017).

Wisner, B., J. C. Gauillard, and I. Kelman. 2012. Handbook of Hazards and Disaster Risk Reduction. London/New York: Routledge.

Wolfers, A. 1952. "National Security" as an Ambiguous Symbol. Political Science Quarterly 67: 481–502.

World Population Review. 2017. New Orleans population 2017. http://worldpopulationreview.com/us-cities/new-orleans-population (accessed June 20, 2017).

Chapter 5 Works Cited

Berger, J. 2016. A dam, small and unsung, is caught up in an Iranian hacking case. New York Times. March 25.

City of Colorado Springs. 2012. Waldo Canyon Fire Initial After Action Report. Colorado Springs, CO: Office of Emergency Management. http://wildfiretoday.com/documents/WaldoCynFireAAR.pdf (accessed April 16, 2016).

Copeland, C. 2005. Hurricane-damaged drinking water and wastewater facilities: Impacts, needs, and response. October 19. CRS Report for Congress. http://www.environmental.lsu.edu/vepr/References/Hurricane%20Damage%20to%20Drinking%20Water.pdf (accessed June 22, 2017).

Department of Homeland Security. n.d. Sector-specific agencies (SSA). https://www.dhs.gov/sector-specific-agencies (accessed October 26, 2017).

Department of Homeland Security. 2013. National infrastructure protection plan 2013: Partnering for critical infrastructure security and resilience. Washington, DC: US Department of Homeland Security.

Department of Homeland Security. 2015. Private sector clearance program for critical infrastructure. DHS/NPPD/PIA-020(a). February 11. https://www.dhs.gov/sites/default/files/publications/privacy-pia-nppd-pscp-february2015.pdf (accessed June 23, 2017).

Eidinger, J., and C. A. Davis. 2012. Recent Earthquakes: Implications for US Water Utilities (Rep.). Denver, CO: Water Research Foundation. http://www.waterrf.org/ExecutiveSummaryLibrary/4408_ProjectSummary.pdf (accessed April 16, 2016).

Electricity Sharing and Analysis Center (E-ISAC). 2016. Analysis of the Cyber Attack on the Ukrainian Power Grid (Rep.). Washington, DC: Electricity Sharing and Analysis Center.

Feder, B. 2005. Hurricane Katrina: The power grid; utility workers come from afar to help their brethren start restoring service. New York Times. September 1. http://query.nytimes.com/gst/fullpage.html?res=9805E2DB1731F932A3575AC0A9639C8B63&mcubz=1 (accessed June 22, 2017).

Federal Bureau of Investigation. n.d. The Insider Threat: An Introduction to Detecting and Deterring an Insider Spy. Washington, DC: US Department of Justice.

Federal Bureau of Investigation. 2014. Active shooter: Quick reference guide. Report. Washington, DC: US Department of Justice.

Food and Drug Administration. 2014. Memorandum of understanding between the National Health Information Sharing & Analysis Center, Inc. (NH-ISAC) and the US Food and Drug Administration Center for devices and radiological health. 225-14-0019. https://www.fda.gov/AboutFDA/PartnershipsCollaborations/Memorandaof UnderstandingMOUs/OtherMOUs/ucm412565.htm (last updated September 3, 2014, accessed October 2017).

Fusion Centers. n.d. National network of fusion centers fact sheet. https://www.dhs.gov/national-network-fusion-centers-fact-sheet (accessed December 3, 2016).

Goodman, M. 2015. Future Crimes: Everything Is Connected, Everyone Is Vulnerable and What We Can Do about It. New York: Anchor Books.

Interagency Security Committee. 2013. Violence in the Federal Workplace: A Guide to Prevention and Response, 1st ed.. Washington, DC: US Department of Homeland Security.

Kemp, R. 2007. Homeland Security for the Private Sector. Jefferson, NC: McFarland.

Knabb, R., J. Rhome and D. Brown, D. 2005. Tropical Cyclone Report – Hurricane Katrina. Miami, FL: National Hurricane Center.

Miller, R. n.d. Hurricane Katrina: Communications & Infrastructure Impacts. Washington, DC: National Defense University.

National Conference of State Legislatures. 2016. Drones and critical infrastructure. September 22. http://www.ncsl.org/research/energy/drones-and-critical-infrastructure.aspx (accessed October 1, 2016).

National Hurricane Center. n.d. Saffir-Simpson hurricane wind scale. http://www.nhc.noaa.gov/aboutsshws.php (accessed April 16, 2016).

National Infrastructure Advisory Council. 2008. The insider threat to critical infrastructures.

National SCADA Test Bed (NSTB). 2006. Lessons learned from cyber security assessments of SCADA and energy management systems. Rep. No. INL/CON-06-116655. Washington, DC: Department of Energy.

National Weather Service. n.d. Glossary. http://w1.weather.gov/glossary/index.php?word=nor%92easter (accessed June 22, 2017).

National Weather Service. n.d. Severe weather definitions. http://www.weather.gov/bgm/severedefinitions (accessed June 22, 2017).

Noonan, T. and E. Archuleta. 2008. The Insider Threat to Critical Infrastructures. Washington, DC: The National Infrastructure Advisory Council.

North American Electric Reliability Corporation. n. d. Electricity ISAC. Electricity. http://www.nerc.com/pa/ci/esisac/Pages/default.aspx (accessed December 2, 2016).

Office of Cyber and Infrastructure Analysis. 2016. Non-Traditional Aviation Technology Risk Assessment for the National Capital Region. Washington, DC: US Department of Homeland Security.

Presidential Policy Directive 21. 2013. Critical infrastructure security and resilience. The White House. February 12. https://obamawhitehouse.archives.gov/the-press-office/2013/02/12/presidential-policy-directive-critical-infrastructure-security-and-resil (accessed June 23, 2017).

San Francisco Public Utilities Commission. 2014. Rim Fire After 2013 Action Report. San Francisco, CA: Hetch Hetchy Regional Water System.

Smith, R. 2014. Assault on California power station raises alarm on potential for terrorism. *Wall Street Journal*. February 5. http://www.wsj.com/articles/SB10001424052702304851104579359141941621778 (accessed June 19, 2016).

Southwire. 2012. A hurricane's effect on electricity. November 7. http://www.southwireblog.com/residential-construction/a-hurricanes-effect-on-electricity/ (accessed April 16, 2016).

Stephens, A. 2016. Photograph [Bureau of Land Reclamation Multimedia: Hoover Dam] Washington, DC: US Department of the Interior. https://www.usbr.gov/lc/region/g5000/photolab/gallery_detail.cfm?PICIDTYPE=77758 (accessed July 31, 2017).

The Weather Channel. 2009. Katrina's statistics tell story of its wrath. August 21. https://weather.com/newscenter/topstories/060829katrinastats.html (accessed November 7, 2017).

Townsend, F. 2006. The Federal Response to Hurricane Katrina – Lessons Learned. Washington, DC: The White House.

US Department of Homeland Security. 2013. National infrastructure protection plan.

US Department of Justice. 2013. A Study of Active Shooter Incidents in the United States Between 2000 and 2013. Report. Washington, DC: Federal Bureau of Investigation.

USA PATRIOT ACT. 42 USC 5195c (1016(e)).

Virginia Department of Emergency Management. 2014. Continuity plan template for executive agencies and institutions of higher education. http://www.vaemergency.gov/emergency-management-community/emergency-management-plans/continuity-planning/ (accessed June 23, 2017).

Water Information Sharing and Analysis Center. n.d. https://www.waterisac.org/ (accessed December 2, 2016).

Water Information Sharing and Analysis Center. 2016. https://www.waterisac.org/about-us (accessed November 16, 2016).

Chapter 6 Works Cited

9/11 Commission. 2004. 9/11 Commission report. Washington, DC. https://9-11commission.gov/report/ (accessed March 14, 2017).

Abrahms, M. 2008. What Terrorists Really Want: Terrorism Motives and Counterterrorism Strategy. International Security, 32 (4), 78–105.

African Union Peace and Security. 2015. The African Union counter terrorism framework. 23 November. http://www.peaceau.org/en/page/64-counter-terrorism-ct (accessed January 20, 2017).

Ahram, A. I. 2016. Pro-government Militias and the Repertoires of Illicit State Violence. Studies in Conflict & Terrorism, 39 (3), 207–226.

Anderson, B. 1991. Imagined Communities. London: Verso.

Andrew, C. and V. Mitrokhin. 1999. The Sword and the Shield: The Mitrokhin Archive and the Secret History of the KGB. New York: Basic Books.

Arendt, H. 1948. The Origins of Totalitarianism. San Diego, CA: Harvest Book.

Ayres, R. W. 2000. A World Flying Apart? Violent Nationalist Conflict and the End of the Cold War. Journal of Peace Research, 37, 105–117.

Azani, E. 2013. The Hybrid Terrorist Organization: Hezbollah as a Case Study. Studies in Conflict & Terrorism, 36 (11), 899–916.

BBC. 2013. Hezbollah condemned for "attack on Syrian villages." February 18. http://www.bbc.com/news/world-middle-east-21496735 (accessed January 20, 2017).

Biersteker, T. J. and S. E. Eckert, eds. 2008. Countering the Financing of Terrorism. New York: Routledge.

Bolger, D. P. 2015. Why We Lost. New York: Mariner Books.

Branch, J. 2014. The Cartographic State: Maps, Territory, and the Origins of Sovereignty. Cambridge: Cambridge University Press.

British Broadcasting Service. 2011. Carlos the Jackal convicted for 1980s French attacks. http://www.bbc.com/news/world-europe-16210927 (accessed March 16, 2017).

British Pathé, 1942. On the chin! https://www.youtube.com/watch?v=to4djmDqJRI (accessed January 1, 2017.

Buzan, B. 2002. Who may we bomb? In Worlds in Collision: Terror and the Future of Global Order, eds. K. Booth and T. Dunne. London: Palgrave.

Byman, D. 2005. Deadly Connections: States that Sponsor Terrorism. Cambridge: Cambridge University Press.

Chase, E. 2013. Defining Terrorism: A Strategic Imperative. Small Wars Journal, 9 (1). http://smallwarsjournal.com/jrnl/art/defining-terrorism-a-strategic-imperative (accessed January 1, 2017).

Chenoweth, E. 2010. Democratic pieces: Democratization and the origins of terrorism. In Coping with Terrorism: Origins, Escalation, Counterstrategies, and Responses, eds. R. Reuveny and W. R. Thompson. Albany, NY: SUNY Press.

Cole, J. S. 2015. Assad: Syria has "no relation" with Hamas, will never trust it again. Informed Comment. April 20, 2015. http://www.juancole.com/2015/04/assad-relation-hamas.html (accessed January 20, 2017).

Coll, S. 2004. Ghost Wars. New York: Penguin.

Congress of the United States. 2002. Public law 107-296. https://www.dhs.gov/xlibrary/assets/hr_5005_enr.pdf (accessed January 1, 2017).

Congress of the United States. 2016. Report of the US Senate Select Committee on intelligence with additional views. http://apps. washingtonpost.com/g/documents/politics/read-the-long-classified-28-pages-on-alleged-saudi-ties-to-911/2079/ (accessed January 1, 2017).

Coolsaet, R. 2010. EU Counterterrorism Strategy: Value Added or Chimera? International Affairs, 86 (4), 857–873.

Crawford, N. 2016. US Budgetary Costs of Wars through 2016: $4.79 Trillion and Counting. Brown University: Watson Institute for International Studies.

Cronin, A. K. 2002. Behind the Curve: Globalization and International Terrorism. International Security, 27 (3), 30–58.

Cronin, A. K. 2009. How Terrorism Ends: Understanding the Decline and Demise of Terrorist Campaigns. Princeton, NJ: Princeton University Press.

Department of Defense. 2014. Joint Publication 3-26, Counterterrorism. Washington, DC. www.dtic.mil/doctrine/new_pubs/jp3_26.pdf (accessed January 1, 2017).

Department of Homeland Security. 2012. Strategic Plan, FY 2012–2016. Washington, DC. https://www.dhs.gov/xlibrary/assets/dhs-strategic-plan-fy-2012-2016.pdf (accessed on May 22, 2017).

Department of State. 2015. Country Reports on Terrorism. Washington, DC. https://www.state.gov/j/ct/rls/crt/2015/index.htm (accessed January 1, 2017).

Department of State. 2017. Report on Human Rights Abuses or Censorship in North Korea, Washington, DC. January 11. https://www.state.gov/j/drl/rls/266853.htm (accessed January 17, 2017).

Donnelly, S. B. and D. Waller. 2005. Ten questions with Peter Schoomaker. Time April 22. http://www.time.com/time/nation/article/0,8599,1053555,00.html (accessed January 1, 2017).

Evans, R. J. 2003. The Coming of the Third Reich. New York: Penguin.

Fair, C. C. 2011. Lashkar-e-Tayiba and the Pakistani State, Survival, 53 (4), 29–52.

Finnemore, M. 1996. National Interests in International Society. Ithaca, NY: Cornell University Press.

Freeman, M. 2011. The Sources of Terrorist Financing: Theory and Typology. Studies in Conflict & Terrorism, 34 (6), 461–475.

Gellner, E. 1983. Nations and Nationalism. Ithaca, NY: Cornell University Press.

Gilbert, M. 1994. The First World War: A Complete History. New York: Henry Holt and Company.

Global Initiative to Combat Nuclear Terrorism. 2017. http://www.gicnt. org/ (accessed January 20, 2017).

Goodarzi, J. M. 2006. Syria and Iran: Diplomatic Alliance and Power Politics in the Middle East. London: Taurus.

Grigas, A. 2015. The New Russian Empire. New Haven, CT: Yale University Press.

Hall, R.B. 1999. National Collective Identity. New York: Columbia University Press.

Hegghammer, T. 2010. Jihad in Saudi Arabia: Violence and Pan-Islamism since 1979. Cambridge: Cambridge University Press.

Heller, J. 1995. The Stern Gang: Ideology, Politics, and Terror, 1940–49. London: Routledge.

Hoffman, B. 2006. Inside Terrorism. New York: Columbia University Press.

Homeland Security Committee, US House of Representatives. 2016. A National Strategy to Win the War Against Islamist Terror. Washington, DC. https://homeland.house.gov/national-strategy-win-war-islamist-terror/ (accessed on May 22, 2017).

Horchem, H. J. 1991. The Decline of the Red Army Faction. Terrorism and Political Violence, 3 (2), 61–75.

Human Security Report Project. 2013. Human Security Report 2013: The Decline in Global Violence: Evidence, Explanation, and Contestation. Vancouver: Human Security Press.

Ikenberry, G. J. 2000. After Victory. Princeton, NJ: Princeton University Press.

Jamieson, A. 1990. Entry, Discipline and Exit in the Italian Red Brigades. Terrorism and Political Violence, 2 (1), 1–21.

Juergensmeyer, M. 2000. Terror in the Mind of God. Berkeley, CA: University of California Press.

Keegan, J. 1983. The Face of Battle. New York: Penguin.

Kepel, G. and A. Roberts, trans. 2003. Jihad: The Trail of Political Islam. Boston, MA: Belknap Press.

Korten, T. and K. Nielsen. 2008. The coddled "terrorists" of South Florida. Salon, http://www.salon.com/2008/01/14/cuba_2/ 14 January (accessed January 4, 2017).

Laquer, W. 2000. The New Terrorism: Fanaticism and Arms of Mass Destruction. New York: Oxford University Press.

Lebow, R. N. 2010. Why Nations fight: Past and Future Motivations for War. Cambridge: Cambridge University Press.

Leverett, F. 2005. Inheriting Syria: Bashar's Trial by Fire. Washington, DC: Brookings.

Levi, M. 1988. Of Rule and Revenue. Berkeley, CA: University of California Press.

Mann, M. 2005. The Dark Side of Democracy: Explaining Ethnic Cleansing. Cambridge: Cambridge University Press.

Mattern, S. P. 1999. Rome and the Enemy: Imperial Strategy in the Principate. Berkeley, CA: University of California Press.

Mazetti, M. and T. Shanker. 2006. Arming of Hezbollah reveals US and Israeli blind spots. The New York Times, July 19. http://www.nytimes.com/2006/07/19/world/middleeast/19missile.html (accessed January 17, 2017).

McNeill, W. H. 1982. The Pursuit of Power. Chicago, IL: University of Chicago Press.

Moseley, R. 1991. Syria's support of US in Gulf War paying dividends. Chicago Tribune, March 12, http://articles.chicagotribune.com/1991-03-12/news/9101220963_1_syria-president-hafez-assad-peacekeeping-force (accessed January 17, 2017).

Mueller, J. 2007. The Remnants of War. Ithaca, NY: Cornell University Press.

Mueller, J. and M. G. Stewart. 2010. Hardly existential: Thinking rationally about terrorism. *Foreign Affairs*. April 2. https://www.foreignaffairs.com/articles/north-america/2010-04-02/hardly-existential (accessed January 17, 2017).

Mueller, J. and M. G. Stewart. 2016. How safe are we?: Asking the right questions about terrorism. *Foreign Affairs*. August 15. https://www.foreignaffairs.com/articles/united-states/2016-08-15/how-safe-are-we (accessed January 17, 2017).

Naji, O. B. 2005. W. McCants, trans. The management of savagery: The most critical stage through which the Umma will pass. Boston, MA: John M. Olin Institute for Strategic Studies.

National Institute of Justice. 2011. Terrorism. https://www.nij.gov/topics/crime/terrorism/Pages/welcome.aspx (accessed on January 1, 2017).

National Security Strategy of the United States. 2002. Washington, DC. https://www.state.gov/documents/organization/63562.pdf (accessed January 1, 2017).

National Security Strategy of the United States. 2015. Washington, DC. http://nssarchive.us/wp-content/uploads/2015/02/2015.pdf (accessed November 7, 2017).

National Strategy for Combating Terrorism. 2003. Washington, DC. https://www.cia.gov/news-information/cia-the-war-on-terrorism/Counter_Terrorism_Strategy.pdf (accessed November 7, 2017)

National Strategy for Counterterrorism. 2011. Washington, DC. http://obamawhitehouse.archives.gov/sites/default/files/counterterrorism_strategy.pdf (accessed April 13, 2017).

National Strategy for Homeland Security. 2002. Washington, DC. https://www.dhs.gov/sites/default/files/publications/nat-strat-hls-2002.pdf (accessed on May 22, 2017).

National Strategy for Homeland Security. 2007. Washington, DC. https://www.dhs.gov/national-strategy-homeland-security-october-2007 (accessed on May 22, 2017).

North, D. C. 1981. Structure and Change in Economic History. New York: W.W. Norton.

North Atlantic Treaty Organization. 2016a. Collective defense—Article 5. http://www.nato.int/cps/en/natohq/topics_110496.htm# (accessed January 20, 2017).

North Atlantic Treaty Organization. 2016b. Countering terrorism. September 5. http://www.nato.int/cps/en/natohq/topics_77646.htm (accessed January 20, 2017).

Olson, M. 1993. Dictatorship, Democracy, and Development. American Political Science Review, 87 (3), 567–76.

Pedahzur, A. and A. Perliger. 2009. Jewish Terrorism in Israel. Cambridge: Cambridge University Press.

Picarelli, J. T. 2012. "Osama bin Corleone? Vito the Jackal?" Framing Threat Convergence through an Examination of Transnational

Organized Crime and International Terrorism. Terrorism and Political Violence, 24 (2), 180–198.

Pinker, S. 2011. The Better Angels of our Nature: Why Violence has Declined. New York: Viking.

Pollard, N. A. 2009. On counterterrorism and intelligence. In National Intelligence Systems, eds. G. Treverton and W. Agrell. Cambridge: Cambridge University Press.

Pushpanathan, S. 2003. ASEAN efforts to combat terrorism. http://asean.org/?static_post=asean-efforts-to-combat-terrorism-by-spushpanathan (accessed on January 20, 2017).

Rapoport, D. C. 2004. The four waves of modern terrorism. In Attacking Terrorism: Elements of a Grand Strategy, eds. A. K. Cronin and J. M. Ludes. Washington, DC: Georgetown University Press, 46–73

Rault, C. 2010. The French approach to counterterrorism. CTC Sentinel 3 (1), 22–25.

Rohter, L. 1998. 4 Salvadorans say they killed US nuns on orders from the military. The New York Times. April 3.

Roskin, M. G. 1994. The National Interest: From Abstraction to Strategy. Carlisle, PA: Strategic Studies Institute, US Army War College.

Rudner, S. 2010. Hizbullah: An Organizational and Operational Profile. International Journal of Intelligence and Counterintelligence. 23 (2), 226–246.

Schevchenko, V. 2014. "Little green men" or "Russian invaders"? BBC. March 11. http://www.bbc.com/news/world-europe-26532154 (accessed January 17, 2017).

Schroefl, J. and S. Kaufman. 2014. Hybrid Actors, Tactical Variety: Rethinking Asymmetric and Hybrid War. Studies in Conflict & Terrorism, 37 (10), 862–880.

Scott, C. R. 2013. Anonymous Agencies, Backstreet Businesses, and Covert Collectives: Rethinking Organizations in the 21st Century. Stanford, CA: Stanford University Press.

Senate Government Affairs Permanent Subcommittee on Investigations. 1995. Global proliferation of Weapons of Mass Destruction: A case study on the Aum Shinrikyo. October 31. Federation of American Scientists, https://fas.org/irp/congress/1995_rpt/aum/part04.htm (accessed January 17, 2017).

Tilly, C. 1990. Coercion, Capital, and European States, AD 1990–1992. Cambridge: Blackwell.

United Nations. 2001. Security Council adopts wide-ranging counter-terrorism resolution. September 28. http://www.un.org/press/en/2001/sc7158.doc.htm (accessed January 20, 2017).

United Nations Counterterrorism Implementation Task Force. 2017. https://www.un.org/counterterrorism/ctitf/en/about-task-force (accessed January 20, 2017).

United Nations Security Council. 2005. Report of the independent investigation commission established pursuant to Security Council Resolution 1595. http://www.un.org/news/dh/docs/mehlisreport/ (accessed January 18, 2017).

United Nations Security Council 1540 Committee. 2017. http://www. un.org/en/sc/1540/ (accessed January 20, 2017).

Vielhaber, D. 2013. The Stasi-Meinhof Complex? Studies in Conflict & Terrorism, 36 (7), 533–546.

Walton, C. 2014. Empire of Secrets: British Intelligence, the Cold War, and the Twilight of Empire. New York: The Overlook Press.

Warner, M. 2014. The Rise and Fall of Intelligence. Washington, DC: Georgetown University Press.

Weber, M. 1946. Politics as a vocation. In From Max Weber: Essays in Sociology, eds. and trans. H. H. Gerth and C. W. Mills. Oxford: Oxford University Press.

Weinberg, L., A. Padahzur, and S. Hirsch-Hoefler. 2008. The Challenges of Conceptualizing Terrorism. Terrorism and Political Violence. 16 (4), 777–794.

Whitaker, B. 2002. Mystery of Abu Nidal's death deepens. *The Guardian*, August 22, https://www.theguardian.com/world/2002/aug/22/iraq. israel (accessed January 1, 2017).

Wright, L. 2006. The Looming Tower: Al Qaeda and the Road to 9/11. New York: Knopf.

Zanchetta, B. 2016. Between Cold War Imperatives and State-sponsored Terrorism: The United States and "Operation Condor." Studies in Conflict & Terrorism, 39 (12), 1084–1102.

Zenko, M. 2013. Most. Dangerous. World. Ever: The ridiculous hyperbole about government budget cuts. *Foreign Policy*. February 26. http://foreignpolicy.com/2013/02/26/most-dangerous-world-ever/ (accessed January 17, 2017).

Chapter 7 Works Cited

Al-Hout, B. N. 2004. Sabra and Shatila: September 1982. London: Pluto Press.

Amos, D. 2010. Eclipse of the Sunnis: Power, Exile, and Upheaval in the Middle East. New York: Public Affairs.

Anderson, S. K. 2009. Historical Dictionary of Terrorism. Lanham, MD: The Scarecrow Press.

Atkins, S. E. 2011. Encyclopedia of Right-wing Extremism in Modern American History. Santa Barbara: ABC-CLIO.

Ayadinli, E. 2016. Violent Non-state Actors: From Anarchists to Jihadists. Abingdon: Routledge.

Baer, R. B. 2015. The Perfect Kill: 21 Laws for Assassins. New York: Random House.

Bailey, B. and R. H. Immerman. 2015. Understanding the US Wars in Iraq and Afghanistan. New York: New York University Press.

Bakshi, S. R. 1983. Gandhi and the Non-cooperation Movement, 1920–22. Detroit: Capital Publishers.

Balz, H. 2015. Militant organizations in Western Europe in the 1970s and 1980s. In The Routledge History of Terrorism, ed. R. D. Law. Abingdon: Routledge.

Bauer, Y. 2014. The Jews: A Contrary People. Zurich: Lit Verlag.

Baumann, C. E. 1973. The Diplomatic Kidnappings: A Revolutionary Technique of Urban Terrorism. The Hague: Martinus Nijhoff.

Beinin, J. 1998. The Dispersion of Egyptian Jewry: Culture, Politics, and the Formation of a Modern Diaspora. Berkeley, CA: The University of California Press.

Berger, D. 2006. Outlaws of America: The Weather Underground and the Politics of Solidarity. Edinburgh: AK Press.

Berger, J. M. 2016. Nazis vs. ISIS on Twitter: A Comparative Study of White Nationalist and IS Online Social Media Networks. George Washington Program on Extremism, September. Washington, DC: George Washington University.

Besier, G., and M. Stokłosa, 2014. European Dictatorships: A Comparative History of the Twentieth Century. Newcastle upon Tyne: Cambridge Scholars Publishing.

Bradbury, M. 2008. Becoming Somaliland. Martlesham: James Currey.

Branch, A. 2010. Exploring the roots of LRA violence: Political crisis and ethnic politics in Acholiland. In The Lord's Resistance Army: Myth and Reality, eds. T. Allen and K. Vlassenroot. New York: Zed Books.

Breckenridge, J. N., and P. G. Zimbardo. 2007. The strategy of terrorism and the psychology of mass-mediated fear. In Psychology of Terrorism, eds. B. Bongar, L. M. Brown, L. E. Beutler, J. N. Breckenridge, and P. G. Zimbardo. Oxford: Oxford University Press.

British Broadcasting Corporation. 2016a. Editorial Guidelines. London: British Broadcasting Corporation.

British Broadcasting Corporation. 2016b. Russian ambassador to Turkey Andrei Karlov shot dead in Ankara. BBC. http://www.bbc.com/news/world-europe-38369962 (accessed December 19, 2016).

Brodzinsky, S. 2016. Splits form among Colombia's FARC rebels after commanders expelled. The Guardian, December 14. https://www.theguardian.com/world/2016/dec/14/colombia-farc-commanders-expelled (accessed December 14, 2016).

Buhari-Gulmez, D. 2015. The clash between Putin and Erdoğan represents a turning point in Russian-Turkish relations. LSE US Centre. http://blogs.lse.ac.uk/usappblog/2015/12/12/the-clash-between-putin-and-erdogan-represents-a-turning-point-in-russian-turkish-relations/ (accessed December 14, 2016).

Carter, J. 2010. White House Diary. New York: Farrar, Straus and Giroux.

Celso, A. 2014. Al Qaeda's post-9/11 Devolution: The Failed Jihadist Struggle against the Near and Far Enemy. New York: Bloomsbury.

Chaliand, G., and A. Blin, 2007. The invention of modern terror. In The History of Terrorism: From Antiquity to Al Qaeda, eds. G. Chaliand and A. Blin. Berkeley, CA: The University of California Press.

Chalmers, D. M. 1987. Hooded Americanism: The History of the Ku Klux Klan. Durham, NC: Duke University Press.

Chandrasekaran, R. 2012. Little America: The War Within the War for Afghanistan. London: Bloomsbury.

Cioffi-Revilla, C. 2012. A complexity method for assessing counterterrorism policies. In Evidence-based Counterterrorism Policy, eds. C. Lum and L. W. Kennedy. New York: Springer.

Climent, J. 2015. World Terrorism: An Encyclopedia of Political Violence from Ancient Times to the Post-9/11 Era. Abingdon: Routledge.

Cockburn, P. 2014. Rise of Islamic State: ISIS and the New Sunni Revolution. London: Verso.

Coker, M. 2015. How Islamic State's Win in Ramadi Reveals New Weapons, Tactical Sophistication and Prowess. The Wall Street Journal, May 25.

Crenshaw, M., and J. Pimlott. 2015. International Encyclopedia of Terrorism. Abingdon: Routledge.

Cronin, A. K. 2010. How al-Qaida ends: The decline and demise of terrorist groups. In Contending with Terrorism: Roots, Strategies, and Responses, eds. M. E. Brown, O. R. Cote Jr., S. M. Lynn-Jones, and S. E. Miller. Cambridge: The MIT Press.

Cruz-del Rosario, T., and J. M. Dorsey. 2016. Comparative Political Transitions between Southeast Asia and the Middle East and North Africa: Lost in Transition. New York: Palgrave Macmillan.

Debata, M. R. 2007. China's Minorities: Ethnic-religious Separatism in Xinjiang. New Delhi: Pentagon Press.

Deeb, D. J. 2013. Israel, Palestine, and the Quest for Middle East Peace. Lanham, MD: University Press of America.

Dingley, J. 2012. The IRA: The Irish Republican Army. Santa Barbara: Praeger.

Dolnik, A. 2007. Understanding Terrorist Innovation: Technology, Tactics and Global Trends. Abingdon: Routledge.

Dolnik, A., and H. Butime. 2016. Understanding the Lord's Resistance Army Insurgency. Singapore: World Scientific Publishing Europe Limited.

Dolnik, A., and K. M. Fitzgerald. 2008. Negotiating Hostage Crises with the New Terrorists. Westport, CT: Praeger.

Dzikansky, M., G. Kleiman, and G. Slater. 2012. Terrorist Suicide Bombings: Attack, Interdiction, Mitigation and Response. Boca Raton, FL: CRC Press.

Elias, B. 2009. Airport and Aviation security: US Policy and Strategy in the Age of Global Terrorism. Santa Barbara, CA: CRC Press.

Engeland, A. V. 2008. Hezbollah From a terrorist group to a political party: Social work as a key to politics. In From Terrorism to Politics, eds. A. V. Engeland and R. M. Rudolph. Aldershot: Ashgate.

Engene, J. O. 2004. Terrorism in Western Europe: Explaining the Trends since 1950. Cheltenham: Edward Elgar.

Feste, K. A. 2015. Terminate Terrorism: Framing, Gaming and Negotiating Conflicts. Abingdon: Routledge.

Fielitz, M., and L. L. Laloire. 2016. Introductory remarks. In Trouble on the Far Right: Contemporary Right-wing Strategies and Practices in Europe, eds. M. Fielitz and L. L. Laloire. Bielefeld: Transcript Verlag.

Fitsanakis, J. 2016. Taliban-Haqqani alliance marks new phase in Afghan war. intelNews, May 10. https://intelnews.org/2016/05/10/01-1898/ (accessed December 1, 2016).

Forest, J. J. F. 2012. The Terrorism Lectures. Santa Ana, CA: Nortia Press.

Gardell, M. 2003. Gods of the Blood: The Pagan Revival and White Separatism. Durham, NC: Duke University Press.

Garland, J., and M. Rowe. 2001. Racism and Anti-racism in Football. Basingstoke, DE: Palgrave.

Garternstein-Ross, D. and D. Trombly.2012. The Tactical and Strategic Use of Small Firearms by Terrorists. Washington, DC: FDD Press.

Gilligan, E. 2010. Terror in Chechnya: Russia and the Tragedy of Civilians in War. Princeton, NJ: Princeton University Press.

Golani, M. 2013. Palestine between Politics and Terror, 1945–1947. Waltham, MA: Brandeis University Press.

Goodrick-Clarke, N. 2003. Black Sun: Aryan Cults, Esoteric Nazism and the Politics of Identity. New York: New York University Press.

Guanaratna, R. 2010. Al-Qaeda is an example of a new terrorism. In Debating Terrorism and Counterterrorism, ed. S. Gottlieb. Washington, DC: CQ Press.

Guardian. 2000. Red Army members expelled by Lebanon. *The Guardian*, March 17. https://www.theguardian.com/world/2000/mar/18/terrorism (accessed October 10, 2016).

Gunaratna, R., and J. Ramirez. 2011. Colombia: Guerrilla warfare and narco-terrorism, 1960s–present. In World Terrorism: An Encyclopedia of Political Violence from Ancient Times to the Post-9/11 Era, ed. J. Climent. London: Routledge.

Gunneflo, M. 2016. Targeted Killing: A Legal and Political History. Cambridge: Cambridge University Press.

Hall, S. G. F. 2016. Reconsidering western concepts of the Ukrainian conflict: The rise to prominence of Russia's 'soft force' policy. In Vocabularies of International Relations after the Crisis in Ukraine, eds. A. Makarychev and A. Yatsyk. Abingdon: Routledge.

Hamm, M.S. 2002. In Bad Company: America's Terrorist Underground. Boston, MA: Northeastern University Press.

Haqqani, H. 2005. Pakistan: Between Mosque and Military. Washington, DC: Carnegie Endowment for International Peace.

Hashim, A. S. 2009. Iraq's Sunni Insurgency. New York: Routledge.

Hashim, A. S. 2013. When Counterinsurgency Wins: Sri Lanka's Defeat of the Tamil Tigers. Philadelphia, PA: University of Pennsylvania Press.

Haynes, J., P. Hough, S. Malik and L. Pettiford. 2017. World Politics: International Relations and Globalisation in the 21st Century. London: Sage.

Heistein, A. 2016. IS's fight with Al Qaeda is making both stronger. *The National Interest*, January 7.

Heller, J. 2012. The Stern Gang: Ideology, Politics and Terror, 1940–1949. Abingdon: Routledge.

Herbst, P. 2003. Talking Terrorism: A Dictionary of the Loaded Language of Political Violence. Westport, CT: Greenwood Press.

Hewitt, C. 2005. Political Violence and Terrorism in Modern America: A Chronology. Westport, CT: Praeger.

Hingley, R. 1967. Nihilists: Russian Radicals and Revolutionaries in the Reign of Alexander II, 1855–81. New York: Delacorte Press.

Hirai-Baun, N. 2004. Country report on Japan. In Terrorism as a Challenge for National and International Law: Security versus Liberty? eds. C. Walter, S. Vöneky, V. Röben and F. Schorkopf. Berlin: Springer.

Homer, F. D. 1988. Terror in the United States: Three perspectives. In The Politics of Terrorism, ed. M. Stohl. New York: Marcel Dekker, Inc..

Hroub, K. 2006. Hamas: A Beginner's guide. London: Pluto Press.

Jackson, P. 2014. 2083 – A European declaration of independence: A license to kill. In Doublespeak: The Rhetoric of the Far Right since 1945, eds. M. Feldman and P. Jackson. Stuttgart: ibidem-Verlag.

Jackson, R., J. Gunning and M. B. Smyth. 2011. Terrorism: A Critical Introduction. Basingstoke: Palgrave Macmillan.

Jensen, R. B. 2016. An overview of early anarchism and lone actor terrorism. In Understanding Lone Actor Terrorism: Past Experience, Future Outlook, and Response Strategies, ed. M. Fredholm. New York: Routledge.

Johnson, T. 2009. Humanist terrorism in the political thought of Robespierre and Sartre. In Engaging Terror: A Critical and Interdisciplinary Approach, eds. M. Vardalos, G. K. Letts, H. M. Teixeira, A. Karzai and J. Haig. Boca Raton, FL: Brown Walker Press.

Johnson, R. 2013. Antiterrorism and Threat Response: Planning and Implementation. Boca Raton, FL: CRC Press.

Jones, S. G., and M. C. Libicki. 2008. How Terrorist Groups End: Lessons for Countering al Qa'ida, Santa Monica, CA: RAND Corporation, National Security Research Division.

Kassimeris, G. 2013. Inside Greek Terrorism. London: C. Hurst & Co.

Kilcullen, D. 2009. The Accidental Guerrilla: Fighting Small Wars in the Midst of a Big One. New York: Oxford University Press.

Kilcullen, D. 2013. Understanding Terrorism: Challenges, Perspectives, and Issues. Thousand Oaks, CA: Sage.

Kilcullen, D. 2016. Blood Year: The Unraveling of Western Counterterrorism. Oxford: Oxford University Press.

Koch, B. 2016. Terror, violence, coercion: States and the use of (il)legitimate Force. In State Terror, State Violence: Global Perspectives, ed. B. Koch. Wiesbaden: Springer.

Kornbluh, P. and M. Byrne. 1993. The Iran-Contra Scandal: The Declassified History. New York: The New Press.

Kushner, H. 2002. Encyclopedia of Terrorism. Thousand Oaks, CA: Sage.

Kushner, H. 2011. Basque separatists. In The SAGE Encyclopedia of Terrorism, ed. G. Martin, Los Angeles, CA: Sage, 94.

Law, R. 2016. Terrorism: A History. Cambridge: Polity Press.

Lowen, M. 2016. Is Turkey still a democracy? BBC, November 5. http://www.bbc.com/news/world-europe-37883006 (accessed November 5, 2016).

Lutz, M. J. and B. J. Lutz. 2005. Terrorism: Origins and Evolution. New York: Palgrave Macmillan.

Mahan, S. and P.L. Griset. 2008. Terrorism in Perspective. Los Angeles, CA: Sage.

Mammone, A. 2015. Transnational Neofascism in France and Italy. Cambridge: Cambridge University Press.

Marshall, R. D. 2012. Introduction. In The Psychology of Terrorism Fears, eds. S. J. Sinclair and D. Antonius. Oxford: Oxford University Press.

Martin, G. 2011. Terrorism and Homeland Security. London: Sage.

Mattingly, D. and H. Schuster, 2005. Rudolph reveals motives. *CNN*, April 19. http://www.cnn.com/2005/LAW/04/13/eric.rudolph/ (accessed on November 12, 2016).

McCann, J. T. 2006. Terrorism on American soil: A Concise History of Plots and Perpetrators from the Famous to the Forgotten. Boulder, CO: Sentient Publications.

McKittrick, D., and D. McVea. 2002. Making Sense of the Troubles: The Story of the Conflict in Northern Ireland. Chicago, IL: Ivan R. Dee, Publisher.

Meghelli, S. 2009. From Harlem to Algiers: Transnational solidarities between the African American freedom movement and Algeria, 1962–1978. In Black Routes to Islam, ed. M. Marable. New York: Palgrave Macmillan.

Meho, L. I. 2004. The Kurdish Question in US Foreign Policy: A Documentary Sourcebook. Westport, CT: Praeger.

Mendelsohn, B. 2016. The Al-Qaeda Franchise: The Expansion of Al-Qaeda and its Consequences. New York: Oxford University Press.

Michael, G. 2009. Theology of Hate: A History of the World Church of the Creator. Miami, FL: University Press of Florida.

Mukhimer, T. 2013. Hamas Rule in Gaza: Human Rights Under Constraint. New York: Palgrave Macmillan.

Mumford, A. 2012. The Counter-insurgency Myth: The British Experience of Irregular Warfare. Abingdon: Routledge.

Myers, L. and R. Windrem. 2007. CIA warned of risks of war in the Mideast. *NBC*, May 25. http://www.nbcnews.com/id/18854414/ns/nbc_nightly_news_with_brian_williams-nbc_news_investigates/t/nbc-cia-warned-risks-war-mideast (accessed December 12, 2016).

Nance, M. W. 2015. The Terrorists of Iraq: Inside the Strategy and Tactics of the Iraqi Insurgency, 2003–2014. Boca Raton, FL: CRC Press.

Nance, M. W. 2016. Defeating IS: Who They are, How they Fight, What they Believe. New York: Skyhorse Publishing.

Newton, M. 2002. The Encyclopedia of Kidnappings. New York: Facts on File, Inc.

Norman, T. L. 2016. Risk Analysis and Security Countermeasure Selection. Boca Raton, FL: CRC Press.

O'Leary, B., and J. Tirman. 2007. Thinking about durable political violence. In Terror, Insurgency and the State: Ending Protracted

Conflicts, eds. B. O'Leary and J. Tirman. Philadelphia, PA: University of Pennsylvania Press.

Parsons, E. F. 2015. Ku Klux: The Birth of the Klan during Reconstruction. Chapel Hill, NC: The University of North Carolina Press.

Perdue, W. D. 1989. Terrorism and the State: A Critique of Domination through Fear. Westport, CT: Praeger.

Perliger, A. 2006. Middle Eastern Terrorism. New York: Chelsea House Publishers.

Plaw, A. 2008. Targeting Terrorists: A License to Kill? Aldershot: Ashgate.

Powell, J. 2014. Terrorists at the Table: Why Negotiating is the Only Way to Peace. New York: The Bodley Head.

Powell, B. 2016. As IS's caliphate crumbles, jihadist tactics are evolving. *Newsweek*, October 11.

Prakash, V. 2008. Terrorism in India's North-east: A Gathering Storm, volume 1. Delhi: Kalpaz Publications.

Pringle, R. W. 2015. Historical Dictionary of Russian and Soviet Intelligence. Lanham, MD: Rowman & Littlefield.

Purpura, P. P. 2016. Security: An Introduction. Boca Raton, FL: CRC Press.

Rabasa, A., R. D. Blackwill, P. Chalk, K. Cragin, C. C. Fair, B. A. Jackson, B. M. Jenkins, S. G. Jones, N. Shestak, A. J. Telliset. 2009. The Lessons of Mumbai. Santa Monica, CA: RAND Corporation.

Raghavan, S. 2013. The Central African Republic descending into complete chaos. *The Washington Post*, November 26.

Rahe, P. A. 2016. The Spartan Regime: Its Character, Origins and Grand Strategy. New Haven, CT: Yale University Press.

Ranstorp, M. and M. Normark. 2015. Understanding Terrorism Innovation and Learning: Al-Qaeda and Beyond. Abingdon: Routledge.

Rapoport, D. C. 2001. Introduction. In Inside Terrorist Organizations, ed. D. C. Rapoport. Portland, OR: Frank Cass Publishers.

Rapoport, D. C. 2017. Reflections on the third or new left wave: 17 years later. In Revolutionary Violence and the New Left: Transnational Perspectives, eds. A. M. Alvarez and E. Ray. New York: Routledge.

Richardson, L. 2006. What Terrorists Want: Understanding the Enemy, Containing the Threat. New York: Random House.

Roy, S. 2011. Hamas and Civil Society in Gaza: Engaging the Islamist Social Sector. Princeton, NJ: Princeton University Press.

Saito, N. T. 2012. Meeting the Enemy: American Exceptionalism and International Law. New York: New York University Press.

Schaefer, R. W. 2010. The insurgency in Chechnya and the North Caucasus: From gazavat to jihad. Santa Barbara: Praeger.

Schiff, Z., and E. Ya'ari, 1984. Israel's Lebanon War, ed. I. Friedman. New York: Simon and Schuster.

Seth, A. 2003. Burma's Muslims: Terrorists or Terrorized? Canberra: Strategic and Defence Studies Centre, Australian National University.

Shah, A. 2015. The intimacy of insurgency: Beyond coercion, greed or grievance in Maoist India. In The Underbelly of the Indian Boom, eds. S. Corbridge and A. Shah. Abingdon: Routledge.

Silverman, M. E. 2011. Awakening Victory: How Iraqi Tribes and American Troops Reclaimed Al Anbar Province and Defeated Al Qaeda in Iraq. Philadelphia, PA: Casemate.

SITE. 2014. Islamic State leader Abu Bakr al-Baghdadi encourages emigration, worldwide action. *SITE Intelligence Group*, 1 July. https://news.siteintelgroup.com/Jihadist-News/islamic-state-leader-abu-bakr-al-baghdadi-encourages-emigration-worldwide-action.html (accessed December 12, 2016).

Skaine, R. 2013. Suicide Warfare: Culture, the Military, and the Individual as a Weapon. Santa Barbara: Praeger.

Sloan, S. 1992. Beating International Terrorism: An Action Strategy for Preemption and Punishment. Collingdale: Diane Publishing Co.

Smith, P. J. 2002. Transnational Terrorism and the Al Qaeda Model: Confronting New Realities. Parameters (Summer), 33–46.

Smith, A. 2005. Conquest: Sexual Violence and American Indian Genocide. Cambridge: South End Press.

Smith, R. 2007. The Utility of force: The Art of War in the Modern World. New York: Knopf Doubleday Publishing Group.

Smith, P. J.. 2015. The Terrorism Ahead: Confronting Transnational Violence in the Twenty-first Century. Abingdon: Routledge.

Sofer, S. 1998. Zionism and the Foundations of Israeli Diplomacy. Cambridge: Cambridge University Press.

Southers, E. 2014. Homegrown Violent Extremism. Abingdon: Routledge.

Stechel, I. 1972. Terrorist Kidnapping of Diplomatic Personnel. Cornell International Law Journal, 5 (2) (Spring), 189–217.

Steed, B. 2016. IS: An Introduction and Guide to the Islamic State, Boca Raton, FL: ABC-CLIO.

Stepanova, E. A. 2008. Terrorism in Asymmetrical Conflict: Ideological and Structural Aspects. Oxford: Oxford University Press.

Stepinska, A. 2010. 9/11 and the transformation of globalized media events. In Media Events in a Global Age, eds. A. Hepp and F. Krotz. London: Routledge.

Steven, G. C. S., and Gunaratna, R. 2004. Counterterrorism: A Reference Handbook. Santa Barbara: ABC-CLIO.

Tanham, G. K. 2006. Communist Revolutionary Warfare: From the Vietminh to the Viet Cong. Westport, CT: Praeger Security International.

Thackrah, J. R. 2004. Dictionary of Terrorism. London: Routledge.

Thomas, B. 2011. The Dark Side of Zionism: Israel's Quest for Security through Dominance. Lanham, NC: Lexington Books.

Truman, J. S. 2010. Communicating Terror: The Rhetorical Dimensions of Terrorism. Los Angeles: Sage.

Ünal, M. C. 2012. Counterterrorism in Turkey: Policy Choices and Policy Effects toward the Kurdistan Workers' Party (PKK). New York: Routledge.

United States Army. 2007. A Military Guide to Terrorism in the Twenty-first Century. Fort Leavenworth: United States Army Training and Doctrine Command.

Various. 2011. The brown army faction: A disturbing new dimension of far-right terror. *Der Spiegel*, 14 November.

Varon, J. P. 2004. Bringing the War Home: The Weather Underground, the Red Army Faction, and Revolutionary Violence in the Sixties and Seventies. Berkeley, CA: University of California Press.

Wahnich, S. 2012. In Defence of the Terror: Liberty or Death in the French Revolution. London: Verso Books.

Weimann, G. 2016. Why do terrorists migrate to social media? In Violent Extremism Online: New Perspectives on Terrorism and the Internet, eds. A. Aly, S. Macodnald, L. Jarvis, and T. Chen. Abingdon: Routledge.

Weiss, G. 2012. The Cage: The Fight for Sri Lanka and the Last Days of the Tamil Tigers. New York: Random House.

Wexler, S. 2015. America's Secret Jihad: The Hidden History of Religious Terrorism in the United States. Berkeley, CA: Counterpoint.

Widmaier, W. W. 2015. Presidential Rhetoric from Wilson to Obama. Abingdon: Routledge.

Williams, B. G. 2017. Counter Jihad: America's Military Experience in Afghanistan, Iraq and Syria. Philadelphia, PA: University of Pennsylvania Press.

Wright-Neville, D. 2010. Dictionary of Terrorism. Cambridge: Polity Press.

Zafirovski, M. and D. G. Rodeheaver. 2013. Modernity and Terrorism: From Anti-modernity to Modern Global Terror. Leiden: Brill.

Zunes, S. and J. Mundy. 2010. Western Sahara: War, Nationalism and Conflict Irresolution. New York: Syracuse University Press.

Chapter 8 Works Cited

Anderson, R. and A. C. Hearn. 1996. The day after … in Cyberspace. In An Exploration of Cyberspace Security R&D Investment Strategies for DARPA. Washington, DC: Rand Corporation/Rand Monograph Report.

Armistead, L., ed. 2004. Information Operations: Warfare and the Hard Reality of Soft Power. Washington, DC: Potomoc Books, Brassey's Inc.

Astahost. 2006. Computer glitch causes massive budget shortfalls in Indiana. *Astahost*. February 11, http://www.astahost.com/info.php/computer-glitch-causes-massive-budget-shortfalls-indiana_t10545.html (accessed May 10, 2006).

Bayles, W. 2001. The Ethics of Computer Network Attacks. Parameters, US Army War College Quarterly, XXXI (Spring), 44–58.

Becker, B. 2017. The truth about Russia, 'hacking' and the 2016 election. *The Hill*. June 25. http://thehill.com/blogs/pundits-blog/national-party-news/339225-what-we-know-about-russian-hacking-and-the-2016 (accessed June 25, 2017).

Browne, R. 2016. Top military official warns of IS attacks. *CNN*. April 5. http://www.cnn.com/2016/04/05/politics/isis-cyberattacks-michael-rogers/index.html (accessed June 27, 2017).

Canadian Broadcast Company. 1999. Military prepares for Y2K. *CBC News*. http://www.cbc.ca/news/canada/military-prepares-for-y2k-1.183459 (last updated November 10, 2000, accessed October 24, 2017).

Carnegie Mellon University. 1988. DARPA establishes Computer Emergency Response Team. http://www.cert.org/about/1988press-rel.html (accessed May 17, 2006).

Clashman, B. 2015. Photograph [DoD Cyber Security Strategy: Cyber Protection Team]. Washington, DC: Department of Defense. https://www.defense.gov/Portals/1/features/2015/0415_cyber-strategy/Final_2015_DoD_CYBER_STRATEGY_for_web.pdf (accessed October 24, 2017).

Cuthbertson, A. 2016. Hackers hijack ISIS Twitter accounts with gay porn after Orlando attack. *Newsweek*. June 14. http://www.newsweek.com/isis-twitter-accounts-gay-porn-orlando-attacks-anonymous-470300 (accessed June 30, 2017).

Defense Science Board. 1996. Report of the Task Forces on Information Warfare – Defense (IW-D). Washington, DC: Department of Defense, Office of the Under Secretary of Defense for Acquisition and Technology.

Denning, D. 2004. Information technology and security, in Grave New World: Security Challenges in the 21st Century, ed. M. E. Brown. Washington, DC: Georgetown University Press.

Department of Defense. 1998. Joint Publication (JP) 3-13, Joint Doctrine for Information Operations, October. Washington, DC: US Government Printing Office.

Department of Defense. 2015. The Department of Defense Cyber Strategy. Washington, DC: US Government Printing Office.

Department of Homeland Security. 2006. Cyber Storm Exercise Report. Washington, DC: Department of Homeland Security, National Cyber Security Division.

Department of Homeland Security. 2013. DHS cyber table top exercise (TTX) for the health care industry. https://www.hsdl.org/?abstract&did=789781 (accessed July 28, 2017).

Department of Homeland Security. 2016. Cyber Storm V After Action Report. Washington, DC: Department of Homeland Security, National Cyber Security Division.

Department of Homeland Security. 2017. President's executive order will strengthen cybersecurity for federal networks and critical infrastructure. May 11. Office of the Press Secretary. https://www.dhs.gov/news/2017/05/11/president-s-executive-order-will-strengthen-cybersecurity-federal-networks-and (accessed June 28, 2017).

Department of the Army. 2003. Field Manual (FM) 3-13, Information Operations: Doctrine, Tactics, Techniques and Procedures, November 28. Washington, DC: Headquarters Department of the Army.

Doman, C. 2016. The first cyber espionage attacks: How operation moonlight maze made history. Medium.com. July 7. https://medium.com/@chris_doman/the-first-sophistiated-cyber-attacks-how-operation-moonlight-maze-made-history-2adb12cc43f7 (accessed June 28, 2017).

Donnelly, J. and V. Crawley. 1999. Hamre to Hill—We're in a cyber-war. Defense Week. March 1. http://jya.com/dod-cyberwar.htm (accessed May 17, 2006).

Doran, L. 2017. Ransomware attacks force school districts to shore up—or pay up. *Education Week.* January 10. http://www.edweek. org/ew/articles/2017/01/11/ransomware-attacks-force-school-districts-to.html (accessed June 26, 2017).

Frenkel, S. 2017. Here's the latest evidence that Russian hackers are targeting Europe's elections. *Buzzfeed.* April 24. https://www. buzzfeed.com/sheerafrenkel/heres-the-latest-evidence-that-russian-hackers-are?utm_term=.lc7vy5nJl#.plqBYzn42 (accessed June 30, 2017).

Fung, B. 2013. How many cyberattacks hit the United States last year? *National Journal.* March 8. http://www.nextgov.com/cybersecurity/ 2013/03/how-many-cyberattacks-hit-united-states-last-year/61775/ (accessed June 27, 2017).

Gellman, B. 2002. Cyber-attacks by Al Qaeda feared. *The Washington Post,* June 27. http://www.washingtonpost.com/wp-dyn/content/ article/2006/06/12/AR2006061200711.html (accessed May 17, 2006).

Global Security. n.d. Solar sunrise. http://www.globalsecurity.org/ military/ops/solar-sunrise.htm (accessed May 11, 2006).

Grant, K. 2017. A global cyber attack could be as costly as hurricane Katrina. *The Street.* July 18. https://news.thestreet.com/independent/ story/14232452/1/a-global-cyber-attack-could-be-as-costly-as-hurricane-katrina.html (accessed July 25, 2017).

Greenberg, A. 2017. How and entire nation became Russia's test lab for cyberwar. *Wired.* June 20. https://www.wired.com/story/russian-hackers-attack-ukraine/ (accessed June 26, 2017).

Hamre, J. 2015. The 'electronic pearl harbour'. *Politico.* December 9. https://www.politico.com/agenda/story/2015/12/pearl-harbor-cyber-security-war-000335 (accessed November 9, 2017).

Hollis, D. 2011. Cyberwar case study: Georgia 2008. *Small Wars Journal.* http://smallwarsjournal.com/blog/journal/docs-temp/639-hollis. pdf (accessed June 26, 2017).

Information Warfare Site. 2003. Joint task force-computer network operations. IWAR. February. http://www.iwar.org.uk/iwar/ resources/jtf-cno/factsheet.htm (accessed November 9, 2017).

Internet Security Threat Report. 2017. Internet security threat report. Volume 22, April. Mountain View, CA: Symantec Corporation.

Kessem, L. 2016. Year in review: top three cyber crime threats in 2016. *Security Intelligence.* December 20. https://securityintelligence.com/ year-in-review-top-three-cybercrime-threats-of-2016/ (accessed June 27, 2017).

Kessler, G. C. 2004. An Overview of Steganography for the Computer Forensics Examiner. Forensic Science Communications, 6 (3 July).

Kessler, G. C. 2014. The impact of cyber-security on critical infrastructure protection, in Critical Issues in Homeland Security, ed. J. D. Ramsay and L. Kiltz. Boulder, CO: Westview Press.

Kilroy, R. J. Jr. 2008. Cyber terrorism and cyber warfare. In Threats to Homeland Security: An All-Hazards Perspective, 1st ed. R. Kilroy. Hoboken, NJ: John Wiley & Sons.

Kumar, M. 2014. US charges five Chinese military officials with economic espionage. *The Hacker News.* http://thehackernews.com/2014/05/us-charges-five-chinese-military.html (accessed June 30, 2017).

Liang, Q. and W. Xiangsui. 1999. Unrestricted Warfare. Beijing: PLA Literature and Arts Publishing House. FBIS translation of selected chapters.

Lipton, E., D. Sanger, and S. Shane. 2016. The perfect weapon: How Russian cyberpower invaded the US. December 13. *The Washington Post.* https://www.nytimes.com/2016/12/13/us/politics/russia-hack-election-dnc.html?rref=collection%2Fnewseventcollection%2Fruss ian-election-hacking&action=click&contentCollection=politics&re gion=rank&module=package&version=highlights&contentPlacem ent=1&pgtype=collection (accessed June 30, 2017).

Mims, C. 2017. In cyberwarfare, everyone is a combatant. *Wall Street Journal,* July 23. https://www.wsj.com/articles/how-cyberwarfare-makes-cold-wars-hotter-1500811201 (accessed July 24, 2017).

Morgan, S. 2016. Cyber crime report. *Cybersecurity Ventures.* http://cybersecurityventures.com/hackerpocalypse-cybercrime-report-2016/ (accessed June 26, 2017).

Muhammad. 2017. Anonymous hacks ISIS website and infects users with malware. *Techworm.net.* April 2. https://www.techworm.net/2017/04/anonymous-hacks-isis-website-infects-users-malware.html (accessed June 28, 2017).

National Crime Prevention Council. 2012. Cyber crime. September. http://www.ncpc.org/resources/files/pdf/internet-safety/13020-Cybercrimes-revSPR.pdf (accessed June 26, 2017).

National Institute of Standards and Technology. 2017. Framework for Improving Critical Infrastructure Cybersecurity. Version 1.1. Washington, DC: National Institute of Standards and Technology, Office of the Director National Intelligence. n.d. Ref Book: *The Cybersecurity Act of 2015.* https://www.dni.gov/index.php/ic-legal-reference-book/cybersecurity-act-of-2015 (accessed June 28, 2017).

Peterson, A. 2014. The Sony pictures hack, explained. *The Washington Post.* December 18. https://www.washingtonpost.com/news/the-switch/wp/2014/12/18/the-sony-pictures-hack-explained/?utm_term=.73ac8a1b4450 (accessed June 30, 2017).

Presidential Decision Directive 63. 1998. Critical Infrastructure Protection. Washington, DC: The White House.

Public Broadcasting Service. 2006. Frontline: Interview with Richard Clarke. January 23. http://www.pbs.org/wgbh/pages/frontline/darkside/interviews/clarke.html (accessed July 24, 2017).

Public Intelligence. 2012. National level exercise 2012 will focus on cyber attacks against critical infrastructure. April 10. https://publicintelligence.net/national-level-exercise-2012-critical-infrastructure/ (accessed June 28, 2017).

Ranger, S. 2017. US intelligence: 30 countries building cyber attack capabilities. *ZDNet*. January 5. http://www.zdnet.com/article/us-intelligence-30-countries-building-cyber-attack-capabilities/ (accessed June 27, 2017).

Ranum, M. 2004. Myths of cyberwarfare. *Information Security*. April. http://infosecuritymag.techtarget.com/ss/0,295796,sid6_iss366_art692,00.html (accessed May 19, 2006).

Reed, D. and D. L. Wilson. 1998. Whiz kid hacker caught. *San Jose Mercury News*. March 19. https://web.archive.org/web/20001007150311/http://www.mercurycenter.com/archives/reprints/hacker110698.htm (accessed May 19, 2006).

Riley, M. and J. Robertson. 2017. Russian cyber hacks on US electoral system far wider than previously known. *Bloomberg Politics*. https://www.bloomberg.com/news/articles/2017-06-13/russian-breach-of-39-states-threatens-future-u-s-elections (accessed June 27, 2017).

Robinson, C. 2002. Military and cyber defense: Reactions to the threat. Center for Defense Information. November 8. http://www.cdi.org/terrorism/cyberdefense-pr.cfm (accessed September 10, 2005).

Rogers, M. 2017. Statement before the Senate Committee on the Armed Services. Ft. Meade, MD: US Cyber Command.

Rumsfeld, D. 2006. Remarks by Secretary Rumsfeld at Southern Center for International Studies. Atlanta, GA: Department of Defense News Transcript. http://www.defenselink.mil/transcripts/2006/tr20060504-12979.html (accessed May 19, 2006).

Sanger, D. 2013. Confront and Conceal: Obama's Secret Wars and Surprising Use of American Power. New York: Broadway Books.

Securities and Exchange Commission. 2015. SEC Charges 32 Defendants in Scheme to Trade on Hacked News Releases. Washington, DC: Securities and Exchange Commission.

Shiloach, G. 2015. IS hackers threaten "message to America" cyber attack. *Vocativ*. May 11. https://themeshreport.com/2015/05/isis-hackers-plan-message-to-america-attack-today/ (accessed November 9, 2017).

Song, J. 2006. 5 nations left off tsunami warning list. *Yahoo News*. May 5. Associated Press. http://news.yahoo.com/s/ap/20060505/ap_on_re_us/tonga_earthquake_warning&printer=1;_ylt=Alj21h9cZbEFwGtf8TV6PElH2ocA;_ylu=X3oDMTA3MXN1bHE0BHNlYwN0bWE- (accessed May 10, 2006).

Stoll, C. 2005. The Cuckoo's Egg: Tracking a Spy Through the Maze of Computer Espionage. New York: Pocket Books.

Sullivan, B. 2005. Bank crime theft on rise. *MSNBC*, June 26. http://msnbc.msn.com/id/3078568/ (accessed May 11, 2006).

Sun, T. n.d. The art of war. Goodreads.com. http://www.goodreads.com/quotes/17976-if-you-know-the-enemy-and-know-yourself-you-need (accessed June 28, 2017).

The Times of India. 2000. I love you virus this 45 million PCs. May 8. http://archive.is/P4p7b (accessed November 9, 2017).

The White House. 2003. National Strategy to Secure Cyberspace. Washington, DC: The White House.

The White House. 2016. Fact sheet: Cybersecurity national action plan. February 9. Office of the Press Secretary. https://obamawhitehouse.archives.gov/the-press-office/2016/02/09/fact-sheet-cybersecurity-national-action-plan (accessed June 28, 2017).

Thompson Reuters. 2017. 'It's like WannaCry all over again': New ransomware attack infects computers across Europe. *CBC News*. June 27. http://www.cbc.ca/news/technology/ransomware-europe-russia-ukraine-petya-bitcoin-1.4179683 (accessed June 27, 2017).

US CERT. n.d. National cybersecurity and communications integration center. US Department of Homeland Security. https://www.us-cert.gov/nccic (accessed June 27, 2017).

US Department of State. n.d. Top officials (TOPOFF). Archived. https://2001-2009.state.gov/s/ct/about/c16661.htm (accessed June 28, 2017).

US Strategic Command. 2016. US cyber command (USCYBERCOM). September 16. http://www.stratcom.mil/Media/Factsheets/Factsheet-View/Article/960492/us-cyber-command-uscybercom/ (accessed June 28, 2017).

Wallace, R. 2001. It's an all out cyber war as US hackers fight back at china. *Fox News*, May 1, http://www.foxnews.com/story/0,2933,19337,00.html (accessed May 18, 2006).

Watson, J. 2017. Sun Tzu's art of war. https://suntzusaid.com/ (accessed July 24, 2017).

Webb, R. 2016. Horry County pays nearly $10k to 'ransomware' hackers. *WBTW News*. March 7. http://wbtw.com/2016/03/07/horry-county-pays-nearly-10k-to-ransomware-hackers/ (accessed June 26, 2017).

Wikiquotes. n.d. Sneakers (1992 Film). https://en.wikiquote.org/wiki/Sneakers_(1992_film) (accessed June 27, 2017).

Winerip, M. 2013. Revisiting Y2K: Much ado about nothing? *New York Times*. May 27. http://www.nytimes.com/2013/05/27/booming/revisiting-y2k-much-ado-about-nothing.html?mcubz=1 (accessed June 27, 2017).

Woolf, N. 2016. DDoS attack that disrupted internet was largest of its kind in history, experts say. *The Guardian*. October 26. https://www.theguardian.com/technology/2016/oct/26/ddos-attack-dyn-mirai-botnet (accessed June 27, 2017).

Zero Days. 2016. Official movie site. http://www.zerodaysfilm.com/ (accessed October 23, 2016).

Zetter, K. 2014. Countdown to zero day: Stuxnet and the launch of the world's first digital weapon. New York: Crown. Kindle Edition.

Chapter 9 Works Cited

ABC News. 2006. List of Saddam's crimes is long. http://abcnews.go.com/WNT/IraqCoverage/story?id=2761722&page=1 (accessed April 14, 2017).

Anderson, A. 2008. Weapons of mass destruction. In Threats to Homeland Security: An All-Hazards Perspective, 1st ed, ed. R. Kilroy. Hoboken, NJ: John Wiley & Sons.

Arms Control Association. 2014. Chemical and biological weapons status at a glance. https://www.armscontrol.org/factsheets/cbwprolif (accessed November 30, 2016).

Arms Control Association. 2016a. Nuclear weapons: Who has what at a glance. https://www.armscontrol.org/factsheets/Nuclearweaponswhohaswhat (accessed November 30, 2016).

Arms Control Association. 2016b. Timeline of Syrian chemical weapons activity, 2012–2016. https://www.armscontrol.org/factsheets/Timeline-of-Syrian-Chemical-Weapons-Activity (accessed November 30, 2016).

Atomic Archive, n.d. Timeline of the nuclear age. http:/www.atomicarchive.com/Timeline/Timeline.shtml (accessed January 7, 2008).

Bunn, M. 2009. Reducing the Greatest Risks of Nuclear Theft and Terrorism. Daedalus, Fall, 112–123.

Couch, D. 2003. US Armed Forces Nuclear, Biological, and Chemical Survival Manual. New York: Basic.

Derbis, V. J. 1996. De Mussis and the Great Plague of 1348: A Forgotten Episode of Bacteriological Warfare. Journal of American Medical Association, 19 (1), 180.

Doornbos, H. and J. Moussa. 2016. How the Islamic State seized a chemical weapons stockpile. Foreign Policy, August 17. http://foreignpolicy.com/2016/08/17/how-the-islamic-state-seized-a-chemical-weapons-stockpile/ (accessed December 7, 2016).

Fackler, M. 2012. Japan arrests fugitive wanted in 1995 gas attack. New York Times, June 3. http://www.nytimes.com/2012/06/04/world/asia/japan-arrests-fugitive-from-1995-subway-gas-attack.html (accessed April 14, 2017)

Federation of American Scientists. n.d.a. Biological threat agents information. https://fas.org/programs/bio/agents.html (accessed December 9, 2016).

Federation of American Scientists. n.d.b. Chemical weapons delivery. https://fas.org/programs/bio/chemweapons/delivery.html (accessed December 9, 2016).

Federation of American Scientists. n.d.c. Introduction to biological weapons. https://fas.org/programs/bio/bwintro.html (accessed December 9, 2016).

Federation of American Scientists. n.d.d. Introduction to chemical weapons. https://fas.org/programs/bio/chemweapons/introduction.html (accessed December 9, 2016).

Federation of American Scientists. n.d.e. Types of chemical weapons. https://fas.org/programs/bio/chemweapons/cwagents.html (accessed December 9, 2016).

Fox News. 2016. Syria, ISIS responsible for chemical weapons attacks, UN inquiry finds. http://www.foxnews.com/world/2016/08/24/syria-isis-responsible-for-chemical-weapons-attacks-un-inquiry-finds.html (accessed December 7, 2016).

Garrett, L. 2013. Biology's Brave New World. Foreign Affairs, November/December, 28–46.

Guardian. 2016. Libya hands over last stockpile of chemical weapons ingredients. https://www.theguardian.com/world/2016/sep/01/libya-hands-over-last-stockpile-of-chemical-weapon-ingredients (accessed December 7, 2016).

International Panel on Fissile Materials. 2015. Global fissile material report 2015. http://fissilematerials.org/library/gfmr15.pdf (accessed November 7, 2016).

Jones, D. 2007. Poison Arrows: North American Indian Hunting and Warfare. Arlington, TX: University of Texas Press.

Kilroy, R. J. Jr. 2006. Photograph [Chernobyl Nuclear Site, Ukraine], personal collection.

Malsin, J. 2016. Assad's regime is still using chemical weapons in Syria. *Time*, September 14. http://time.com/4492670/syria-chemical-weapon-aleppo-assad-regime/ (accessed December 7, 2016).

Mayo Clinic. n.d. Radiation sickness symptoms. http://www.mayoclinic.org/diseases-conditions/radiation-sickness/basics/symptoms/con-20022901 (accessed December 13, 2016).

National Public Radio. 2011. Timeline: How the anthrax terror unfolded. http://www.npr.org/2011/02/15/93170200/timeline-how-the-anthrax-terror-unfolded (accessed May 18, 2017).

Noble, R. 2013. Keeping Science in the Right hands. Foreign Affairs, November/December, 47–53.

Nuclear Threat Initiative. 2012. Iraq: Biological weapons. http://www.nti.org/learn/countries/iraq/chemical/ (accessed December 9, 2016).

Nuclear Threat Initiative. 2014. Syria: Chemical weapons. http://www.nti.org/learn/countries/syria/chemical/ (accessed December 7, 2016).

Nuclear Threat Initiative. 2015a. Iraq: Chemical weapons. http://www.nti.org/learn/countries/iraq/chemical/ (accessed December 7, 2016).

Nuclear Threat Initiative. 2015b. Russia: Chemical weapons. http://www.nti.org/learn/countries/russia/chemical/ (accessed December 7, 2016).

Omand, D. 2016. Keeping Europe Safe. Foreign Affairs, September/October, 83–93.

Organization for the Prohibition of Chemical Weapons. 2016a. Eliminating chemical weapons and chemical weapons facilities. https://www.opcw.org/fileadmin/OPCW/Fact_Sheets/English/Fact_Sheet_6_-_destruction.pdf (accessed December 6, 2016).

Organization for the Prohibition of Chemical Weapons. 2016b. Monitoring chemicals with possible chemical weapons applications.

https://www.opcw.org/fileadmin/OPCW/Fact_Sheets/English/
Fact_Sheet_7_-_Schedule_of_chemicals.pdf (accessed December 6,
2016).

Osborne, S. 2017. Syria chemical attack: Sarin gas was used in Khan
Sheikhoun strike, says UK ambassador to UN. *The Independent.*
April 12. http://www.independent.co.uk/news/world/middle-east/
syria-chemical-attack-sarin-gas-khan-sheikhoun-assad-strike-uk-
ambassador-to-un-british-scientists-a7680556.html (accessed May
9, 2017).

Sanger, D. and A. Kramer. 2015. Iran hands over stockpile of enriched
uranium to Russia. *New York Times*, December 28, A4.

Syrian American Medical Society. 2016. A new normal: Ongoing chemical weapons attacks in Syria. https://www.sams-usa.net/wp-content/
uploads/2016/09/A-New-Normal_Ongoing-Chemical-Weapons-
Attacks-in-Syria.compressed.pdf (accessed April 14, 2017).

Takakura, A. 2010. This is how it feels to be under a nuclear attack.
Gizmodo. August 6. http://gizmodo.com/5606053/this-it-how-it-
feels-to-be-under-a-nuclear-attack (accessed May 18, 2017).

Texas City Disaster. n.d. The Texas City Disaster: April 16, 1947. http:/
www.local1259iaff.org/disaster.html (accessed January 8, 2007).

Vicinanzo, A. 2015. "Biological terrorist attack on US an urgent and
serious threat. *Homeland Security Today*, April 23. http://www.
hstoday.us/single-article/biological-terrorist-attack-on-us-an-
urgent-and-serious-threat/0ce6ebf3524d83c537b1f4f0cc578547.
html (accessed May 8, 2017).

White House. 2002. National Security Strategy. www.state.gov/
documents/organization/63562.pdf (accessed April 14, 2017).

White House. 2015. National security strategy. https://www.whitehouse.
gov/sites/default/files/docs/2015_national_security_strategy.pdf
(accessed November 22, 2016).

Chapter 10 Works Cited

Adams, J. 1987. The financing of terror. In Contemporary Research on
Terrorism, eds. P. Wilkinson and A. Stewart. Aberdeen: Aberdeen
University Press.

Alakoc, B. P. 2015. Competing to Kill: Terrorist Organizations Versus
Lone Wolf Terrorists. Terrorism and Political Violence 27: 1–24.

Alda, E. and J. L. Sala. 2014. Links Between Terrorism, Organized
Crime and Crime: The Case of the Sahel Region. International
Journal of Security & Development, 3 (1), 1–9.

Aldrich, D. P. 2014. First Steps Towards Hearts and Minds? USAID's
Countering Violent Extremism Policies in Africa. Terrorism and
Political Violence, 26, 532–546.

Bartlett, J. and C. Miller. 2012. The Edge of Violence: Towards Telling
the Difference Between Violent and Non-violent Radicalization.
Terrorism and Political Violence, 24, 1–21.

Borum, R. 2011. Radicalization into Violent Extremism II: A Review of Conceptual Models and Empirical Research. Journal of Strategic Studies, 4 (4), 37–62.

Carlson, J. R. 1995. The Future Terrorists in America. American Journal of Police, 14 (3/4), 71–91.

Chalk, P. 1995. The Liberal Democratic Response to Terrorism. Terrorism & Political Violence, 7 (4), 10–44.

Chalk, P. and W. Rosenau. 2004. Confronting the "Enemy Within": Security Intelligence, the Police, and Counterterrorism in Four Democracies. Santa Monica, CA: Rand.

CNN. 2005. Hezbollah pushes Prada? CNN.Money.com. May 26. http://money.cnn.com/2005/05/26/news/terror_knockoffs/index.htm?cnn=yes (accessed November 9, 2017).

Connor, J. and C. R. Flynn. 2015. Report: Lone wolf terrorism. Report prepared by Security Studies Program, National Security Critical Issue Task Force. Washington, DC: Georgetown University.

Crenshaw, M. 1990. The logic of terrorism: Terrorist behavior as a product of strategic choice. In Origins of Terrorism: Psychologies, Theologies, States of Mind, ed. W. Reich. Cambridge: Cambridge University Press.

Danzell, O. and S. Zidek. 2013. Does Counterterrorism Spending Reduce the Incidence and Lethality of Terrorism? A Quantitative Analysis of 34 Countries. Defense & Security Analysis, 29 (3), 218–233.

Dishman, C. 2005. The Leaderless Nexus: When Crime and Terror Converge. Studies in Conflict & Terrorism, 28, 237–252.

Donohue, L. K. 2001. In the Name of National Security: US Counterterrorist Measures, 1960–2000. Terrorism and Political Violence, 13 (1), 15–60.

Donohue, L. K. and J. N. Kayyem. 2002. Federalism and the Battle over Counterterrorist Law: State Sovereignty, Criminal Law Enforcement, and National Security. Studies in Conflict & Terrorism, 25, 1–18.

Doornbos, C. 2016. Transcripts of 911 calls reveal pulse shooter's terrorist motives. Orlando Sentinel. September 23.

Eisenhower, D. D. (n.d.) Dwight D. Eisenhower quotes. https://www.brainyquote.com/quotes/quotes/d/dwightdei149102.html (accessed May 30, 2017).

Emerson, S. 2003. American Jihad: The Terrorists Living Among Us. New York: The Free Press.

Enders, W. and T. Sandler. 2000. Is Transnational Terrorism becoming more Threatening? Journal of Conflict Resolution, 44 (3), 307–332.

Fernandez, M. and A. Blinder. 2014. At Fort Hood, wrestling with label of terrorism. New York Times. p. A11.

Fitzpatrick, K. M., J. Gruenewald, B. L. Smith, and P. Roberts. 2017. A Community-level Comparison of Terrorism Movements in the United States. Studies in Conflict & Terrorism, 40 (5), 399–418.

Freilich, J. D., S. M. Chermak, and R. Belli. 2014. Introducing the United States Extremis Crime Database. Terrorism and Political Violence, 26, 372–384.

Gill, P., J. Horgan, and P. Deckert. 2014. Bombing Alone: Tracing the Motivations and Antecedent Behaviors of Lone-Actor Terrorists. Journal of Forensic Sciences, 59 (2), 425–435.

Griset, P. L. and S. Mahan. 2003. Terrorism in Perspective. Thousand Oaks, CA: Sage Publications.

Gruenewald, J., S. Chermak, and J. D. Freilich. 2013. Distinguishing "Loner" Attacks from Other Domestic Extremist Violence: A Comparison of Far-Right Homicide Incident and Offender Characteristics. Criminology & Public Policy, 12 (1), 65–91.

Hewitt, C. 2000. Patterns of American Terrorism 1955–1998: An Historical Perspective on Terrorism-Related Fatalities. Terrorism & Political Violence, 12 (1), 1–14.

Hewitt, C. 2003. Understanding Terrorism in America: From the Klan to Al-Qaeda. New York: Routledge.

Hewitt, C. 2005. Political Violence and Terrorism in Modern America: A Chronology. Westport, CT: Praeger Security International.

Hoffman, B. 1998. Inside Terrorism. New York: Columbia University Press.

Hoffman, B. 2008. The Myth of Grass-Roots Terrorism. Foreign Affairs, 87 (3), 133–138.

Jensen, R. 2010. The United States, International Policing and the War Against Anarchist Terrorism, 1900-1914. Terrorism and Political Violence, 13 (1), 15–46.

Kaplan, J. 1997. Leaderless Resistance. Terrorism and Political Violence, 9 (3), 80–95.

Karber, P. A. and R. W. Mengla, 1983. Political and economic forces affecting terrorism. In Managing Terrorism: Strategies for the Corporate Executive, eds. P. J. Montana and G. S. Roukis. Westport, CT: Quorum Books.

Kiras, J. D. 2013. Irregular warfare: Terrorism and insurgency. In Strategy in the Contemporary World, 5th ed, eds. J. Byalis, J. J. Wirtz, and C. S. Gray. New York: Oxford University Press.

Lankford, A. 2016. Are America's Public Mass Shooters Unique? A Comparative Analysis of Offenders in the United States and Other Countries. International Journal of Comparative and Applied Criminal Justice, 40 (2), 171–183.

Lichbach, M. I. 1995. The Rebel's Dilemma. Ann Arbor, MI: University of Michigan Press.

Long, D. E. 1990. The Anatomy of Terrorism. New York: The Free Press.

Lutz, J. M. and B. Lutz. 2013. Islamic extremism in the United States. In Extremism in America, ed. L. T. Sargent. Gainesville, FL: University of Florida Press.

Makarenko, T. 2004. The Crime-Terror Continuum: Tracing the Interplay between Transnational Organized Crime and Terrorism. Global Crime, 6 (1), 129–145.

Malthaner, S. and P. Waldmann. 2014. The Radical Milieu: Conceptualizing the Supportive Social Environment of Terrorist Groups. Studies in Conflict & Terrorism, 37, 979–998.

McCauley, C. and S. Moskalenko. 2014. Toward a Profile of Lone Wolf Terrorists: What Moves an Individual from Radical Opinion to Radical Action. Terrorism and Political Violence, 26, 69–85.

Memorial Institute for the Prevention of Terrorism (MIPT). 2006. Terrorism knowledge base. http://tkb.org/Home.jsp (accessed December 7, 2006).

Mullins, S. and J. K. Wither. 2016. Terrorism and Organized Crime. Connections: The Quarterly Journal, 15 (3), 65–82.

National Counterterrorism Center (NCTC). 2006. Worldwide incidents tracking system. http://wits.nctc.gov/ (accessed November 27, 2006).

Neumann, P. R. 2013. The Trouble with Radicalization. International Affairs, 89 (4), 873–893.

Phillips, B. J. 2015. Deadlier in the US? On Lone Wolves, Terrorist Groups, and Attack Lethality. Terrorism and Political Violence, 27, 1–17.

Picarelli, J. T. 2006. The Turbulent Nexus of Transnational Organized Crime and Terrorism: A Theory of Malevolent International Relations. Global Crime, 7 (1), 1–24.

Powers, R. G. 2004. A bomb with a long fuse: 9/11 and the FBI 'reforms' of the 1970s. American History. December, pp. 43–47.

Rabbie, J. M. 1991. A Behavioral Interaction Model: Toward a Social-Psychological Framework for Studying Terrorism. Terrorism & Political Violence, 3 (4), 134–163.

Raphaeli, N. 2003. Financing of Terrorism: Sources, Methods, and Channels. Terrorism & Political Violence, 15 (4), 59–82.

Roberts, S. (2012). The Port Huron statement at 50. The New York Times, SR5. http://www.nytimes.com/2012/03/04/sunday-review/the-port-huron-statement-at-50.html (accessed November 9, 2017).

Sageman, M. 2008. Does Osama Still Call the Shots? Debating the Containment of Al Qaeda's Leadership. Foreign Affairs, 87 (3), 163–166.

Schiller, D. Th. 1987. The police response to terrorism: A critical overview. In Contemporary Research on Terrorism, eds. P. Wilkinson and A. Stewart. Aberdeen: Aberdeen University Press.

Siqueira, K. 2005. Political and Militant Wings within Dissident Movements and Organizations. Journal of Conflict Resolution, 49 (2), 218–236.

Taylor, M. and J. Horgan. 2012. A conceptual framework for addressing psychological process in the development of the terrorist. In Terrorism Studies: A Reader, eds. J. Horgan and K. Braddock. New York: Routledge.

Turkewitz, J. and B. Mueller. 2015. Couple kept tight lid on plans for San Bernardino shooting. The New York Times. December 3. https://

www.nytimes.com/2015/12/04/us/san-bernardino-shooting-syed-rizwan-farook.html?_r=0 (accessed on March 3, 2017).

Vidino, L. 2009. Homegrown Jihadist Terrorist in the United States: New and Occasional Phenomenon? Studies in Conflict & Terrorism, 32, 1–17.

Walker, C. 2000. Briefing on the Terrorism Act 2000. Terrorism & Political Violence, 12 (2), 1–36.

Webb, J. J. and S. L. Cutter. 2009. The Geography of US Terrorist Incidents, 1970–2004. Terrorism and Political Violence, 21, 428–449.

Weimann, G. 2012. Lone Wolves in Cyberspace. Journal of Terrorism Research, 3 (2), 75–90.

Weinberg, L. 1991. Turning to Terror: The Conditions under Which Political Parties Turn to Terrorist Activities. Comparative Politics, 23 (4), 423–438.

Weinberg, L. and W. Eubank. 1990. Political Parties and the Formation of Terrorist Groups. Terrorism & Political Violence, 2 (2), 125–144.

Weinstein, J. M. 2005. Resources and the Information Problem in Rebel Recruitment. Journal of Conflict Resolution, 49 (4), 598–624.

Wessinger, C. 2000. How the Millenium Comes Violently: From Jonestown to Heaven's Gate. New York: Seven Bridges Press.

Wilkinson, P. 2000. Terrorism Versus Democracy: The Liberal State Response. London: Frank Cass.

Chapter 11 Works Cited

Allen, T. 2006. Leadership in disaster. Comments made at the annual Federal Emergency Management Agency Emergency Management Institute, Emmitsburg, MD. June 6. https://training.fema.gov/hiedu/06conf/06papers/adm%20thad%20allen%20-%20leadership%20in%20disaster.doc (accessed November 22, 2016).

Almond, G. and J. Coleman, eds. 1960. The Politics of the Developing Areas Princeton, NJ: Princeton University Press.

Anthony, M. G. and R. J. Thomas. 2010. 'This is Citizen Journalism at its Finest:' YouTube and the Public Sphere in the Oscar Grant Shooting Incident. New Media & Society, 12 (8), 1280–1296.

Armanios, F. 2003. Islamic Religious Schools, Madrasas. Background Report #RS21654, October 29. Washington, DC: Congressional Research Service.

Associated Press. 2014. Is it IS, ISIS, ISIL or maybe Daesh? Ynet News. December 9. http://www.ynetnews.com/articles/0,7340,L-4570385,00.html (accessed December 27, 2016).

AWDNews.com. 2016. Israeli Defense Minister: If Pakistan send ground troops into Syria on any pretext, we will destroy this country with nuclear attack. AWD News. December 20. http://awdnews.com/political/israeli-defense-minister-if-pakistan-send-ground-troops-into-syria-on-any-pretext,-we-will-destroy-them-with-a-nuclear-attack (accessed December 26, 2016).

Baele, S. 2016. Lone-Actor Terrorists' Emotions and Cognition: An Evaluation beyond Stereotypes. *Political Psychology*. http://onlinelibrary.wiley.com/doi/10.1111/pops.12365/full (accessed December 29, 2016).

Baran, Z. 2005. Fighting the War of Ideas. *Foreign Affairs*. November/December. https://www.foreignaffairs.com/articles/europe/2005-10-01/fighting-war-ideas (accessed December 22, 2016).

Benoliel, S. 2003. Strengthening Education in the Moslem World. Issue Paper #2. Washington, DC: United States Agency for International Development.

Bergen, P. 2002. Holy War, Inc. New York: Touchstone.

Bishop, B. 2008. The Big Sort: Why the Clustering of Like-Minded America is Tearing Us Apart. Boston, MA: Houghton Mifflin Harcourt.

Bonikowski, B. 2016. Nationalism in Settled Times. Annual Review of Sociology, 42, 427–449.

Brooking, E. and P. W. Singer. 2016. War Goes Viral: How Social Media is being Weaponized. The Atlantic, November, 70–83.

Bureau of Educational and Cultural Affairs. 2002. Evaluation summary: Edmund S. Muskie/FSA graduate program. http://exchanges/state/gov/education/evaluations/one-pagers/Muskie-FSA.pdf (accessed March 16, 2007).

Cigainero, J. 2016. A Belgian woman explains why she joined ISIS, and why she came back. *PRI*. December 19. http://www.pri.org/stories/2016-12-19/belgian-woman-explains-why-she-joined-isis-and-why-she-came-back (accessed December 22, 2016).

Dauber, C. and M. Robinson. 2015. ISIS and the Hollywood Visual Style. *Jihadology*. http://jihadology.net/2015/07/06/guest-post-isis-and-the-hollywood-visual-style/ (accessed December 28, 2016).

Davis, J. 2015. Obama Urges Global United Front against Extremist Groups like IS. *The New York Times*, February 18.

DHS. 2016. Entry/exit overstay report: Fiscal year 2015. https://www.dhs.gov/sites/default/files/publications/FY%2015%20DHS%20Entry%20and%20Exit%20Overstay%20Report.pdf (accessed December 28, 2016).

Dunleavy, P. 2012. The myth of self-radicalization: investigative project on terrorism. April 4. http://www.investigativeproject.org/3520/the-myth-of-self-radicalization# (accessed December 22, 2016).

Feeney, N. 2014. Feds say ISIS may target US military at home. *Time*. December 2. http://time.com/3612970/isis-military-social-media/ (accessed February 28, 2017).

Ford, P. 2001. Europe cringes at bush 'crusade' against terrorism. *Christian Science Monitor*, September 19. http://www.csmonitor.com/2001/0919/p12s2-woeu.html (accessed December 29, 2016).

GAO 2004. Overstay tracking: A key component of homeland security and a layered defense. http://www.gao.gov/new.items/d0482.pdf (accessed December 26, 2016).

Gellman, B. 2002. Cyber-attacks by Al-Qaeda feared. *Washington Post*, June 27. http://www.washingtonpost.com/wp-dyn/content/article/2006/06/12/AR2006061200711.html (accessed December 26, 2016).

Gerbaudo, P. 2012. Tweets and the Streets: Social Media and Contemporary Activism. London: Pluto Press.

Gladwell, M. 2000. The Tipping Point: How Little Things Can Make a Big Difference. Boston, MA: Little, Brown.

Gotttfried, J. and E. Shearer. 2016. News use across social media platforms 2016. Pew Research Center, May 26. http://www.journalism.org/2016/05/26/news-use-across-social-media-platforms-2016/ (accessed November 9, 2017).

Grodzins, M. 1958. The Metropolitan Area as a Racial Problem. Pittsburgh, PA: University of Pittsburgh Press.

Hirschfield Davis, J. 2015. Obama urges global united front against extremist groups like ISIS. *New York Times*. February 18. http://www.nytimes.com/2015/02/19/us/obama-to-outline-nonmilitary-plans-to-counter-groups-like-isis.html?_r=0 (accessed December 27, 2016).

Houston, J. B., J. Hawthorne, M. F. Perreault, E. H. Park, M. Goldstein Hode, M. R. Halliwell, and S. E. Turner McGowen. 2015. Social Media and Disasters: A Functional Framework for Social Media Use in Disaster Planning, Response, and Research. Disasters, 39 (1), 1–22.

Huntington, S. 1996. The Clash of Civilizations and the Remaking of World Order. New York: Simon and Schuster.

Independent. 2016. Fake 'pizzagate' news story alleging Hillary Clinton ran a child sex ring led man to open fire in Washington pizza parlour. *Independent*. http://www.independent.co.uk/news/world/americas/hillary-clinton-fake-news-conspiracy-theory-child-sex-ring-edgar-maddison-welch-open-fire-comet-ping-a7456021.html (accessed December 26, 2016).

Inglehart, R. and W. Baker. 2000. Modernization, Cultural Change, and the Persistence of Traditional Values. American Sociological Review, 65 (1), 19–51.

Inglehart, R. and C. Welzel. 2015. Inglehart-Wezel cultural map. http://www.worldvaluessurvey.org//WVSContents.jsp (accessed December 27, 2016).

Inspire. 2016. The successful pressure cooker bomb. November 22. https://isdacenter.org/al-qaeda-magazine-inspire-issue-16/ (accessed December 22, 2016).

Irshaid, F. 2014. How ISIS is spreading its message online. *BBC*. June 19. http://www.bbc.com/news/world-middle-east-27912569 (accessed December 22, 2016).

Johnson, N. 2016. Disrupting Pro-ISIS online 'ecosystems' could help thwart real-world terrorism. June 16. https://theconversation.com/disrupting-pro-isis-online-ecosystems-could-help-thwart-real-world-terrorism-60995 (accessed December 23, 2016).

Joint Publication 3-53. 2003. Doctrine for Joint Psychological Operations. Washington, DC: US Joint Chiefs of Staff, September 5.

Kahneman, D. and A. Tversky. 1973. On the Psychology of Prediction, Psychology Review, 80, 237–251.

Kang, C. 2016. Fake News Onslaught Targets Pizzeria as Nest of Child-Trafficking. *New York Times*. November 21. http://www.nytimes.com/2016/11/21/technology/fact-check-this-pizzeria-is-not-a-child-trafficking-site.html?_r=0 (accessed December 26, 2016).

Kingdon, J. 1984. Agendas, Alternatives, and Public Policies. Boston, MA: Little, Brown.

Klausen, J. 2015. Tweeting the Jihad: Social Media Networks of Western Foreign Fighters in Syria and Iraq. Studies in Conflict & Terrorism, 38 (1), 1–22.

Knabb, R. J. Rhome, and D. Brown. 2011. Tropical cyclone report: hurricane Katrina; 23–30 August 2005. National Hurricane Center. http://www.nhc.noaa.gov/data/tcr/AL122005_Katrina.pdf (accessed February 28, 2017).

Mallet, V. 2015. Madrassas: Behind closed doors: Are south Asia's Islamic schools causing a surge in extremism? *Financial Times*, October 30. https://www.ft.com/content/d807f15a-7db0-11e5-98fb-5a6d4728f74e (accessed December 30, 2016).

Matheson, D. 2014. History of citizen journalism. *Oxford Bibliographies*, http://www.oxfordbibliographies.com/view/document/obo-9780199756841/obo-9780199756841-0145.xml (accessed December 29, 2016).

McCauley, C. and S. Moskalenko. 2008. Mechanisms of Political Radicalization: Pathways toward Terrorism. Terrorism and Political Violence, 20 (3), 415–433.

McGray, D. 2005. San Francisco Dispatch: After Shock. The New Republic, 26 (September), 19–21.

Mendelsohn, B. 2016. ISIS' lone-wolf strategy: And how the west should respond. *Foreign Affairs*. August 25. https://www.foreignaffairs.com/articles/2016-08-25/isis-lone-wolf-strategy (accessed December 29, 2016).

Moghaddam, F. 2005. The Staircase to Terrorism. American Psychologist, 60 (2), 161–169.

Moore, D. and T. Rid. 2016. Cryptopolitik and the Darknet. Survival, 58 (1), 7–38.

National Hurricane Center. 2017a. Hurricane preparedness—Hazards. http://www.nhc.noaa.gov/prepare/hazards.php (accessed February 27, 2017).

National Hurricane Center. 2017b. Saffir-Simpson hurricane wind scale, http://www.nhc.noaa.gov/aboutsshws.php (accessed February 27, 2017).

Neumann, P. (2013) The Trouble with Radicalization. International Affairs. 89 (4): 873–893.

Nielsen, R. and R. Sambrook 2016. What is happening to television news. Reuters Institute for the Study of Journalism. http://www.digitalnewsreport.org/publications/2016/what-is-happening-to-television-news/ (accessed December 27, 2016).

Nisbett, R. and L. Ross. 1980. Human Inference: Strategies and Shortcomings of Social Judgment. New York: Prentice-Hall.

Nixon, R. 2016. US doesn't know how many foreign visitors overstay visas. *New York Times*, January 1. https://www.nytimes.com/2016/01/02/us/politics/us-doesnt-know-how-many-foreign-visitors-overstay-visas.html (accessed December 22, 2016).

NS. 2016. The dark secrets of the Internet that will dread you. *NS*. http://nsonline.in/the-dark-secrets-of-the-internet-that-will-dread-you/ (accessed February 27, 2017).

Open Doors. 2016. International Students: Primary Source of Funding. Institute for International Education. http://www.iie.org/research-and-publications/open-doors/data/international-students/primary-source-of-funding#.WGavxbmMDHk (accessed December 30, 2016).

Paganini, P. and R. Amores. 2012. The Deep Dark Web: The Hidden World. Providence, RI: Paganini-Amores.

Parsons, P. 2003. The Evolution of the Cable-Satellite Distribution System. Journal of Broadcasting & Electronic Media, 47 (1), 1–17.

Passoni, L. and C. Lorsignol. 2016. Au Coeur de Daesh avec mons Fils [In the Heart of Daesh with my Son]. Paris: Pandora's Box.

Perrin, A. 2015. Social media usage: 2005–2015. Pew Research Center. http://www.pewinternet.org/2015/10/08/social-networking-usage-2005-2015/ (accessed December 27, 2016).

Podobnik, B., M. Jusup, and H. E. Stanley. 2016. predicting the rise of right-wing populism in response to unbalanced immigration. *Arxiv*. https://arxiv.org/abs/1612.00270 (accessed December 28, 2016).

Politico. 2016. Full text: Donald trump's speech on fighting terrorism. *Politico.* http://www.politico.com/story/2016/08/donald-trump-terrorism-speech-227025 (accessed December 28, 2016).

Project Atlas. 2016. International Students in the United States. Institute of International Education. http://www.iie.org/Services/Project-Atlas/United-States/International-Students-In-US#.WGat77mMDHk (accessed December 30, 2016).

Reilly, R. 2015. If you're trying to join is through Twitter, the FBI probably knows about it. *Huffington Post.* July 9. http://www.huffingtonpost.com/2015/07/09/isis-twitter-fbi-islamic-state_n_7763992.html (accessed December 23, 2016).

Rumiyah. 2016. Just terror tactics. November. https://pietervanostaeyen.files.wordpress.com/2016/11/rumiyah3en.pdf (accessed December 29, 2016).

Russell Goldman. 2016. Reading Fake News, Pakistani Minister Directs Nuclear Threat at Israel. *New York Times*, December 24, 2016.

Schelling, T. 1978. Micromotives and Macrobehavior. New York: W. W. Norton.

Silber, M and A. Bhatt. 2007. Radicalization in the West: The Homegrown Threat. New York: New York Police Department. http://moonbattery.com/graphics/NYPD_Report-Radicalization_in_the_West.pdf (accessed December 23, 2016).

Soufan Group. 2015. Foreign fighters: An updated assessment of the flow of foreign fighters into Syria and Iraq. December. http:// soufangroup.com/wp-content/uploads/2015/12/TSG_ForeignFighters Update_FINAL3.pdf (accessed December 28, 2016).

Statista. 2016a. Number of monthly active Facebook users worldwide as of 3rd quarter 2016 (in millions). *Statista.* https://www.statista. com/statistics/264810/number-of-monthly-active-facebook-users-worldwide/ (accessed December 26, 2016).

Statista. 2016b. Number of monthly Twitter users worldwide from 1st quarter 2010 to 3rd quarter 2016 (in millions). https://www.statista. com/statistics/282087/number-of-monthly-active-twitter-users/ (accessed December 26, 2016).

Teich, S. 2013. Trends and developments in lone wolf terrorism in the western world: an analysis of terrorist attacks and attempted attacks by Islamic extremists. International Institute for Counter-Terrorism. http://s3.amazonaws.com/academia.edu.documents/39623318/ Lone_Wolf_-_S.Teich_2013.pdf?AWSAccessKeyId=AKIAIWOWYY GZ2Y53UL3A&Expires=1488414703&Signature=jXkW%2 BNFfQN4ME8cimGyw%2Bfm3JwE%3D&response-content-disposition=inline%3B%20filename%3DTrends_and_Developments_ in_Lone_Wolf_Ter.pdf (accessed February 27, 2017).

TOR. 2016. Anonymity online. *TOR.* https://www.torproject.org/ (accessed December 28, 2016).

Turner, C. 2015. US colleges see a big bump in international students. *National Public Radio*, November 18. http://www.npr.org/sections/ ed/2015/11/18/456353089/u-s-colleges-see-a-big-bump-in-international-students (accessed February 26, 2017).

Veldhuis, T. and S. J. Staun. 2009. Islamic Radicalization: A Root Cause Model. Clingendael: Netherlands Institute of International Relations.

Vidino, L. and S. Hughes. 2015. ISIS in America: From Retweets to Raqqa. Washington, DC: The Program on Extremism/The George Washington University.

Wallace-Williams, B. 2006. Private Jihad: How Rita Katz got into the spying business. *The New Yorker*. May 29. http://www.newyorker. com/magazine/2006/05/29/private-jihad (accessed December 27, 2016).

Weimann, G. 2004. www.terror.net: How Modern Terrorism uses the Internet. Washington, DC: United States Institute of Peace.

Weimann, G. 2006. Terror on the Internet: The New Arena, the New Challenges. Washington, DC: United States Institute of Peace Press.

Williams, J., R. Anthes, S. Abrams, and J. Cantore. 2015. The AMS Weather Book: The Ultimate Guide to America's Weather. Chicago, IL: University of Chicago Press.

Zhou, Y., E. Reid, J. Qin, H. Chen, and G. Lai. 2005. US Domestic Extremist Groups on the Web: Link and Content Analysis. IEEE Intelligent Systems, 20 (5), 44–51.

Zong, J. and J. Batalova. 2016. International Students in the United States. Migration Information Source. May 12. http://www.migrationpolicy.org/article/international-students-united-states (accessed February 25, 2017).

Chapter 12 Works Cited

Al Qaeda. 2001. Training Manual: Eleventh Lesson –Espionage. Air University. http://www.au.af.mil/au/awc/awcgate/terrorism/alqaida_manual/manualpart1_3.pdf (accessed April 15, 2017).

Apuzzo, M. and A. Goldman. 2012. NYPD: Muslim spying led to no leads, terror cases. Associated Press, 21 February. https://www.ap.org/ap-in-the-news/2012/nypd-muslim-spying-led-to-no-leads-terror-cases (accessed November 9, 2017).

Apuzzo, M. and J. Goldstein. 2014. New York drops unit that spied on Muslims. *New York Times*, 15 April.

Bazelon, E. 2013. Why should I care that no one's reading Dzhokhar Tsarnaev his Miranda rights? *Slate*. 19 April. http://www.slate.com/articles/news_and_politics/jurisprudence/2013/04/dzhokhar_tsarnaev_and_miranda_rights_the_public_safety_exception_and_terrorism.html (accessed May 1, 2017).

Bluemel, D. 2013. Does LAPD's reporting on our 'suspicious behavior' protect us from terrorism? *LA Progressive*. 2 April. https://www.laprogressive.com/suspicious-behavior/ (accessed February 2, 2017).

Breglio, N. 2003. Leaving FISA Behind: The Need to Return to Warrantless Foreign Intelligence Surveillance. Yale Law Journal, 113, 179–217.

Bullock, J., G. Haddow, and D. Coppola. 2013. Introduction to Homeland Security, 4th ed. New York: Butterworth-Heinemann.

Buxbaum, P. 2010. Full Motion Progress. GIF, 8 (8). http://www.usma.edu/cegs/siteassets/sitepages/research%20ipad/full%20motion%20video.pdf (accessed December 12, 2016).

Carter, D. 2004. Law Enforcement Intelligence: A Guide to State, Local, and Tribal Law Enforcement Agencies. Washington, DC: US Department of Justice, Office of Community Oriented Policing Services.

Carter, J. 2016. Law Enforcement Fusion Centers: Cultivating an Information Sharing Environment while Safeguarding Privacy. *Journal of Police and Criminal Psychology*. http://phys.org/news/2016-07-violations-privacy-rights-fusion-centers.html (accessed March 1, 2017).

Central Intelligence Agency. 2012. Factbook on Intelligence. Washington, DC: Central Intelligence Agency.

Coble, M. 2009. National Guard Support to Domestic Intelligence Operations. Fort Leavenworth, KS: Army Command and General Staff College.

Collier, K. 2016. Inside the controversial government centers where the FBI shares Intel with police. *The Week*. http://theweek.com/

articles/643783/inside-controversial-government-centers-where-fbi-shares-intel-police (accessed November 10, 2016).

Department of Homeland Security. 2004. US Department of Homeland Security, Fiscal Year 2005 Homeland Security Grant Program: Program Guidelines and Application Kit. Washington, DC: Government Printing Office.

Department of Homeland Security. 2016. Our Mission. Washington, DC: Department of Homeland Security. https://www.dhs.gov/our-mission (accessed April 2, 2017).

Department of Justice. 2016. State and Major Urban Area Fusion Centers. Washington, DC: Department of Justice Bureau of Justice Assistance. https://www.dhs.gov/sites/default/files/publications/Fusion%20Centers%20Handout_0.pdf (accessed January 15, 2017).

Dharapak, C. 2012. NYPD built secret files on Newark mosques. *CBS News*, February 15.

Director of National Intelligence. 2011. Intelligence Consumers Guide. Washington, DC: Director of National Intelligence.

Epstein, J. 2011. James Jesus Angleton: Was He Right? New York: Fast Track Press.

Federal Bureau of Investigation. 2009. Fusion centers. March 12. https://archives.fbi.gov/archives/news/stories/2009/march/fusion_031209 (accessed August 1, 2017).

Federal Bureau of Investigation. 2015. Model partnership: The New York joint terrorism task force celebrates 35 years. Federal Bureau of Investigation. https://www.fbi.gov/news/stories/new-york-jttf-celebrates-35-years (accessed October 20, 2016).

Federal Emergency Management Agency. 2013. National Incident Management System: Intelligence/Investigations Function Guidance and Field Operations Guide. Washington, DC: Government Printing Office.

Gellman, B. and A. Soltani. 2013. NSA infiltrates links to Yahoo, Google Data Centers Worldwide, Snowden documents say. *Washington Post*, October 30.

German, M. and J. Stanley. 2007. What's Wrong with Fusion Centers. Washington, DC: American Civil Liberties Union.

Gerringer, A. and J. Bart. 2014. Law Enforcement Intelligence. The Intelligencer, 21 (1), 74–78.

Goodwin, B. 2016. Interview: James Bamford on surveillance, Snowden, and technology companies. *ComputerWeekly.com*. January. http://www.computerweekly.com/feature/Interview-James-Bamford-on-surveillance-Snowden-and-technology-companies (accessed November 10, 2017).

Goren, D. 1981. Communication Intelligence and the Freedom of the Press. The Chicago Tribune's Battle of Midway Dispatch and the Breaking of the Japanese Naval Code. Contemporary History, 16 (4), 663–690.

Greaney, T. 2009. Fusion center data draws fire over assertions: Politics, banners seen as suspect. *Columbia Daily Tribune* (Missouri), March 14.

Greenwald, G. 2013. NSA collecting phone records of millions of verizon customers daily. *The Guardian*, June 6.

Gregory, A. 2016. American Surveillance: Intelligence, Privacy and the Fourth Amendment. Madison, WI: University of Wisconsin Press.

Higgins, P. 2014. Releasing a public domain image of the NSA's Utah data center. Electronic Freedom Foundation. July 9. https://www.eff.org/deeplinks/2014/07/releasing-public-domain-image-nsas-utah-data-center (accessed July 31, 2017).

Horgan, J. 2013. Unmanned flight. *National Geographic*. http://ngm.nationalgeographic.com/2013/03/unmanned-flight/horgan-text (accessed November 22, 2016).

Hulnick, A. 2015. The intelligence cycle. In Intelligence: The Secret World of Spies, 4th ed, eds. L. Johnson and J. Wirtz. New York: Oxford University Press.

Internet Live Stats. 2016. Total number of web sites. *Internet Live Stats*. http://www.internetlivestats.com/total-number-of-websites/ (accessed January 10, 2017).

Internet World Stats. 2016. Internet growth statistics. *Internet World Stats*. http://www.internetworldstats.com/emarketing.htm (accessed January 10, 2017).

Jeffreys-Jones, R. 1989. The CIA and American Democracy. New Haven, CT: Yale University Press.

Jehl, D. 1993. CIA nominee wary of budget cuts. *New York Times*, February 3.

Jensen, C., D. McElreath, and M. Graves. 2013. Introduction to Intelligence Studies. New York: CRC Press.

Joachim, D. 2003. What is intelligence chatter, anyway? *Slate*, September 12. http://www.slate.com/articles/news_and_politics/explainer/2003/09/what_is_intelligence_chatter_anyway.html (accessed November 10, 2016).

Jones, J. 1986. Explosives linked to 1984 terrorism case. *Los Angeles Times*. August 23. http://articles.latimes.com/1986-08-23/local/me-15849_1_los-angeles (accessed April 7, 2017).

Kang, C. 2011. Number of cellphones exceeds US population: CTIA Trade Group. *Washington Post*, October 11.

Kean, T. H. and L. Hamilton. 2004. The 9/11 Commission Report: Final report of the National Commission on terrorist attacks upon the United States. Washington, DC: National Commission on Terrorist Attacks upon the United States.

Khan, A. 2012. Senate Report: Massive Post-9/11 Surveillance Apparatus a 'Waste'. *Frontline*. Washington, DC: Public Broadcasting System. http://www.pbs.org/wgbh/frontline/article/senate-report-massive-post-911-surveillance-apparatus-a-waste/ (accessed March 12, 2017).

Kojm, C. 2016. Global change and megatrends: Implications for intelligence and its oversight. *Lawfare Blog*. May 12. https://www.lawfareblog.com/global-change-and-megatrends-implications-intelligence-and-its-oversight (accessed March 5, 2017).

Larence, E. 2007. Homeland Security: Federal Efforts Are Helping to Alleviate Some Challenges Encountered by State and Local Information Fusion Centers, GAO-08-35. Washington, DC: Government Accountability Office.

Larence, E. 2014. DHS Intelligence Analysis: Additional Actions Needed to Address Analytic Priorities and Workforce Challenges, GAO-14-397. Washington, DC: Government Accountability Office.

Lindsay, B. 2011. Social Media and Disasters: Current Uses, Future Options, and Policy Considerations. Washington, DC: Congressional Research Service.

Lowenthal, M. 2015. Intelligence: From Secrets to Policy, 6th ed. Washington, DC: CQ Press.

Maclin, T. 2012. The Supreme Court and the Fourth Amendment's Exclusionary Rule. London: Oxford University Press.

Magnuson, S. 2010. Military swimming in sensors and drowning in data. *National Defense Magazine*, January. http://www.nationaldefensemagazine.org/archive/2010/January/Pages/Military%E2%80%98SwimmingInSensorsandDrowninginData%E2%80%99.aspx (accessed January 12, 2017).

Mayer, M. 2016. Consolidate Domestic Intelligence Entities Under FBI. Washington, DC: American Enterprise Institute.

Metz, C. 2016. How Facebook is transforming disaster response. *Wired Magazine*, November 10. https://www.wired.com/2016/11/facebook-disaster-response/ (accessed October 12, 2016).

National Counter Terrorism Center. 2016. National counter-terrorism center: Who we are. https://www.dni.gov/index.php/about/organization/national-counterterrorism-center-who-we-are (accessed October 15, 2016).

Office of the Director of National Drug Control Policy. 2001. The High Intensity Drug Trafficking Area Program: An Overview. White House Office of National Drug Control Policy. https://www.ncjrs.gov/ondcppubs/publications/enforce/hidta2001/overview.html#3 (accessed September 25, 2016).

Office of the Director of National Drug Control Policy. 2016. High Intensity Drug Trafficking Areas (HIDTA) Program. The White House. https://www.whitehouse.gov/ondcp/high-intensity-drug-trafficking-areas-program (accessed October 22, 2016).

Office of the Director of National Intelligence. 2006. Intelligence Community Directive 301: National Open Source Enterprise. Office of the Director of National Intelligence. https://fas.org/irp/dni/icd/icd-301.pdf (accessed October 12, 2016).

Office of the Director of National Intelligence. 2017. Fact Sheet. February 24. https://www.dni.gov/files/documents/FACTSHEET_ ODNI_History_and_Background_2_24-17.pdf (accessed November 9, 2017).

O'Harrow, R., Jr. 2012. DHS 'fusion centers' portrayed as pools of ineptitude, civil liberties intrusions. *Washington Post*, October 2.

Palantir. 2017. Supporting relief efforts. *Palantir Industries*. https://www. palantir.com/wp-assets/wp-content/uploads/2014/03/Impact-Study-Supporting-Relief-Efforts-DRI.pdf/ (accessed April 17, 2017).

Peteritas, B. 2013. Fusion centers struggle to find their place in the post-9/11 world. *Governing*. http://www.governing.com/topics/public-justice-safety/gov-fusion-centers-post-911-world.html (accessed October 10, 2016).

Petitjean, M. 2013. Intelligence Support to Disaster Relief and Humanitarian Assistance. The Intelligencer, 19 (Winter), 57–60.

Posner, R. 2006. Uncertain Shield: The US Intelligence System in the Throes of Reform. Lanham, MD: Rowman and Littlefield Publishers.

Portnoy, J. 2012. Christie slams NYPD over Muslim spying program in N.J. *Star-Ledger*, 29 February.

Priest, D. and W. Arkin. 2012. Top Secret America: The Rise of the New American Security State. New York: Back Bay Books.

Randol, M. 2010. The Department of Homeland Security Intelligence Enterprise: Operational Overview and Oversight Challenges for Congress, R40602. Washington, DC: Congressional Research Service.

Richelson, J. 2015. The US Intelligence Community. New York: Westview Press.

Rittgers, D. 2011. We're All Terrorists Now. The CATO Institute. http:// www.cato.org/blog/were-all-terrorists-now (accessed October 15, 2016).

Rosen, J. 2013. Column: Palmer raids Redux: the NSA versus civil liberties. *Reuters*, June 12. http://www.reuters.com/article/us-rosen-nsa-idUSBRE95B12M20130612 (accessed October 23, 2016).

Rubin, J. 2016. Apple vs. FBI: iPhone encryption battle likely to continue even after San Bernardino. *Los Angeles Times*, March 22.

Savasta, M. 2015. The FBI joint terrorism task force. *Law and Order*. http://www.hendonpub.com/resources/article_archive/results/ details?id=5505 (accessed September 5, 2016).

Schmitt, E. 2009. Surveillance effort draws civil liberties concern. *New York Times*, April 29.

Seng, A. 2007. MASINT: The Future of Intelligence. Singapore: Defense Science and Technology Agency.

Sheldon, R. 1986. Tradecraft in Ancient Greece. Studies in Intelligence, 30, 39–47.

Shorrock, T. 2013. Put the spies back under one roof. *New York Times*, June 17.

Smith, R. 2014. Law Enforcement Intelligence: Its Evolution and Scope Today. The Intelligencer, 20 (3), 28–32.

Spracher, W. 2014. Homeland Security and Intelligence: Fusing Sometimes Incompatible Missions. The Intelligencer, 20 (1), 19–24.

Steiner, J. 2015. Homeland Security Intelligence. Washington, DC: CQ Press.

Steiner, J. 2016. Evaluating and Teaching Homeland Security Intelligence. Guide to the Study of Intelligence. Washington, DC: Association of Former Intelligence Officers: 353–362.

Stentiford, B. 2002. The American Home Guard: The State Militia in the Twentieth Century. College Station, TX: Texas A & M Press.

Streams, K. 2012. Palantir's terrorist tracking technology used for hurricane sandy relief. The Verge, November 27. https://www.theverge.com/2012/11/27/3698266/palantir-team-rubicon-hurricane-sandy (accessed April 17, 2017).

The Holy Bible, New International Version. 1984. Numbers (Ch. 13, Vers. 17-20). Grand Rapids: Zondervan Publishing.

The Onion. 2011. CIA's 'Facebook' program dramatically cuts agency's costs. The Onion. http://www.theonion.com/video/cias-facebook-program-dramatically-cut-agencys-cos-19753 (accessed November 10, 2016).

The White House. 1981. Executive Order 12333: United States Intelligence Activities. Washington, DC: Government Printing Office. https://www.archives.gov/federal-register/codification/executive-order/12333.html (accessed September 20, 2016).

The White House. 2006. The Federal Response to Hurricane Katrina: Lessons Learned. Washington, DC: Government Printing Office.

Turner, M. 2005. Intelligence Reform and the Politics of Entrenchment. International Journal of Intelligence and Counterintelligence, 18, 383–397.

United States Constitution. 1789. Amendment I.

United States Supreme Court. 1967. Katz v. United States, 389 US 347.

US Customs and Border Protection. n.d. Fact sheet MQ-9 predator B. https://www.cbp.gov/sites/default/files/documents/FS_2015_UAS_FINAL_0.pdf (accessed July 13, 2017).

US Navy. 2006. Infrared image of a ship at sea. February 4. http://www.navy.mil/view_image.asp?id=31723 (accessed August 1, 2017).

Walton, T. 2010. Challenges in Intelligence Analysis: Lessons from 1300 BCE to the Present. New York: Cambridge University Press.

Warner, M. 2007. Wanted: A Definition of Intelligence. Studies in Intelligence, 46 (3), 15–22.

Weisner, B. 2015. Lawsuit over New York police surveillance of Muslims is revived. New York Times, October 13.

Whitlock, C. and C. Timberg. 2014. Border-patrol drones being borrowed by other agencies more often than previously known. Washington Post, January 14.

Young, J. 2012. Drugstores struggle to fill prescriptions in areas hard-hit by hurricane sandy. The Huffington Post, November 1.

Chapter 13 Works Cited

Brusset, E., J. Cosgrove, and W. MacDonald. 2010. Real-time evaluation. In Humanitarian Emergencies in Enhancing Disaster and Emergency Preparedness, Response and Recovery Through Evaluation, eds. L. Ritchie and W. MacDonald. Vancouver, BC: Josey Bass.

Carafano, J., J. Zuckerman, M. Mayer, P. Rosenzweig, and B. Slattery. 2013. The Second Quadrennial Homeland Security Review: Setting Priorities for the Next Four Years. The Heritage Foundation. http://www.heritage.org/homeland-security/report/the-second-quadrennial-homeland-security-review-setting-priorities-the (accessed July 26, 2017).

CHDS. 2017. University and agency partnership initiative: Partners list. https://www.uapi.us/partners-list (accessed June 18, 2017).

Congressional Research Service. 2016. Transportation security: Issues for the 114th congress. https://fas.org/sgp/crs/homesec/RL33512.pdf (accessed July 26, 2017).

Department of Homeland Security. n.d. Science and technology. Welcome to centers of excellence. https://www.dhs.gov/science-and-technology/centers-excellence (accessed July 26, 2017).

Department of Homeland Security. 2011. Presidential policy directive #8: National preparedness. https://www.dhs.gov/presidential-policy-directive-8-national-preparedness (accessed July 26, 2017).

Department of Homeland Security. 2014a. The 2014 quadrennial homeland security review. June 18. https://www.dhs.gov/sites/default/files/publications/2014-qhsr-final-508.pdf (accessed June 17, 2017).

Department of Homeland Security. 2014b. FY 14–18 strategic plan. https://www.dhs.gov/sites/default/files/publications/FY14-18%20Strategic%20Plan_0_0.PDF (accessed June 17, 2017).

Department of Homeland Security. 2015. National preparedness goal. https://www.fema.gov/national-preparedness-goal (accessed July 26, 2017).

Department of Homeland Security. 2016. The 2018 quadrennial homeland security review. November 17. https://www.dhs.gov/2018-quadrennial-homeland-security-review (accessed June 17, 2017).

Doran, G. 1981. There's a S.M.A.R.T way to write management's goals and objectives. Management Review 70 (11), 35–36.

Eastern Kentucky University. 2017. Homeland Security Program Guide, 2017–2018. Richmond, KY: Eastern Kentucky University.

Federal Emergency Management Agency. 2010. Comprehensive preparedness guide (CPG) 101. Version 2.0. November. https://www.fema.gov/media-library-data/20130726-1828-25045-0014/cpg_101_comprehensive_preparedness_guide_developing_and_maintaining_emergency_operations_plans_2010.pdf (accessed June 17, 2017).

Federal Emergency Management Agency. 2013. Emergency management institute: Introduction to homeland security planning. https://emilms.fema.gov/IS453/HSPPrint.htm (accessed July 26, 2017).

Federal Emergency Management Agency. 2016a. Alphabetical listing of programs in the US. August 5. https://training.fema.gov/hiedu/collegelist/alphabetical_programs_by_type_8_5_16.pdf (accessed June 18, 2017).

Federal Emergency Management Agency. 2016b. Response federal interagency operational plan (FIOP). https://www.fema.gov/media-library-data/1471452095112.../Response_FIOP_2nd.pdf (accessed July 26, 2017).

Federal Emergency Management Agency. 2016c. The national preparedness report. March 30. https://www.fema.gov/media-library-data/1476817353589-987d6a58e2eb124ac6b19ef1f7c9a77d/2016NPR_508c_052716_1600_alla.pdf (accessed June 17, 2017).

Fleming, M. H. and E. Goldstein. 2012. Metrics for Measuring the Efficacy of Critical Infrastructure-Centric Cybersecurity Information Sharing Efforts. March 31. Falls Church, VA: Homeland Security Studies and Analysis Institute.

Frost, B. 2000. Measuring Performance. Dallas, TX: Measurement International.

Goodykoontz, E., J. Carbonette, K. Klein, S. Nashed, and A. Smith. 2014. Measuring for results: Key concepts for understanding the performance of DHS programs and activities. 1 October. Homeland Security Studies and Analysis Institute. https://www.anser.org/Docs/Performance-Measurement-Guidebook_508_final.pdf (accessed July 26, 2017).

Harrison, G. 2002. Any road. Brainwashed album. *AZLyrics.com*. http://www.azlyrics.com/lyrics/georgeharrison/anyroad.html (accessed June 17, 2017).

Jackson, B. 2008. The Problem of Measuring Emergency Preparedness: The Need for Assessing "Response Reliability" as Part of Homeland Security Planning. Rand Corporation www.rand.org/content/dam/rand/pubs/occasional_papers/2008/RAND_OP234.pdf (accessed July 26, 2017).

National Center for Education Statistics.n.d. Integrated postsecondary education data system. https://nces.ed.gov/ipeds/ (accessed June 18, 2017).

National Security Education Program.n.d. Critical languages. https://www.nsep.gov/content/critical-languages (accessed June 18, 2017).

Nixon, R. M. 1962. Six Crises. New York: Doubleday and Company.

Oklahoma Government (OKGOV). n.d. Documents. SMART objectives. https://ok.gov/odmhsas/documents/Handout%20-%20SMART%20Objectives.docx (accessed November 9, 2017).

Pennsylvania State University World Campus. n.d. Master of professional studies in homeland security. https://www.worldcampus.psu.edu/degrees-and-certificates/homeland-security/overview (accessed July 26, 2017).

Public Safety Canada. 2012. 2011–2012 evaluation of the emergency prevention/mitigation and preparedness initiative – Final report.

https://www.publicsafety.gc.ca/cnt/rsrcs/pblctns/vltn-mrgnc-prvntn-mtgtn-2011-12/index-en.aspx (accessed July 29, 2017).

Richards, L. 2012. Planning Is Bringing The Future Into the Present. *The MHEDA Journal.* October 14. http://www.themhedajournal. org/2012/10/14/planning-is-bringing-the-future-into-the-present/ (accessed June 17, 2017).

University of Wisconsin Extension. n.d. Logic models. http://fyi.uwex. edu/programdevelopment/logic-models/ (accessed July 26, 2017).

Willis, H. 2014. Building on the Quadrennial Homeland Security Review to Improve the Effectiveness and Efficiency of the Department of Homeland Security. Rand Corporation. http://www. rand.org/content/dam/rand/pubs/testimonies/CT400/CT412/ RAND_CT412.pdf (accessed July 26, 2017).

W.K. Kellogg Foundation. 2004. Logic model development guide. https:// www.wkkf.org/resource-directory/resource/2006/02/wk-kellogg-foundation-logic-model-development-guide (accessed July 26, 2017).

Zantal-Weiner, K. and T. Horwood. 2010. Logic modeling as a tool to prepared to evaluate disaster and emergency preparedness, response, and recovery in schools. In Enhancing Disaster and Emergency Preparedness, Response and Recovery Through Evaluation, eds. L Ritchie and W MacDonald. Vancouver, BC: Josey Bass.

INDEX

Threats to Homeland Security: Reassessing the All-Hazards Perspective, Second Edition.
Edited by Richard J. Kilroy, Jr.
© 2018 John Wiley & Sons, Inc. Published 2018 by John Wiley & Sons, Inc.
Companion website: www.wiley.com/go/Kilroy/Threats_to_Homeland_Security

Printed and bound by CPI Group (UK) Ltd, Croydon, CR0 4YY

17/04/2025

14658914-0001